INTEGRATED PATHOLOGY

From Concepts to Diagnosis

FRCPATH AND INTERNATIONAL RESIDENTS

Vishal Tayade

INTEGRATED PATHOLOGY

From Concepts to Diagnosis

Volume 2A

General Pathology and Major Organ Systems

FRCPATH AND INTERNATIONAL RESIDENTS

Vishal Tayade

MD Pathology · FRCPath (Part 1)

VAYDEN ACADEMIC PRESS

First Edition, 2026

ISBN (Paperback): 978-81-686730-0-7

Published by Vayden Academic Press, Mumbai

www.vaydenpress.com

Disclaimer

This book is intended as an educational reference for FRCPath candidates, international pathology residents, and early-career pathologists. Diagnostic thresholds, immunohistochemistry panels, molecular criteria, and therapeutic recommendations reflect WHO 5th Edition classifications and AJCC 8th Edition staging current to April 2026. Clinical and laboratory practice evolves; the reader is responsible for verifying current standards before applying any information from this volume to patient care.

A Note on This Volume

Volume 2 of *Integrated Pathology: From Concepts to Diagnosis* is published in two physical volumes for printing accessibility. The volume in your hand — Volume 2A — contains Chapters 1 through 24, covering general pathology and the major organ systems through to the male genital tract. The companion volume, Volume 2B, contains Chapters 25 through 43, covering the female genital tract, breast, endocrine, dermatopathology, bone and soft tissue, neuropathology, cytopathology, and applied laboratory pathology.

Each volume carries its own ISBN and is independently bound. Cross-references between volumes are kept to a minimum; where a topic crosses a volume boundary, the discussion is self-contained within its primary chapter. Readers requiring the complete text are encouraged to acquire both volumes; readers focused on a single domain may use either volume in isolation without loss of conceptual continuity.

The two-volume division is editorial, not conceptual. The full integrated framework — biology to morphology to immunohistochemistry to molecular workup — is preserved across the set.

Dedication

...

For my parents,

whose patience built the quiet behind every page.

...

For my teachers at the Tata Memorial Centre,

who taught me to look again.

...

And for my students,

who keep me reading the slide once more.

Preface

This book started at the multiheaded microscope at Tata Memorial Centre. That is where I understood that pathology is not a subject you memorise. It is a discipline you reason through. Every slide tells a story. The pathologist's job is to read it, correlate it, and report it clearly.

That belief runs through all 43 chapters of this book. Each chapter is built around five elements: THE BIG PICTURE boxes that set the conceptual framework before any detail, Quick Recall boxes for rapid revision, Exam Pitfall boxes that flag the traps examiners actually set, Pathologist's Eye boxes that show how a practising pathologist thinks at the microscope, and International Frameworks blocks that consolidate WHO, AJCC, and equivalent reference standards across organ systems.

WHO 5th Edition classifications are integrated wherever applicable — CNS tumours (2021), Female Genital Tract (2020), Urinary and Male Genital (2022), Endocrine (2022), Soft Tissue and Bone (2020), Breast (2019). Where the 5th Edition has not yet superseded the 4th, the current authoritative classification is used. AJCC 8th Edition staging is integrated throughout. Diagnostic criteria, IHC panels, and molecular profiles are woven into every chapter rather than appended. Sixteen original diagnostic algorithms provide stepwise approaches to biopsies from every major organ system. Over 300 figures include real photomicrographs sourced under Creative Commons licences alongside original diagrams.

This book does not try to replace Robbins. It occupies a different space: examination-focused, algorithm-driven, and calibrated to the standards of the FRCPath syllabus, international fellowship programmes, and contemporary diagnostic practice. Every chapter integrates current WHO 5th Edition classifications and AJCC 8th Edition staging.

I hope it serves you well at the reading desk, in the examination hall, and at the microscope.

— From the Author

May 2026

About the Author

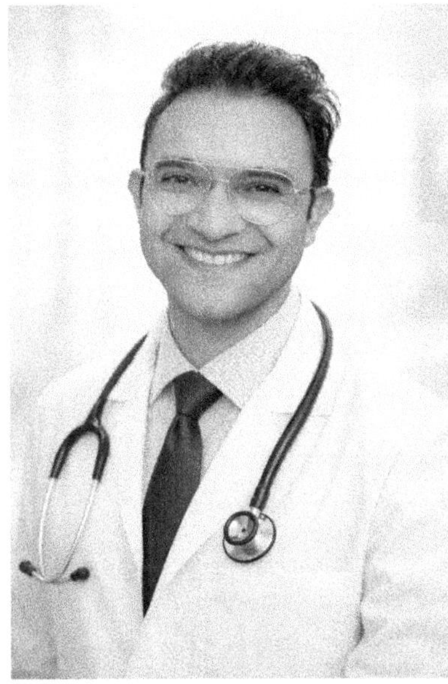

Vishal Tayade

MD Pathology · FRCPath Part 1

Vishal Tayade is Assistant Professor of Pathology at Grant Government Medical College and Sir J.J. Group of Hospitals, Mumbai, where he trains residents in surgical pathology, haematopathology, and cytopathology. He completed his MD in Pathology at Grant Government Medical College and trained in oncopathology at Tata Memorial Centre, Mumbai. He holds the FRCPath Part 1 (Histopathology and Haematology) of the Royal College of Pathologists, London.

His academic interests sit at the intersection of pattern recognition, integrated diagnostics, and pathology education. He has published in peer-reviewed journals on haematopathology, cytology artefacts, and laboratory diagnostics, and contributes images to the ASH Image Bank.

He is the founder of Vayden Academic Press, dedicated to writing focused, examination-grade textbooks for postgraduate pathology and laboratory medicine. Pathology in Patterns is the USMLE rapid-revision companion to his Pathway to USMLE series, alongside his FRCPath First Paper preparation volumes and the two-volume Integrated Pathology textbook.

Outside the laboratory, he writes literary fiction. His published novels include Love in Chaos, Resonance, the Dr Vishal Sarkar Mystery trilogy, and the literary novels The Chalk Line and No One Was Responsible.

He lives in Mumbai.

Table of Contents

Abbreviations

The following abbreviations appear throughout the text. Specialised abbreviations of limited scope are defined in their respective chapters at first use.

AFB — Acid-fast bacilli

AJCC — American Joint Committee on Cancer

AKI — Acute kidney injury

ALK — Anaplastic lymphoma kinase

ALL — Acute lymphoblastic leukaemia

AML — Acute myeloid leukaemia

ANA — Antinuclear antibody

ANCA — Antineutrophil cytoplasmic antibody

ARDS — Acute respiratory distress syndrome

ATN — Acute tubular necrosis

BCC — Basal cell carcinoma

BRAF — B-Raf proto-oncogene

BRCA — Breast cancer susceptibility gene

CAP — College of American Pathologists

CD — Crohn disease (in GI context)

CDX2 — Caudal-type homeobox 2

CIS — Carcinoma in situ

CK — Cytokeratin

CKD — Chronic kidney disease

CLL — Chronic lymphocytic leukaemia

CML — Chronic myeloid leukaemia

CMV — Cytomegalovirus

CNB — Core needle biopsy

CNS — Central nervous system

CRP — C-reactive protein

CSF — Cerebrospinal fluid

DCIS — Ductal carcinoma in situ

DIC — Disseminated intravascular coagulation

DLBCL — Diffuse large B-cell lymphoma

DVT — Deep vein thrombosis

EBV — Epstein–Barr virus

EGFR — Epidermal growth factor receptor

EM — Electron microscopy

ER — Oestrogen receptor

ESR — Erythrocyte sedimentation rate

ESRD — End-stage renal disease

FFPE — Formalin-fixed paraffin-embedded

FIGO — International Federation of Gynecology and Obstetrics

FISH — Fluorescence in situ hybridisation

FL — Follicular lymphoma

FNAC — Fine needle aspiration cytology

FRCPath — Fellow of the Royal College of Pathologists (UK)

FSGS — Focal segmental glomerulosclerosis

FTC — Follicular thyroid carcinoma

GERD — Gastro-oesophageal reflux disease

GIST — Gastrointestinal stromal tumour

GN — Glomerulonephritis

H&E — Haematoxylin and eosin

HBV — Hepatitis B virus

HCC — Hepatocellular carcinoma

HCV — Hepatitis C virus

HER2 — Human epidermal growth factor receptor 2

HGSC — High-grade serous carcinoma

HIER — Heat-induced epitope retrieval

HIV — Human immunodeficiency virus

HL — Hodgkin lymphoma

HPV — Human papillomavirus

HSV — Herpes simplex virus

IBD — Inflammatory bowel disease

IDH — Isocitrate dehydrogenase

IgAN — IgA nephropathy

IHC — Immunohistochemistry

ILC — Invasive lobular carcinoma

ISH — In situ hybridisation

ITP — Immune thrombocytopenic purpura

Ki-67 — Proliferation marker (MIB-1)

KRAS — Kirsten rat sarcoma viral oncogene

LBC — Liquid-based cytology

LCIS — Lobular carcinoma in situ

MASLD — Metabolic dysfunction-associated steatotic liver disease

MCD — Minimal change disease

MCL — Mantle cell lymphoma

MD — Doctor of Medicine

MDS — Myelodysplastic syndrome

MM — Multiple myeloma

MMR — Mismatch repair

MN — Membranous nephropathy

MPN — Myeloproliferative neoplasm

MSI — Microsatellite instability

NGS — Next-generation sequencing

NHL — Non-Hodgkin lymphoma

NSCLC — Non-small cell lung carcinoma

NST — No special type (breast)

OSCC — Oral squamous cell carcinoma

PAS — Periodic acid–Schiff

PBC — Primary biliary cholangitis

PCR — Polymerase chain reaction

PD-L1 — Programmed death ligand 1

PDAC — Pancreatic ductal adenocarcinoma

PE — Pulmonary embolism

PR — Progesterone receptor

PSA — Prostate-specific antigen

PSC — Primary sclerosing cholangitis

PTC — Papillary thyroid carcinoma

RCC — Renal cell carcinoma

ROSE — Rapid on-site evaluation

SCC — Squamous cell carcinoma

SCLC — Small cell lung carcinoma

SLE — Systemic lupus erythematosus

TB — Tuberculosis

TNM — Tumour-Node-Metastasis (staging)

TTF-1 — Thyroid transcription factor 1

UC — Ulcerative colitis

WHO — World Health Organization

ZN — Ziehl-Neelsen

Chapter 1: Cell Injury, Adaptation, and Cell Death

THE BIG PICTURE

Cell injury produces characteristic morphological changes that form the basis of histopathological diagnosis. Swollen hepatocytes indicate ATP-dependent pump failure (hydropic change). Shrunken eosinophilic bodies with condensed nuclear fragments indicate caspase-mediated apoptosis. Preserved tissue outlines with nuclear loss indicate coagulative necrosis. This chapter covers the mechanisms of cellular adaptation, reversible and irreversible cell injury, necrosis, apoptosis, and other forms of regulated cell death. These concepts are foundational to all subsequent chapters in systemic pathology.

High-yield topics in this chapter: Apoptosis (intrinsic and extrinsic pathways, dysregulation), free radical mechanisms and antioxidant defence, ischaemia-reperfusion injury, necrosis (types and morphology), dystrophic versus metastatic calcification, newer forms of regulated cell death (pyroptosis, necroptosis, ferroptosis), cellular adaptations, autophagy, and telomere biology.

Cells continuously monitor their environment and respond through adaptation, injury, or death. Cell injury occurs when stress exceeds the cell's adaptive capacity or when the cell is exposed to inherently damaging agents. The morphological correlates of cell injury—swollen hepatocytes in hydropic change, shrunken eosinophilic bodies in apoptosis, ghost outlines in coagulative necrosis—are the foundation of histopathological diagnosis. This chapter covers the mechanisms and morphology of cellular adaptation, reversible and irreversible cell injury, and the principal forms of cell death.

Cellular Adaptations

When cells encounter persistent changes in their environment, they respond not by dying but by adapting. These adaptations are controlled, reversible alterations in cell size, number, phenotype, metabolic activity, or function. They represent a new, altered steady state that preserves viability while adjusting to the changed demand. The four principal adaptive responses are hypertrophy, hyperplasia, atrophy, and metaplasia. A fifth response, dysplasia, occupies the uncertain territory between adaptation and early neoplasia.

Hypertrophy

Hypertrophy is an increase in cell size resulting in an increase in organ size, without an increase in cell number. It occurs in cells with limited replicative capacity, notably cardiac myocytes and skeletal muscle fibres. The mechanisms differ between physiological and pathological hypertrophy.

Physiological hypertrophy, such as that seen in the exercising athlete or the gravid uterus, is driven primarily through the PI3K/Akt/mTOR signalling axis, which promotes protein synthesis and cell growth in a balanced, sustainable manner. Pathological hypertrophy, by contrast, is driven largely by neurohumoral activation. In the pressure-overloaded heart, angiotensin II and endothelin-1 activate the calcineurin-NFAT and GATA4 transcription factor pathways, producing a pattern of growth that is initially compensatory but ultimately maladaptive, predisposing to cardiac failure.

The key clinical distinction is this: physiological hypertrophy does not carry a risk of functional decompensation; pathological hypertrophy does. The PI3K/Akt pathway of physiological hypertrophy maintains normal sarcomere organisation and angiogenesis. The calcineurin-NFAT pathway of pathological hypertrophy promotes fibrosis and re-expression of foetal gene programmes (beta-myosin heavy chain, atrial natriuretic peptide), which are markers of a failing heart.

Hyperplasia

Hyperplasia is an increase in cell number resulting from increased cell division. It can only occur in cells capable of mitosis and therefore does not occur in cardiac muscle or neurons. Physiological hyperplasia takes two forms: hormonal hyperplasia, exemplified by proliferation of glandular breast epithelium at puberty and during pregnancy; and compensatory hyperplasia, exemplified by liver regeneration after partial hepatectomy.

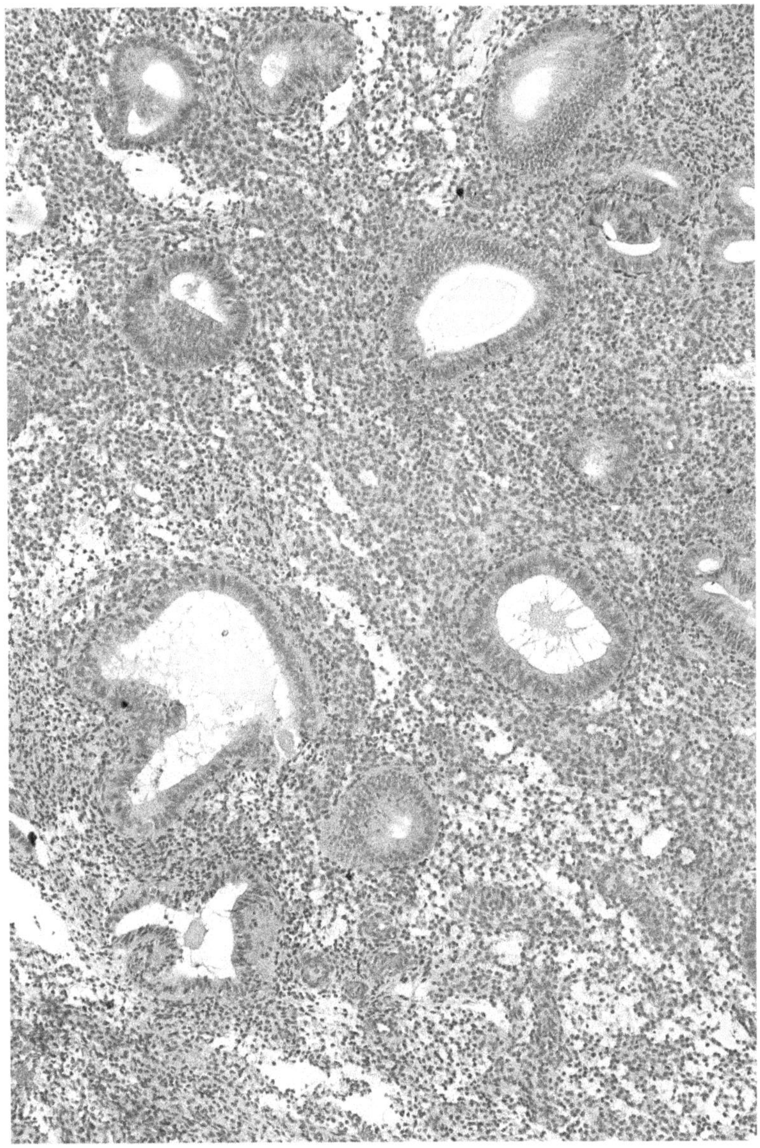

Figure 1.1: Simple endometrial hyperplasia. H&E showing increased endometrial glands with cystic dilation and abundant stroma. *(Source: Nephron, Wikimedia Commons, CC BY-SA 3.0.)*

Atrophy

Atrophy is the shrinkage of a cell by loss of cell substance, resulting in decreased organ size. The causes include disuse, denervation, diminished blood supply, inadequate nutrition, loss of endocrine stimulation, and pressure atrophy. Two principal degradation systems drive atrophy: the ubiquitin-proteasome pathway, which tags cytoplasmic proteins with ubiquitin chains for degradation; and autophagy, which degrades organelles through lysosomal digestion.

In skeletal muscle atrophy, transcription factors such as FoxO drive expression of E3 ubiquitin ligases atrogin-1 and MuRF1. The residual undigested lipofuscin granules accumulate as brown pigment in atrophic cells, producing brown atrophy, characteristically seen in the heart and liver of elderly or malnourished patients.

Clinical Pearl

Lipofuscin is the wear-and-tear pigment: insoluble brown-yellow granules of oxidised lipid-protein complexes, accumulated through decades of incomplete autophagic digestion. Brown atrophy of the heart in cachectic patients, brown discolouration of the liver in chronic illness, and pigmented neurons in the substantia nigra all reflect the same process. Lipofuscin is not pathological in itself, but its presence in unexpected quantity in a young patient signals chronic oxidative stress; in autopsy practice, brown atrophy is a useful corroborative finding for chronic systemic disease.

Metaplasia

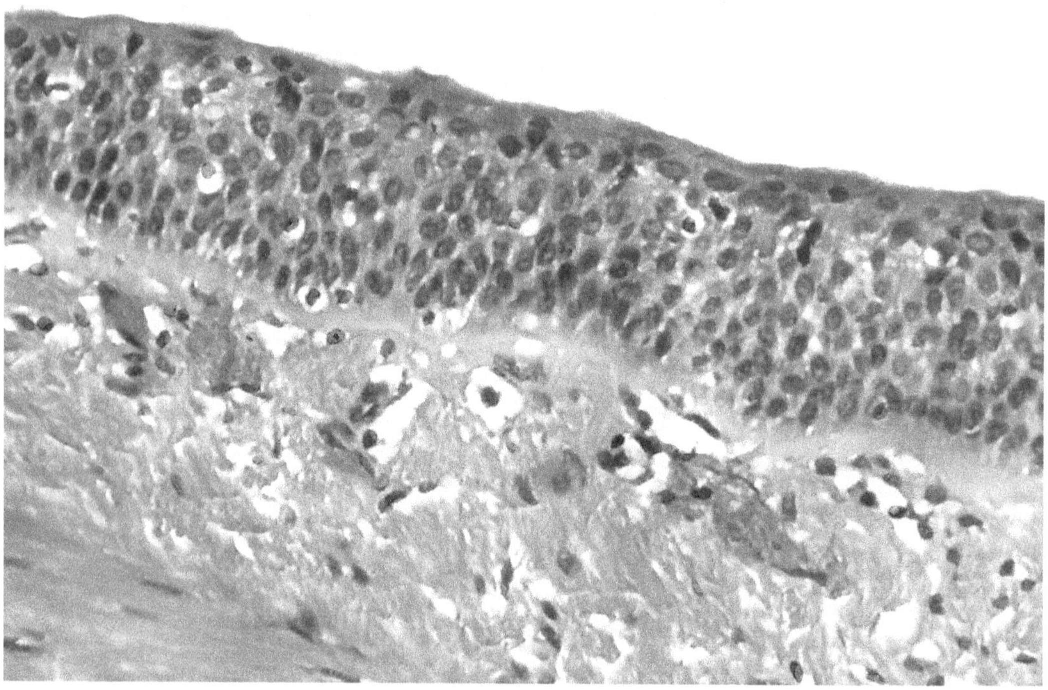

Figure 1.2: Squamous metaplasia of bronchial epithelium. H&E showing stratified squamous epithelium replacing pseudostratified ciliated columnar epithelium. *(Source: Yale Rosen, Wikimedia Commons, CC BY-SA 2.0.)*

Clinical Pearl

Metaplasia is reversible: remove the irritant (cessation of smoking, reflux control) and the normal epithelium can regenerate. However, metaplastic epithelium is not inherently premalignant. The danger is that the same chronic irritation driving metaplasia, if sustained, can drive the metaplastic epithelium into dysplasia, which IS the red flag that crosses the line toward neoplasia.

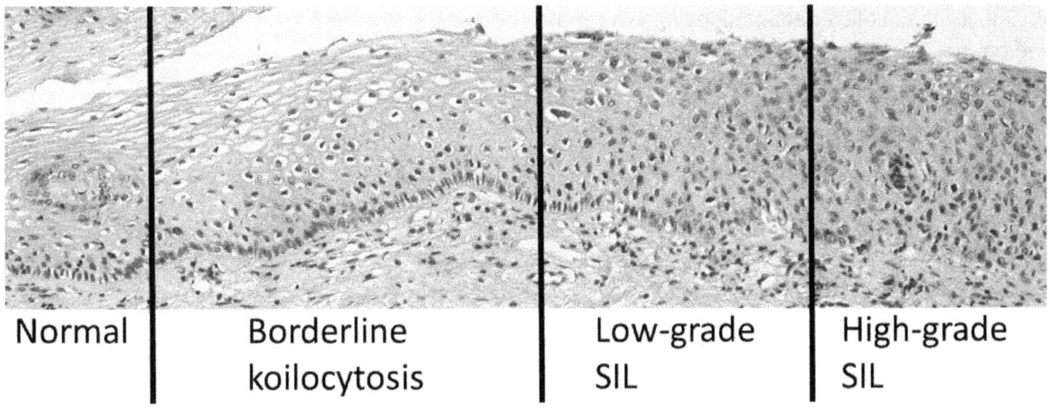

Figure 1.3: Spectrum of cervical squamous intraepithelial lesion (SIL). Comparison of normal, borderline koilocytosis, LSIL, and HSIL. *(Source: Mikael Häggström, Wikimedia Commons, CC0.)*

Dysplasia refers to disordered, premalignant epithelial growth characterised by loss of uniformity and architectural orientation. Dysplastic cells exhibit pleomorphism, hyperchromatic nuclei, increased nuclear-to-cytoplasmic ratio, disordered maturation, and increased mitotic figures including atypical mitoses. High-grade dysplasia (carcinoma in situ) involves the full thickness of the epithelium and, if untreated, carries significant risk of progression to invasive carcinoma. The biology and molecular basis of the dysplasia-carcinoma sequence are discussed in Chapter 6 (Figure 1.4).

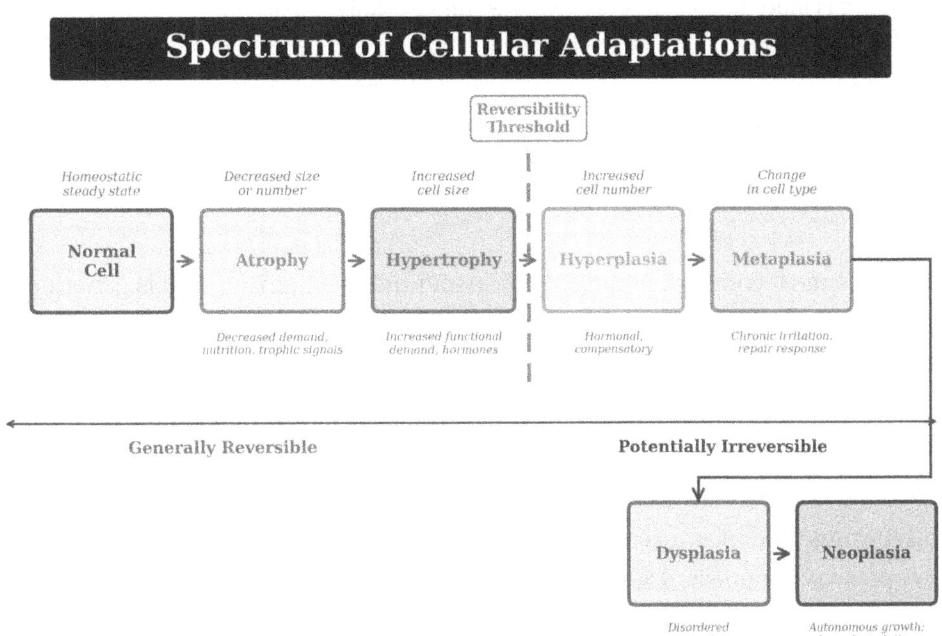

Figure 1.4: Spectrum of cellular adaptations from normal to neoplasia, showing reversibility thresholds. (Source: Author's original.)

Quick Recall: Cellular Adaptations

Hypertrophy: ↑ cell size (not number). Physiological = PI3K/Akt/mTOR.

Hyperplasia: ↑ cell number. Only in mitosis-competent cells.

Atrophy: ↓ cell size. Ubiquitin-proteasome + autophagy.

Metaplasia: Reversible switch in cell type. Stem cell reprogramming.

Dysplasia: Disordered growth. Premalignant.

Causes and Mechanisms of Cell Injury

Cell injury results when cells are stressed beyond their ability to adapt, exposed to inherently damaging agents, or deprived of essential substrates. The principal causes are hypoxia and ischaemia, physical agents, chemical agents, infectious agents, immunological reactions, genetic derangements, and nutritional imbalances.

Exam Pitfall

Ischaemia is worse than hypoxia. Hypoxia is reduced oxygen with preserved blood flow; the cell can still receive glucose and remove waste via anaerobic glycolysis. Ischaemia is reduced blood flow itself, depriving the cell of both oxygen and substrates while allowing toxic metabolites to accumulate. This is why ischaemic injury is more rapid and severe. Why is this clinically important?

Biochemical Mechanisms of Cell Injury

Regardless of the inciting cause, cell injury converges on a limited number of biochemical mechanisms. These are not mutually exclusive; in most forms of injury, several operate simultaneously in a self-amplifying cascade.

ATP depletion is the most common and most consequential mechanism. ATP is generated primarily by oxidative phosphorylation in mitochondria. Ischaemia, hypoxia, and mitochondrial damage all reduce ATP synthesis. The consequences unfold in a predictable sequence:

Ischaemia → ↓ATP → Na^+/K^+ pump failure → Na^+ + H_2O influx → cell swelling → anaerobic glycolysis → ↓pH (acidosis) → chromatin clumping → ribosome detachment → ↓protein synthesis

At this stage, the injury is still reversible. Restore blood flow, and the cell can recover.

Mitochondrial damage occupies a central role because mitochondria are both the major source of ATP and the gatekeepers of apoptosis. Damage can open the mitochondrial permeability transition pore (MPTP), a high-conductance channel in the inner mitochondrial membrane. Opening of the MPTP collapses the membrane potential, halts oxidative phosphorylation, and releases cytochrome c into the cytoplasm, triggering the intrinsic pathway of apoptosis.

Calcium influx is both a consequence and an amplifier of cell injury. Cytosolic calcium is normally maintained at very low concentrations (~0.1 μM) by active pumping. When pumps fail or membranes are damaged, cytosolic calcium rises dramatically, activating phospholipases (membrane damage), proteases (cytoskeletal degradation), endonucleases (DNA fragmentation), and ATPases (further ATP depletion). Calcium accumulation in mitochondria promotes MPTP opening, creating a vicious cycle.

The Point of No Return: Reversible versus Irreversible Injury

The Two Critical Points of No Return

Two events mark the transition from reversible to irreversible cell injury:

1. Mitochondrial permeability transition pore opening: collapses membrane potential, releases pro-apoptotic factors. Once this pore opens, the cell cannot regenerate its ATP supply.

2. Severe plasma membrane damage: loss of membrane phospholipids, cytoskeletal disruption, generation of lipid breakdown products. Once the membrane is breached, extracellular calcium floods in, lysosomal enzymes leak out, and intracellular contents escape (triggering inflammation).

The morphological correlates: reversible injury = cell swelling, fatty change, ER dilation. Irreversible injury = membrane blebs, mitochondrial dense bodies (calcium phosphate), nuclear changes (pyknosis, karyorrhexis, karyolysis) (Figure 1.5).

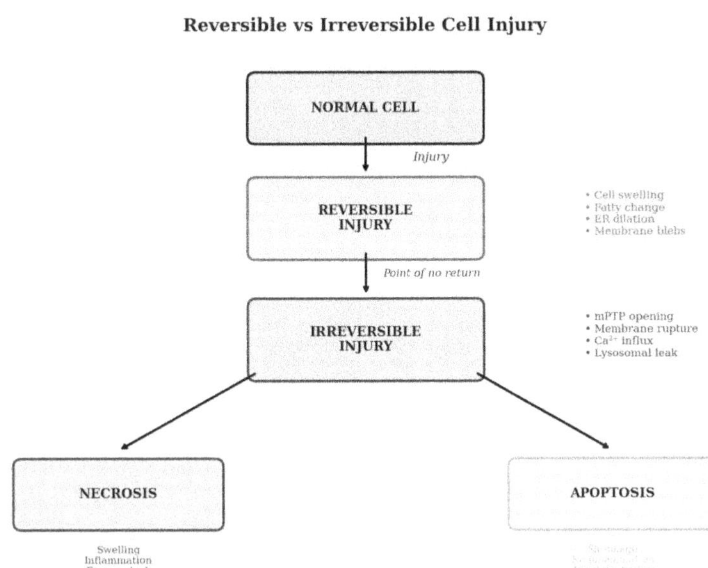

Figure 1.5: Reversible vs Irreversible Cell Injury. *(Source: Author's original.)*

If ischaemia persists beyond the reversible phase, the critical transition is marked by severe mitochondrial dysfunction (MPTP opening), massive calcium influx, and progressive membrane damage. Lysosomal enzymes leak into the cytoplasm and begin autodigestion. The cell undergoes necrosis (Figures 1.6–1.7).

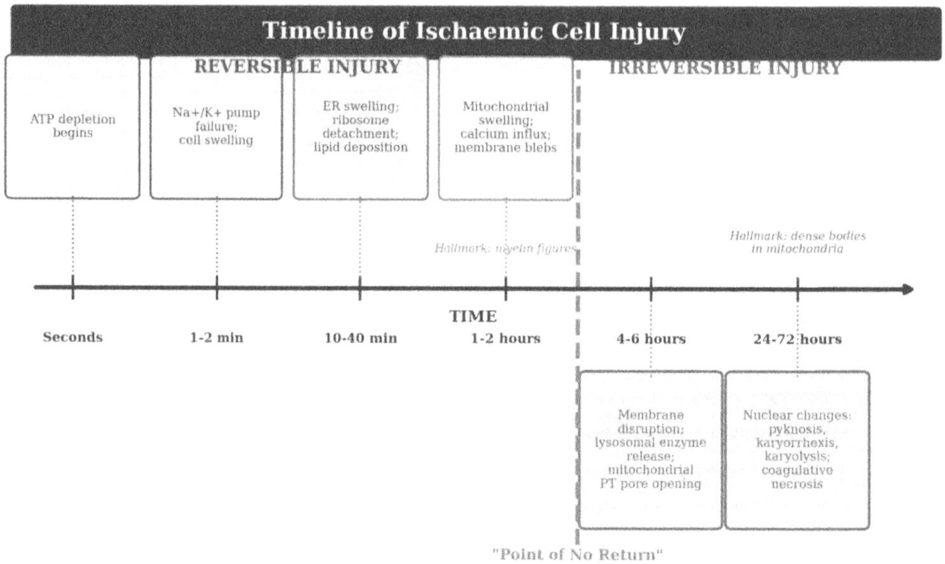

Figure 1.6: Timeline of ischaemic cell injury showing reversible and irreversible phases. (Source: Author's original.)

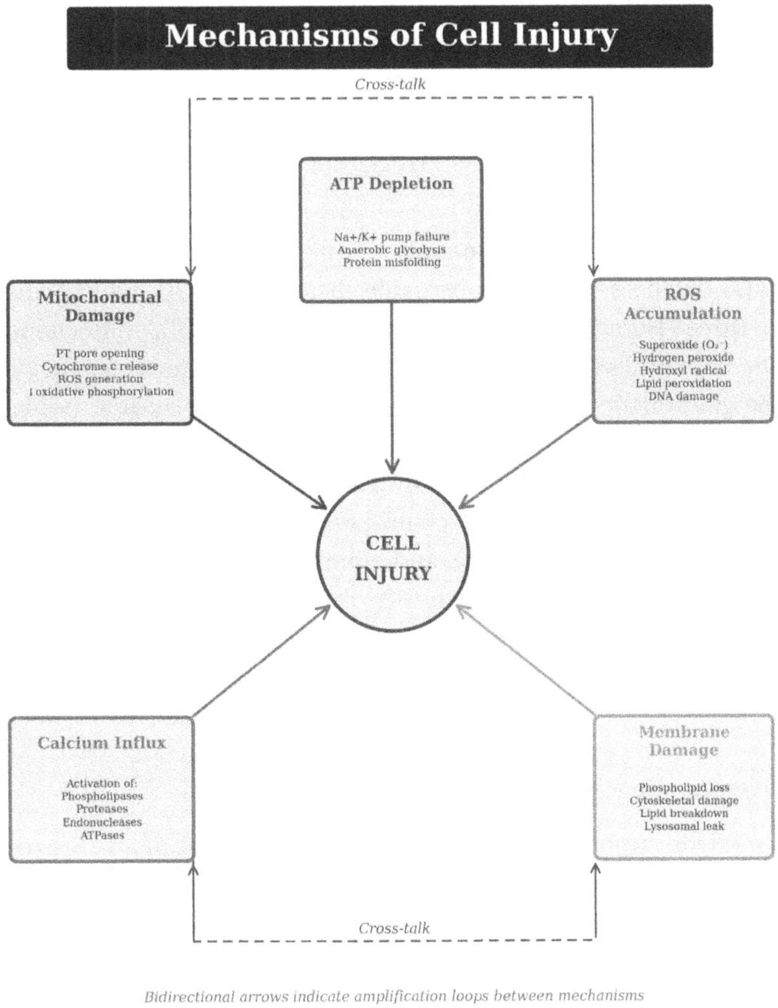

Figure 1.7: Mechanisms of cell injury: hub diagram with five major pathways. (Source: Author's original.)

Quick Recall: Mechanisms of Cell Injury

ATP depletion: pump failure → swelling → acidosis → ribosome detachment.

Mitochondrial damage: MPTP → ↓ATP + cytochrome c release → apoptosis.

Calcium influx: activates phospholipases, proteases, endonucleases, ATPases.

ROS: lipid peroxidation, protein oxidation, DNA damage.

Membrane damage: irreversible → necrosis.

Reversible: swelling, fatty change. Irreversible: membrane blebs, mitochondrial dense bodies, nuclear changes.

Free Radicals and Oxidative Stress

Free radicals are chemical species with a single unpaired electron in their outer orbital, making them highly reactive. The most important in biological systems are the reactive oxygen species (ROS): superoxide anion ($O_2 \bullet^-$), hydroxyl radical ($\bullet OH$), and hydrogen peroxide (H_2O_2, which generates hydroxyl radicals through the Fenton reaction). Reactive nitrogen species, particularly peroxynitrite ($ONOO^-$), also contribute.

The cellular antioxidant defence system operates at multiple levels and is essential for maintaining redox homeostasis. Enzymatic defences include superoxide dismutase (SOD, which converts superoxide to hydrogen peroxide; three isoforms exist: cytoplasmic Cu/Zn-SOD, mitochondrial Mn-SOD, and extracellular EC-SOD), catalase (which converts hydrogen peroxide to water and oxygen, primarily in peroxisomes), and the glutathione peroxidase/glutathione reductase system (which reduces hydrogen peroxide and lipid peroxides using reduced glutathione as a cofactor, with NADPH from the hexose monophosphate shunt regenerating oxidised glutathione). Non-enzymatic antioxidants include vitamin E (alpha-tocopherol, the principal lipid-soluble chain-breaking antioxidant in membranes), vitamin C (ascorbic acid, a water-soluble ROS scavenger), and glutathione itself (the most abundant intracellular thiol antioxidant). The Fenton reaction, in which Fe2+ catalyses conversion of hydrogen peroxide to the highly reactive hydroxyl radical, explains why iron overload states (haemochromatosis, transfusional siderosis, see Volume 1) are associated with oxidative tissue damage in the liver, heart, and endocrine organs.

Sources of Reactive Oxygen Species

The mitochondrial electron transport chain is the major endogenous source: during oxidative phosphorylation, a small proportion of electrons leak from complexes I and III and react with O_2 to form superoxide. Under ischaemia-reperfusion, this leakage increases dramatically.

Other enzymatic sources include xanthine oxidase (important in reperfusion injury), NADPH oxidase in phagocytic leukocytes (the respiratory burst for microbial killing), and the cytochrome P450 system (drug and xenobiotic metabolism). Exogenous sources include ionising radiation, ultraviolet light, cigarette smoke, and certain drugs.

Mechanisms of ROS-Mediated Cell Injury

Lipid peroxidation: free radicals attack double bonds in polyunsaturated fatty acids of membrane phospholipids, generating lipid peroxyl radicals that propagate chain reactions. By-products include malondialdehyde and 4-hydroxynonenal. This destabilises both plasma and organelle membranes.

Protein oxidation: oxidation of amino acid side chains, protein-protein cross-links, and backbone fragmentation lead to loss of enzymatic activity and enhanced proteasomal degradation.

DNA damage: single-strand and double-strand breaks, base modifications (particularly 8-hydroxydeoxyguanosine, a widely used biomarker of oxidative DNA damage), and cross-links. Such damage drives mutagenesis, ageing, and carcinogenesis.

The pathologist suspects oxidative stress as a driver of disease not by seeing ROS directly, but by recognising its footprints: increased lipofuscin (the wear-and-tear pigment of oxidative damage), Mallory-Denk bodies (oxidatively damaged cytokeratins in steatohepatitis), or iron accumulation in tissues (the Fenton reaction waiting to happen).

> **Clinical Pearl**
>
> **The Fenton reaction ($Fe^{2+} + H_2O_2 \rightarrow Fe^{3+} + \bullet OH + OH^-$)** is why iron overload causes tissue damage. This single reaction links haemochromatosis, transfusion siderosis, and iron-mediated cell injury. It explains why free iron is always bound to carrier proteins (transferrin in plasma, ferritin intracellularly): the body treats free iron as a toxin.

Antioxidant Defence Mechanisms

The cell maintains elaborate antioxidant defences, both enzymatic and non-enzymatic, to neutralise ROS before they cause damage.

Table 1.4: Antioxidant Defence Systems

Enzyme/Molecule	Reaction/Action	Location	Cofactor	Clinical Note
Superoxide dismutase (SOD)	$2O_2\bullet^- \rightarrow H_2O_2 + O_2$	Mitochondria (Mn-SOD), cytoplasm (Cu/Zn-SOD)	Mn, Cu, Zn	First line of defence
Catalase	$2H_2O_2 \rightarrow 2H_2O + O_2$	Peroxisomes	Fe (haem)	Especially important in hepatocytes
Glutathione peroxidase (GPx)	$H_2O_2 + 2GSH \rightarrow GSSG + 2H_2O$	Cytoplasm, mitochondria	Selenium	Also reduces lipid peroxides; selenium deficiency impairs this
Glutathione reductase	$GSSG + NADPH \rightarrow 2GSH$	Cytoplasm	NADPH (G6PD)	Links to G6PD deficiency
Vitamin E (α-tocopherol)	Lipid peroxyl radical quenching	Cell membranes (lipid phase)	Dietary	Major chain-breaking antioxidant in membranes
Vitamin C (ascorbate)	Regenerates vitamin E; scavenges aqueous ROS	Cytoplasm (aqueous phase)	Dietary	Pro-oxidant at high concentrations with free iron

Ferritin, transferrin, ceruloplasmin	Sequester free iron and copper	Intracellular, plasma	N/A	Prevent Fenton reaction (Figure 1.8)

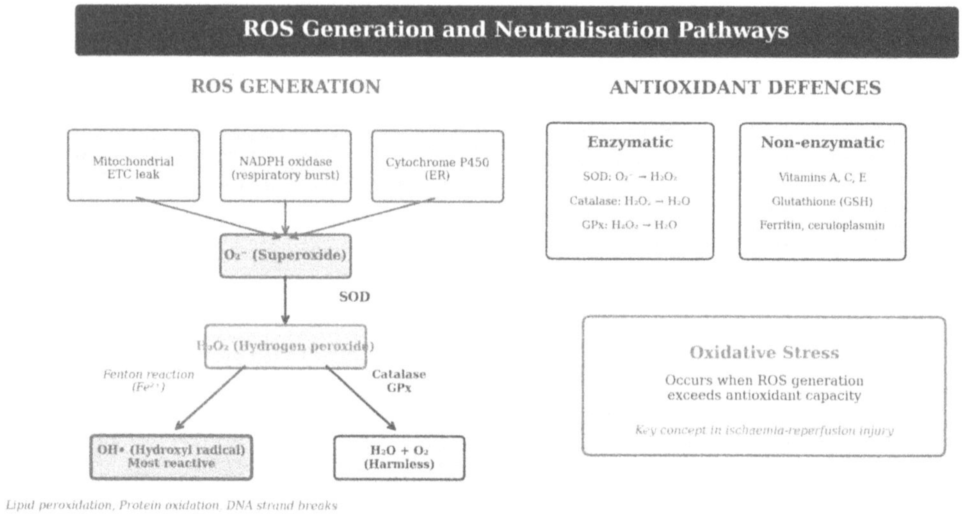

Figure 1.8: Generation and neutralisation of reactive oxygen species (ROS). (Source: Author's original.)

Integration: Oxidative stress is not confined to this chapter. It is a recurring theme linking cell injury to ageing (telomere damage, Section 12), carcinogenesis (DNA mutations, Chapter 6), atherosclerosis (LDL oxidation, Chapter 13), and inflammation (neutrophil respiratory burst, Chapter 2). Recognising oxidative stress as a unifying mechanism across organ systems is a hallmark of sophisticated pathological thinking.

Ischaemia-Reperfusion Injury

One of the most clinically important manifestations of oxidative stress is ischaemia-reperfusion injury: the paradox that restoration of blood flow to ischaemic tissue can cause additional damage beyond that produced by the ischaemia itself. This is relevant in myocardial reperfusion after thrombolysis, organ transplantation, and restoration of circulation after shock.

The mechanisms involve interconnected pathways. Reoxygenation of damaged mitochondria generates a burst of ROS from the electron transport chain. Xanthine oxidase, converted from xanthine dehydrogenase during ischaemia, uses accumulated hypoxanthine as substrate to generate superoxide upon reoxygenation. The damaged endothelium expresses adhesion molecules (P-selectin, ICAM-1) that recruit neutrophils, which release additional ROS and proteases. The complement system is activated, generating C3a, C5a, and the membrane attack complex. In severely damaged cells, reoxygenation triggers the mitochondrial permeability transition, converting recoverable cells into ones that undergo necrosis.

Ischaemia: ↓ATP → XD → XO conversion → hypoxanthine accumulation || Reperfusion: O_2 returns → XO + hypoxanthine → ROS burst → complement activation → neutrophil recruitment → tissue damage (Figure 1.9)

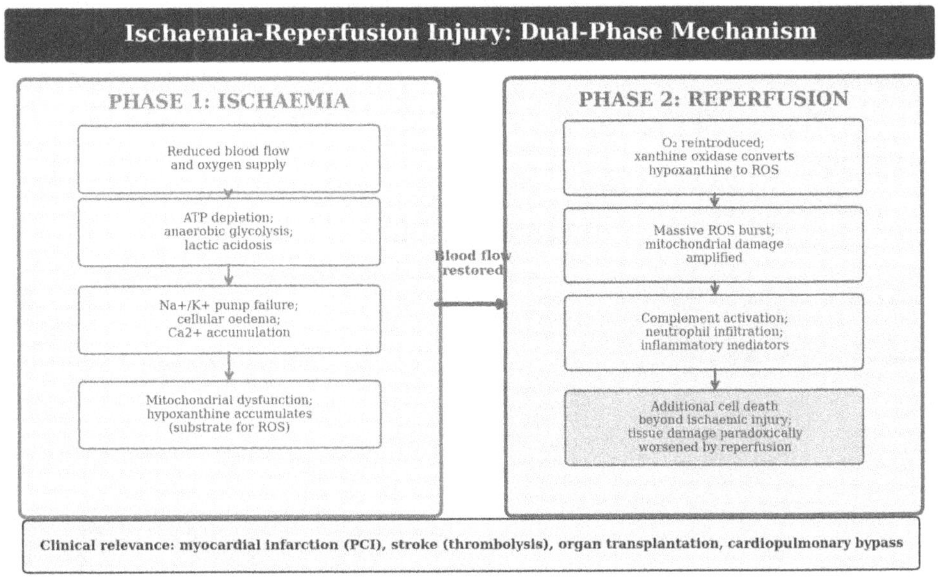

Figure 1.9: Mechanism of ischaemia-reperfusion injury. (Source: Author's original.)

Quick Recall: Free Radicals and Reperfusion

ROS sources: mitochondrial ETC, xanthine oxidase, NADPH oxidase, cytochrome P450, radiation.

ROS damage: lipid peroxidation, protein oxidation, DNA damage (8-OHdG).

Defence: SOD → catalase/GPx. Vitamin E (membranes), C (cytoplasm).

Fenton: Fe^{2+} + H_2O_2 → •OH. Why iron overload = tissue damage.

Reperfusion: ROS burst (XO + mitochondria) + complement + neutrophils → paradoxical damage.

IRI is clinically significant across cardiology (reperfusion injury after PCI accounts for up to 50% of infarct size), nephrology (principal mechanism of ATN in renal transplantation; see Chapter 23), and neurology. Experimental mitigation strategies include ischaemic preconditioning and postconditioning. Molecularly, IRI involves ATP depletion, calcium overload, mPTP opening during ischaemia, followed by ROS burst (xanthine oxidase, mitochondrial dysfunction), complement activation, neutrophil recruitment, and NLRP3 inflammasome activation upon reperfusion.*This finding, when seen alongside reperfusion injury in exam questions, points strongly towards:* a question about the paradox of oxygen as both essential for survival and a source of additional damage. The examiners expect candidates to articulate the specific molecular mechanisms (xanthine oxidase, mitochondrial ROS burst, complement activation, neutrophil-mediated injury) rather than simply stating that reperfusion causes damage.

Necrosis

Necrosis is the morphological pattern of cell death resulting from severe, irreversible injury. It is characterised by cellular swelling, protein denaturation, and organelle breakdown. Unlike apoptosis, necrosis is always pathological and always provokes inflammation, because the disrupted membrane releases intracellular contents (damage-associated molecular patterns, DAMPs) into the surrounding tissue.

Morphological Features

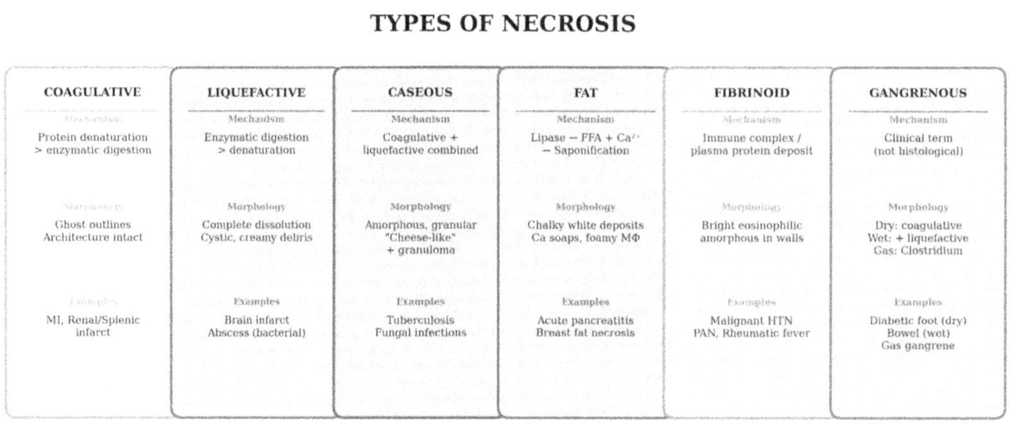

Figure 1.10: Types of necrosis — morphological classification comparing coagulative, liquefactive, caseous, fat, fibrinoid, and gangrenous patterns. (Source: Author's original.)

Figure: Types of Necrosis: Comparative Overview. (Source: Author's original.)

The nuclear changes are the most reliable indicators on histopathology. Three patterns are recognised: pyknosis (nuclear shrinkage with chromatin condensation into a dark basophilic mass), karyorrhexis (fragmentation of the pyknotic nucleus), and karyolysis (dissolution of the nucleus by DNase activity, leaving a faint ghost outline). These progress sequentially. Cytoplasmic changes include increased eosinophilia (denatured proteins, lost RNA basophilia), a glassy homogeneous appearance, and vacuolation as organelle membranes are digested.

> **The Pathologist's Eye**
>
> **Artefact versus true cell death:** "Dark neurons" in brain biopsies, crush artefact in small biopsies, and drying artefact in frozen sections can mimic necrosis or apoptosis. The key distinction: artefactual damage is spatially random and does not respect anatomical boundaries, whereas true necrosis follows vascular territories (infarcts) or surrounds an inflammatory focus (abscess). Nuclear changes of true necrosis (pyknosis, karyorrhexis, karyolysis) progress in an orderly sequence; artefactual darkening is uniform and does not show this progression. This is a common pitfall for junior residents examining surgical pathology specimens.

Types of Necrosis

Table 1.5: Types of Necrosis

Type	Mechanism	Classic Sites	Morphology	Clinical Example
Coagulative	Protein denaturation > enzymatic digestion; architecture preserved	Most organs (heart, kidney, spleen); ischaemic injury	Ghost outlines of cells; no nuclei; architecture maintained	Myocardial infarction, renal infarction
Liquefactive	Enzymatic digestion > protein denaturation; tissue liquefied	Brain; also bacterial abscess	Creamy liquid; no architecture	Cerebral infarction, abscess (Figure 1.14)
Caseous	Combination of coagulative and liquefactive; amorphous debris	Centre of granulomas (TB)	Structureless, granular, eosinophilic	Tuberculosis, fungal infections
Fat necrosis	Lipase digests adipose; fatty acids + calcium = saponification	Peripancreatic (enzymatic); breast (traumatic)	Chalky white; basophilic Ca deposits	Acute pancreatitis
Fibrinoid	Fibrin-like material in vessel walls	Vessel walls in vasculitis, malignant hypertension	Bright pink, smudgy, homogeneous in vessel wall (Figure 1.13)	PAN, malignant HTN

A question that reveals diagnostic understanding: why is brain infarction liquefactive when virtually all other organ infarcts are coagulative? The answer lies in the high lipid content of neural tissue and the abundance of hydrolytic enzymes, which favour enzymatic digestion over protein denaturation. Additionally, the brain parenchyma lacks the firm stromal framework that preserves architecture in coagulative necrosis of solid organs like the kidney or spleen.

> **Exam Pitfall**
>
> **Gangrenous necrosis is not a separate histological type.** Dry gangrene = coagulative necrosis + desiccation (peripheral vascular disease of a limb). Wet gangrene = coagulative + liquefactive from bacterial superinfection (bowel infarction, diabetic feet) (Figure 1.16). Gas gangrene = wet gangrene + Clostridium perfringens.

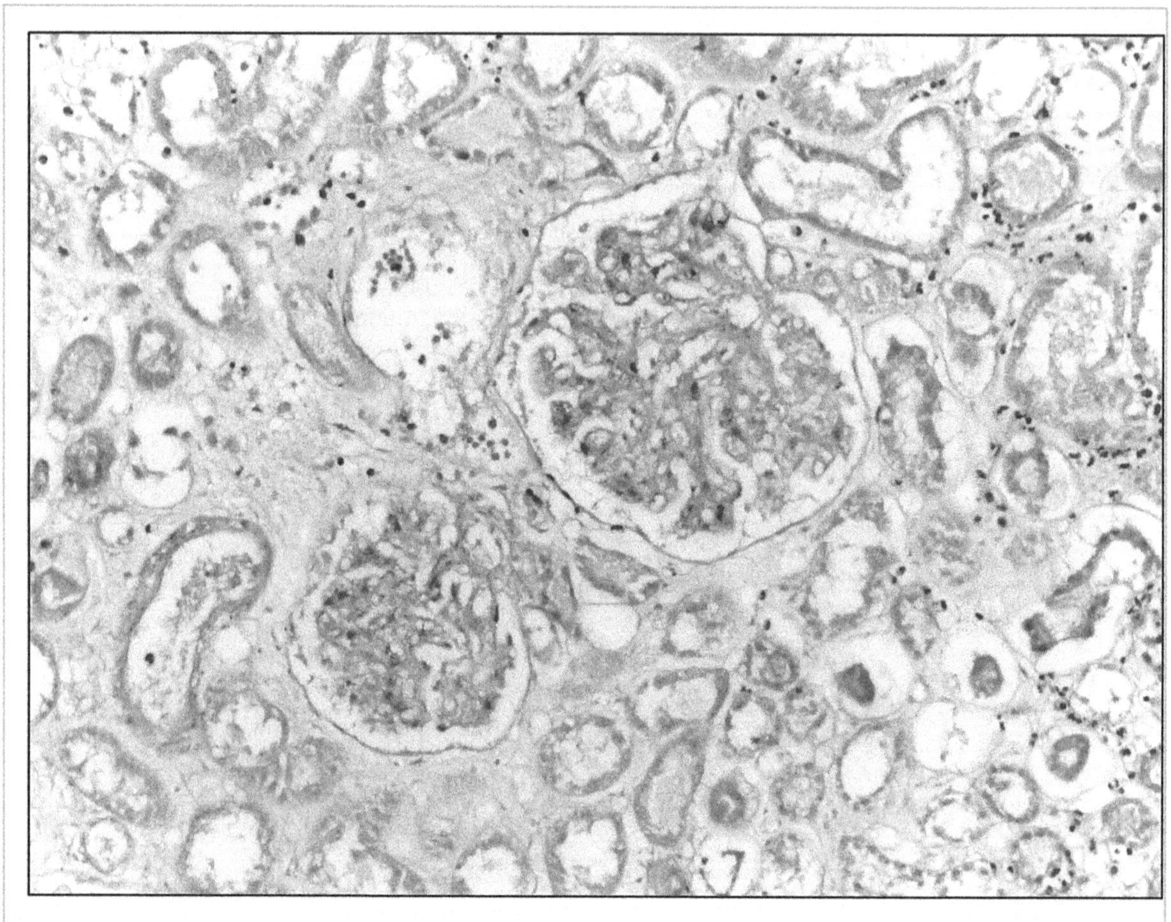

Diagnostic thinking: preserved architecture + absent nuclei → coagulative necrosis (Figure 1.11)

Diagnostic thinking: amorphous debris + epithelioid rim + Langhans cells → caseous necrosis (TB until proven otherwise) (Figures 1.12 and 1.15)

Figure 1.11: Coagulative necrosis of kidney. Preserved tissue architecture with ghost outlines of tubules; nuclei absent. H&E, 200×. (Source: Patho, Wikimedia Commons, CC BY-SA 4.0.)

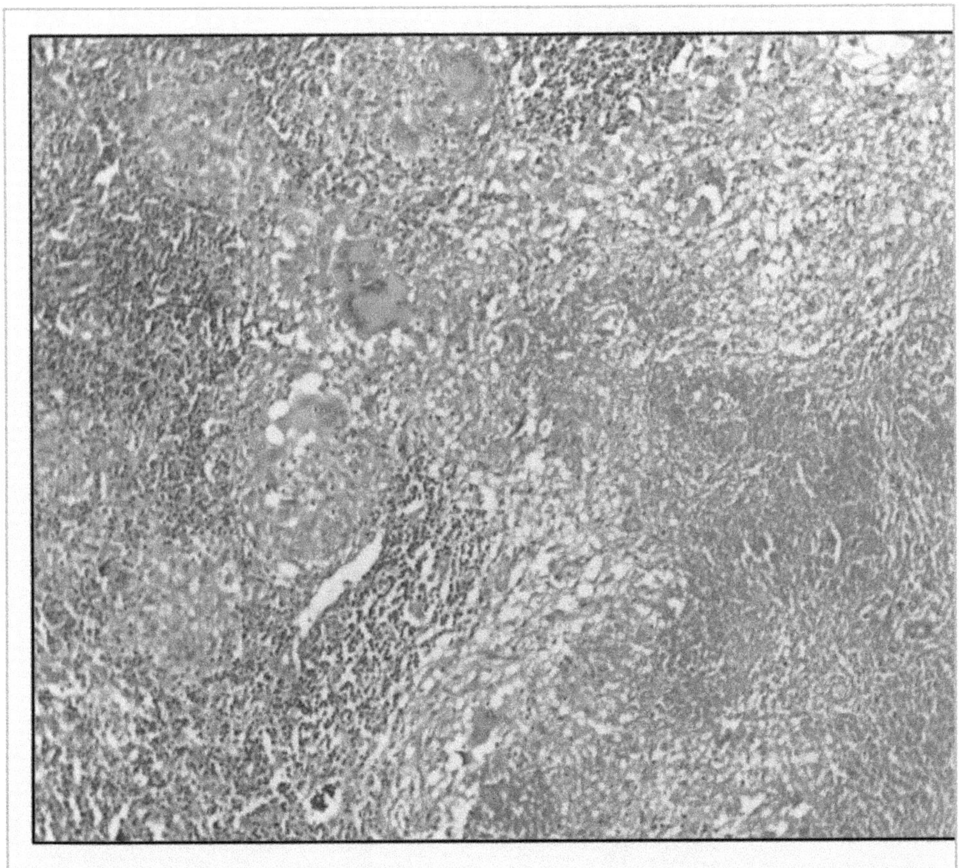

Figure 1.12: Caseous necrosis in a lymph node. Amorphous, granular, eosinophilic debris without preserved cellular outlines, surrounded by epithelioid histiocytes. H&E, 100×. (Source: Patho, Wikimedia Commons, CC BY-SA 4.0.)

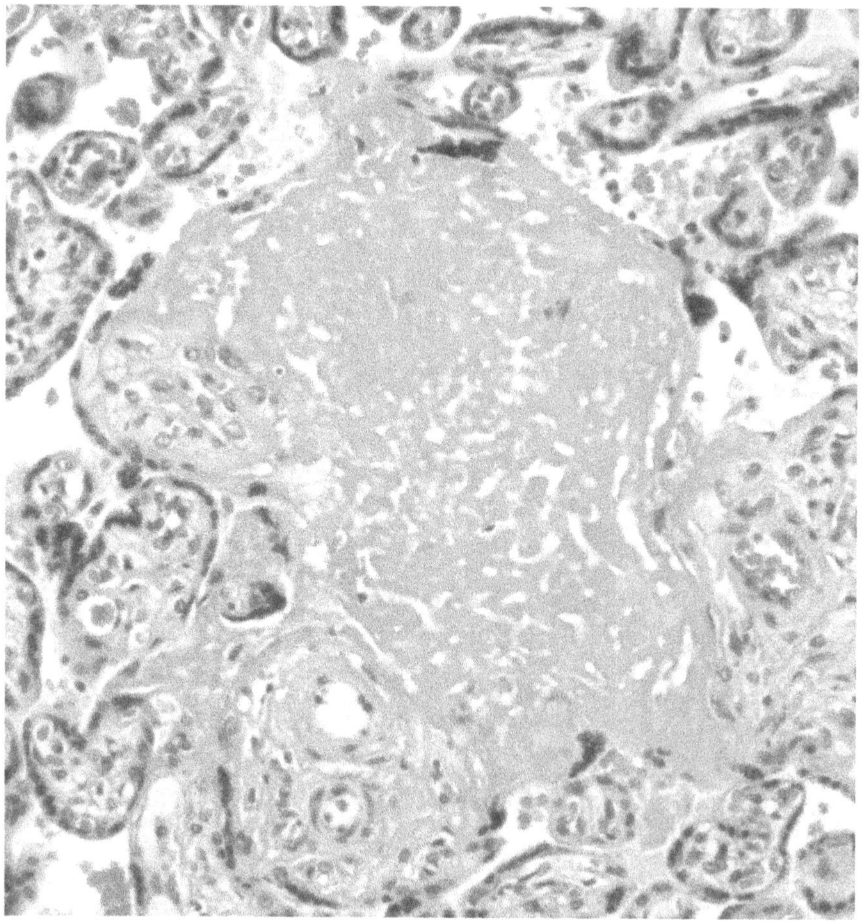

Figure 1.13: Fibrinoid necrosis of placental villi. Brightly eosinophilic, smudgy deposits replacing normal villous architecture; H&E, high magnification. (Source: Mikael Häggström, Wikimedia Commons, CC BY-SA 4.0.)

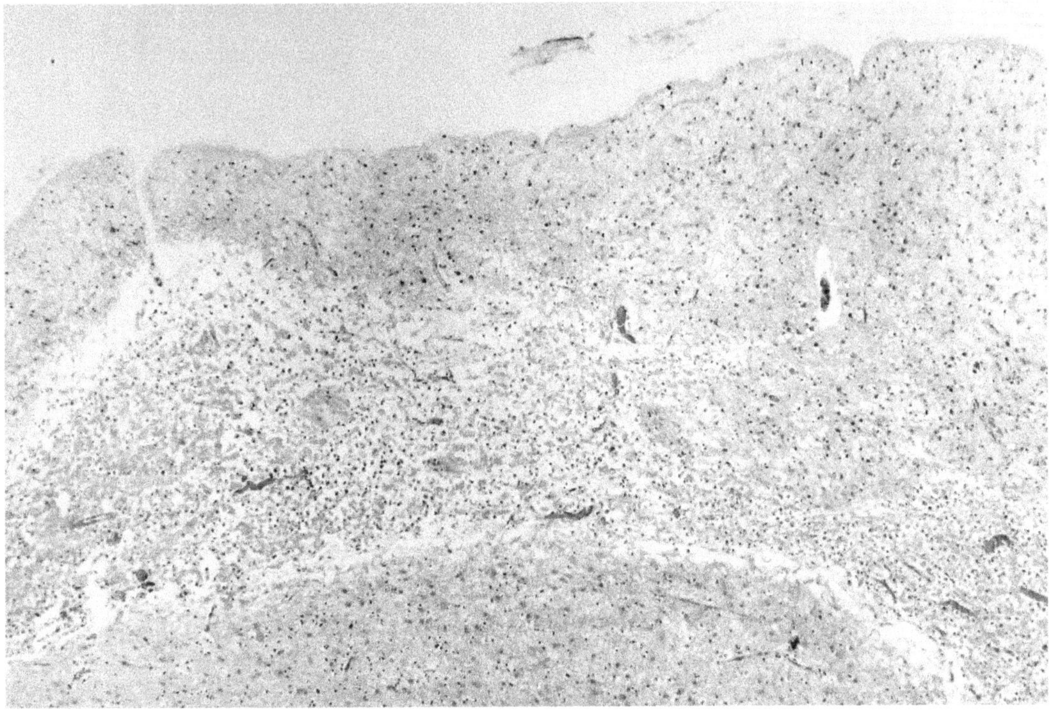

Figure 1.14: Liquefactive necrosis — ischaemic cerebral infarct (~24 hours). H&E showing tissue dissolution, red neurons, and neutrophilic infiltration. (Source: Patho, Wikimedia Commons, CC BY-SA 3.0.)

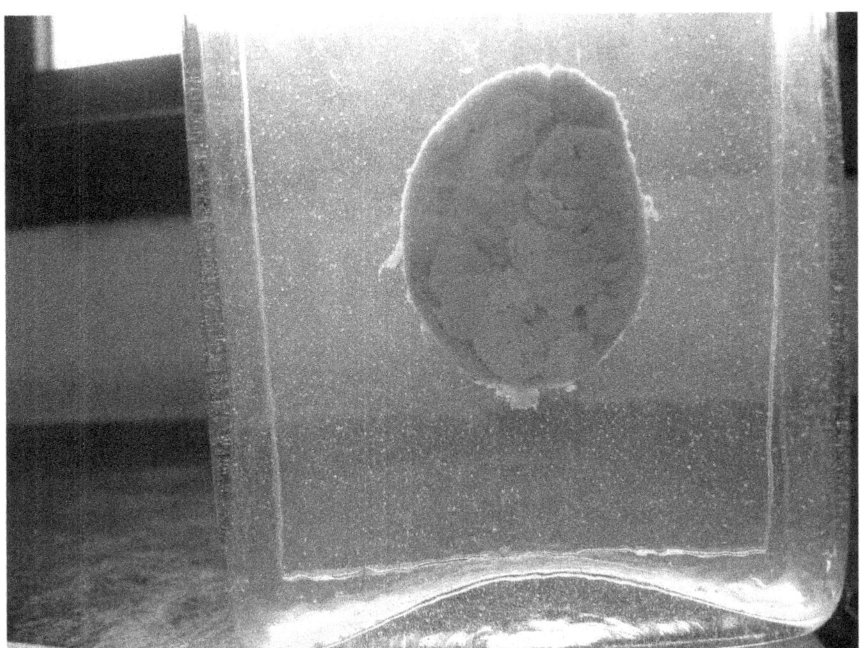

Figure 1.15: Caseous necrosis (lymph node, gross). Friable, cheese-like central necrosis in granulomatous tuberculosis. (Source: Yale Rosen, Wikimedia Commons, CC BY-SA 2.0.)

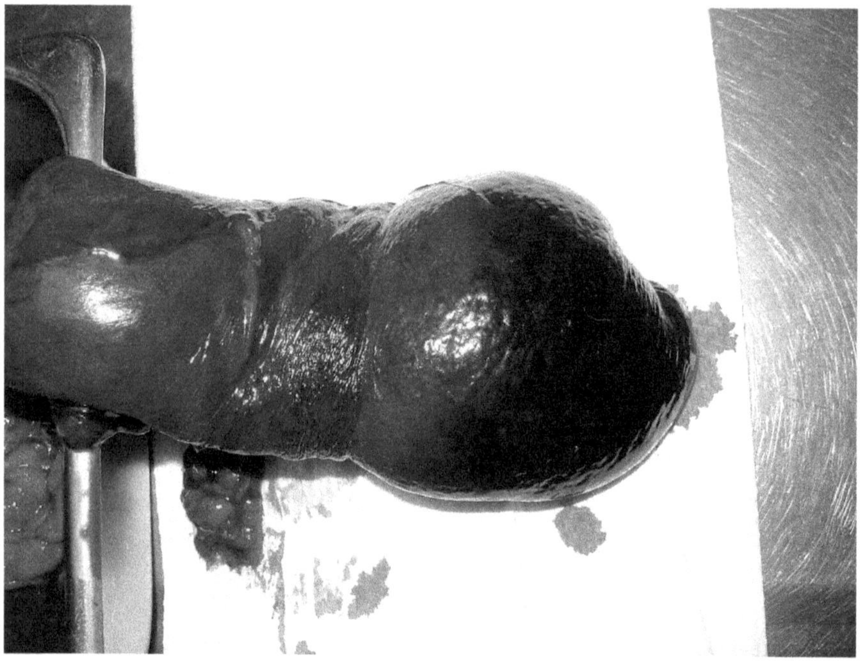

Figure 1.16: Gangrenous necrosis (spleen, gross). Gross specimen of splenic necrosis demonstrating haemorrhagic/ischaemic mechanisms. (Source: KGH, Wikimedia Commons, CC BY-SA 3.0.)

Apoptosis

Apoptosis is a pathway of cell death in which the cell activates an internally encoded suicide programme, resulting in orderly dismantling without eliciting inflammation. The term, from the Greek for "falling off" (as leaves from a tree), was coined by Kerr, Wyllie, and Currie in 1972. Apoptosis is not merely passive; it is an active, energy-requiring process essential for embryogenesis, tissue homeostasis, and immune regulation. Its dysregulation is implicated in cancer (insufficient apoptosis), autoimmune diseases (insufficient elimination of self-reactive lymphocytes), and neurodegenerative diseases (excessive apoptosis).

Necrosis versus Apoptosis

Figure: Apoptosis versus Necrosis. (Source: Author's original.)

Table 1.6: Necrosis versus Apoptosis

Feature	Necrosis	Apoptosis
Cell size	Enlarged (swelling)	Reduced (shrinkage)
Nucleus	Pyknosis → karyorrhexis → karyolysis	Condensation, fragmentation into discrete fragments

Plasma membrane	Disrupted early	Intact until late; blebs form but do not rupture
Cellular contents	Released (DAMPs)	Retained in apoptotic bodies
Inflammation	Always present (neutrophilic)	Absent (immunologically silent)
Mechanism	Passive, energy-independent	Active, ATP-dependent, caspase-mediated
Physiological?	Always pathological	Both physiological and pathological
DNA pattern	Random degradation (smear on gel)	Internucleosomal cleavage (DNA ladder)
Detection	LDH release, vital dye uptake	Annexin V (PS), TUNEL, caspase assays

Morphological Features of Apoptosis

The apoptotic cell shrinks, with dense eosinophilic cytoplasm and tightly packed organelles. Chromatin condenses along the nuclear membrane in crescentic or globular masses. The cell fragments into membrane-bound apoptotic bodies, each containing cytoplasm with or without nuclear fragments. These are rapidly phagocytosed by neighbouring cells and macrophages.

On a histology slide, the diagnostic clue to apoptosis is not just the presence of dying cells, but the absence of surrounding inflammation. Finding an eosinophilic body with a condensed nuclear fragment in a background of intact, uninflamed liver parenchyma points to apoptosis (Councilman body in viral hepatitis). A similar cell in a sea of neutrophils points to necrosis. This distinction is fundamental and is the first question the pathologist should ask when encountering cell death on a biopsy.

The Intrinsic (Mitochondrial) Pathway

The intrinsic pathway is triggered by intracellular signals: DNA damage, ER stress, growth factor withdrawal, oxidative stress. The central regulators are the Bcl-2 family of proteins, which govern mitochondrial outer membrane permeability.

Three functional groups: anti-apoptotic members (Bcl-2, Bcl-xL, Mcl-1) guard the mitochondrial membrane; pro-apoptotic effectors (Bax, Bak), when activated, oligomerise in the outer membrane to form channels; and BH3-only sensors (Bid, Bim, Bad, Puma, Noxa) detect stress signals and tip the balance towards death.

The decision to live or die depends on the ratio of pro-apoptotic to anti-apoptotic members. When BH3-only proteins are activated, they neutralise anti-apoptotic members and activate Bax/Bak. The activated effectors form pores in the outer mitochondrial membrane, releasing cytochrome c into the cytoplasm.

Cytochrome c binds APAF-1 and, with dATP, assembles the apoptosome (a heptameric wheel-shaped structure) that recruits and activates caspase-9 (initiator caspase of the intrinsic pathway). Activated caspase-9 cleaves executioner caspases (caspase-3, -6, -7). Other mitochondrial proteins released include Smac/DIABLO (neutralises IAPs) and AIF (caspase-independent DNA fragmentation).

Stress signal → BH3-only activation → Bax/Bak pore formation → cytochrome c release → apoptosome (APAF-1 + caspase-9) → caspase-3 activation → execution

The Extrinsic (Death Receptor) Pathway

The extrinsic pathway is initiated by engagement of cell surface death receptors: FasL/Fas (CD95), TNF/TNFR1, TRAIL/DR4-DR5. These receptors contain a cytoplasmic death domain (DD) essential for signalling.

When Fas is engaged by FasL (on cytotoxic T cells and NK cells), its death domain recruits FADD, which recruits procaspase-8 via death effector domain (DED) interactions. The resulting DISC (death-inducing signalling complex) activates caspase-8 by induced proximity. Caspase-8 then either directly activates executioner caspases (type I cells, e.g. thymocytes) or cleaves Bid to truncated Bid (tBid), which translocates to mitochondria and activates the intrinsic pathway (type II cells, e.g. hepatocytes). This cross-talk via Bid links both pathways and amplifies the signal.

FasL → Fas → FADD → DISC → caspase-8 || Type I: caspase-8 → caspase-3 directly || Type II: caspase-8 → Bid cleavage → mitochondrial pathway

The Execution Phase

The Caspase Cascade

Initiator caspases (caspase-8 from extrinsic, caspase-9 from intrinsic) activate **executioner caspases** (caspase-3, -6, -7). Caspase-3 is the convergence point:

- Cleaves ICAD → releases CAD → internucleosomal DNA fragmentation (DNA ladder)
- Cleaves lamins → nuclear envelope dissolution
- Cleaves cytoskeletal proteins → cell shrinkage and blebbing

Clearance of Apoptotic Bodies

Apoptotic cells expose phosphatidylserine (PS) on the outer membrane leaflet (normally confined to the inner leaflet by flippases). PS acts as an "eat-me" signal recognised by macrophage receptors (TIM-4, BAI1, stabilin-2). Additional signals include thrombospondin and oxidised lipids. The phagocyte engulfs the apoptotic body before its membrane ruptures, preventing release of pro-inflammatory contents. This immunologically silent clearance is the defining difference from necrosis.

Dysregulated Apoptosis in Disease

Insufficient apoptosis: in cancer, overexpression of anti-apoptotic proteins (Bcl-2 in follicular lymphoma from t(14;18), Mcl-1 in myeloma) or loss of pro-apoptotic signalling (TP53 mutations eliminating Puma/Noxa) enables tumour cell accumulation. In autoimmune diseases, defective Fas/FasL signalling (autoimmune lymphoproliferative syndrome, ALPS) allows self-reactive clones to persist.

Excessive apoptosis: in neurodegenerative diseases (Alzheimer, Parkinson), neurons undergo apoptosis from misfolded protein accumulation and mitochondrial dysfunction. In AIDS, CD4+ T cells are depleted by both direct viral killing and bystander apoptosis. Post-ischaemic apoptosis in the penumbral zone of cerebral infarcts contributes to infarct expansion.

> **Clinical Pearl**
>
> **Venetoclax** (a selective Bcl-2 inhibitor) is the clinical proof that apoptosis pathways are druggable. By blocking Bcl-2, venetoclax restores the ability of CLL cells and AML blasts to undergo apoptosis. Its success has validated decades of basic apoptosis research. For venetoclax in CLL and AML treatment protocols, see Volume 1 (Figures 1.17–1.18).

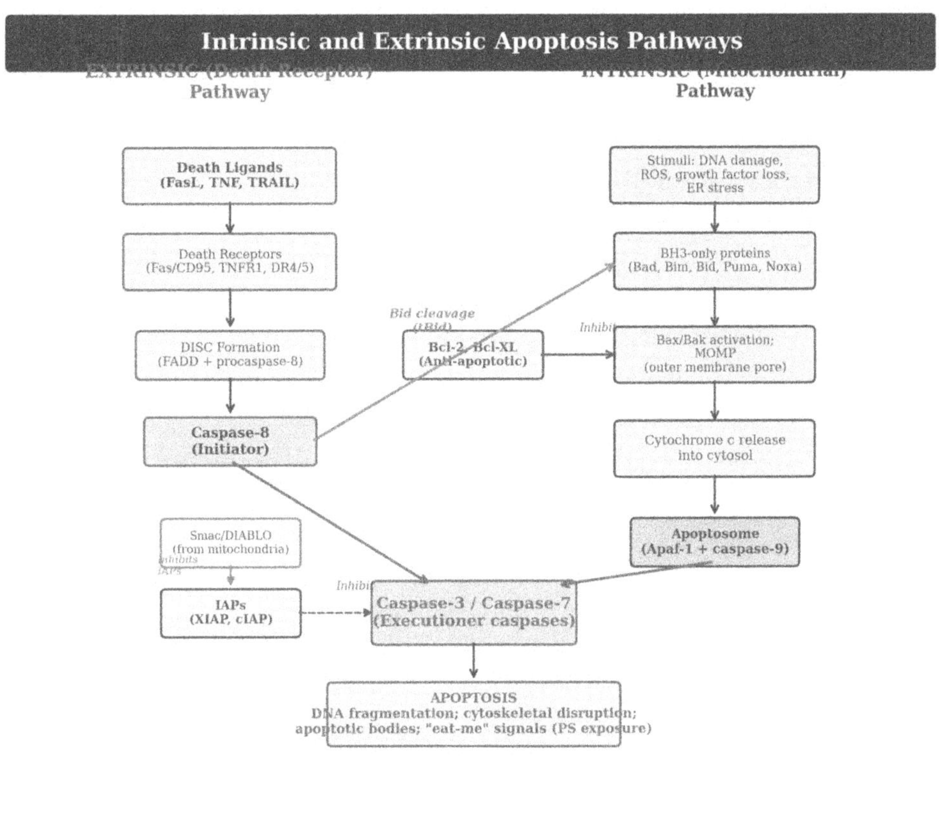

Figure 1.17: Intrinsic and extrinsic pathways of apoptosis. (Source: Author's original.)

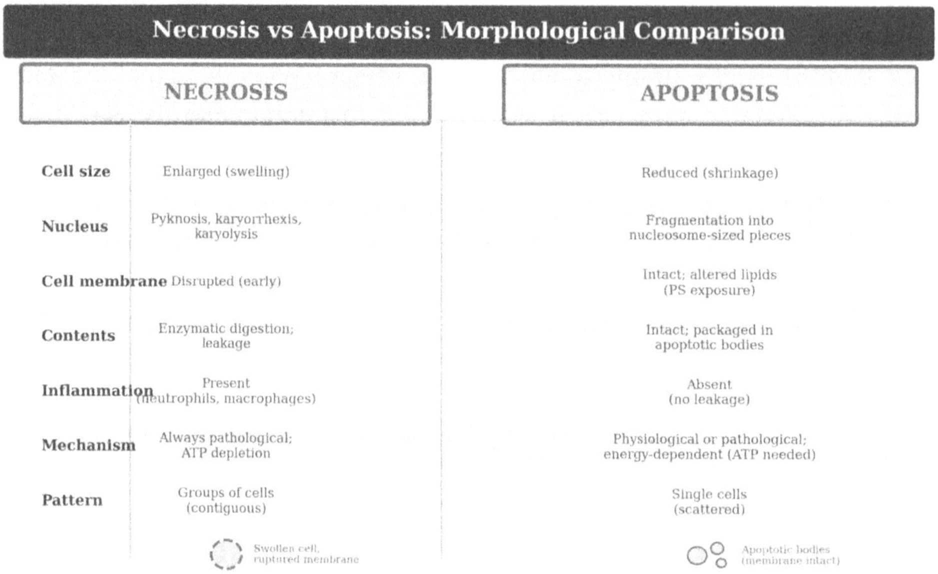

Figure 1.18: Necrosis versus apoptosis: morphological comparison. (Source: Author's original.)

Quick Recall: Apoptosis

Intrinsic (mitochondrial): stress → BH3-only → Bax/Bak pores → cytochrome c → apoptosome → caspase-9 → caspase-3.

Extrinsic (death receptor): FasL/Fas → FADD → DISC → caspase-8 → caspase-3 (or Bid → intrinsic).

Convergence: caspase-3 → ICAD → DNA ladder; lamins → nuclear dissolution.

Clearance: PS exposure → eat-me signal → silent phagocytosis.

↓ **Apoptosis:** cancer (Bcl-2), autoimmunity (ALPS).

↑ **Apoptosis:** neurodegeneration, AIDS, post-ischaemic injury.

Other Forms of Regulated Cell Death

The traditional necrosis/apoptosis dichotomy is an oversimplification. Several additional forms of regulated cell death share features of both and are increasingly relevant to examination and clinical practice.

Necroptosis

Necroptosis produces necrotic morphology (swelling, membrane rupture, inflammation) but is initiated by a regulated signalling pathway. When caspase-8 is inhibited (as in certain viral infections where viral proteins block caspase-8), TNF receptor signalling is diverted from apoptosis to necroptosis.

TNF + caspase-8 blocked → RIPK1 → RIPK3 → MLKL phosphorylation → MLKL oligomerisation → membrane pores → DAMPs release → inflammation

Necroptosis serves as a "backup" death pathway ensuring virus-infected cells are eliminated even when caspase-dependent apoptosis is blocked. It also plays a role in inflammatory bowel disease, pancreatitis, and kidney injury.

Pyroptosis

Pyroptosis is an inflammatory cell death mediated by inflammasome activation and gasdermin family proteins. The canonical pathway involves pattern recognition receptors (NLRP3 is the most studied) detecting danger signals. The activated inflammasome recruits and activates caspase-1, which cleaves both pro-IL-1β/pro-IL-18 into their active forms and gasdermin D (GSDMD). The N-terminal GSDMD fragment oligomerises in the plasma membrane to form large pores (~10–20 nm), through which mature IL-1β and IL-18 are released, and through which the cell lyses.

A non-canonical pathway exists in which caspase-4/5 (caspase-11 in mice) is directly activated by cytoplasmic LPS from Gram-negative bacteria, cleaving GSDMD independently of inflammasome formation. Gasdermin D pore formation has been implicated in the cytokine storm of severe COVID-19, making this an emerging topic in recent postgraduate examinations.

> **Clinical Pearl**
>
> Pyroptosis is the immune system's fire alarm. Unlike apoptosis (quiet, immunologically silent), pyroptosis deliberately releases IL-1β and IL-18 through gasdermin D pores, actively recruiting innate immune cells. This makes pyroptosis essential for host defence against intracellular pathogens but also a driver of pathological inflammation in sepsis, autoinflammatory syndromes (familial Mediterranean fever, CAPS), atherosclerosis, and the cytokine storm of severe COVID-19.

Ferroptosis

Ferroptosis is driven by iron-dependent lipid peroxidation. The central event is the overwhelming accumulation of lipid peroxides in membranes. GPX4 (glutathione peroxidase 4), the key protective enzyme, reduces lipid hydroperoxides using glutathione as cofactor. GPX4 depends on cysteine via the system Xc^- cystine/glutamate antiporter.

System Xc^- inhibition (erastin) or GPX4 inhibition (RSL3) → lipid peroxide accumulation → membrane damage → ferroptotic death

Morphologically, ferroptotic cells show shrunken mitochondria with increased membrane density and reduced cristae, distinct from both apoptosis and necrosis. Ferroptosis is implicated in neurodegeneration (Parkinson, Alzheimer), acute kidney injury, and, paradoxically, may be therapeutically exploited: tumour cells with high iron content and RAS mutations are particularly susceptible.

NETosis

NETosis is a neutrophil-specific death in which the cell releases neutrophil extracellular traps (NETs): web-like structures of decondensed chromatin studded with antimicrobial proteins (elastase, myeloperoxidase, histones). PAD4-mediated histone citrullination drives chromatin decondensation. Suicidal NETosis kills the neutrophil; vital NETosis allows continued phagocytic function. NETs trap pathogens but excessive NETosis is pathogenic in SLE (NETs as autoantigen source), thrombosis (scaffold for platelet adhesion), and sepsis (see Volume 1 for neutrophil biology).

Parthanatos

Parthanatos is triggered by hyperactivation of PARP1 in response to severe DNA damage. Excessive PARP1 depletes NAD+ and ATP, generates PAR polymers that trigger AIF (apoptosis-inducing factor) release from mitochondria. AIF translocates to the nucleus causing large-scale DNA fragmentation. Implicated in excitotoxic neuronal death (stroke, traumatic brain injury).

Table 1.7: All Forms of Cell Death Compared

Type	Trigger	Key Molecules	Morphology	Inflammation	Disease	Key Feature	Detection
Apoptosis	Stress signals (intrinsic/extrinsic)	Caspases, Bcl-2 family	Shrinkage, blebbing	None	Cancer, autoimmunity	Caspase-dependent	Annexin V, TUNEL, caspase assays
Necrosis	Severe injury	None (passive)	Swelling, rupture	Marked (DAMPs)	Infarction, toxins	Unregulated	LDH release, vital dyes
Necroptosis	TNF when caspase-8 blocked	RIPK1/3, MLKL	Swelling, rupture	Marked	Viral infection, IBD	Caspase-independent	p-MLKL antibodies
Pyroptosis	PAMPs/DAMPs	Caspase-1, GSDMD	Pores, lysis	Marked (IL-1β)	Sepsis, COVID-19	Caspase-1-dependent	GSDMD cleavage, IL-1β ELISA
Ferroptosis	Iron + lipid perox	GPX4 failure	Shrunken mitochondria	Minimal	Neurodegeneration	Iron-dependent	Lipid peroxidation assays, GPX4 WB
NETosis	Infection,	PAD4	Chromatin	Variable	SLE,	Neutroph	Citrullina

	autoimmune		release		thrombosis	il-specific	ted histone H3, cfDNA (Figure 1.19)
Parthanatos	Severe DNA damage	PARP1, AIF	DNA fragmentation	Variable	Stroke, TBI	PARP1-dependent	PAR polymer assays

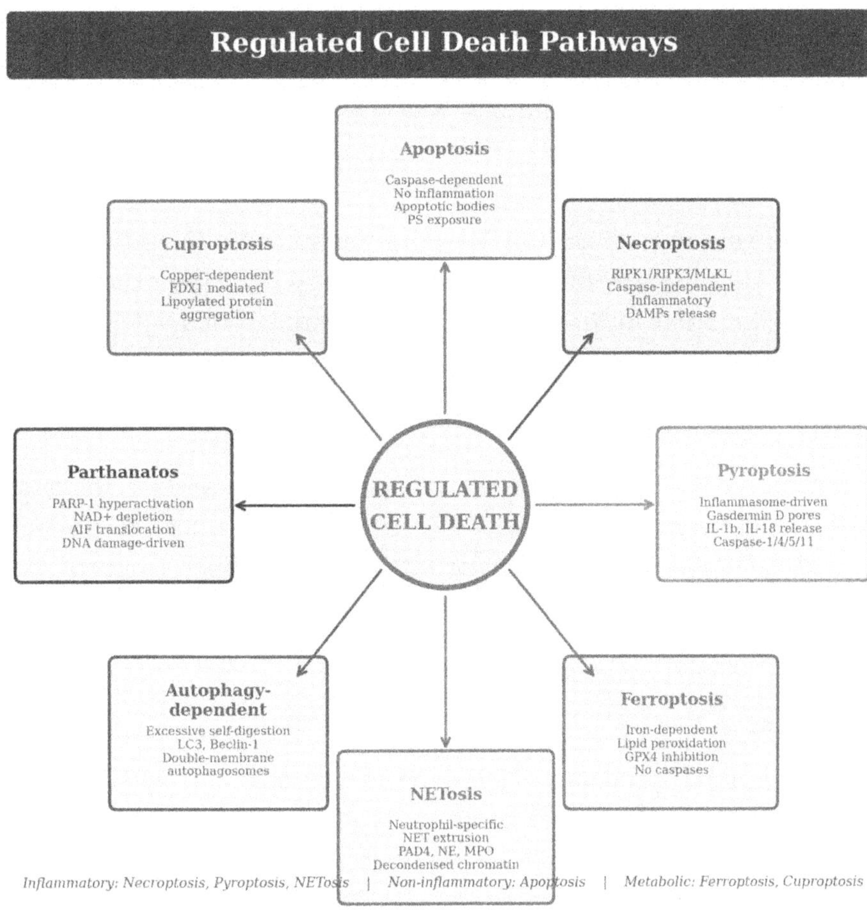

Figure 1.19: Hub-and-spoke summary of regulated cell death pathways. (Source: Author's original.)

Autophagy

Autophagy ("self-eating") is an evolutionarily conserved process by which cytoplasmic components, including damaged organelles and misfolded proteins, are sequestered in autophagosomes and delivered to lysosomes for degradation and recycling. It serves as cellular housekeeping under basal conditions and as a survival strategy under nutrient deprivation.

Three forms exist: macroautophagy (de novo double-membrane phagophore engulfs cargo), microautophagy (direct lysosomal membrane invagination), and chaperone-mediated autophagy (KFERQ-motif proteins delivered to LAMP-2A receptor via Hsc70).

Molecular Mechanism

mTOR active (fed state) → ULK1 inhibited → no autophagy || mTOR inactive (starvation, AMPK) → ULK1 active → Beclin-1/PI3K nucleation → ATG5-12 + LC3 elongation → autophagosome → lysosome fusion → autolysosome → degradation

LC3-II (membrane-bound form of LC3) is the most widely used marker of autophagosome formation.

Autophagy in Disease

Autophagy has a dual role in cancer: tumour-suppressive early (clearing damaged organelles, maintaining genomic stability; Beclin-1 deletions in breast/ovarian cancer) but pro-survival in established tumours. Defective autophagy is also implicated in neurodegenerative diseases and MDS (see Volume 1).

Intracellular Accumulations

Under certain conditions, cells accumulate abnormal amounts of substances in the cytoplasm, organelles, or nucleus. Four mechanisms operate: (1) inadequate metabolism of a normal substance (fatty change); (2) genetic/acquired defects in folding, transport, or secretion (alpha-1 antitrypsin deficiency); (3) inherited enzyme deficiency (lysosomal storage disorders, Chapter 8); (4) inability to degrade exogenous substances (carbon, silica).

Fatty Change (Steatosis)

Fatty change is the abnormal accumulation of triglycerides within parenchymal cells, most commonly the liver. It results from an imbalance between fat influx/synthesis and utilisation/secretion. Mechanisms include excessive delivery of free fatty acids (obesity, diabetes), increased de novo lipogenesis (alcohol), decreased oxidation (mitochondrial damage), and impaired VLDL export (toxin-damaged apolipoprotein B synthesis).

Morphologically, mild steatosis presents as small vacuoles not displacing the nucleus (microvesicular), while advanced steatosis produces a single large vacuole pushing the nucleus peripherally (macrovesicular). The clinical significance lies in progression through steatohepatitis, fibrosis, and cirrhosis, now termed metabolic dysfunction-associated steatotic liver disease (MASLD), discussed in Chapter 20.

Intracellular Protein Accumulations

Important examples include Russell bodies (distended ER with immunoglobulin in plasma cells), Mallory-Denk bodies (aggregated damaged cytokeratins 8 and 18 in steatohepatitis, Wilson disease, and HCC), and alpha-1 antitrypsin globules (PAS-positive, diastase-resistant globules in hepatocytes).

Hyaline and Mucoid Change

Hyaline change is a descriptive, not mechanistic, term for any alteration within cells or in the extracellular space that imparts a homogeneous, glassy, pink (eosinophilic) appearance on H&E. Different substances produce it in different settings; the shared feature is optical, not chemical. The classification that examiners expect is intracellular versus extracellular. Intracellular hyaline includes Russell bodies (discussed above), Mallory-Denk bodies, alpha-1 antitrypsin globules, and protein reabsorption droplets in proximal tubular epithelium seen with heavy proteinuria. Extracellular hyaline includes arteriolar hyalinosis of hypertension and diabetes (homogeneous pink material replacing the arteriolar wall), hyalinised long-standing scars and keloid (cross-linked type I collagen), sclerosed glomeruli of end-stage renal disease, corpora amylacea in the prostate and CNS, and amyloid (hyaline on H&E, but identified by apple-green birefringence on Congo red; see Chapter 5).

Mucoid change (mucoid degeneration) is the accumulation of mucin or mucin-like material, intracellular or stromal. Intracellular (epithelial) mucoid change is physiological in goblet cells and salivary glands, and pathological in mucinous carcinomas — the distended signet-ring cell of gastric and colorectal carcinoma is an intracytoplasmic mucin vacuole that peripheralises the nucleus. Stromal (connective-tissue) mucoid change is the deposition of acidic glycosaminoglycans, principally hyaluronic acid, in loose connective tissue: cystic medial degeneration of the aorta in Marfan syndrome, dermal myxoedema in hypothyroidism, pretibial myxoedema in Graves disease, and the myxoid stroma of soft-tissue neoplasms (myxoid liposarcoma, myxoid leiomyosarcoma, myxoid chondrosarcoma; Chapter 29). Periodic acid–Schiff (PAS) identifies neutral mucin and Alcian blue (at pH 2.5) identifies acidic mucin; the combined PAS–Alcian blue stain is a routine workhorse on gastric and colorectal biopsies.

Table 1.9: Intracellular accumulations — summary

Category	Substance	Mechanism	Classic examples
Lipid	Triglycerides, cholesterol, complex lipids	Inadequate metabolism of a normal substance	Hepatic steatosis (MASLD, alcohol); cholesterolosis of gallbladder; atheromatous plaque; xanthomas; Niemann–Pick, Tay–Sachs (Chapter 8)
Protein	Keratin aggregates; Ig;	Defective folding,	Mallory–Denk bodies (ASH, NASH,

	misfolded AAT; reabsorbed albumin	transport or secretion	Wilson, HCC); Russell bodies (myeloma, chronic inflammation); AAT globules (PiZZ); hyaline reabsorption droplets in PCT (nephrotic proteinuria)
Carbohydrate	Glycogen	Inherited enzyme deficiency; metabolic overload	Glycogen storage diseases (Chapter 8); diabetes mellitus (glycogen in distal tubular cells, hepatocytes, islet β-cells – Armanni–Ebstein lesion)
Pigment (endogenous)	Lipofuscin, haemosiderin, melanin, bile	Oxidative wear; overload; excess synthesis; impaired excretion	Brown atrophy (lipofuscin); haemochromatosis, heart-failure cells (haemosiderin); naevi, melanoma, Addison disease (melanin); canalicular bile plugs (bile); stains: Perl's, Fontana–Masson, PAS/acid-fast (lipofuscin), Fouchet
Pigment (exogenous)	Carbon, silica, asbestos, tattoo, silver, gold, minocycline	Inability to degrade an inhaled, ingested or inoculated substance	Anthracosis, coal-worker's pneumoconiosis; silicotic nodule; asbestos (ferruginous) bodies; tattoo pigment; argyria; chrysiasis; minocycline pigmentation (see Exogenous Pigments below)

Pigments

Pigment Identification Quick Reference

Haemosiderin: Golden-brown, granular. Perl's Prussian blue (blue-green).
Melanin: Brown-black. Fontana-Masson (black).
Lipofuscin: Golden-brown, perinuclear. PAS+, acid-fast, autofluorescent. Wear-and-tear pigment.
Bile: Yellow-green. Fouchet stain (green). Cholestasis.
Carbon: Black, refractile. No special stain.
Ochronosis: Brown-black in cartilage/sclera. Endogenous (alkaptonuria) or exogenous (hydroquinone).

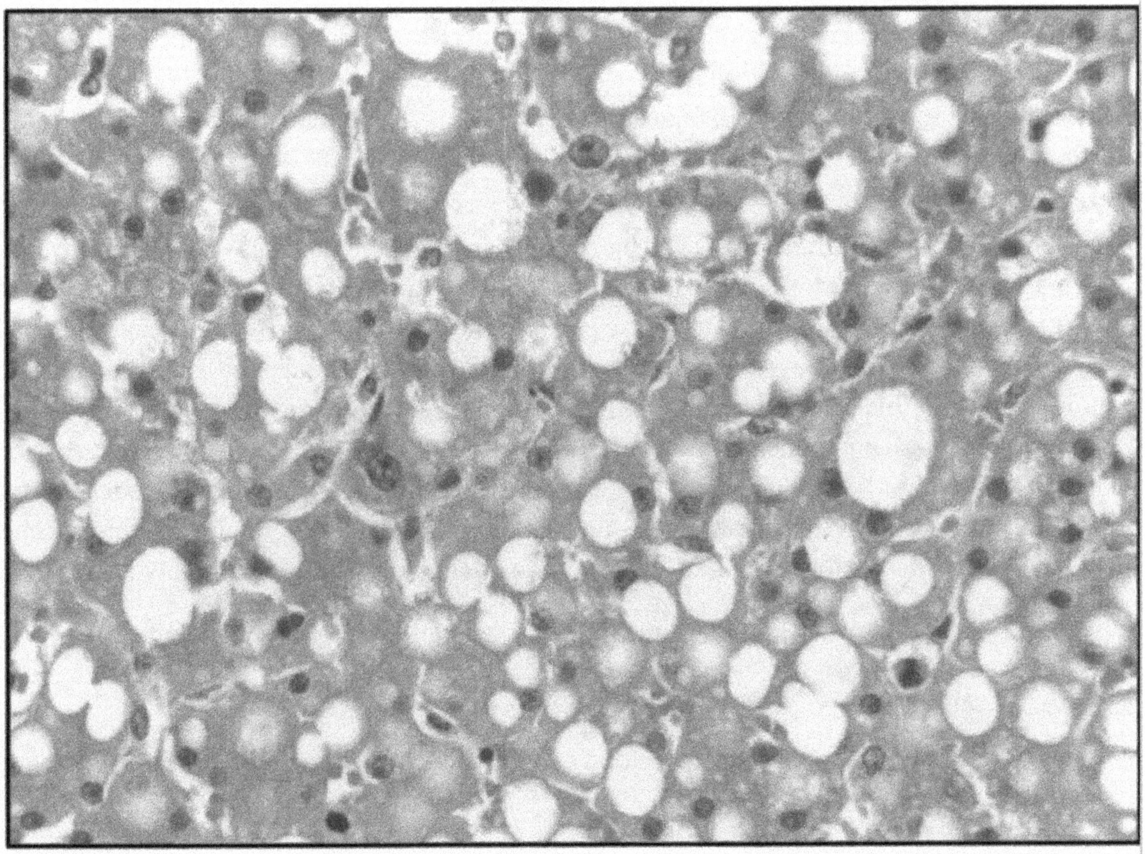

Clinical Pearl

Macrovesicular vs microvesicular steatosis is not a histological curiosity. Macrovesicular fat (single large droplet displacing the nucleus) is the morphology of alcoholic and metabolic dysfunction associated steatotic liver disease (MASLD); it accumulates slowly, signals chronic injury, and is biochemically benign in the short term. Microvesicular fat (multiple small droplets, nucleus retained centrally) is biochemically dangerous: it reflects acute mitochondrial dysfunction and beta-oxidation failure. Its differential is short and urgent: Reye syndrome, acute fatty liver of pregnancy, sodium valproate toxicity, tetracycline injury, HELLP syndrome. Macrovesicular = chronic; microvesicular = metabolic emergency.

Figure 1.20: Hepatic steatosis. Large clear vacuoles displacing nuclei peripherally (macrovesicular steatosis). H&E, 200×. (Source: Patho, Wikimedia Commons, CC BY-SA 4.0.)

Exogenous Pigments

Exogenous pigments are substances taken up from the environment that cells cannot degrade, and that therefore persist in macrophages or interstitium for life. The commonest is carbon. Inhaled carbon from urban air pollution, coal smoke, and cigarette smoke is phagocytosed by alveolar macrophages, transported by lymphatics to peribronchial and hilar lymph nodes, and deposited as jet-black granules — the change is termed anthracosis. In small amounts it is innocuous; heavier occupational exposure produces coal-worker's pneumoconiosis with coal macules and, in the most severe form, progressive massive fibrosis (Chapter 15). Inhaled silica is cytotoxic to the macrophages that engulf it; lysosomal rupture releases proteolytic enzymes and drives formation of the characteristic silicotic nodule — a whorled mass of hyalinised collagen with silica particles birefringent on polarised light. Inhaled asbestos fibres become coated by iron and protein to form asbestos bodies (ferruginous bodies), dumbbell-shaped golden-brown structures seen in lung parenchyma and pleural plaques, and a histological marker of past exposure and future risk for mesothelioma (Chapter 15).

Tattoo pigment is inoculated intradermally and persists in dermal macrophages for life; it is inert and does not require a specific immune response to be retained. Drug- and metal-related exogenous pigments include argyria (slate-grey skin from chronic silver ingestion, historically from colloidal silver preparations marketed as tonics), chrysiasis (grey-blue discolouration from gold therapy, now largely of historical interest since biologics replaced parenteral gold in rheumatoid arthritis), and minocycline-induced black pigmentation of bone, thyroid, and skin — a recognised pitfall when a "black thyroid" is discovered unexpectedly at thyroidectomy. A practical caution for reporting: anthracotic pigment is almost universal in hilar lymph nodes of urban adults and must not be mistaken for metastatic melanoma on frozen section. Cytological atypia and S100/SOX10/HMB-45 immunohistochemistry resolve the differential (Chapter 7).

Pathological Calcification

Pathological calcification is the abnormal deposition of calcium salts in tissues. Two forms are recognised.

Dystrophic Calcification

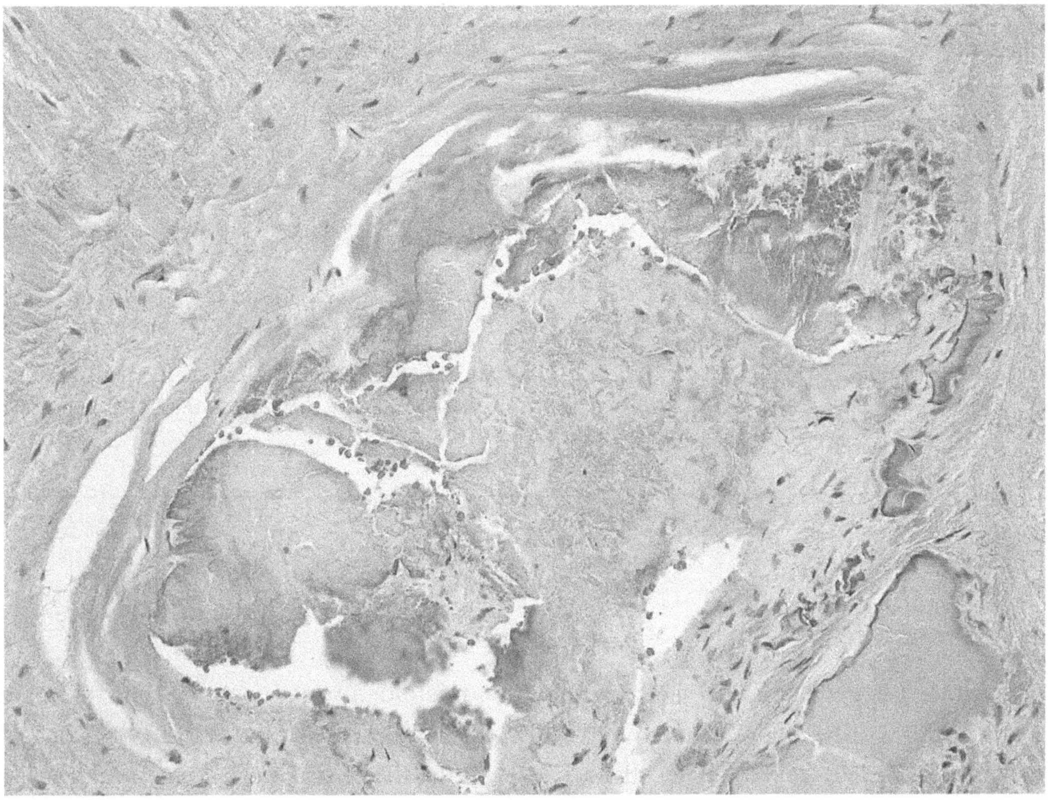

Figure 1.21: Dystrophic calcification in a heart valve. H&E showing basophilic, granular calcium deposits within degenerative valve tissue. *(Source: Mikael Häggström, Wikimedia Commons, CC0.)*

Metastatic Calcification

Metastatic calcification occurs in normal tissues in the setting of hypercalcaemia: primary hyperparathyroidism, osteolytic metastases, excessive vitamin D, chronic renal failure. It preferentially affects tissues with internal alkaline microenvironments: lungs (CO_2 exhalation raises pH), kidneys (bicarbonate generation), gastric mucosa (acid secretion creates lamina propria alkalinity), and blood vessels.

> **Exam Pitfall**
>
> **This is the single most tested distinction in pathological calcification.** Dystrophic = DEAD/DYING tissue + NORMAL serum calcium. Metastatic = NORMAL tissue + ELEVATED serum calcium. Calcification in a TB granuloma? Dystrophic (tissue is necrotic, calcium is normal). Calcification in lungs of a patient with chronic renal failure?

Table 1.8: Dystrophic versus Metastatic Calcification

Feature	Dystrophic	Metastatic

Tissue state	Dead, dying, or damaged	Normal, viable
Serum calcium	Normal	Elevated (hypercalcaemia)
Mechanism	Local: membrane vesicles, phosphatase	Systemic: high Ca × PO_4 product
Common sites	Plaques, valves, TB, tumours (psammoma bodies)	Lungs, kidneys, gastric mucosa, vessels
Reversibility	Irreversible once deposited	May regress if hypercalcaemia corrected
Morphology	Basophilic, granular on H&E; von Kossa stain	Same appearance; distribution is the clue

Cellular Housekeeping and Protein Homeostasis

The Unfolded Protein Response

The unfolded protein response (UPR) is activated when misfolded proteins exceed ER folding capacity. Three sensors—PERK, IRE1, and ATF6—upregulate chaperones and reduce protein translation; failure triggers apoptosis via CHOP (see Quick Recall).If the UPR is insufficient, the cell triggers apoptosis through CHOP (C/EBP homologous protein), linking protein misfolding to programmed cell death (Figure 1.22).

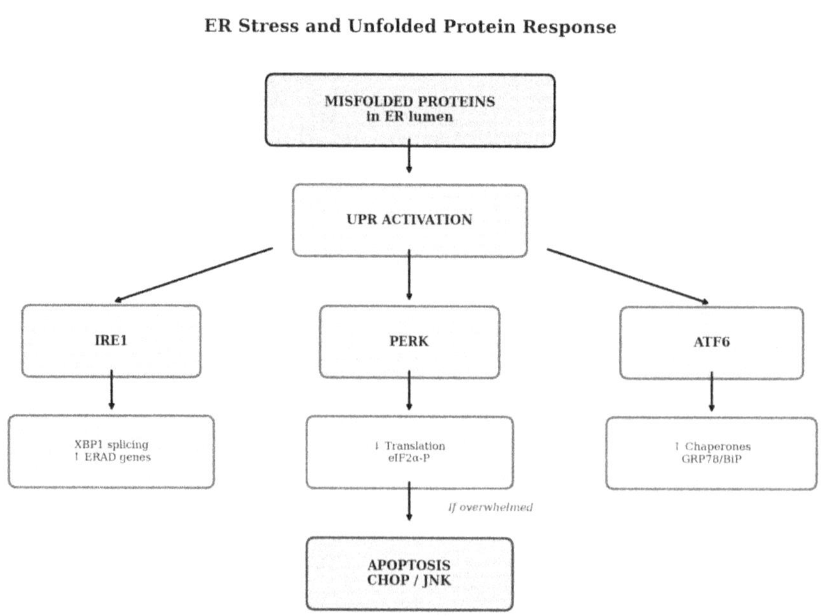

Figure 1.22: ER Stress and Unfolded Protein Response. *(Source: Author's original.)*

The Ubiquitin-Proteasome Pathway

Cytoplasmic proteins are tagged with polyubiquitin chains by E1/E2/E3 enzyme cascades and degraded by the 26S proteasome. This pathway regulates cell cycle progression (cyclin/CDK inhibitor degradation), signal transduction (IκB degradation releasing NF-κB), and antigen presentation (peptide generation for MHC class I).

The ubiquitin-proteasome system explains why certain intracellular inclusions are visible on H&E: Lewy bodies (alpha-synuclein, Parkinson disease), neurofibrillary tangles (hyperphosphorylated tau, Alzheimer disease), and Huntington aggregates (polyglutamine-expanded huntingtin) all represent proteins that have escaped degradation. When this system fails, aggregates accumulate, becoming the histological signatures of neurodegenerative disease. For amyloidosis, see Chapter 5; for prion diseases, see Chapter 30.

Cellular Ageing

Cellular ageing results from progressive decline in function and replicative capacity, driven by interconnected mechanisms: telomere shortening, DNA damage accumulation, epigenetic drift, mitochondrial dysfunction, defective protein homeostasis, stem cell exhaustion, and altered intercellular communication.

Telomere Biology and Replicative Senescence

Telomeres are repetitive TTAGGG sequences at chromosome ends, protected by the shelterin complex (TRF1, TRF2, POT1, TIN2, TPP1, RAP1). With each division, the end-replication problem causes progressive shortening. When critically short, exposed ends activate the ATM/ATR kinases and p53/p21 pathway, arresting the cell in replicative senescence (the Hayflick limit, ~60–70 divisions for human fibroblasts).

Telomerase (hTERT + hTR/TERC) extends telomeres. In somatic cells, it is repressed (enforcing the Hayflick limit). In germ cells, stem cells (at low levels), and ~90% of cancers, it is active. The remaining ~10% use the ALT (alternative lengthening of telomeres) pathway via homologous recombination.

> **Clinical Pearl**
>
> Telomerase is inactive in most somatic cells (hence the Hayflick limit) but reactivated in ~90% of cancers. This dual role makes it both a tumour suppressor (limiting proliferation in normal cells) and a tumour enabler (conferring immortality in cancer cells). Telomeropathies, caused by mutations in telomerase components or telomere maintenance proteins (dyskeratosis congenita, aplastic anaemia, idiopathic pulmonary fibrosis, familial liver cirrhosis), provide clinical evidence that telomere shortening directly drives tissue failure. For telomere biology in haematological disease, see Volume 1.

Cellular Senescence and the SASP

Senescent cells, while permanently growth-arrested, secrete a complex mixture of pro-inflammatory cytokines (IL-6, IL-8), chemokines, metalloproteinases, and growth factors: the senescence-associated secretory phenotype (SASP). SASP contributes to "inflammaging," tissue remodelling, and paradoxically promotes tumour progression in neighbouring cells. This dual nature (tumour-suppressive via arrest, tumour-promoting via SASP) has led to interest in senolytic drugs, discussed below.

Integration: cellular ageing connects to autophagy (defective autophagy accelerates ageing by allowing damaged mitochondria to persist), oxidative stress (telomere shortening is accelerated by ROS-induced DNA damage), and cancer biology (telomerase reactivation is a hallmark of cancer, Chapter 6). Understanding ageing as a convergence of multiple mechanisms discussed in this chapter provides a unified framework.

Recent Advances

Ferroptosis as a therapeutic target. Certain therapy-resistant cancers (mesenchymal-state and RAS-mutant tumours) are highly susceptible to ferroptosis. GPX4 inhibitors and system Xc^- inhibitors can induce ferroptosis in apoptosis-resistant cancer cells. Conversely, ferroptosis inhibitors (liproxstatin-1, ferrostatin-1) are being explored as neuroprotective agents in Parkinson disease and acute kidney injury. Iron chelation therapy, already established in thalassaemia management (see Volume 1), may have broader neuroprotective applications through ferroptosis inhibition.

Inflammasome biology and pyroptosis as drug targets. The CANTOS trial demonstrated that canakinumab (anti-IL-1β monoclonal antibody) reduced cardiovascular events in patients with prior MI and elevated CRP, proving that inflammasome-driven inflammation contributes to atherosclerotic disease. Small-molecule NLRP3 inhibitors (MCC950/CRID3, dapansutrile) are in clinical trials for gout, atherosclerosis, and autoinflammatory syndromes. Gasdermin D inhibitors are under investigation for sepsis-associated organ damage.

Senolytic drugs. Senolytics selectively induce apoptosis in senescent cells. The most studied combination is dasatinib plus quercetin, targeting anti-apoptotic pathways (Bcl-2 family, PI3K/Akt) on which senescent cells depend. Navitoclax (ABT-263), a Bcl-2/Bcl-xL inhibitor, is another potent senolytic. Preclinical studies show improved cardiovascular, renal, and physical function with senolytic clearance. Early-phase human trials are underway for idiopathic pulmonary fibrosis and diabetic kidney disease.

International Frameworks

Nomenclature Committee on Cell Death (NCCD) 2018. The NCCD updated its classification of cell death subroutines in 2018, moving from morphology-based categories (apoptosis, necrosis, autophagy) to mechanism-based definitions of fourteen distinct modalities — intrinsic and extrinsic apoptosis, mitochondrial permeability transition (MPT)-driven necrosis, necroptosis, ferroptosis, pyroptosis, parthanatos, entotic cell death, NETotic cell death, lysosome-dependent cell death, autophagy-dependent cell death, immunogenic cell death, cellular senescence, and mitotic catastrophe. The diagnostic implication is that immunohistochemical and histopathological recognition increasingly relies on mechanism-specific markers — RIPK1/RIPK3/MLKL phosphorylation for necroptosis, GPX4 inactivation and lipid peroxidation for ferroptosis, gasdermin D cleavage for pyroptosis — rather than morphology alone. Citation: Galluzzi L, et al. Cell Death Differ 2018;25(3):486–541. PMID 29362479.

Ultra High-Yield Chapter Summary

This table distils the most-tested concepts from this chapter into a format designed for rapid final revision.

Topic	Must Remember
Reversible injury	Cell swelling, fatty change, ER dilation. Membrane intact.
Irreversible injury	Membrane damage + MPTP opening. Dense mitochondrial bodies.
Free radical defence	SOD → catalase/GPx chain. Vitamin E (lipid), C (aqueous). Ferritin sequesters iron.
Coagulative necrosis	Architecture preserved, nuclei lost. Ghost outlines.
Liquefactive necrosis	Tissue liquefied. Brain infarcts and abscesses.
Caseous necrosis	Amorphous granular debris. TB granulomas.
Apoptosis: intrinsic pathway	Stress → BH3-only → Bax/Bak pores → cytochrome c → apoptosome → caspase-9 → caspase-3.
Apoptosis: extrinsic pathway	FasL → Fas → FADD → DISC → caspase-8 → caspase-3 (or via Bid to mitochondria).
Apoptosis vs necrosis (key)	Apoptosis: shrinkage, no inflammation, caspase-dependent.
Necroptosis	TNF + caspase-8 blocked → RIPK1/RIPK3/MLKL → necrotic

	morphology.
Pyroptosis	Inflammasome → caspase-1 → gasdermin D pores → IL-1β/IL-18 release.
Ferroptosis	Iron + lipid peroxidation. GPX4 is the gatekeeper. Shrunken mitochondria.
Dystrophic vs metastatic calcification	Dystrophic: dead tissue + normal Ca^{2+}. Metastatic: normal tissue + high Ca^{2+}.
Telomeres	TTAGGG repeats, shelterin complex. Telomerase inactive in soma, active in ~90% cancers.
Autophagy	mTOR off → ULK1 → Beclin-1 → LC3-II.
UPR sensors	PERK (↓translation), IRE1 (XBP1/chaperones), ATF6 (chaperones) (Figure 1.22).

Chapter 2: Inflammation: Acute and Chronic

> **THE BIG PICTURE**
>
> Inflammation is the body's first organised response to tissue injury. It is not a disease; it is a defence mechanism. Every red, swollen wound, every febrile illness, every abscess drained in the operating theatre represents inflammation doing its job. The pathologist must understand inflammation at three levels: the vascular events that deliver plasma and cells to the site of injury, the cellular events by which leukocytes recognise and destroy offending agents, and the chemical mediators that orchestrate the entire process. When inflammation succeeds, it is followed by repair (Chapter 3). When it fails or persists, it becomes chronic inflammation, which itself drives fibrosis, tissue destruction, and, in some settings, carcinogenesis.
>
> **High-yield topics in this chapter:** Chemical mediators of acute inflammation (vasoactive amines, arachidonic acid metabolites, cytokines, complement, kinins), leukocyte adhesion and emigration (selectins, integrins, chemotaxis), defects in leukocyte function, phagocytosis and microbicidal mechanisms, chronic inflammation and its causes, granulomatous inflammation, and inflammasomes.

Inflammation is the most ancient and most fundamental host response to tissue damage. Long before adaptive immunity evolved, organisms relied on inflammatory mechanisms to contain infection and clear debris. For the pathologist, inflammation is simultaneously the most commonly encountered process on biopsy material and the most complex to dissect mechanistically. A single inflamed appendix, examined under the microscope, reveals the full repertoire: vascular dilation, oedema, neutrophilic infiltration, fibrin deposition, and tissue destruction. Understanding why each of these occurs, and what mediates each step, is what separates the diagnostician from the descriptor.

Overview: Acute versus Chronic Inflammation

Inflammation is broadly divided into acute and chronic forms, though in practice there is often overlap.

Acute inflammation is the rapid, initial response to injury, lasting hours to days. It is characterised by vascular changes (vasodilation, increased permeability) and cellular events (neutrophil emigration and activation). The hallmark cell is the neutrophil. The cardinal signs, described by Celsus (rubor, tumor, calor, dolor) and Virchow (functio laesa), reflect the underlying vascular and cellular events: redness and heat from vasodilation, swelling from increased permeability and oedema, pain from mediator stimulation of nerve endings, and loss of function from tissue damage and swelling.

Chronic inflammation is a prolonged response (weeks to years) in which tissue destruction and repair proceed simultaneously. The hallmark cells are macrophages, lymphocytes, and plasma cells. Chronic inflammation arises from persistent infections (tuberculosis, viral hepatitis), autoimmune diseases (rheumatoid arthritis, SLE), prolonged toxic exposure (silicosis, atherosclerosis), or transition from acute inflammation when the offending agent is not eliminated.

Cardinal Signs of Inflammation

Celsus described four cardinal signs of inflammation in the first century AD: rubor (redness), calor (heat), tumor (swelling), and dolor (pain). Virchow added a fifth, functio laesa (loss of function), in the nineteenth century. Each has a defined molecular basis that the resident must be able to recite.

Rubor and calor share the same mechanism: vasodilation. Histamine released from mast cells, prostaglandin PGI2 and PGE2 generated by COX, and nitric oxide from endothelial NOS together relax arteriolar smooth muscle. The resulting hyperaemia delivers warm, oxygenated, plasma-rich blood to the injured tissue. This is why the redness of inflammation blanches on pressure: it is engorged but patent vasculature, not extravasated blood.

Tumor reflects the protein-rich exudate that escapes through inflamed endothelium. Histamine, bradykinin, leukotrienes C4/D4/E4, and substance P each increase venular permeability through endothelial contraction or, when injury is direct, endothelial necrosis. VEGF amplifies the response in chronic inflammation. The swelling is interstitial, not intravascular, and contains fibrinogen, immunoglobulins, and complement.

Dolor arises from two parallel mechanisms. Bradykinin and PGE2 lower the threshold of nociceptive sensory neurons (peripheral sensitisation), so that even normal stimuli are perceived as painful. Pressure on those neurons by exudate amplifies the signal. NSAIDs work by blocking the COX-derived contribution, which is why they are most effective when the dominant driver is prostaglandin sensitisation rather than direct mechanical pressure.

Functio laesa is the integrated consequence: a swollen, painful, hyperaemic part cannot function normally. A swollen knee will not bear weight; an inflamed bronchial mucosa cannot ciliate; an inflamed intestinal segment loses motility and absorptive capacity. In every clinical examination, the absence or presence of functio laesa is the simplest gauge of inflammation severity.

Acute Inflammation: Vascular Events

The vascular response is the earliest event in acute inflammation and serves to maximise delivery of plasma proteins and leukocytes to the site of injury.

Vasodilation is one of the earliest responses, occurring within seconds to minutes. It is mediated primarily by histamine and nitric oxide acting on arteriolar smooth muscle. Vasodilation increases blood flow to the injured area, accounting for the redness (erythema) and warmth of inflamed tissue. Initially, blood flow accelerates, but as vessels dilate and permeability increases, the flow slows (stasis), which is critical for allowing leukocytes to marginate along the vessel wall.

Increased vascular permeability is the hallmark of acute inflammation. It results in the escape of protein-rich fluid (exudate) into the extravascular space, producing oedema. The mechanism involves contraction of endothelial cells in postcapillary venules, creating intercellular gaps. This contraction is induced by histamine, bradykinin, leukotrienes, and other mediators. In severe injury, direct endothelial damage (burns, toxins, infections) causes uncontrolled leakage. The distinction between exudate and transudate is clinically important:

Table 2.1: Exudate versus Transudate

Feature	Exudate	Transudate
Mechanism	Increased vascular permeability (inflammation)	Increased hydrostatic or decreased oncotic pressure
Protein content	High (>3 g/dL)	Low (<3 g/dL)
Specific gravity	>1.020	<1.012
Cells	Inflammatory cells present	Few or no cells
LDH	Elevated	Low
Appearance	Often turbid, may clot	Clear, straw-coloured
Clinical examples	Pneumonia, peritonitis, pleuritis	Heart failure, nephrotic syndrome, cirrhosis

The net result of vascular events is the delivery of plasma proteins (complement, antibodies, fibrinogen) and leukocytes to the site of injury. Fibrinogen polymerises to fibrin in the extravascular space, forming a scaffold that limits the spread of infection and provides a framework for repair (Figure 2.1).

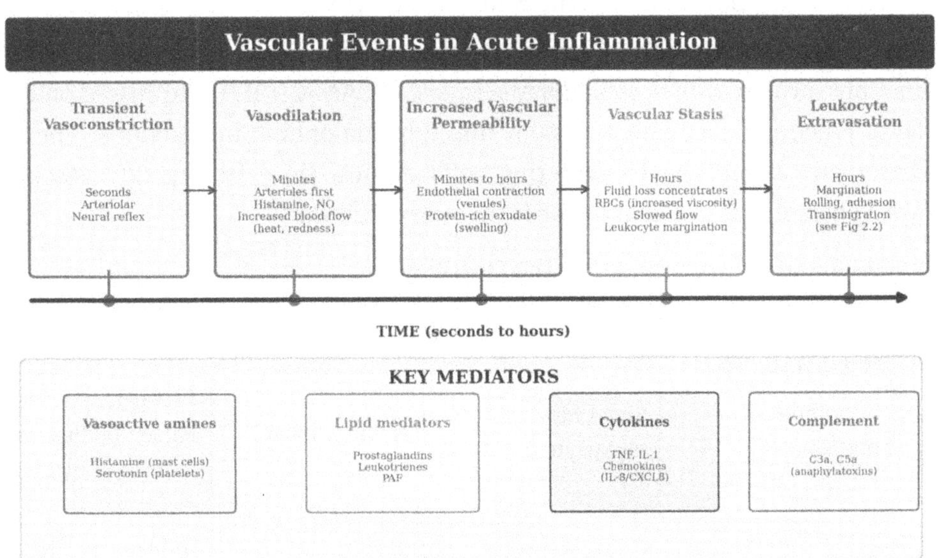

Figure 2.1: Vascular events in acute inflammation. (Source: Author's original.)

Acute Inflammation: Cellular Events

The cellular response of acute inflammation centres on the recruitment of leukocytes, primarily neutrophils, from the blood to the site of injury. This multi-step process, known as the leukocyte adhesion cascade, is one of the most frequently tested topics in postgraduate pathology.

The Leukocyte Adhesion Cascade

Figure: Leukocyte Adhesion Cascade. (Source: Author's original.)

Margination → Rolling (selectins) → Firm adhesion (integrins) → Transmigration (diapedesis, PECAM-1) → Chemotaxis → Activation → Phagocytosis

Margination and rolling: as blood flow slows (stasis), leukocytes move from the central axial stream to the vessel periphery (margination) and begin to roll along the endothelium. Rolling is mediated by selectins, a family of lectins that bind sialylated carbohydrate ligands. E-selectin (expressed on activated endothelium, induced by TNF and IL-1), P-selectin (preformed in Weibel-Palade bodies of endothelium and alpha-granules of platelets, rapidly translocated to the surface by histamine), and L-selectin (constitutively expressed on leukocytes) each contribute to rolling at different phases. The selectin-ligand interactions are low-affinity and transient, producing the characteristic rolling motion.

Firm adhesion: the transition from rolling to firm adhesion requires integrin activation. Integrins are heterodimeric transmembrane receptors on leukocytes (LFA-1/Mac-1 on neutrophils) that normally exist in a low-affinity state. Chemokines displayed on the endothelial surface (bound to proteoglycans) activate integrins via inside-out signalling, converting them to a high-affinity conformation that binds tightly to endothelial ligands ICAM-1 and VCAM-1. ICAM-1 and VCAM-1 are upregulated on activated endothelium by TNF and IL-1. This firm adhesion arrests the rolling leukocyte.

Transmigration (diapedesis): the adherent leukocyte squeezes between endothelial cells at intercellular junctions, primarily in postcapillary venules. PECAM-1 (CD31), expressed on both leukocytes and at endothelial junctions, mediates this step through homophilic interactions. The leukocyte also traverses the basement membrane by secreting collagenases. Once in the extravascular tissue, the leukocyte follows a chemotactic gradient towards the source of injury.

Table 2.2: Adhesion Molecules in Leukocyte Recruitment

Molecule	Location	Ligand	Function	Clinical Note
P-selectin	Endothelium, platelets	Sialyl-Lewis X (on leukocytes)	Rolling (early)	Preformed in Weibel-Palade bodies; rapidly mobilised by histamine
E-selectin	Activated endothelium	Sialyl-Lewis X	Rolling (later)	Induced by TNF, IL-1; transcription-dependent (hours)

L-selectin	Leukocytes	GlyCAM-1, CD34 (on endothelium)	Rolling (initial)	Constitutive; shed after activation
ICAM-1	Activated endothelium	LFA-1, Mac-1 (integrins)	Firm adhesion	Upregulated by TNF, IL-1, IFN-γ
VCAM-1	Activated endothelium	VLA-4 (integrin)	Firm adhesion (monocytes, lymphocytes, eosinophils)	Important in chronic inflammation
PECAM-1 (CD31)	Endothelial junctions, leukocytes	PECAM-1 (homophilic)	Transmigration	Mediates diapedesis

Chemotaxis

Once in the extravascular tissue, leukocytes migrate along a concentration gradient of chemoattractants towards the site of injury. Both exogenous and endogenous chemoattractants exist. Exogenous chemoattractants include bacterial products, particularly N-formyl-methionyl peptides (fMLP). Endogenous chemoattractants include complement fragment C5a, leukotriene B4 (LTB4), and chemokines (IL-8/CXCL8 for neutrophils, MCP-1/CCL2 for monocytes, eotaxin/CCL11 for eosinophils).

The chemotactic signal is transduced through G-protein-coupled receptors (GPCRs) on the leukocyte surface. Binding activates phospholipase C, generating IP3 (calcium release) and DAG (protein kinase C activation). The leukocyte extends pseudopods in the direction of the gradient by polymerising actin at the leading edge and depolymerising at the trailing edge. This directional locomotion requires an intact cytoskeleton and functional signalling machinery.

Defects in Leukocyte Function

Defects at any step of the adhesion cascade or in subsequent leukocyte functions produce immunodeficiency characterised by recurrent, severe infections.

Table 2.3: Leukocyte Function Defects

Disorder	Defect	Mechanism	Clinical Features
Leukocyte adhesion deficiency type 1 (LAD-1)	Defective CD18 (beta-2 integrin subunit)	Absent firm adhesion; leukocytes cannot emigrate	Recurrent bacterial infections; delayed umbilical cord separation; no pus formation; marked leukocytosis

Leukocyte adhesion deficiency type 2 (LAD-2)	Defective fucose metabolism; absent sialyl-Lewis X	Absent selectin-mediated rolling	Similar to LAD-1 but milder; mental retardation
Chédiak-Higashi syndrome	Defective LYST gene; abnormal lysosomal trafficking	Defective phagolysosome fusion; giant granules in leukocytes	Recurrent pyogenic infections; partial oculocutaneous albinism; peripheral neuropathy
Chronic granulomatous disease (CGD)	Defective NADPH oxidase (gp91phox or p47phox)	Absent respiratory burst; cannot generate superoxide	Recurrent infections with catalase-positive organisms (S. aureus, Aspergillus, Serratia); granuloma formation; diagnosed by dihydrorhodamine (DHR) flow cytometry or nitroblue tetrazolium (NBT) test
Myeloperoxidase deficiency	Absent MPO	Defective HOCl generation	Usually clinically silent; increased susceptibility to Candida in immunocompromised
Job syndrome (Hyper-IgE)	STAT3 mutation	Defective Th17 responses; impaired chemotaxis	"Cold" abscesses, eczema, elevated IgE, recurrent staphylococcal infections

Exam Pitfall

Chronic granulomatous disease produces granulomas NOT because of a defect in granuloma formation, but because the neutrophils cannot kill catalase-positive bacteria. The persistent, living bacteria stimulate a chronic inflammatory response with macrophage accumulation and granuloma formation. Catalase-negative organisms (like streptococci) generate their own H_2O_2, which the CGD neutrophil can still use for killing. This is why CGD patients are specifically susceptible to catalase-positive organisms: Staphylococcus aureus, Aspergillus, Serratia, Nocardia, Burkholderia cepacia.

Phagocytosis and Microbicidal Mechanisms

Phagocytosis proceeds in three steps: recognition and attachment, engulfment, and killing/degradation.

Recognition and attachment: phagocytes recognise microbes either directly through pattern recognition receptors (mannose receptors, scavenger receptors, TLRs) or indirectly through opsonins. The major opsonins are IgG (Fc fragment binds Fc receptors on phagocytes), C3b (binds complement receptors CR1), and collectins (mannose-binding lectin, surfactant proteins). Opsonisation dramatically increases phagocytic efficiency.

Engulfment: the phagocyte extends pseudopods around the opsonised particle, fusing to form a phagosome. The phagosome then fuses with lysosomes to form a phagolysosome.

Killing: two principal microbicidal mechanisms operate within the phagolysosome:

(1) Oxygen-dependent killing (respiratory burst): NADPH oxidase assembles on the phagosomal membrane, generating superoxide ($O_2{\bullet}^-$). Superoxide is converted to H_2O_2 by SOD. H_2O_2 alone is not efficient at killing most bacteria. The MPO-H_2O_2-halide system is the most potent microbicidal mechanism: myeloperoxidase (from azurophilic granules) converts H_2O_2 + Cl^- into hypochlorous acid (HOCl), a powerful oxidant that kills bacteria. Reactive nitrogen intermediates (NO, generated by iNOS) also contribute, particularly against intracellular organisms.

(2) Oxygen-independent killing: lysosomal enzymes (lysozyme, defensins, lactoferrin, elastase, bactericidal/permeability-increasing protein) kill microbes in oxygen-poor environments such as anaerobic abscesses. Defensins are cationic peptides that form pores in microbial membranes. Lactoferrin chelates iron, depriving bacteria of an essential nutrient.

NADPH oxidase → $O_2{\bullet}^-$ → SOD → H_2O_2 → MPO + Cl^- → HOCl (most potent bactericidal)

Quick Recall: Cellular Events

Adhesion cascade: rolling (selectins) → firm adhesion (integrins/ICAM) → transmigration (PECAM-1) → chemotaxis.

Chemotaxis: C5a, LTB4, IL-8, fMLP. Via GPCRs.

Opsonins: IgG (Fc receptors), C3b (CR1), collectins. Enhance phagocytosis.

Killing: O_2-dependent: NADPH oxidase → HOCl (MPO system). O_2-independent: defensins, lysozyme, lactoferrin.

LAD-1: no CD18 → no firm adhesion → no pus. CGD: no NADPH oxidase → no respiratory burst → catalase+ infections (Figure 2.2).

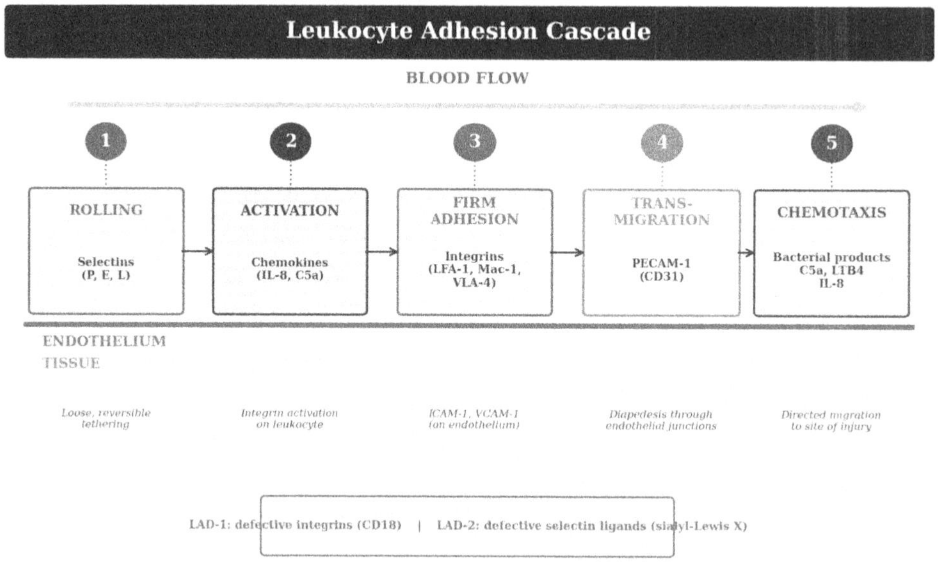

Figure 2.2: Leukocyte adhesion cascade. (Source: Author's original.)

Chemical Mediators of Inflammation (Figure 2.3)

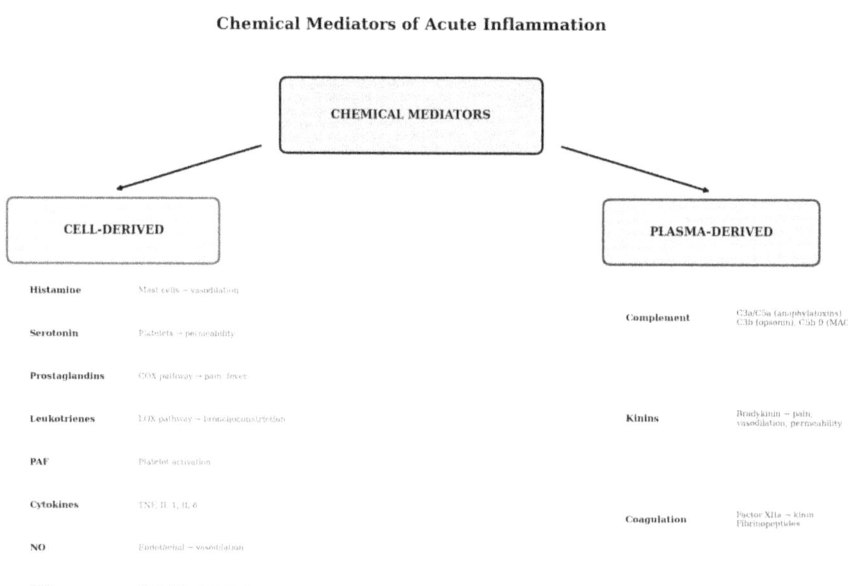

Figure 2.3: Chemical Mediators of Acute Inflammation. *(Source: Author's original.)*

Chemical mediators are the molecular signals that initiate, amplify, and regulate the inflammatory response (Figure 2.13 consolidates all pathways). They may be cell-derived (preformed in granules or synthesised de novo) or plasma-derived (circulating as inactive precursors). Understanding mediators is essential because they are the targets of anti-inflammatory therapy, they explain the clinical features of inflammation, and they are among the most frequently examined topics in pathology.

Cell-Derived Mediators

Vasoactive amines: Histamine, the prototypical mediator of acute inflammation, is stored preformed in mast cell granules, basophils, and platelets. It is released by physical injury, immune reactions (IgE cross-linking), C3a and C5a (anaphylatoxins), and neuropeptides. Histamine causes arteriolar vasodilation (via H1 receptors on smooth muscle) and increased venular permeability (via H1 receptors on endothelial cells). Its action is rapid but transient (minutes), representing the immediate vascular response. Serotonin (5-HT), stored in platelet dense granules, is released during platelet aggregation and produces similar vascular effects.

Arachidonic acid metabolites (eicosanoids): arachidonic acid (AA) is released from membrane phospholipids by phospholipase A2 (activated by mechanical, chemical, or inflammatory stimuli). AA is then metabolised by two major enzymatic pathways:

The cyclooxygenase (COX) pathway generates prostaglandins and thromboxane. COX-1 is constitutive (housekeeping functions: gastric mucosal protection, platelet aggregation, renal perfusion). COX-2 is inducible, upregulated at sites of inflammation by TNF, IL-1, and other stimuli. PGE2 and PGI2 (prostacyclin) cause vasodilation and potentiate oedema by enhancing the permeability effects of histamine and bradykinin. PGE2 also sensitises nociceptors (contributing to pain) and resets the hypothalamic thermostat (producing fever). Thromboxane A2 (TXA2), produced by platelets, causes vasoconstriction and platelet aggregation.

Prostaglandins deserve particular emphasis because they are among the most frequently examined mediators. Cyclooxygenase exists in two isoforms: COX-1 (constitutive, present in most tissues, responsible for physiological prostaglandin production including gastric mucosal protection, platelet aggregation via TXA2, and renal blood flow regulation) and COX-2 (inducible, upregulated at sites of inflammation by IL-1, TNF, and growth factors, responsible for the prostaglandins that mediate pain, fever, and vasodilation in inflammation). Non-steroidal anti-inflammatory drugs (NSAIDs) inhibit both COX-1 and COX-2, explaining their anti-inflammatory efficacy but also their adverse effects (gastric ulceration from loss of COX-1-derived protective prostaglandins, and renal impairment from reduced renal prostaglandin synthesis). Selective COX-2 inhibitors (celecoxib) were developed to minimise gastric toxicity but were found to increase cardiovascular risk because COX-2 in endothelium produces prostacyclin (PGI2, a vasodilator and anti-aggregant), and its inhibition tips the balance toward COX-1-derived TXA2 (pro-aggregant).

The prostaglandin PGE2 is the principal mediator of fever. It is produced in the hypothalamic vascular endothelium in response to circulating IL-1 and TNF, and acts on EP3 receptors in the thermoregulatory centre to raise the temperature set point. Antipyretics (aspirin, paracetamol, ibuprofen) reduce fever by inhibiting COX-mediated PGE2 synthesis. PGD2, produced by mast cells, mediates vasodilation, bronchospasm, and mucus secretion in allergic responses. The leukotriene pathway (5-lipoxygenase) produces LTB4 (a potent neutrophil chemoattractant) and the cysteinyl leukotrienes LTC4, LTD4, and LTE4 (slow-reacting substances of anaphylaxis, causing bronchospasm, vasoconstriction, and increased vascular permeability). Leukotriene receptor antagonists (montelukast) are used in asthma management. Lipoxins, generated by the transcellular lipoxygenase pathway, are anti-inflammatory mediators that inhibit neutrophil recruitment and promote resolution of inflammation.

The lipoxygenase (LOX) pathway generates leukotrienes and lipoxins. 5-lipoxygenase, the dominant enzyme in neutrophils, converts AA to leukotriene A4, which is then converted to LTB4 (a potent chemotactic agent for neutrophils) or to the cysteinyl leukotrienes LTC4, LTD4, and LTE4 (which cause intense vasoconstriction, bronchospasm, and increased vascular permeability; these are the slow-reacting substances of anaphylaxis, SRS-A). Lipoxins, generated by the coordinated action of 5-LOX and 12-LOX in different cell types (transcellular biosynthesis), are anti-inflammatory mediators that inhibit neutrophil recruitment and promote resolution of inflammation.

Why does aspirin reduce inflammation and fever but not the chemotactic recruitment of neutrophils? Because aspirin inhibits COX (blocking PGE2, which mediates vasodilation, pain, and fever) but does not inhibit LOX (LTB4, the neutrophil chemoattractant, is still produced). This explains why NSAIDs reduce the signs of inflammation without eliminating the cellular infiltrate (Figure 2.4).

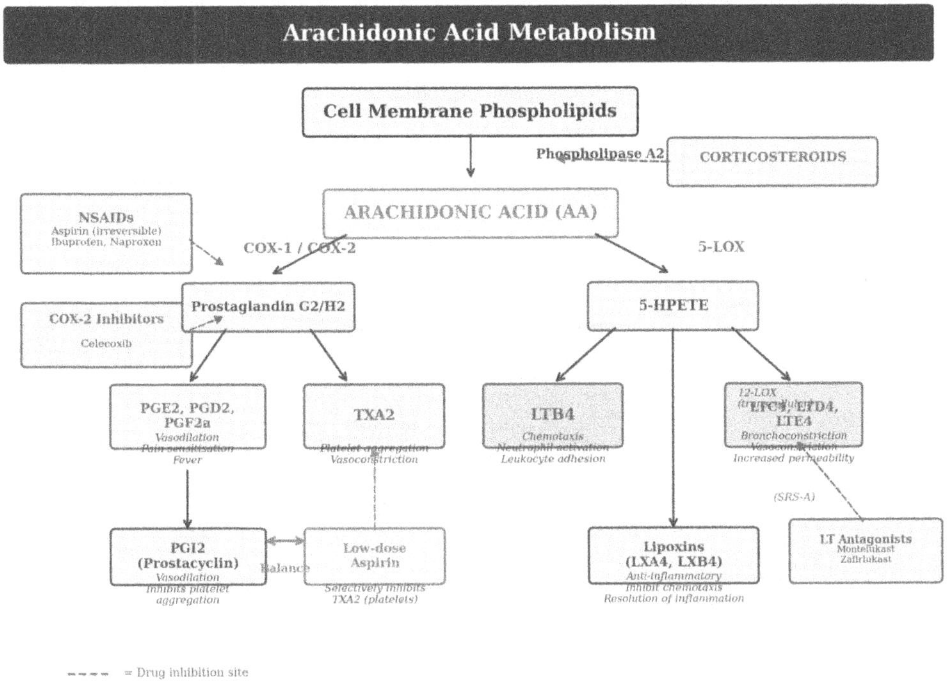

Figure 2.4: Arachidonic acid metabolism: COX and LOX pathways. (Source: Author's original.)

Cytokines: TNF and IL-1 are the major pro-inflammatory cytokines, produced primarily by activated macrophages. They act on endothelium (inducing E-selectin, ICAM-1, VCAM-1 expression; stimulating chemokine and prostaglandin production), on leukocytes (activating neutrophils, priming for enhanced killing), and systemically (inducing fever via hypothalamic PGE2, acute-phase protein synthesis by the liver, leukocytosis via bone marrow stimulation, and, in severe cases, the haemodynamic changes of septic shock). IL-6 is the principal driver of acute-phase protein synthesis (CRP, fibrinogen, SAA). Chemokines are a large family of small proteins that direct leukocyte migration: CXC chemokines (IL-8/CXCL8) recruit neutrophils; CC chemokines (MCP-1, RANTES, eotaxin) recruit monocytes, lymphocytes, and eosinophils.

Plasma-Derived Mediators

The complement system is a cascade of plasma proteins activated by three pathways (classical, alternative, and lectin) that converge on C3 and C5. The critical inflammatory mediators generated are: C3a and C5a (anaphylatoxins; stimulate mast cell histamine release; C5a is also a potent neutrophil chemoattractant and activator), C3b (opsonin; facilitates phagocytosis), and C5b-9 (membrane attack complex; lyses cells, particularly Gram-negative bacteria and enveloped viruses). Complement activation is tightly regulated by inhibitors (C1-INH, factor H, DAF/CD55, protectin/CD59). Deficiency of C1-INH causes hereditary angioedema (recurrent episodes of oedema due to unregulated bradykinin and C2 kinin generation) (Figure 2.5).

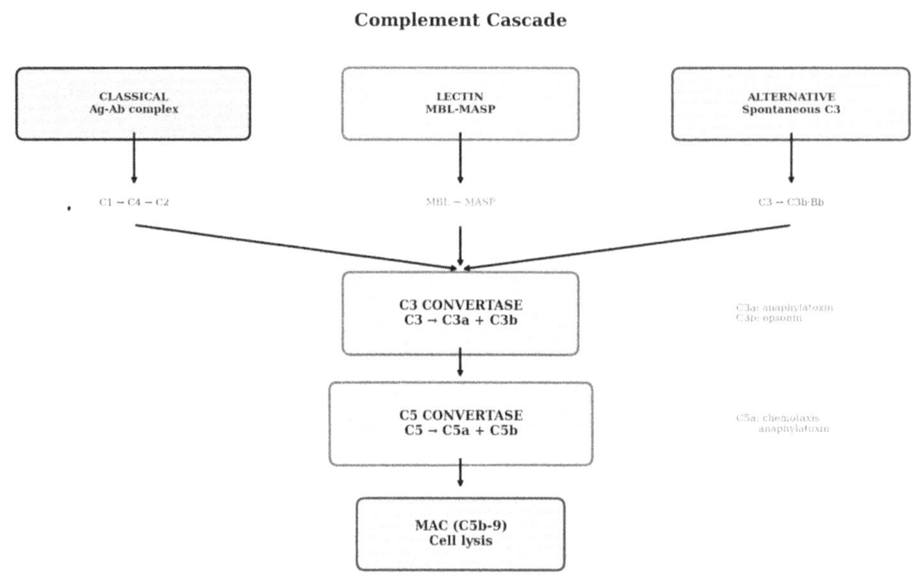

Figure 2.5: Complement Cascade. *(Source: Author's original.)*

The kinin system: Hageman factor (factor XII), activated by contact with collagen, basement membrane, or activated platelets, triggers the kinin cascade. Prekallikrein is converted to kallikrein, which cleaves high-molecular-weight kininogen (HMWK) to generate bradykinin. Bradykinin causes vasodilation, increased vascular permeability, pain, and smooth muscle contraction. It is rapidly inactivated by kininases, including ACE (angiotensin-converting enzyme). This explains why ACE inhibitors can cause angioedema: they prevent bradykinin degradation.

Table 2.4: Major Chemical Mediators of Inflammation

Mediator	Source	Action	Onset	Clinical Note
Histamine	Mast cells, basophils, platelets	Vasodilation, ↑permeability	Immediate (minutes)	H1 receptor mediated; blocked by antihistamines
PGE2, PGI2	All cells (via COX)	Vasodilation, pain, fever	Hours	Blocked by NSAIDs/aspirin
LTB4	Neutrophils (via 5-LOX)	Neutrophil chemotaxis	Hours	Not blocked by NSAIDs (LOX

				pathway)
LTC4/D4/E4	Mast cells, leukocytes	Vasoconstriction, bronchospasm, ↑permeability	Minutes–hours	SRS-A; blocked by montelukast
TNF, IL-1	Macrophages	Endothelial activation, fever, acute-phase response	Hours	Key mediators of systemic effects
IL-8 (CXCL8)	Macrophages, endothelium	Neutrophil chemotaxis	Hours	CXC chemokine
C3a, C5a	Plasma (complement)	Mast cell degranulation; C5a = chemotaxis	Minutes	Anaphylatoxins
C3b	Plasma (complement)	Opsonisation	Minutes	Enhances phagocytosis
Bradykinin	Plasma (kinin system)	Vasodilation, pain, ↑permeability	Minutes	Degraded by ACE; ACEi → angioedema
NO	Endothelium, macrophages	Vasodilation; microbicidal (macrophage iNOS)	Seconds	eNOS = physiological; iNOS = inflammatory
PAF	Mast cells, leukocytes, endothelium	Platelet aggregation, vasodilation, bronchospasm	Minutes	Lipid mediator from membrane phospholipids
Lipoxins	Leukocytes (transcellular)	Anti-inflammatory; inhibit neutrophil recruitment	Hours	Pro-resolution mediators

Quick Recall: Chemical Mediators

Vasodilation: histamine, PGE2, PGI2, NO, bradykinin.

↑ **Permeability:** histamine, bradykinin, LTC4/D4/E4, C3a/C5a, PAF.

Chemotaxis: C5a, LTB4, IL-8, fMLP, chemokines.

Pain: PGE2 (sensitises), bradykinin (direct).

Fever: IL-1, TNF, IL-6 → hypothalamic PGE2.

Opsonisation: C3b, IgG, collectins.

Drug targets: Aspirin = COX. Steroids = PLA2. Zileuton = 5-LOX. Montelukast = CysLT receptor.

Inflammasomes

Inflammasomes are cytoplasmic multiprotein complexes that serve as platforms for activation of caspase-1, linking the detection of danger signals to the production of pro-inflammatory cytokines. The best characterised is the NLRP3 inflammasome, composed of the sensor protein NLRP3, the adaptor ASC, and pro-caspase-1.

NLRP3 is activated by a wide range of stimuli: microbial products, crystals (monosodium urate in gout, cholesterol crystals in atherosclerosis, silica in silicosis), extracellular ATP (released from dying cells), and potassium efflux. Activation triggers assembly of the inflammasome complex, which recruits and activates caspase-1. Caspase-1 cleaves pro-IL-1β and pro-IL-18 into their mature, secreted forms, and also cleaves gasdermin D, triggering pyroptosis (see Chapter 1).

Integration: the inflammasome is the molecular bridge between the innate immune system's danger detection and the inflammatory response. It links sterile inflammation (gout, atherosclerosis) to the same pathway that detects infection. This convergence explains why conditions as different as gout and sepsis share the same downstream mediator (IL-1β) and respond to the same drug (canakinumab, anti-IL-1β). For pyroptosis and gasdermin D biology, see Chapter 1.

Morphological Patterns of Acute Inflammation

The morphological appearance of acute inflammation varies depending on the severity, cause, and tissue involved.

Serous inflammation: characterised by outpouring of thin, protein-rich fluid (serous exudate) derived from plasma or mesothelial cell secretion. Examples include skin blisters from burns and pleural effusion in early tuberculosis.

Fibrinous inflammation: occurs when vascular permeability is sufficiently increased to allow fibrinogen to escape. Fibrinogen polymerises to fibrin in the extravascular space, forming a shaggy, eosinophilic meshwork. Classic examples include fibrinous pericarditis ("bread-and-butter" pericarditis in rheumatic fever and uraemia) and fibrinous pleuritis. If the fibrin is not removed by fibrinolysis or macrophage digestion, it becomes organised by ingrowth of fibroblasts and blood vessels, producing adhesions.

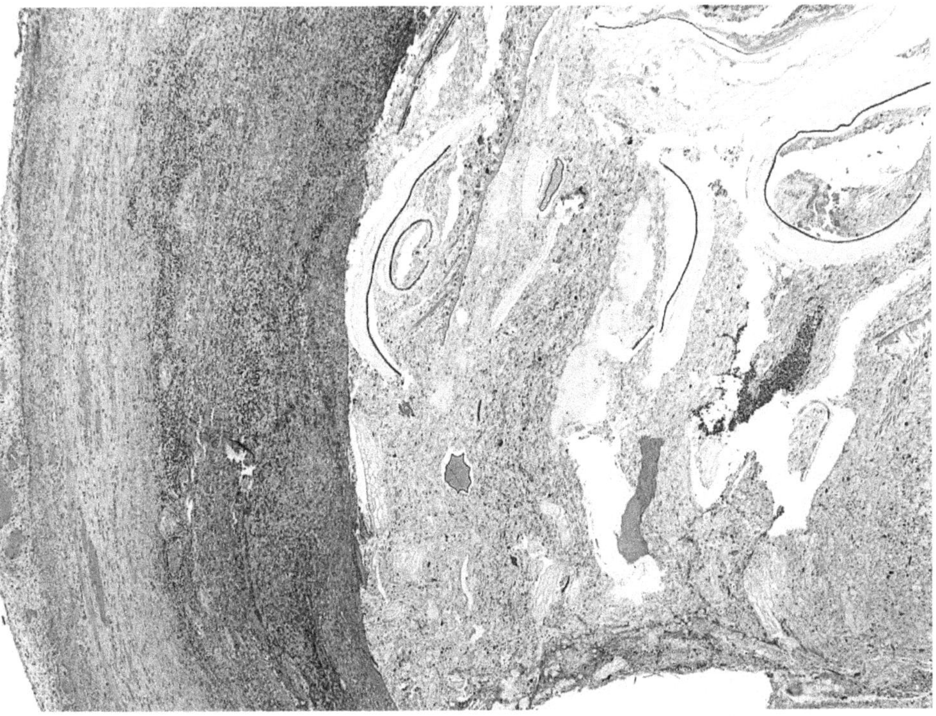

Figure 2.6: Acute suppurative inflammation — appendicitis. H&E showing transmural neutrophilic infiltrate with mucosal ulceration. *(Source: Nephron, Wikimedia Commons, CC BY-SA 3.0.)*

Ulceration: occurs when an inflammatory necrotic surface sloughs, creating a local defect (ulcer). Most commonly seen in the oral mucosa, stomach, duodenum, intestine, and skin.

Pseudomembranous inflammation is a particular form of fibrinopurulent exudate adherent to a denuded mucosal surface, classically caused by Clostridioides difficile colitis (yellow-tan plaques on colonic mucosa) and historically by diphtheritic pharyngitis (grey-white membrane on the tonsils and pharynx). The membrane consists of fibrin, neutrophils, sloughed epithelium, mucin, and bacteria, and lifts off to leave a raw bleeding surface beneath. It is the morphological signature of toxin-mediated mucosal necrosis with brisk acute inflammation.

The five patterns (serous, fibrinous, suppurative or purulent, ulcerative, pseudomembranous) are not mutually exclusive. A perforated peptic ulcer shows ulcerative inflammation at the lesion and fibrinous or suppurative inflammation on the serosa. A bacterial pneumonia evolves from suppurative alveolar exudate to fibrinous pleuritis as the process reaches the pleural surface. Pattern recognition is the first step; cause-pattern correlation is the second.

The Pathologist's Eye

Pattern recognition on biopsy: when a pathologist sees a neutrophilic infiltrate, the first thought is acute inflammation (bacterial infection, early autoimmune flare). When the infiltrate is predominantly lymphocytic, the thought shifts to chronic inflammation or viral infection. When macrophages aggregate into granulomas, the differential narrows to a specific list (TB, sarcoidosis, fungal, foreign body, Crohn). Pattern recognition, not marker memorisation, is the foundation of diagnostic pathology.

Diagnostic thinking: neutrophils + fibrin + oedema → acute inflammation

Clinical Pearl

Pattern recognition at the eyepiece. Serous inflammation looks like an empty space with a thin eosinophilic film; the burn blister and early viral pleurisy are the classic examples. Fibrinous inflammation looks shaggy and stringy, an eosinophilic mat draped across an epithelial surface; fibrinous pericarditis ('bread and butter') and lobar pneumonia in red hepatisation are the prototype lessons. Suppurative inflammation looks dense and basophilic, a sea of neutrophils; appendicitis and abscess are the readily-recognised teaching slides. The distinction matters because it predicts outcome: serous resolves, fibrinous can organise into adhesions, suppurative may form an abscess.

Outcomes of Acute Inflammation

Acute inflammation can resolve in one of four ways: complete resolution (restoration of normal tissue, the ideal outcome), healing by fibrosis (when tissue destruction is substantial, replaced by scar tissue; see Chapter 3), abscess formation (when a localised collection of pus is walled off), or progression to chronic inflammation (when the offending agent is not eliminated).

Outcomes of Acute Inflammation in Detail

Complete resolution is the ideal outcome and the default response to mild, self-limited injury. The inciting agent is neutralised, neutrophils undergo apoptosis and are cleared by tissue macrophages, vascular permeability returns to baseline, lymphatic drainage clears oedema fluid, and tissue architecture is restored. Specialised pro-resolving mediators (resolvins, protectins, maresins) actively orchestrate this clearance; resolution is no longer regarded as passive.

Healing by connective-tissue replacement (fibrosis) occurs when tissue destruction is substantial, when fibrinous exudate cannot be cleared, when an abscess is incompletely drained, or when the parenchyma lacks regenerative capacity (heart, brain, kidney). Granulation tissue replaces the lost tissue and matures into a fibrous scar. This is the subject of Chapter 3.

Abscess formation occurs when neutrophilic exudate is walled off by fibrin and granulation tissue. Pyogenic organisms (Staphylococcus aureus, Klebsiella, anaerobic bacteria) typically drive this outcome. Once formed, an abscess will not resolve without drainage; antibiotics alone cannot penetrate the central necrotic core in adequate concentration. The clinical lesson is that source control precedes antimicrobial therapy.

Progression to chronic inflammation is the fourth outcome. It occurs when the inciting agent is not cleared (intracellular pathogens such as Mycobacterium tuberculosis, persistent foreign material, autoimmune drivers, low-grade chemical irritation), or when the acute response itself becomes self-sustaining through cytokine feedback loops. The cellular composition shifts to mononuclear cells, and tissue destruction and repair occur simultaneously.

Chronic Inflammation

Chronic inflammation is a prolonged inflammatory response (weeks to months to years) in which active inflammation, tissue destruction, and attempted repair proceed simultaneously. The hallmark cells are macrophages, lymphocytes, and plasma cells, in contrast to the neutrophil-dominated infiltrate of acute inflammation.

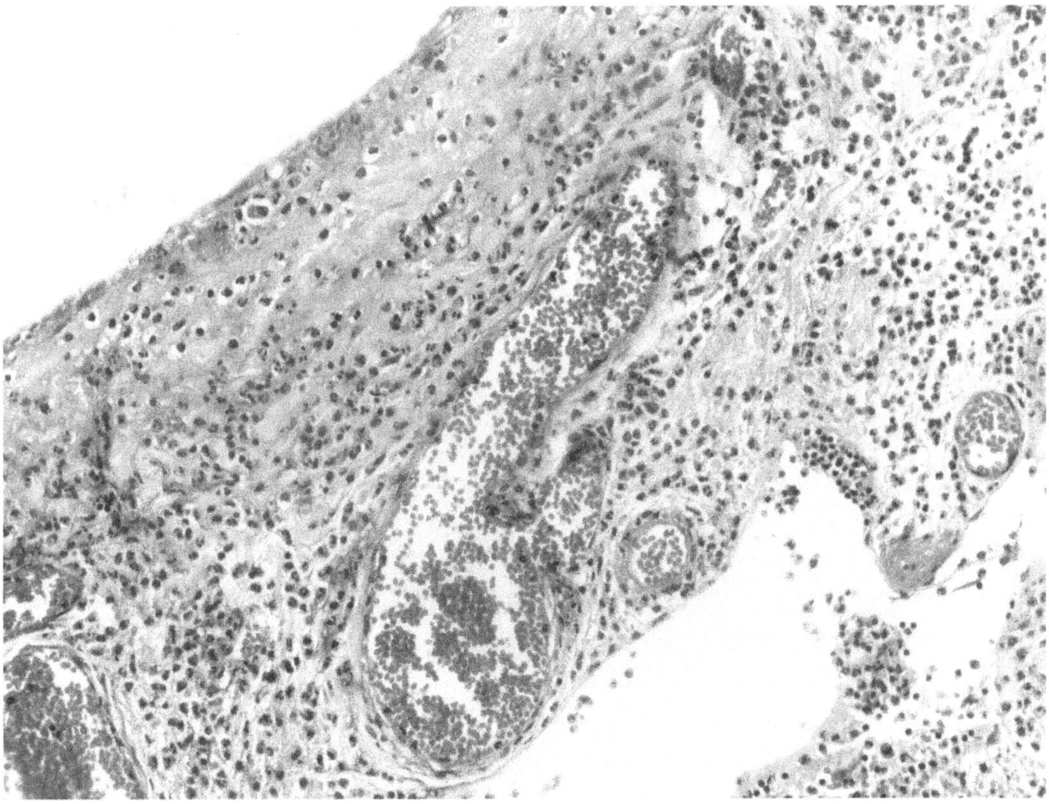

Figure 2.7: Acute inflammatory exudate. H&E showing fibrin-rich exudate with neutrophils and congested vessels. *(Source: Netha Hussain, Wikimedia Commons, CC BY-SA 4.0.)*

When faced with a biopsy showing dense mononuclear infiltrate with fibrosis, the pathologist should consider: the chronicity of the process, the presence or absence of granulomas (which narrows the differential significantly), the type of giant cells (Langhans-type with peripheral nuclei in an arc suggests TB/sarcoid; foreign body type with scattered nuclei suggests exogenous material), and the pattern of fibrosis (bridging fibrosis in hepatitis, interstitial fibrosis in lungs, submucosal fibrosis in Crohn disease).

Causes

Chronic inflammation arises in several settings: persistent infections by organisms that are difficult to eradicate (Mycobacterium tuberculosis, Treponema pallidum, certain viruses and fungi), immune-mediated inflammatory diseases (autoimmune: rheumatoid arthritis, SLE, IBD; allergic: asthma), prolonged exposure to potentially toxic agents (exogenous: silica, asbestos causing silicosis and asbestosis;

endogenous: oxidised lipids in atherosclerosis), and some conditions classified as "autoinflammatory" (related to inflammasome dysregulation rather than adaptive immunity).

The Macrophage: Central Cell of Chronic Inflammation

The macrophage is the dominant cell in chronic inflammation. Circulating monocytes are recruited to the site of inflammation and differentiate into tissue macrophages under the influence of local signals. Once activated, macrophages serve as the workhorses of chronic inflammation through three principal mechanisms: phagocytosis and microbial killing, antigen presentation to T lymphocytes (linking innate and adaptive immunity), and secretion of cytokines, growth factors, and tissue-remodelling enzymes.

Macrophage activation follows two pathways. Classical (M1) activation, driven by IFN-γ from Th1 cells and by TLR signalling, produces macrophages that are microbicidal and pro-inflammatory (secreting TNF, IL-1, IL-12, ROS, NO). Alternative (M2) activation, driven by IL-4 and IL-13 from Th2 cells, produces macrophages that promote tissue repair (secreting TGF-β, PDGF, VEGF, anti-inflammatory IL-10) and fibrosis. In most chronic inflammatory lesions, both M1 and M2 macrophages coexist, and their balance determines whether the tissue moves toward further destruction or toward healing.

> **Quick Recall: Chronic Inflammation**
>
> Definition: inflammation of prolonged duration (weeks to years) in which tissue destruction, inflammation, and repair proceed simultaneously.
>
> Cells: macrophages (dominant), lymphocytes, plasma cells, eosinophils. Macrophage activation: classical (M1, pro-inflammatory, microbicidal) vs alternative (M2, anti-inflammatory, tissue repair).
>
> Causes: persistent infections (TB, viral hepatitis), autoimmune diseases (RA, SLE, IBD), prolonged exposure to toxic agents (silicosis, atherosclerosis).
>
> Systemic effects: acute phase response (CRP, SAA, fibrinogen from liver via IL-6), leukocytosis, ESR elevation. SAA in chronic inflammation can lead to secondary (AA) amyloidosis (see Chapter 5).
>
> Key distinction from acute: acute = vascular changes + neutrophils; chronic = tissue destruction + mononuclear infiltrate + fibrosis.

Granulomatous Inflammation

Granulomatous inflammation is a distinctive pattern of chronic inflammation characterised by aggregates of activated macrophages (epithelioid cells), often with multinucleated giant cells, surrounded by a collar of lymphocytes (types compared in Figure 2.14). The formation of a granuloma is not random; it represents an attempt by the immune system to wall off agents it cannot easily destroy. The clinical significance lies in recognising the pattern, because the differential diagnosis of granulomatous inflammation is itself a high-yield diagnostic exercise.

In TB-endemic regions, tuberculosis dominates the differential, but the pathologist must systematically consider sarcoidosis, fungal infections (histoplasmosis, cryptococcosis), foreign body reactions, Crohn's disease, leprosy, and drug reactions before defaulting to that assumption. The presence or absence of central caseous necrosis is the first branch point: caseating granulomas strongly suggest TB or certain fungal infections; non-caseating granulomas favour sarcoidosis, foreign body, Crohn, or drug reaction.

Clinical Pearl

Caseation is not synonymous with tuberculosis. At least four other entities produce caseating granulomas: deep fungal infection (histoplasmosis, blastomycosis, cryptococcosis), tertiary syphilis (gummas), tularemia, and certain forms of Hodgkin lymphoma necrosis. The morphological clue in fungal disease is the persistence of granuloma architecture with relatively scant Langhans giant cells; ZN-negative, GMS-positive caseating granulomas should always raise the fungal possibility before declaring 'TB on histology, treat empirically.' Always request both ZN and GMS on every caseating granuloma.

TYPES OF GRANULOMAS

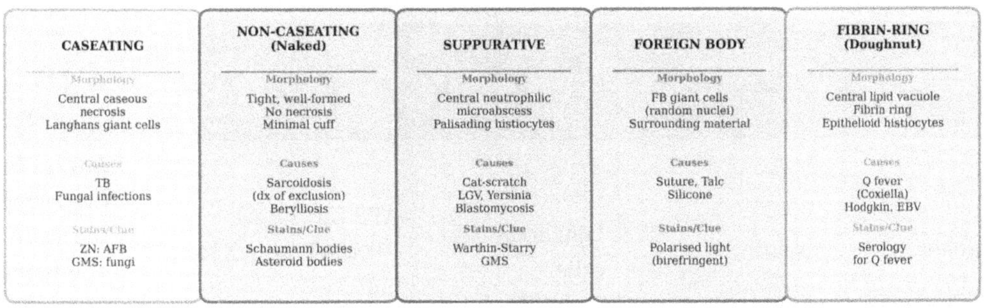

Figure 2.8: Types of granulomas — caseating, non-caseating, suppurative, foreign body, and fibrin-ring patterns with diagnostic features. (Source: Author's original.)

Figure: Types of Granulomas. (Source: Author's original.)

Diagnostic thinking: non-caseating granuloma + bilateral hilar LAP + negative AFB → sarcoidosis

Types of Granulomas

Immune (epithelioid) granulomas: formed when T cell-mediated immunity is directed against persistent, poorly degradable antigens. CD4+ T cells (Th1) secrete IFN-γ, which activates macrophages, transforming them into epithelioid cells (large, pale, elongated cells with abundant eosinophilic cytoplasm, resembling epithelial cells). Epithelioid cells may fuse to form multinucleated giant cells. Langhans giant cells (nuclei arranged in a horseshoe or peripheral arc) are characteristic of tuberculosis but not pathognomonic. Touton giant cells (lipid-laden, with a central ring of nuclei) are seen in fat-processing lesions (xanthogranulomas). The prototype is the caseating granuloma of tuberculosis.

Foreign body granulomas: formed around inert, non-immunogenic foreign material too large for a single macrophage to phagocytose (suture material, talc, silicone, beryllium). Giant cells contain the foreign material and often have randomly arranged nuclei (foreign body type giant cells). These granulomas form without T cell involvement.

The Leprosy Spectrum: Granulomas as Mirrors of Immunity

Leprosy (Hansen disease) provides the most elegant clinical demonstration of how the host immune response determines granuloma morphology. At the tuberculoid pole, a strong Th1/cell-mediated response produces well-formed, epithelioid granulomas with few bacilli (paucibacillary), limited tissue involvement, and a positive lepromin test. At the lepromatous pole, a weak cell-mediated response (Th2-dominant) produces diffuse infiltrates of foamy macrophages (lepra cells/Virchow cells) packed with acid-fast bacilli (multibacillary), widespread tissue involvement, and a negative lepromin test. Between these poles lie borderline forms (borderline tuberculoid, mid-borderline, borderline lepromatous) with intermediate histology and immune responses. The Ridley-Jopling classification captures this spectrum.

Table 2.5: Differential Diagnosis of Granulomatous Inflammation

Cause	Necrosis	Special Features	Diagnosis	Notes
Tuberculosis	Caseating	Langhans giant cells	AFB (ZN stain), CBNAAT/GeneXpert, culture	Always consider first; commonly the leading granulomatous cause in TB-endemic settings
Sarcoidosis	Non-caseating	Asteroid bodies, Schaumann bodies (not specific)	Diagnosis of exclusion; elevated ACE, serum calcium	Must exclude TB before diagnosing sarcoidosis in TB-endemic settings
Fungal infections	May be caseating or non-caseating	Organisms visible on GMS/PAS	Culture, serology	Histoplasmosis, cryptococcosis, coccidioidomycosis
Foreign body reaction	Non-caseating	Foreign body giant cells; polarisable material	Polarised light microscopy	Suture, talc, silicone, starch
Crohn's disease	Non-caseating (small, loose)	Few giant cells	Clinical + endoscopic + histological correlation	Distinguish from intestinal TB (major differential in TB-endemic regions)

Leprosy	Non-caseating (tuberculoid) or foamy macrophages (lepromatous)	Variable	Fite-Faraco stain for AFB	Spectrum: tuberculoid (granulomas, few bacilli) to lepromatous (foamy macrophages, many bacilli)
Drug reaction	Non-caseating (may have eosinophils)	Poorly formed	Temporal relationship to drug	Methotrexate, anti-TNF agents, BCG
Cat-scratch disease	Stellate (star-shaped) microabscesses within granulomas	Suppurative granulomas	Warthin-Starry stain, serology	Bartonella henselae

Exam Pitfall

In TB-endemic regions, non-caseating granulomas on a lymph node biopsy should not be called sarcoidosis until AFB stains, TB culture, and TB PCR (CBNAAT/GeneXpert) are negative. Similarly, distinguishing intestinal TB from Crohn's disease remains one of the most challenging diagnostic problems in gastroenterology and pathology. Features favouring TB: caseation, confluent granulomas, AFB positivity, involvement of ileocaecal region predominantly, peritoneal involvement, and transverse ulcer orientation (along the lymphatic drainage).

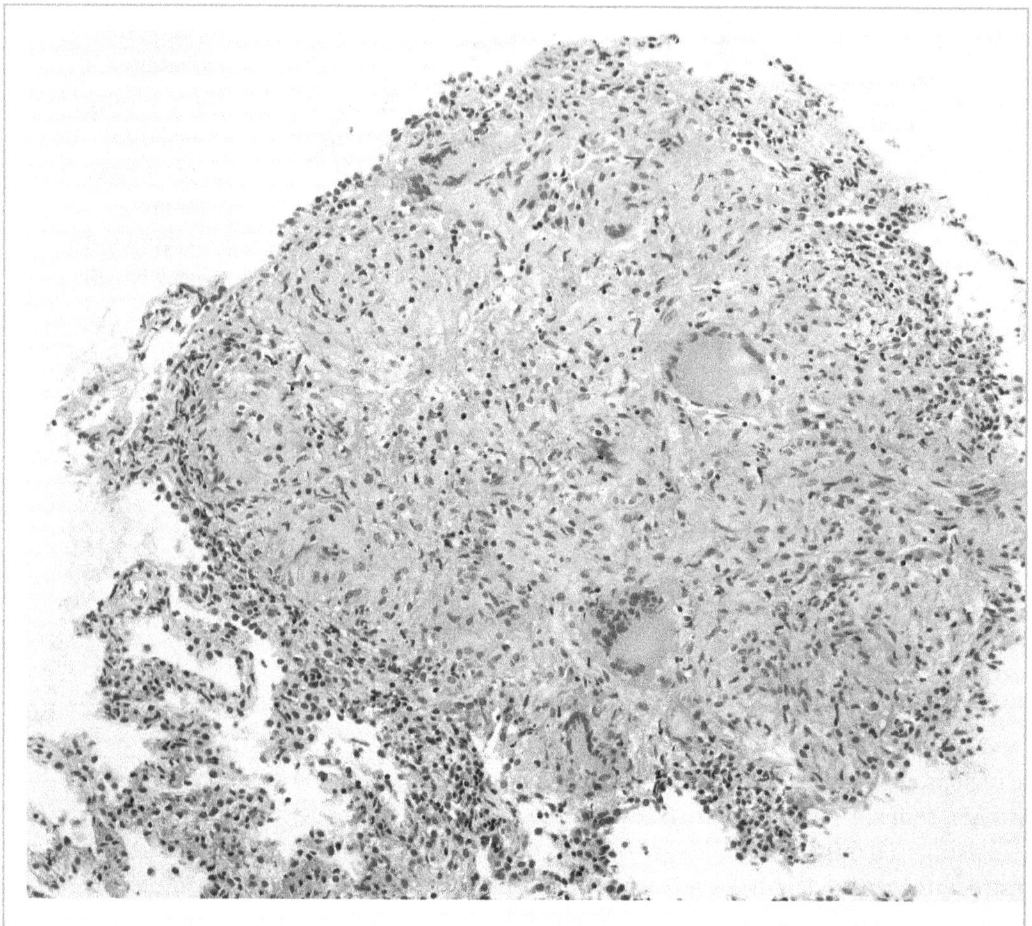

Figure 2.9: Caseating granuloma in tuberculosis. Central amorphous eosinophilic caseous necrosis surrounded by epithelioid histiocytes and Langhans giant cells, with a peripheral collar of lymphocytes. H&E, 100×. (Source: KGH, Wikimedia Commons, CC BY-SA 3.0.)

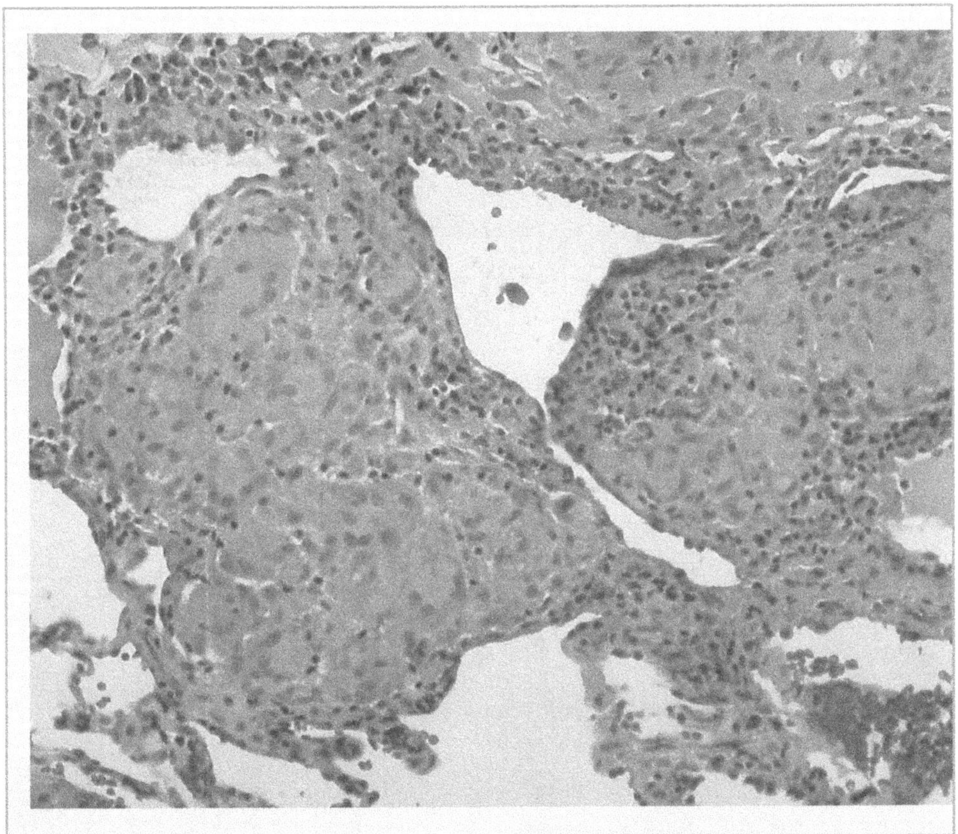

Figure 2.10: Non-caseating granuloma in sarcoidosis. Well-formed, tight epithelioid granuloma without central necrosis. H&E, 200×. (Source: Yale Rosen, Wikimedia Commons, CC BY 2.0.)

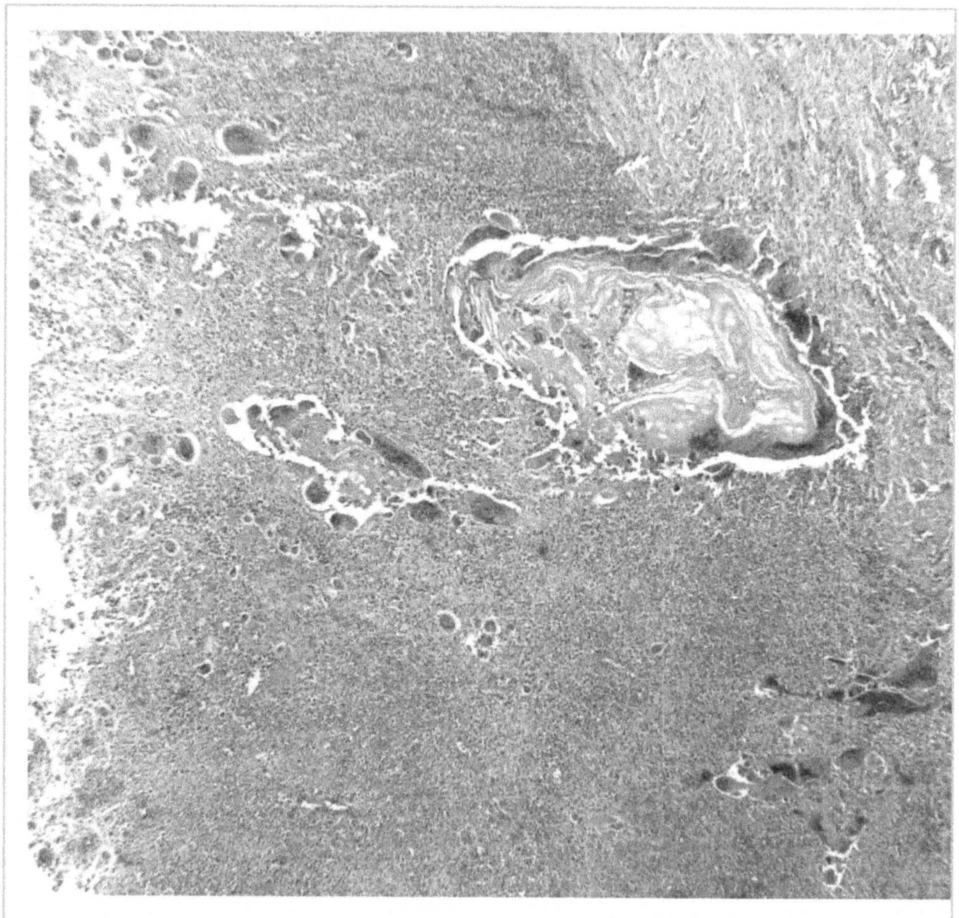

Figure 2.11: Foreign body giant cell reaction. Multinucleated giant cell with randomly arranged nuclei engulfing refractile foreign material (suture). H&E, 400×. (Source: Calicut Medical College, Wikimedia Commons, CC BY-SA 3.0.)

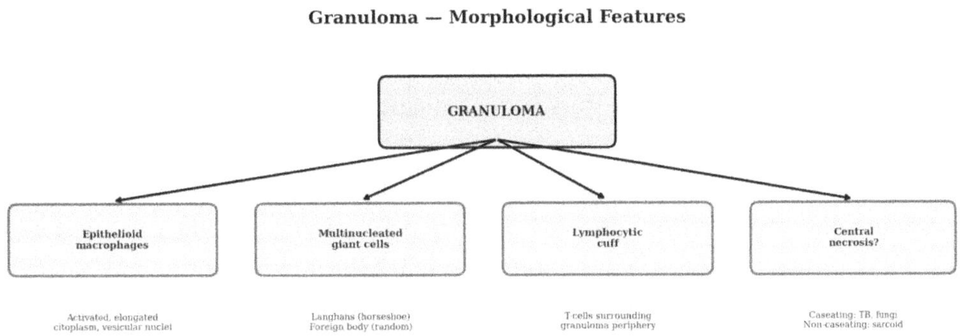

Figure 2.12: Granuloma — Morphological Features. *(Source: Author's original.)*

Integration: Granulomatous inflammation connects to tuberculosis and leprosy (Chapter 9 for detailed organism-specific pathogenesis, including the CBNAAT/Truenat diagnostic algorithm), sarcoidosis (Chapter 15 for pulmonary involvement), Crohn disease versus intestinal TB (Chapter 19 for the critical differential diagnosis), and foreign body reactions in surgical pathology (Chapter 35). The granuloma-forming immune response also links to cell-mediated immunity and type IV hypersensitivity (Chapter 5). Chronic inflammation and the acute phase response connect to amyloidosis (AA amyloid from persistent SAA elevation, Chapter 5) and to anaemia of chronic disease (hepcidin upregulation, see Volume 1).

Systemic Effects of Inflammation

When inflammation is severe or widespread, the local response spills over into systemic effects mediated primarily by TNF, IL-1, and IL-6.

Fever: pyrogenic cytokines (IL-1, TNF, IL-6) act on the hypothalamus, stimulating PGE2 synthesis via COX-2. PGE2 resets the thermoregulatory set point upward. NSAIDs reduce fever by inhibiting hypothalamic COX-2.

Acute-phase response: IL-6 stimulates hepatocytes to synthesise acute-phase proteins. CRP (C-reactive protein) opsonises bacteria and activates complement. Fibrinogen contributes to the elevated ESR (by promoting rouleaux formation). SAA (serum amyloid A) replaces apolipoprotein A-I in HDL; chronic elevation leads to secondary (AA) amyloidosis (see Chapter 5). Hepcidin, induced by IL-6, blocks ferroportin and causes the anaemia of chronic disease (see Volume 1).

The acute-phase response is the systemic, hepatocyte-driven, IL-6-orchestrated counterpart of local inflammation. Six acute-phase proteins are postgraduate-relevant. C-reactive protein (CRP) opsonises bacteria, activates the classical complement pathway, and rises within hours; serum amyloid A (SAA) displaces apoA-I from HDL and primes leukocyte chemotaxis, with chronic elevation predisposing to AA amyloidosis. Fibrinogen and haptoglobin elevate the erythrocyte sedimentation rate (ESR) by promoting rouleaux. Hepcidin, induced by IL-6, sequesters iron in macrophages and reduces duodenal absorption, producing the anaemia of chronic disease. Ferritin, an acute-phase reactant in its own right, becomes unreliable as an iron-stores marker during inflammation; soluble transferrin receptor is preferred in this setting. Ceruloplasmin and complement components C3 and C4 also rise, while albumin and transferrin fall as negative acute-phase reactants. These shifts explain why a low albumin with high CRP in a hospitalised patient signals systemic inflammation, not necessarily malnutrition.

Leukocytosis: TNF and IL-1 stimulate bone marrow production and release of neutrophils (neutrophilia). The type of leukocyte elevation provides a diagnostic clue: neutrophilia in bacterial infections, lymphocytosis in viral infections, eosinophilia in parasitic and allergic conditions. Leukopenia (decreased leukocytes) occurs in some infections (typhoid, certain viral infections) and in overwhelming sepsis (bone marrow exhaustion). In severe infections, the neutrophil count may exceed 40,000–50,000/µL with left shift (leukaemoid reaction), which must be distinguished from chronic myeloid leukaemia by the absence of basophilia, the presence of toxic granulation and Döhle bodies, elevated leukocyte alkaline phosphatase (LAP) score, and absence of the BCR-ABL1 fusion (see Volume 1).

Sepsis and septic shock: when TNF and IL-1 are produced in overwhelming quantities (as in severe Gram-negative sepsis), they cause systemic vasodilation, increased vascular permeability, myocardial depression, DIC, and multi-organ dysfunction (MODS). This represents the most lethal consequence of dysregulated inflammation and is discussed in detail in Chapter 4.

Recent Advances

Pulmonary pathology of COVID-19 — Bergamo–Milan series. The first systematic post-mortem series of fatal COVID-19 from the early Lombardy outbreak documented the dominant histological signature of severe SARS-CoV-2 pneumonia (Carsana et al. Lancet Infectious Diseases 2020; 20: 1135–1140; PMID 32526193). Lung tissue from 38 patients who died at two centres between 29 February and 24 March 2020 was examined with haematoxylin–eosin, immunohistochemistry, and electron microscopy. All cases showed exudative and proliferative phases of diffuse alveolar damage, with capillary congestion, pneumocyte necrosis, type II pneumocyte hyperplasia, hyaline membranes (33/38), interstitial and intra-alveolar oedema (37/38), squamous metaplasia with cytological atypia (21/38), and platelet–fibrin microthrombi in small pulmonary arterial vessels (33/38). The inflammatory infiltrate was macrophage-rich within alveolar lumina and lymphocytic in the interstitium. Electron microscopy localised viral particles principally to pneumocytes. The series established diffuse alveolar damage with pulmonary microvascular thrombosis as the histological hallmark of fatal COVID-19 and supplied the mechanistic rationale for early anticoagulant strategies.

Resolution of inflammation and specialised pro-resolving mediators (SPMs). Resolution is now understood to be an active, programmed process, not merely the passive dissipation of pro-inflammatory signals. SPMs, including resolvins (derived from omega-3 fatty acids EPA and DHA), protectins, and maresins, actively promote resolution by inhibiting neutrophil recruitment, enhancing macrophage efferocytosis (clearance of apoptotic cells), and promoting tissue repair. This has therapeutic implications: failure of resolution may underlie chronic inflammatory diseases, and SPM-based therapies are in early-stage clinical trials for conditions including periodontitis, dry eye, and inflammatory bowel disease.

Trained immunity. The classical view held that only adaptive immunity has memory. Recent evidence shows that innate immune cells, particularly monocytes and macrophages, can undergo epigenetic reprogramming (histone methylation and acetylation changes) after initial stimulation, producing a heightened response to subsequent, unrelated stimuli. This "trained immunity" is mediated by metabolic rewiring (shift from oxidative phosphorylation to glycolysis) and is the mechanistic basis for the non-specific protective effects of BCG vaccination. Trained immunity may also contribute to the sustained inflammation of atherosclerosis and autoinflammatory diseases.

NLRP3 inflammasome inhibitors. Following the success of canakinumab (anti-IL-1β) in the CANTOS trial for cardiovascular risk reduction, small-molecule NLRP3 inhibitors (MCC950/CRID3, dapansutrile) are in clinical trials for gout, atherosclerosis, Alzheimer disease, and autoinflammatory syndromes. These represent a new class of anti-inflammatory drugs targeting the upstream sensor rather than the downstream cytokine.

International Frameworks

Sepsis-3 (2016) — SIRS deprecated. The Third International Consensus redefined sepsis as life-threatening organ dysfunction caused by a dysregulated host response to infection, and explicitly deprecated the systemic inflammatory response syndrome (SIRS) criteria as inadequately specific. Organ dysfunction is now operationalised by an increase of two or more points in the Sequential Organ Failure Assessment (SOFA) score. For rapid bedside identification outside the intensive care unit, qSOFA flags suspected sepsis when at least two of three criteria are present: respiratory rate ≥22/min, altered mentation, or systolic blood pressure ≤100 mm Hg. Septic shock requires a vasopressor requirement to maintain mean arterial pressure ≥65 mm Hg and serum lactate >2 mmol/L despite adequate volume resuscitation, with an associated in-hospital mortality exceeding 40%. The term "severe sepsis" was retired as redundant. Citation: Singer M, et al. JAMA 2016;315(8):801–810. PMID 26903338.

Ultra High-Yield Chapter Summary

Topic	Must Remember
Acute vs chronic	Acute: neutrophils, vascular changes, hours–days.
Cardinal signs	Rubor (vasodilation), tumor (oedema), calor (vasodilation), dolor (PGE2, bradykinin), functio laesa.
Exudate vs transudate	Exudate: high protein (>3 g/dL), inflammatory.
Rolling	Selectins: P-selectin (rapid, histamine), E-selectin (hours, TNF/IL-1), L-selectin (constitutive on leukocytes).
Firm adhesion	Integrins (LFA-1, Mac-1) bind ICAM-1/VCAM-1.
Transmigration	PECAM-1 (CD31) homophilic interactions at endothelial junctions.
Chemotaxis	C5a, LTB4, IL-8, fMLP. GPCRs → actin polymerisation.
LAD-1	No CD18 (beta-2 integrin) → no firm adhesion → no pus formation → leukocytosis.
CGD	No NADPH oxidase → no respiratory burst → catalase-positive infections → granulomas.
Most potent bactericidal	MPO-H_2O_2-halide system → HOCl. Oxygen-dependent.

Vasodilation mediators	Histamine, NO, PGE2, PGI2, bradykinin.
Chemotactic mediators	C5a, LTB4, IL-8 (CXCL8), fMLP.
Fever pathway	IL-1/TNF/IL-6 → hypothalamic PGE2 (COX-2) → raised set point.
COX vs LOX	COX: PGs, TXA2. LOX: LTs, lipoxins. Aspirin blocks COX only.
Granuloma formation	T cell (Th1) → IFN-γ → macrophage activation → epithelioid cells ± giant cells.
Caseating granuloma	TB, fungi.
Acute-phase proteins	CRP (opsonin), fibrinogen (ESR), SAA (amyloid precursor), hepcidin (anaemia of chronic disease).
Inflammasome	NLRP3 → caspase-1 → IL-1β/IL-18 + gasdermin D (pyroptosis).
Trained immunity	Epigenetic reprogramming of monocytes/macrophages. Metabolic shift to glycolysis.
Patterns of acute inflammation	Serous (blister, early effusion), fibrinous (bread-and-butter pericarditis), suppurative/purulent (abscess, cellulitis), ulcerative (mucosal defect from sloughing).
Leprosy spectrum	Tuberculoid: granulomas, few bacilli, strong CMI. Lepromatous: foamy macrophages, many bacilli, weak CMI (Figures 9.3 and 9.4).

Chemical Mediators of Inflammation: Master Map

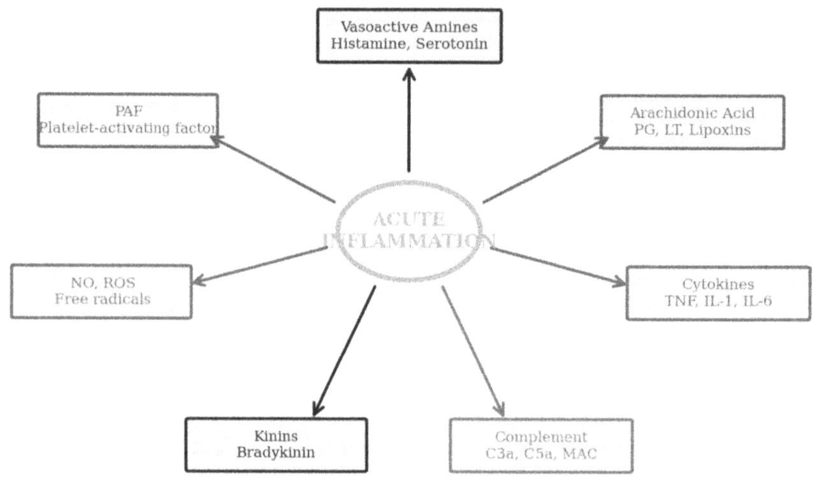

Figure 2.13: Chemical Mediators of Inflammation: Master Map. (Source: Author's original.)

Granuloma Types Composite

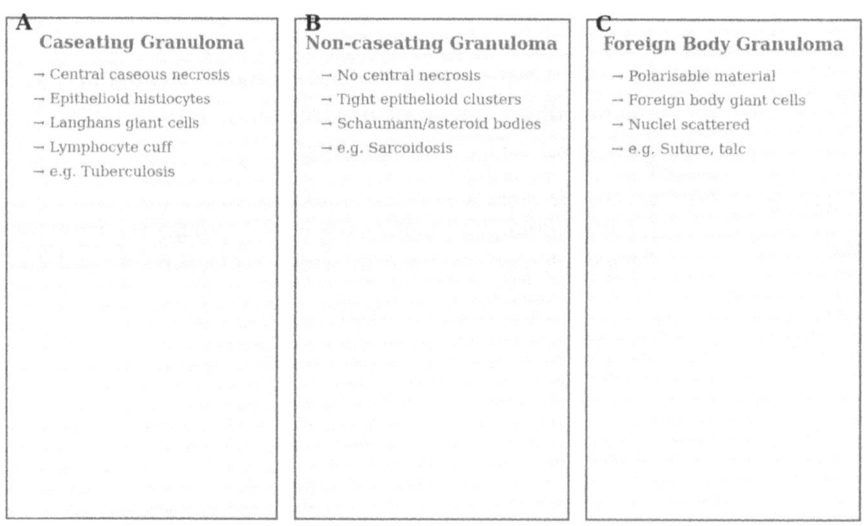

Figure 2.14: Granuloma Types Composite. (Source: Author's original.)

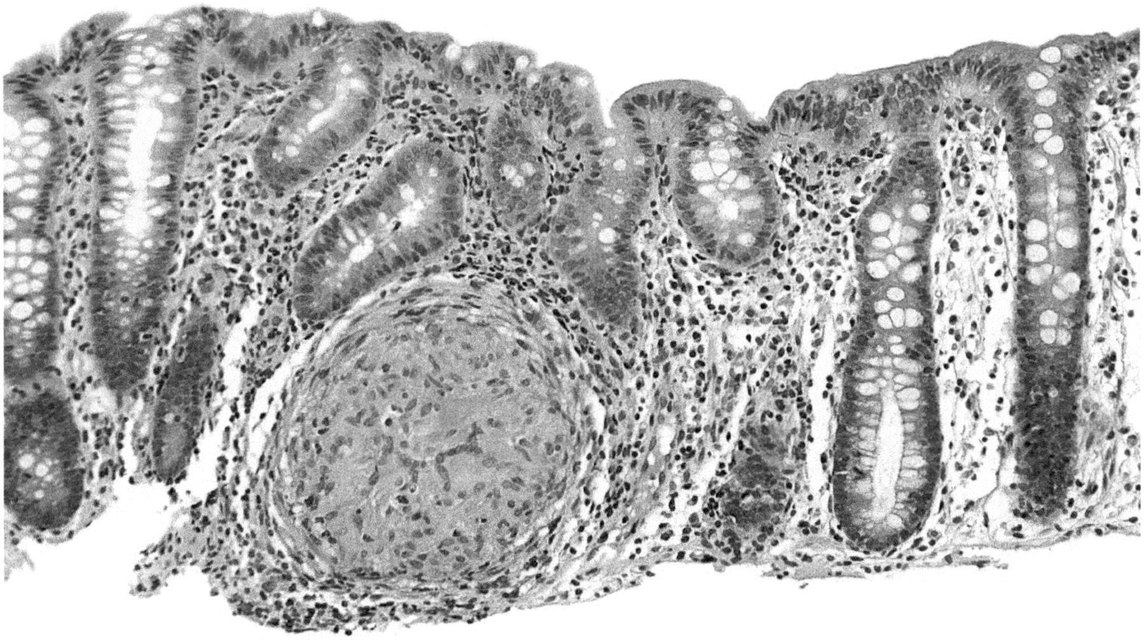

Figure 2.14B: Non-caseating granuloma (Crohn disease, duodenum). See Figure 19.2A (Chapter 19) for photomicrograph. (Source: Nephron, Wikimedia Commons, CC BY-SA 3.0.)

Chapter 3: Tissue Repair, Regeneration, and Wound Healing

THE BIG PICTURE

When tissue is damaged, the body responds with one of two fundamental processes: regeneration, in which destroyed cells are replaced by identical functional cells, or repair, in which the defect is filled by connective tissue (scar). In practice, most healing involves both processes in varying proportions. The outcome depends on three variables: the regenerative capacity of the injured tissue, the severity and extent of damage, and the integrity of the extracellular matrix scaffold. Organs composed of labile or stable cells (liver, bone marrow, epithelial surfaces) can regenerate substantially; those composed of permanent cells (myocardium, neurons) heal predominantly by scarring. Understanding these principles is essential for interpreting wound pathology, transplant biology, and the fibrotic complications that underlie cirrhosis, pulmonary fibrosis, and post-myocardial infarction remodelling.

High-yield topics in this chapter: angiogenesis (mechanism and regulators); growth factors in tissue repair (VEGF, PDGF, TGF-β, FGF, EGF); extracellular matrix components (collagens, proteoglycans, adhesive glycoproteins); wound healing by primary and secondary intention; granulation tissue; abnormalities of tissue repair (keloid, contracture, dehiscence); stem cells and regenerative capacity; fracture healing.

Diagnostic thinking: capillary proliferation + fibroblasts + loose stroma + inflammation → granulation tissue (proliferative phase)

Tissue repair involves two fundamental processes: regeneration (replacement of damaged cells by identical functional cells) and repair by scarring (replacement by connective tissue). Most healing involves both processes in varying proportions. The outcome depends on the regenerative capacity of the injured tissue, the severity of damage, and the integrity of the extracellular matrix scaffold. This chapter covers cell proliferation, growth factors, angiogenesis, wound healing by primary and secondary intention, and abnormalities of tissue repair.

Cell Proliferation and the Cell Cycle

Figure: Wound Healing Phases. (Source: Author's original.)

Tissue repair depends on cell proliferation, which is governed by the cell cycle. Cells in the body exist in one of three proliferative states, and this classification is central to understanding which tissues can regenerate and which cannot.

Labile cells are continuously dividing. They cycle from one mitosis to the next with only brief pauses, replacing cells that are constantly being shed. Examples include surface epithelia (skin, oral mucosa, gastrointestinal tract, uterine endometrium), haematopoietic cells of the bone marrow, and the transitional epithelium of the urinary tract. These tissues contain stem cell populations that fuel continuous turnover and can regenerate rapidly after injury, provided the stem cell niche and basement membrane remain intact.

Stable (quiescent) cells reside in G0, the resting phase, under normal conditions. They have low baseline replication rates but can be stimulated to re-enter the cell cycle in response to injury or growth factor signals. The best example is the hepatocyte: after partial hepatectomy or toxic injury, the liver can regenerate its original mass within weeks. Other stable cells include renal tubular epithelium, pancreatic acinar cells, fibroblasts, smooth muscle cells, vascular endothelial cells, and resting lymphocytes.

Permanent cells have left the cell cycle irreversibly and cannot divide. Cardiac myocytes, skeletal muscle fibres, and most neurons fall into this category. Injury to tissues composed of permanent cells results in scar formation rather than regeneration. emerging evidence suggests limited regenerative capacity in cardiac myocytes and certain neuronal populations (see Recent Advances), but for practical clinical and examination purposes, these remain classified as permanent.

Table 3.1: Classification of cells by proliferative capacity

Cell Type	Cell Cycle Status	Examples	Regenerative Capacity
Labile	Continuously dividing	Epidermis, GI epithelium, bone marrow, cervical epithelium	High; rapid regeneration if stem cells intact
Stable (quiescent)	G0; re-enter cycle on stimulation	Hepatocytes, renal tubular cells, fibroblasts, endothelium, smooth muscle	Moderate to high; regeneration driven by growth factors
Permanent	Left cell cycle irreversibly	Cardiac myocytes, skeletal muscle, neurons	Minimal; injury heals by scarring

The key diagnostic clue when evaluating tissue repair on biopsy is the proliferative status of the damaged cell population: if the tissue is composed of labile or stable cells and the extracellular matrix framework is preserved, regeneration can restore normal architecture. If the matrix is destroyed or the cells are permanent, scarring is inevitable.

Stem Cells in Tissue Homeostasis and Repair

Stem cells are the reservoir from which tissues replace worn-out or damaged cells. Two properties define a stem cell: self-renewal (the ability to produce at least one daughter cell that remains a stem cell) and asymmetric division (the ability to generate differentiated progeny). These properties are maintained by the stem cell niche, a specialised microenvironment of stromal cells, extracellular matrix, and paracrine signals that regulates stem cell quiescence, activation, and fate.

Embryonic stem cells (ESCs) are derived from the inner cell mass of the blastocyst and are totipotent (or, strictly, pluripotent), capable of generating all cell lineages of the body. Their clinical use is limited by ethical concerns and the risk of teratoma formation.

Adult (tissue) stem cells reside in specific niches in postnatal tissues. They are multipotent, generating the differentiated cell types of the tissue in which they reside. Well-characterised examples include haematopoietic stem cells in bone marrow (see Volume 1), intestinal crypt stem cells (Lgr5-positive cells at the crypt base), epidermal stem cells in the bulge region of the hair follicle, and hepatic progenitor cells (oval cells) in the canals of Hering. Tissue stem cells have limited plasticity; under normal conditions, they do not cross lineage boundaries.

Induced pluripotent stem cells (iPSCs) are somatic cells reprogrammed to a pluripotent state by introduction of defined transcription factors (Yamanaka factors: Oct4, Sox2, Klf4, c-Myc). Shinya Yamanaka received the Nobel Prize in 2012 for this discovery. iPSCs bypass the ethical concerns of ESCs and offer the possibility of patient-specific cell therapies, though clinical translation remains limited by reprogramming efficiency and residual tumorigenic risk.

Integration: *Stem cell biology connects to haematopoietic stem cell transplantation (see Volume 1, Chapter 38), intestinal regeneration (see Chapter 19), and hepatic regeneration (see Chapter 20).*

Growth Factors and Signalling in Tissue Repair

Growth factors are polypeptide signals that stimulate cell proliferation, migration, differentiation, and survival. In tissue repair, they are produced by activated platelets, macrophages, endothelial cells, fibroblasts, and the injured parenchymal cells themselves. Growth factors act through receptor tyrosine kinases (RTKs) or serine/threonine kinase receptors, activating downstream signalling cascades including the RAS-MAP kinase, PI3K-AKT, and JAK-STAT pathways.

Table 3.2: Major growth factors in tissue repair

Growth Factor	Principal Source	Key Functions in Repair
EGF (Epidermal Growth Factor)	Platelets, macrophages, saliva	Epithelial cell and fibroblast proliferation and migration
TGF-β (Transforming Growth Factor-β)	Platelets, macrophages, lymphocytes, fibroblasts	Fibroblast chemotaxis, collagen synthesis, inhibits inflammation; master regulator of fibrosis
PDGF (Platelet-Derived Growth Factor)	Platelets, macrophages, endothelium, smooth muscle	Fibroblast and smooth muscle chemotaxis and proliferation; stimulates collagen and ECM production
VEGF (Vascular	Mesenchymal cells,	Angiogenesis (endothelial proliferation and

Endothelial Growth Factor)	macrophages (hypoxia-induced)	migration); vascular permeability
FGF (Fibroblast Growth Factor) family	Macrophages, mast cells, endothelium, many other cells	Angiogenesis, fibroblast proliferation, skeletal muscle repair, wound contraction
HGF (Hepatocyte Growth Factor)	Fibroblasts, stellate cells, endothelium	Hepatocyte proliferation, epithelial repair; acts via c-MET receptor
KGF (Keratinocyte Growth Factor; FGF-7)	Fibroblasts	Keratinocyte proliferation and migration in wound re-epithelialisation

Among these, TGF-β deserves particular emphasis. It is the most important cytokine in fibrosis, driving the transition of fibroblasts to myofibroblasts and stimulating the production of collagen, fibronectin, and proteoglycans. Excessive or prolonged TGF-β signalling is implicated in the pathogenesis of keloid scars, pulmonary fibrosis, hepatic cirrhosis, and the desmoplastic stroma of many carcinomas. Conversely, inadequate growth factor signalling contributes to chronic non-healing wounds, as seen in diabetic foot ulcers.

Tissue injury → platelet degranulation (PDGF, TGF-β) → macrophage recruitment → growth factor amplification (VEGF, FGF, EGF) → fibroblast/endothelial proliferation → granulation tissue → scar remodelling (Figure 3.1)

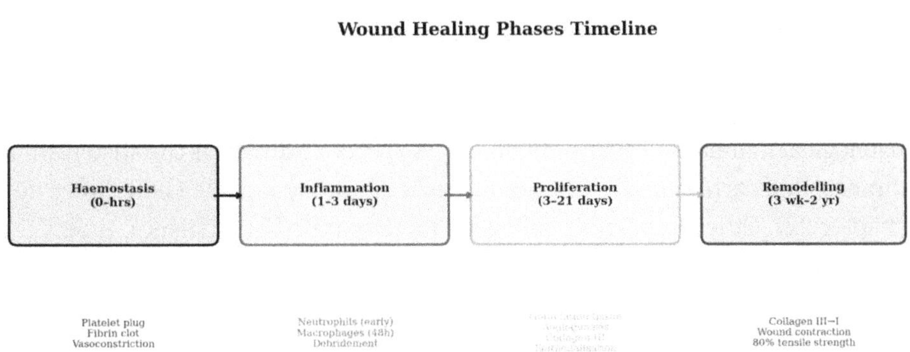

Figure 3.1: Wound Healing Phases Timeline. *(Source: Author's original.)*

> Quick Recall: Growth Factors in Repair
>
> **Master regulator of fibrosis:** TGF-β (drives fibroblast-to-myofibroblast transition and collagen synthesis).
> **Key angiogenic factor:** VEGF (induced by hypoxia via HIF-1α).
> **First growth factor at wound site:** PDGF (released from platelet α-granules within minutes of injury).
> **Hepatocyte regeneration:** HGF (acts via c-MET receptor).
> **Keratinocyte migration:** KGF (FGF-7), produced by dermal fibroblasts.

Extracellular Matrix: Components and Functions

The extracellular matrix (ECM) is not merely structural scaffolding; it is a dynamic, signalling-rich environment that regulates cell behaviour during repair. The ECM sequesters growth factors, presents adhesive substrates for cell migration, transmits mechanical signals, and provides the architectural template that determines whether healing produces regeneration or scar. Two broad forms of ECM exist: the basement membrane (a thin, specialised sheet underlying epithelia and surrounding vessels, muscle, and Schwann cells) and the interstitial matrix (the connective tissue stroma that fills the space between cells in all organs).

Collagens

Collagens are the most abundant structural proteins in the body, comprising about 30% of total body protein. At least 28 types have been identified. **Type I collagen** is the dominant collagen of skin, bone, tendon, and mature scar tissue and provides tensile strength. **Type III collagen** is prominent in early granulation tissue and is progressively replaced by type I during scar maturation; this transition from type III to type I is the histological hallmark of scar remodelling. **Type IV collagen** is the structural backbone of all basement membranes. Defects in type IV collagen underlie Alport syndrome (hereditary nephritis with hearing loss; see Chapter 22). Other important collagens include type II (cartilage), type VII (anchoring fibrils at the dermal-epidermal junction; defective in dystrophic epidermolysis bullosa), and type XVII (hemidesmosomes).

Adhesive Glycoproteins

Fibronectin is the principal adhesive glycoprotein of the ECM. It exists in two forms: plasma fibronectin (circulating, incorporated into the provisional matrix of wounds) and cellular fibronectin (produced by fibroblasts and deposited in the interstitial matrix). Fibronectin contains RGD (Arg-Gly-Asp) sequences that bind integrins on cell surfaces, mediating cell adhesion and migration. **Laminin** is the most abundant glycoprotein of basement membranes and is critical for cell adhesion, differentiation, and migration on the basement membrane scaffold.

Proteoglycans and Hyaluronan

Proteoglycans consist of a core protein linked to glycosaminoglycans (GAGs) such as heparan sulphate, chondroitin sulphate, and keratan sulphate. They form a hydrated gel that resists compressive forces (important in cartilage) and serves as a reservoir for growth factors. Heparan sulphate proteoglycans on cell surfaces (syndecans) and in the basement membrane (perlecan) bind and present FGF and VEGF to their receptors, modulating angiogenic and mitogenic signalling. **Hyaluronan (hyaluronic acid)** is a non-sulphated GAG that does not bind a core protein. It creates a hydrated, viscous matrix that facilitates cell migration in early wounds and embryonic development. Notably, fetal wounds heal without scarring in part because of the hyaluronan-rich ECM environment.

Integrins and Cell-Matrix Interactions

Integrins are transmembrane heterodimeric receptors (composed of α and β subunits) that mediate cell-ECM and cell-cell adhesion. They transduce signals bidirectionally: outside-in signalling from the ECM regulates cell survival, proliferation, and differentiation; inside-out signalling from the cell modifies integrin affinity for ECM ligands. In wound healing, integrins on migrating keratinocytes, fibroblasts, and endothelial cells bind fibronectin, fibrinogen, and collagen in the provisional matrix, enabling the coordinated cell migration that rebuilds tissue architecture.

> **Quick Recall: Extracellular Matrix**
>
> **Type I collagen:** mature scar, bone, tendon; provides tensile strength.
> **Type III collagen:** early granulation tissue; replaced by type I during remodelling.
> **Type IV collagen:** all basement membranes; defective in Alport syndrome.
> **Fibronectin:** principal ECM adhesive glycoprotein; RGD motif binds integrins.
> **Laminin:** major basement membrane glycoprotein.
> **Integrins:** αβ heterodimers; mediate cell-ECM adhesion and bidirectional signalling.

Angiogenesis

Angiogenesis, the formation of new blood vessels from pre-existing vessels, is one of the most frequently examined topics in tissue repair. It is essential for delivering oxygen and nutrients to healing tissue, and its dysregulation underlies conditions ranging from diabetic retinopathy to tumour growth. The process is distinct from vasculogenesis, which is the de novo formation of blood vessels from endothelial precursor cells (angioblasts) during embryonic development.

Steps of Angiogenesis

Angiogenesis proceeds through a stereotyped sequence of events. First, nitric oxide (NO) and VEGF increase vascular permeability and cause vasodilation in the existing vessel. Second, proteolytic degradation of the basement membrane by matrix metalloproteinases (MMPs), particularly MMP-2 and

MMP-9, creates space for endothelial cell migration. Third, endothelial cells proliferate and migrate toward the angiogenic stimulus, guided by a chemotactic gradient of VEGF. Fourth, a solid sprout of endothelial cells extends into the extracellular matrix, with a specialised tip cell at the leading edge and proliferating stalk cells behind it. Fifth, the sprout acquires a lumen (canalisation) and forms a capillary tube. Sixth, pericytes and smooth muscle cells are recruited to stabilise the new vessel and regulate blood flow. Finally, the immature vessel matures and remodels, with some branches regressing and others enlarging to meet functional demand.

VEGF/hypoxia → vasodilation + ↑ permeability → MMP-mediated basement membrane degradation → endothelial migration (tip cell) → sprouting and proliferation (stalk cells) → lumen formation → pericyte recruitment (PDGF-B/Ang1) → vessel maturation

Molecular Regulators of Angiogenesis

The balance between pro-angiogenic and anti-angiogenic factors determines whether new vessel formation proceeds or is suppressed.

Table 3.3: Regulators of angiogenesis

Pro-angiogenic Factors	Anti-angiogenic Factors
VEGF (VEGF-A most important; binds VEGFR-2/Flk-1)	Thrombospondin-1 (TSP-1; induced by p53)
FGF-2 (bFGF; potent mitogen for endothelial cells)	Angiostatin (plasminogen fragment)
Angiopoietin 1 (Ang1; stabilises vessels via Tie2 receptor)	Endostatin (collagen XVIII fragment)
Angiopoietin 2 (Ang2; destabilises vessels, permits sprouting)	Tumstatin (collagen IV fragment)
PDGF-B/PDGFR-β (recruits pericytes)	Vasculostatin
HIF-1α (master transcriptional regulator under hypoxia)	Interferons (α and β)
Notch signalling (Delta-like ligand 4 / DLL4; tip vs stalk cell fate)	VEGF-trap (soluble Flt-1)

VEGF is the single most important driver of angiogenesis. Under hypoxic conditions, the transcription factor HIF-1α (hypoxia-inducible factor 1α) accumulates because the prolyl hydroxylase enzymes that normally target it for proteasomal degradation (via the VHL pathway) are oxygen-dependent and inactive in hypoxia. Stabilised HIF-1α translocates to the nucleus and induces transcription of VEGF, VEGF receptors, and other pro-angiogenic genes.

The Notch-DLL4 pathway determines tip versus stalk cell fate during sprouting. The tip cell at the leading edge of the sprout expresses high levels of DLL4, which activates Notch receptors on adjacent cells, suppressing their tip cell phenotype and converting them into stalk cells. This mechanism prevents excessive, disorganised sprouting and is an active target for anti-angiogenic drug development.

The VHL-HIF-VEGF axis is one of the most clinically significant signalling cascades in angiogenesis. Under normoxic conditions, prolyl hydroxylase domain (PHD) enzymes hydroxylate HIF-1α at specific proline residues, targeting it for ubiquitination by the von Hippel-Lindau (VHL) E3 ligase complex and subsequent proteasomal degradation. Under hypoxic conditions, PHD activity is inhibited, HIF-1α accumulates, translocates to the nucleus, heterodimerises with HIF-1β, and activates transcription of VEGF-A and other target genes including erythropoietin, GLUT1, and glycolytic enzymes. Loss-of-function mutations in VHL (as in clear cell renal cell carcinoma, see Chapter 23) result in constitutive HIF stabilisation and VEGF overproduction, explaining the characteristic hypervascularity of these tumours.

Matrix metalloproteinases (MMPs) play critical roles in all phases of tissue repair. During early wound healing, MMP-1 (collagenase-1) and MMP-9 (gelatinase B) facilitate keratinocyte migration by cleaving type I and type IV collagen respectively at the wound edge. During angiogenesis, MMP-2 and MMP-9 degrade the basement membrane of parent vessels, allowing endothelial cell sprouting. During remodelling, MMP-1, MMP-8, and MMP-13 (collectively the collagenases) cleave native triple-helical collagen, enabling its replacement. MMP activity is tightly regulated by tissue inhibitors of metalloproteinases (TIMPs); imbalance between MMPs and TIMPs underlies pathological fibrosis (excess TIMPs leading to matrix accumulation) and chronic non-healing wounds (excess MMPs causing matrix degradation).

Why is angiogenesis essential in wound healing but detrimental in tumours? In wound healing, angiogenesis provides oxygen and nutrients to the provisional matrix and is self-limited by the restoration of tissue oxygenation. In tumours, persistent angiogenesis (driven by constitutive VEGF production and loss of anti-angiogenic factors such as TSP-1) enables tumour growth beyond the 1–2 mm diffusion limit and facilitates haematogenous metastasis (see Chapter 6).

Quick Recall: Angiogenesis

Master angiogenic factor: VEGF-A (induced by HIF-1α under hypoxia, binds VEGFR-2).

Tip vs stalk cell fate: Notch-DLL4 pathway (DLL4 on tip cell activates Notch on neighbours → stalk cell fate).

Pericyte recruitment: PDGF-B (secreted by endothelium) and Ang1/Tie2 signalling.

Key anti-angiogenic factor: Thrombospondin-1 (TSP-1); its production is induced by wild-type p53.

Clinical application: Bevacizumab (anti-VEGF antibody); ranibizumab (for macular degeneration).

Repair by Connective Tissue: Scarring and Fibrosis

When injury is severe, when the tissue framework is destroyed, or when the damaged cells are permanent, repair proceeds by deposition of connective tissue (scar) rather than regeneration. This process involves four overlapping phases: inflammation (to remove dead tissue and debris), proliferation (formation of granulation tissue), remodelling (maturation of scar), and contraction (reduction of wound size by myofibroblasts).

The steps of connective tissue repair follow a stereotyped sequence that mirrors and overlaps with the inflammatory response. The initial event is the formation of a fibrin-fibronectin provisional matrix within the wound, derived from plasma proteins that leak through damaged blood vessels. This provisional matrix serves as a scaffold for cell migration and a reservoir for growth factors. Platelets trapped within this matrix degranulate, releasing PDGF and TGF-β, which recruit inflammatory cells and fibroblasts. Macrophages, which replace neutrophils as the dominant inflammatory cell by 48 to 72 hours, are the pivotal cell in the transition from inflammation to repair. M2 (alternatively activated) macrophages secrete growth factors (VEGF, FGF, PDGF), anti-inflammatory cytokines (IL-10, TGF-β), and matrix metalloproteinases that collectively orchestrate angiogenesis, fibroblast activation, and matrix remodelling.

Fibroblasts migrate into the wound along the fibronectin gradient, proliferate under the influence of PDGF and FGF, and begin synthesising new ECM. Initially, they deposit type III collagen (the collagen of granulation tissue), which is subsequently replaced by the stronger type I collagen during the remodelling phase. Under the influence of TGF-β, a subset of fibroblasts differentiates into myofibroblasts expressing alpha-smooth muscle actin, which generate the contractile force responsible for wound contraction and are the key effector cells in fibrosis. The entire sequence from provisional matrix through granulation tissue to mature scar represents a continuous process in which each phase overlaps with and modulates the next.

Granulation Tissue

Granulation tissue is the hallmark of active healing. It appears grossly as a pink, soft, granular tissue (the name derives from the tiny granule-like projections on the wound surface, each representing a loop of new capillaries). Microscopically, granulation tissue consists of three components: (1) newly formed, thin-walled capillaries (angiogenesis), (2) proliferating fibroblasts and myofibroblasts, and (3) loose extracellular matrix rich in hyaluronan, fibronectin, and type III collagen, with a variable inflammatory infiltrate of macrophages and occasional neutrophils.

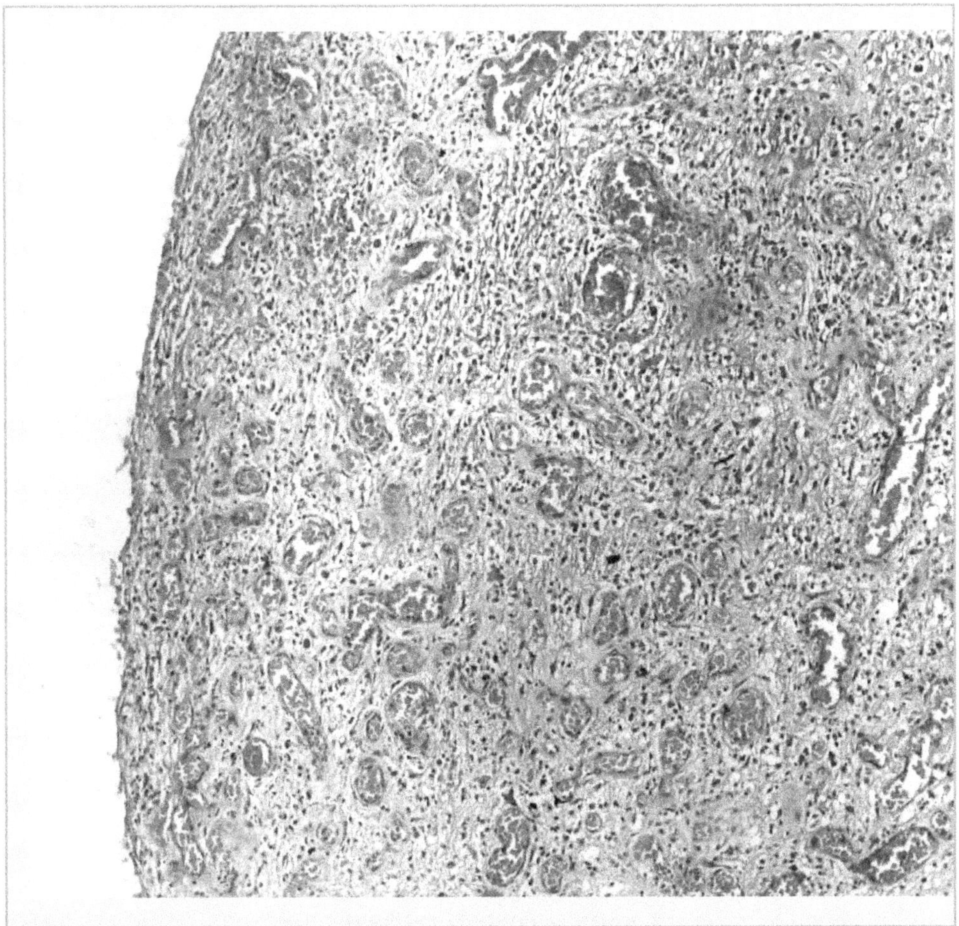

Figure 3.2: Granulation tissue showing proliferating capillaries, plump fibroblasts, and loose oedematous stroma with scattered inflammatory cells. H&E, 200×. (Source: Patho, Wikimedia Commons, CC BY-SA 4.0.)

The distinction from [differential] rests on three features: granulation tissue must be distinguished from granulomatous inflammation. Granulation tissue is a repair process characterised by capillary proliferation and fibroblasts; granulomatous inflammation is a pattern of chronic inflammation characterised by epithelioid macrophages and giant cells. The two are unrelated despite the confusingly similar names.

Myofibroblasts and Wound Contraction

Myofibroblasts are modified fibroblasts that express alpha-smooth muscle actin (α-SMA) and generate contractile force. They are recruited by TGF-β and PDGF and are responsible for wound contraction, the process by which the edges of an open wound are drawn together, reducing the surface area that must be covered by new epithelium. Wound contraction is beneficial in open wounds (reducing scar size) but pathological when excessive, producing contractures across joints or in hollow organs. Myofibroblasts also play a central role in organ fibrosis: they are the principal collagen-producing cells in hepatic cirrhosis (activated stellate cells are myofibroblasts; see Chapter 20), pulmonary fibrosis, and renal fibrosis.

The Pathologist's Eye

On biopsy, granulation tissue can be mistaken for a vascular neoplasm by the unwary. The key features that identify granulation tissue are: (1) lobular arrangement of small capillaries with plump endothelial cells, (2) accompanying fibroblasts and inflammatory cells in a loose, oedematous stroma, (3) mitotic figures in fibroblasts and endothelial cells (reactive, not atypical), and (4) clinical context of a healing wound or ulcer base. The absence of cytological atypia and the presence of a maturation gradient (more mature tissue at the base, more vascular tissue at the surface) distinguish granulation tissue from angiosarcoma or Kaposi sarcoma.

Wound Healing

Cutaneous wound healing is the classic model for understanding tissue repair. Two patterns are described based on the nature of the wound and the method of closure.

Healing by Primary Intention (First Intention)

This occurs in clean, uninfected surgical incisions that are closed by sutures, staples, or adhesive strips. The wound edges are closely approximated, and the gap to be filled is minimal. The sequence of events is as follows. Within 24 hours, neutrophils appear at the wound margins and a thin fibrin clot fills the narrow incisional space. Within 24 to 48 hours, epithelial cells from both wound edges begin to migrate along the cut dermal surfaces, meeting in the midline to form a thin, continuous epithelial layer. By day 3, neutrophils are largely replaced by macrophages, granulation tissue begins to invade the incision space, and collagen fibres appear. By the end of the first week, the wound is bridged by granulation tissue, collagen deposition is well established, and the epidermis has regained its normal thickness. During the second week, collagen accumulation continues, fibroblast proliferation diminishes, and the wound blanches as blood vessels regress. By the end of the first month, the scar consists of a dense connective tissue devoid of inflammatory cells, covered by intact epidermis. Dermal appendages (hair follicles, sweat glands) are permanently lost within the scar.

Healing by Secondary Intention (Second Intention)

This occurs when wounds involve extensive tissue loss, are infected, or are left open deliberately (e.g., abscess cavities, large ulcers). The same fundamental processes operate as in primary intention, but three features differ quantitatively. First, the inflammatory response is more intense and prolonged because of the larger volume of necrotic debris and potential contamination. Second, much greater quantities of granulation tissue are formed to fill the wound defect. Third, wound contraction by myofibroblasts plays a major role in reducing wound size, a phenomenon that is minimal in primary intention. The resulting scar is larger, irregular, and cosmetically inferior compared with healing by primary intention.

Table 3.4: Comparison of healing by primary and secondary intention

Feature	Primary Intention	Secondary Intention

Wound type	Clean incision, edges approximated	Large defect, edges separated
Inflammation	Minimal	Intense and prolonged
Granulation tissue	Small amount	Abundant (fills defect)
Wound contraction	Minimal	Significant (myofibroblast-driven)
Epithelial regeneration	Rapid (thin gap)	Slow (covers large surface) (Figures 3.3–3.4)
Scar	Thin, linear	Large, irregular
Time to heal	Shorter	Longer
Risk of infection	Low	Higher

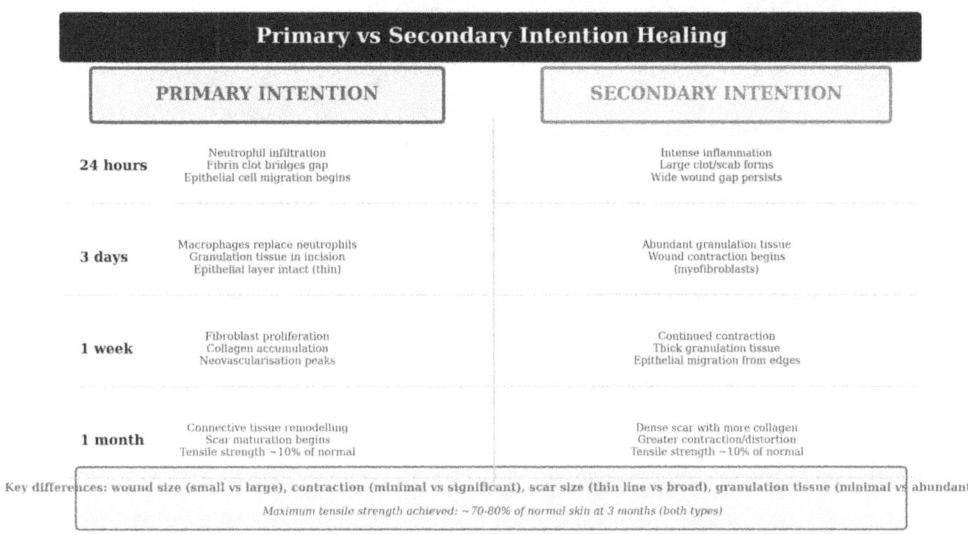

Figure 3.2 : Comparison of primary and secondary intention healing at key time points

Figure 3.3: Comparison of healing by primary and secondary intention. (Source: Author's original.)

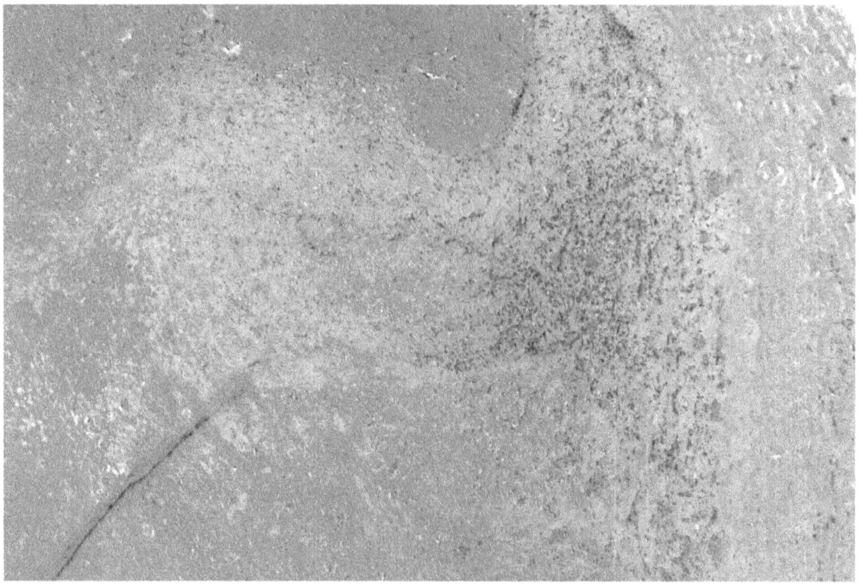

Figure 3.4: Organising deep vein thrombosis. Vessel lumen occluded by fibrin with early fibroblastic ingrowth and recanalisation channels (H&E, low magnification). (Source: Patho, Wikimedia Commons, CC BY-SA 3.0.)

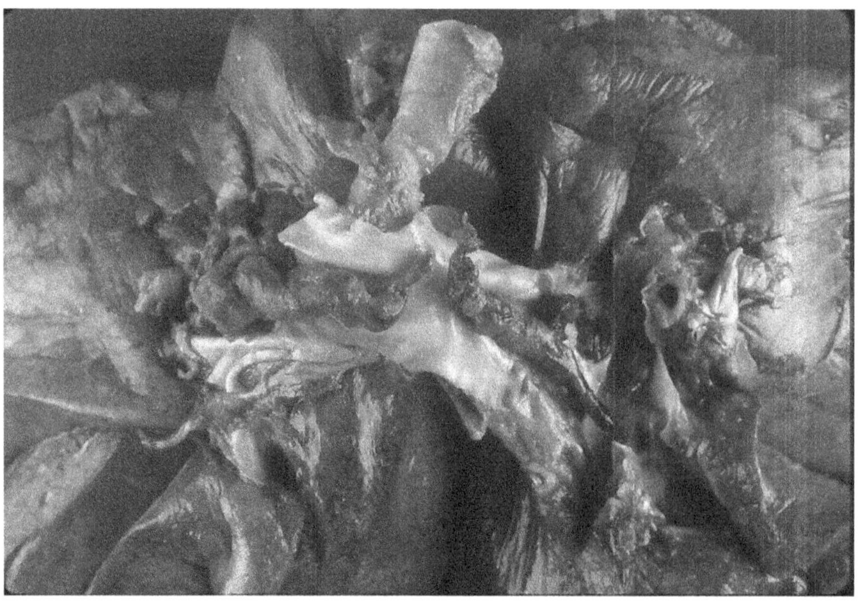

Figure 3.5: Saddle pulmonary embolism (gross). Large thromboembolus straddling the bifurcation of the main pulmonary artery. (Source: Wikimedia Commons, public domain.)

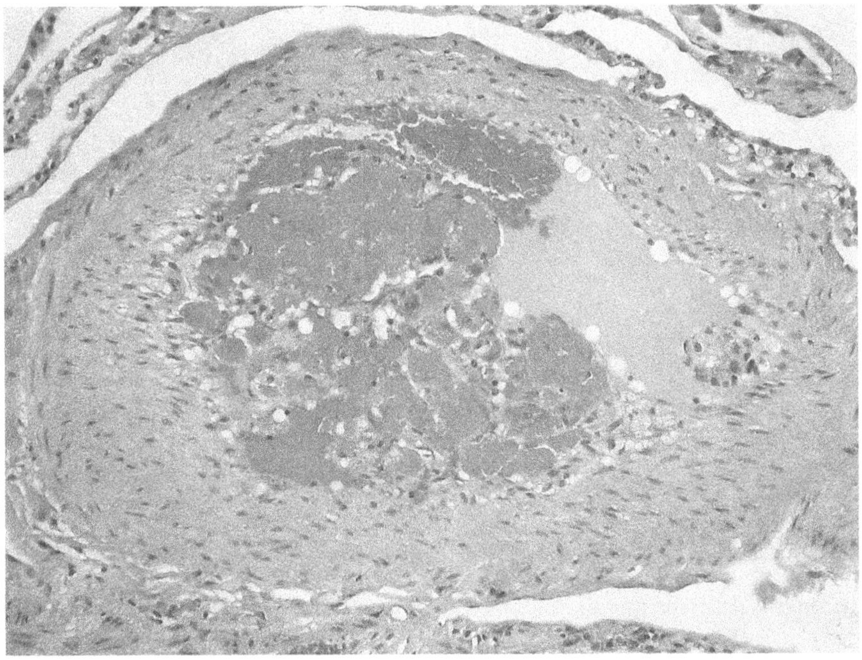

Figure 3.6: Organising pulmonary thromboembolus. Vessel wall with attached thrombus showing fibroblastic organisation and partial recanalisation (H&E). (Source: Yale Rosen, Flickr/Wikimedia Commons, CC BY-SA 2.0.)

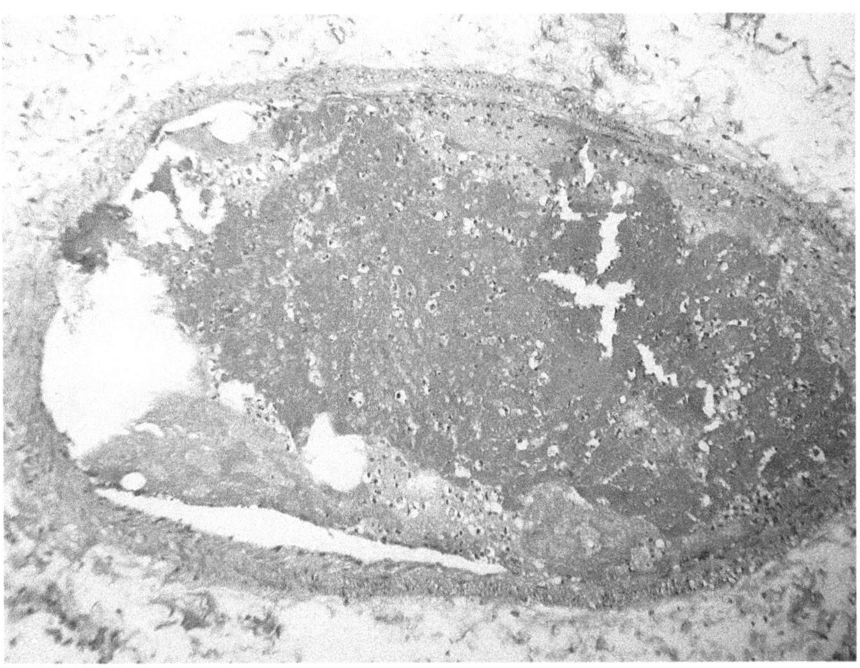

Figure 3.7: Recent pulmonary thromboembolus. Fresh thrombus with layered fibrin, entrapped red blood cells, and early neutrophilic infiltration (H&E). (Source: Yale Rosen, Flickr/Wikimedia Commons, CC BY-SA 2.0.)

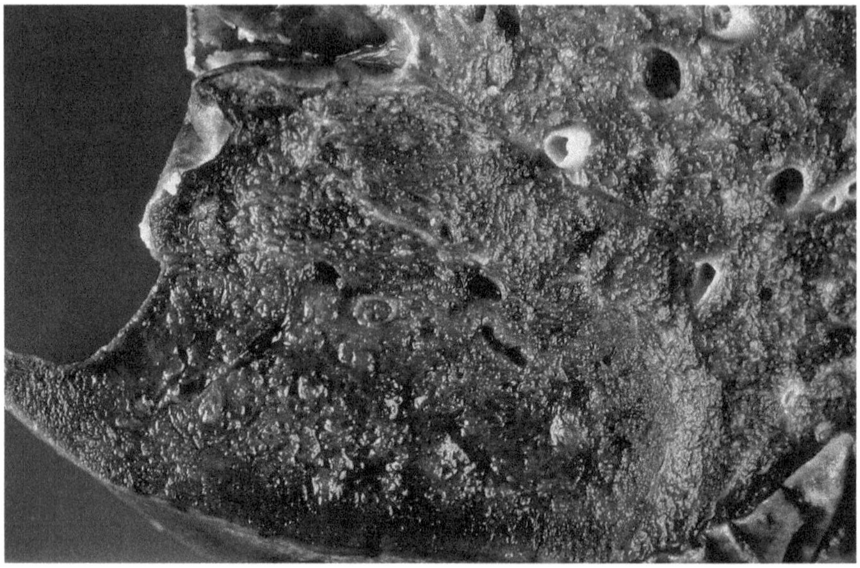

Figure 3.8: Recent haemorrhagic infarct (gross). Wedge-shaped area of dark-red haemorrhagic necrosis in lung parenchyma. (Source: Yale Rosen, Flickr/Wikimedia Commons, CC BY-SA 2.0.)

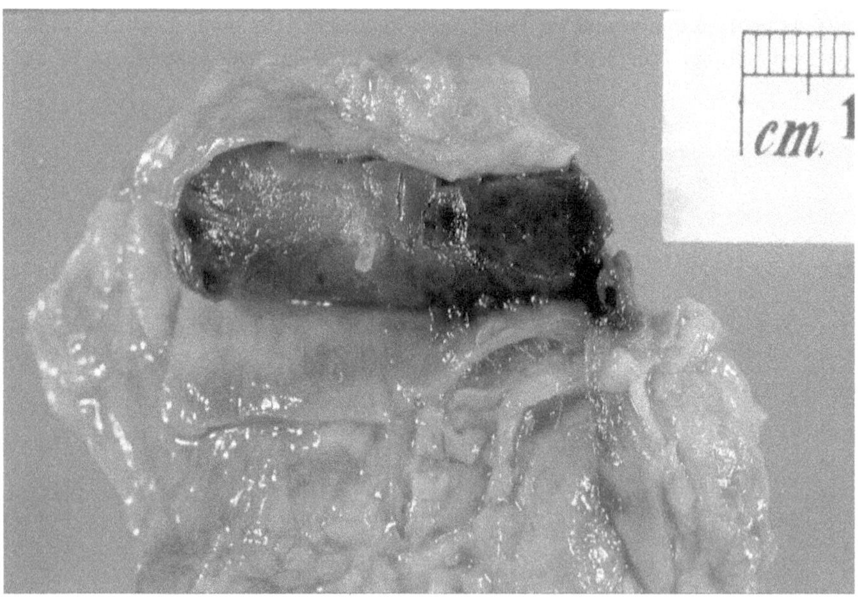

Figure 3.9: Portal vein thrombosis (gross). Opened portal vein showing occlusive dark-red thrombus adherent to the vessel wall. (Source: Wikimedia Commons, public domain.)

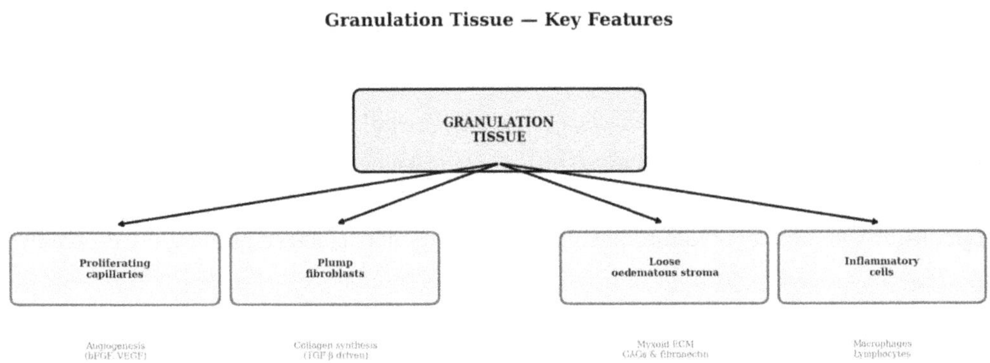

Figure 3.10: Granulation Tissue — Key Features. *(Source: Author's original.)*

Phases of Wound Healing

Regardless of the type of healing, wound repair follows three overlapping phases.

The inflammatory phase (day 0 to day 3) begins with haemostasis. Platelet aggregation and activation of the coagulation cascade form a fibrin clot that serves as both a haemostatic plug and a provisional matrix for cell migration. Platelets release PDGF and TGF-β from their alpha-granules, initiating the repair cascade. Neutrophils are recruited within hours to debride the wound, followed by macrophages (from day 2), which are essential for the transition to the proliferative phase. Macrophages phagocytose debris, secrete growth factors (VEGF, FGF, PDGF, TGF-β), and recruit fibroblasts and endothelial cells.

The proliferative phase (day 3 to day 21) is characterised by three concurrent processes: angiogenesis (new vessel formation to supply the healing tissue), fibroplasia (fibroblast proliferation and collagen deposition), and re-epithelialisation (epithelial cells migrate across the wound surface, restoring the epithelial barrier). Granulation tissue fills the wound bed during this phase.

The remodelling (maturation) phase (week 3 onward, lasting months to years) involves the progressive replacement of type III collagen by type I collagen, cross-linking of collagen fibres, regression of blood vessels, and contraction of the scar. The net result is a scar with increasing tensile strength. A wound regains approximately 70–80% of the tensile strength of unwounded skin by 3 months; it never regains 100%.

Haemostasis (minutes) → Inflammation (hours to days) → Proliferation (days to weeks: angiogenesis + fibroplasia + re-epithelialisation) → Remodelling (weeks to months: collagen III → I, cross-linking, ↑ tensile strength)

Quick Recall: Wound Healing Phases

Inflammatory phase (0–3 days): Haemostasis, neutrophils, then macrophages (the critical cell for transition to proliferative phase).

Proliferative phase (3–21 days): Angiogenesis, fibroplasia, re-epithelialisation, granulation tissue.

Remodelling phase (3 weeks onward): Collagen III → I replacement, cross-linking, scar contraction, max 70–80% tensile strength.

Key cell of proliferative phase: Myofibroblast (wound contraction, collagen production; driven by TGF-β).

Factors Influencing Wound Healing

Multiple local and systemic factors influence the quality and speed of wound healing. Recognition of these factors is essential for clinical management and is a commonly tested examination topic.

Table 3.5: Factors affecting wound healing

Local Factors	Systemic Factors
Infection (most important local cause of delayed healing)	Nutrition: protein and vitamin C deficiency impair collagen synthesis; zinc deficiency impairs immune function
Blood supply: ischaemic tissues heal poorly (e.g., lower limb in peripheral vascular disease)	Diabetes mellitus: microangiopathy, neuropathy, impaired neutrophil function
Foreign bodies (sutures, glass, dirt): provoke persistent inflammation	Glucocorticoids: inhibit TGF-β production, reduce collagen synthesis, suppress inflammation
Mechanical factors: early mobilisation, pressure, torsion	Age: elderly heal more slowly (reduced growth factor production)
Size, location, and type of wound	Anaemia and hypoxia
Radiation damage to local tissue	Immunosuppression

Abnormalities of Tissue Repair

The repair process can go awry in two broad directions: deficient repair (inadequate scar formation or insufficient healing) and excessive repair (overproduction of repair components).

Deficient Healing

Wound dehiscence (rupture of a closed wound) occurs most commonly in abdominal surgical wounds and is precipitated by increased abdominal pressure (coughing, vomiting, ileus), wound infection, poor nutrition, or systemic disease. **Ulceration** results when a wound fails to heal because of inadequate blood supply or persistent tissue damage. The classic examples are diabetic foot ulcers (neuropathy and microangiopathy), venous leg ulcers (chronic venous insufficiency), and decubitus ulcers (pressure sores). **Incisional hernia** develops when weak scar tissue in an abdominal wound fails to withstand intra-abdominal pressure.

Excessive Healing

Hypertrophic scars form when excessive collagen is deposited at the wound site but the scar remains confined within the boundaries of the original wound. They tend to develop after burns or in wounds subject to mechanical tension and usually regress partially over time.

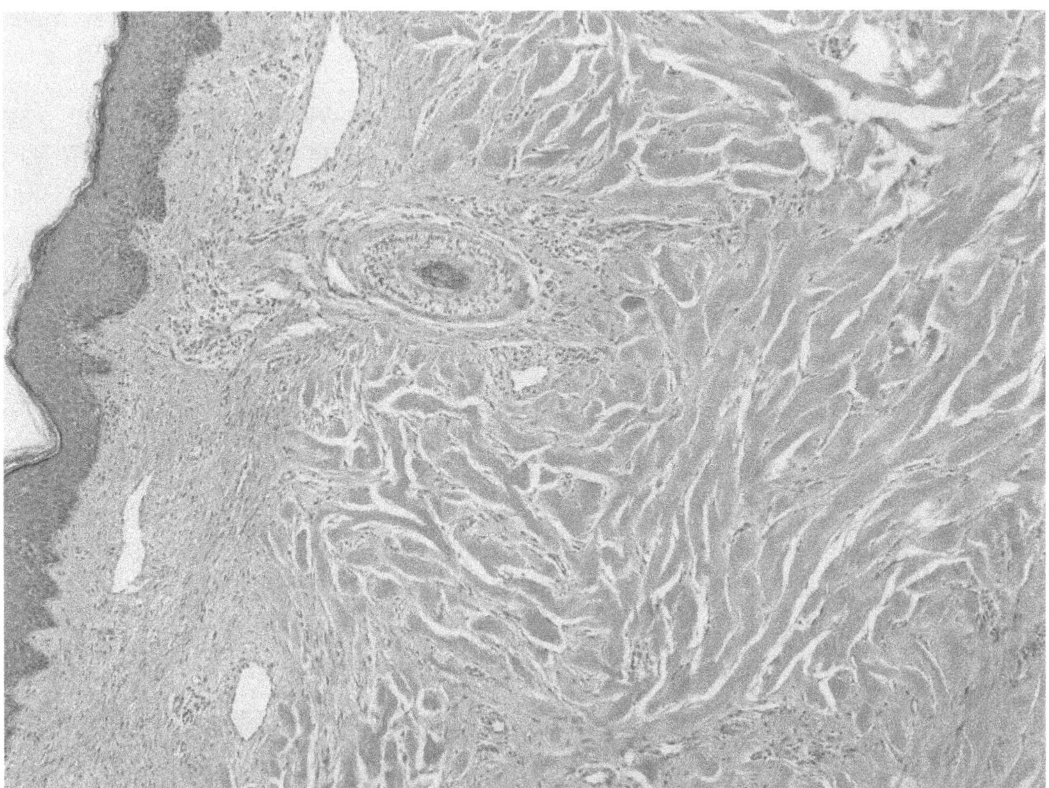

Figure 3.11: Keloid scar. H&E showing thick, hyalinised collagen bundles arranged haphazardly with scattered fibroblasts. *(Source: Mikael Häggström, Wikimedia Commons, CC0.)*

Exuberant granulation tissue ("proud flesh") occurs when granulation tissue grows excessively, protruding above the wound surface and preventing re-epithelialisation. It is managed by cauterisation or surgical excision.

Desmoid tumours (aggressive fibromatosis) represent a neoplastic extreme of excessive fibroblastic proliferation. They arise from fascial or musculoaponeurotic structures, often at sites of previous surgery, and may be associated with familial adenomatous polyposis (Gardner syndrome). Despite being classified as benign (they do not metastasise), they are locally aggressive and difficult to eradicate. Most harbour activating mutations in CTNNB1 (beta-catenin).

Contractures develop when wound contraction is excessive, particularly across joint surfaces, in burn wounds, or in the palms (Dupuytren contracture).

Chronic non-healing wounds represent a major clinical burden, particularly where diabetic foot ulcers, pressure sores, and post-operative wound complications are common. The pathophysiology involves persistent inflammation with elevated MMP levels (especially MMP-2, MMP-8, MMP-9) that degrade newly formed ECM faster than it can be deposited; a biofilm of bacteria that maintains the inflammatory state; reduced growth factor activity (proteolytic degradation of PDGF, VEGF, and EGF by excess MMPs); and impaired keratinocyte migration at the wound edge. Negative pressure wound therapy (NPWT), growth factor application (becaplermin, a recombinant PDGF), and bioengineered skin substitutes represent current therapeutic approaches, though their availability in resource-limited settings remains variable.

When faced with a biopsy from a chronic wound edge, the pathologist should evaluate for: adequacy of granulation tissue (should have vertically oriented capillaries and plump fibroblasts), evidence of re-epithelialisation at the margins, presence of biofilm or invasive infection, foreign body granulomas, and, critically, the presence of malignant transformation (Marjolin ulcer: squamous cell carcinoma arising in chronic wounds, burns, or sinuses, typically well-differentiated but with a high rate of regional metastasis).

Clinical Pearl

Marjolin ulcer: never miss a malignant transformation in a chronic wound. Squamous cell carcinoma arising in a chronic burn scar, sinus tract, or non-healing leg ulcer is the classical Marjolin lesion, named after the French surgeon who described it in 1828. The interval from injury to malignancy is typically decades. Histological clues: dyskeratosis at the wound edge, downward bulbous epithelial proliferation, individual cell keratinisation, and stromal desmoplastic response. Any chronic ulcer biopsied for 'non-healing' deserves multiple deep biopsies from the edge, not the centre, and explicit evaluation for malignant transformation.

Table 3.6: Hypertrophic scar vs keloid

Feature	Hypertrophic Scar	Keloid
Extent	Stays within wound margins	Extends beyond wound margins
Regression	Often regresses with time	Does not regress; tends to recur

Collagen pattern	Parallel, organised fibres	Thick, hyalinised, haphazard ("keloidal collagen")
Genetic predisposition	Less prominent	Strong; more common in African and South Asian descent
Response to excision	Low recurrence	High recurrence
Mechanism	Excess collagen deposition at wound	Excessive TGF-β, altered myofibroblast apoptosis

Exam Pitfall

Do not confuse a keloid with a hypertrophic scar. The single most reliable distinguishing feature is extension beyond the wound margins: keloids grow into surrounding normal tissue, while hypertrophic scars remain within the original wound boundary. Examiners frequently test this distinction.

Clinical Pearl

Keloid versus hypertrophic scar is a distinction examiners enjoy. The single reliable feature is extension beyond the original wound margins: keloids invade adjacent normal skin; hypertrophic scars stay within the wound boundary. Histologically, keloids show thick, glassy, eosinophilic 'keloidal' collagen bundles oriented haphazardly; hypertrophic scars show normal-calibre collagen oriented parallel to the skin surface. Keloids recur after simple excision in 50-100% of cases; hypertrophic scars typically do not. The pre-sternal area, deltoid, earlobes, and darker skin types are the high-risk anatomical and demographic substrates.

Quick Recall: Abnormalities of Tissue Repair

Keloid: extends beyond wound, does not regress, high recurrence, keloidal collagen, genetic predisposition.

Hypertrophic scar: stays within wound, may regress, parallel collagen.

Wound dehiscence: rupture of closed wound; abdominal pressure, infection, malnutrition.

Contracture: excessive myofibroblast contraction; burn scars, Dupuytren.

Proud flesh: exuberant granulation tissue protruding above wound surface.

Fracture Healing

> **Quick Recall: Pathological Aspects of Wound Healing**
>
> Deficient healing: dehiscence (abdominal wounds, increased IAP, infection), ulceration (chronic wounds, impaired blood supply), non-healing wounds (diabetes, excess MMPs degrading ECM).
>
> Excessive healing: hypertrophic scar (within wound, may regress, parallel collagen), keloid (extends beyond wound, does not regress, keloidal collagen, genetic predisposition), exuberant granulation tissue (proud flesh), desmoid tumour (aggressive fibromatosis, beta-catenin mutation).
>
> Contractures: excessive myofibroblast contraction, especially burn scars and across joints. Dupuytren contracture: palmar fascia.
>
> Marjolin ulcer: SCC arising in chronic wound/burn scar; well-differentiated but high metastatic rate.

Fracture healing is a specialised form of tissue repair in which bone regenerates rather than forming a fibrous scar. It proceeds through three overlapping stages.

The inflammatory phase begins immediately after fracture. A haematoma forms at the fracture site from ruptured periosteal and intramedullary vessels. Inflammatory cells (neutrophils, then macrophages) infiltrate the haematoma, removing debris and releasing cytokines (IL-1, IL-6, TNF) and growth factors (PDGF, TGF-β, BMPs) that recruit mesenchymal stem cells from the periosteum, endosteum, and bone marrow.

The reparative phase involves the formation of a soft callus composed of cartilage and fibrous tissue (by mesenchymal cells undergoing chondrogenesis), followed by its replacement with a hard (bony) callus through endochondral ossification. Osteoblasts at the periphery of the callus deposit woven bone directly (intramembranous ossification), bridging the fracture gap.

The remodelling phase involves the gradual replacement of woven bone by lamellar bone and resorption of excess callus by osteoclasts, ultimately restoring the normal cortical and medullary architecture. Bone morphogenetic proteins (BMPs), particularly BMP-2 and BMP-7, are critical regulators of osteoblast differentiation and are used therapeutically in recalcitrant non-union fractures.

Fracture haematoma → Inflammatory phase (cytokines, BMPs) → Soft callus (cartilage) → Hard callus (woven bone via endochondral ossification) → Remodelling (lamellar bone)

Complications of fracture healing include delayed union (healing takes longer than expected), non-union (healing fails to occur, often due to interposition of soft tissue, infection, or inadequate immobilisation), malunion (healing in a malaligned position), and avascular necrosis (ischaemic death of bone, particularly in the femoral head and scaphoid where blood supply is tenuous).

Integration: *Fracture healing connects to bone morphogenetic proteins and osteoblast biology (see Chapter 29) and to metabolic bone diseases that impair healing (osteoporosis, hyperparathyroidism, vitamin D deficiency; see Chapter 27).*

Fibrosis in Parenchymal Organs

Integration: Pathological wound healing connects to diabetic microangiopathy (Chapter 27), keloid genetics and dermatopathology (Chapter 28), Marjolin ulcer and SCC biology (Chapter 28), and the role of TGF-β in organ fibrosis (see below and Chapters 15, 20, 22 for pulmonary, hepatic, and renal fibrosis respectively). Wound healing principles are directly tested as both LAQ and SAQ questions (S-2025 LAQ on connective tissue repair steps; W-2025 SAQ on pathological aspects of repair).

Fibrosis is the pathological accumulation of extracellular matrix, primarily collagen, in a parenchymal organ. It results from the same repair mechanisms that operate in wound healing, but the stimulus is chronic and repetitive rather than self-limited. Fibrosis is the final common pathway of chronic injury in the liver (cirrhosis), lung (idiopathic pulmonary fibrosis), kidney (chronic kidney disease), and heart (post-infarction scarring). The key mediator is TGF-β, which activates tissue-resident fibroblasts and recruits bone marrow-derived fibrocytes. Myofibroblasts are the effector cells, producing abundant collagen I and III. In the liver, the stellate cell (Ito cell) is the principal myofibroblast precursor (see Chapter 20).

Unlike wound healing, organ fibrosis is generally irreversible once advanced, although recent evidence suggests that early fibrosis in the liver may regress if the inciting stimulus is removed (e.g., successful antiviral therapy for hepatitis B or C). This has shifted the clinical paradigm toward early intervention to prevent irreversible fibrosis.

Recent Advances

Mechanotransduction and fibrosis. Research has established that mechanical forces within the ECM activate fibroblasts through integrin-mediated signalling and the YAP/TAZ pathway, a key mechanosensitive transcriptional programme. Stiff ECM activates YAP/TAZ, which promotes fibroblast proliferation and collagen production, creating a positive feedback loop that perpetuates fibrosis. Targeting YAP/TAZ signalling is being explored as a therapeutic strategy in pulmonary and hepatic fibrosis.

Single-cell transcriptomics of wound healing. Single-cell RNA sequencing (scRNA-seq) studies have revealed that wound macrophages exist in multiple transcriptionally distinct states, with specific subpopulations driving fibrosis (pro-fibrotic macrophages expressing TREM2 and SPP1) and others promoting resolution (restorative macrophages expressing MerTK and CD163). This heterogeneity explains why bulk analysis of macrophage markers has yielded contradictory results in wound healing studies and opens the door to subpopulation-targeted therapies.

Scarless healing and fetal wound repair. Fetal wounds heal without scarring, a property attributed to a hyaluronan-rich ECM, a reduced inflammatory response, and a distinct fibroblast transcriptional programme (Engrailed-1-negative fibroblasts). Efforts to recapitulate fetal-type healing in adults include the topical application of hyaluronan-based scaffolds and the selective inhibition of TGF-β signalling. Clinical trials of anti-TGF-β therapies (e.g., pirfenidone, nintedanib) in idiopathic pulmonary fibrosis have demonstrated reduced fibrosis progression, though neither agent reverses established fibrosis.

Ultra High-Yield Chapter Summary

Topic	Must Remember
Labile cells	Continuously dividing; epidermis, GI epithelium, bone marrow; regenerate readily
Stable cells	G0 (quiescent); hepatocytes, renal tubular cells; re-enter cycle on stimulation
Permanent cells	Cannot divide; cardiac myocytes, skeletal muscle, neurons; heal by scarring
VEGF	Master angiogenic factor; induced by HIF-1α under hypoxia; binds VEGFR-2 (Flk-1)
TGF-β	Master regulator of fibrosis; drives fibroblast → myofibroblast transition; stimulates collagen synthesis
PDGF	First growth factor at wound (platelet α-granules); fibroblast chemotaxis and proliferation
HGF / c-MET	Hepatocyte regeneration; acts via c-MET receptor
Type I collagen	Mature scar, bone, tendon; provides tensile strength
Type III collagen	Early granulation tissue; replaced by type I during remodelling
Type IV collagen	All basement membranes; defective in Alport syndrome
Fibronectin	Principal ECM adhesive glycoprotein; RGD motif binds integrins
Integrins	αβ heterodimers; cell-ECM adhesion; bidirectional signalling
Granulation tissue	Capillaries + fibroblasts + loose ECM; hallmark of active healing; not granulomatous inflammation
Myofibroblast	α-SMA positive; wound contraction; driven by TGF-β; key effector in organ fibrosis
Primary intention	Clean incision, edges approximated, minimal scar; sutures

Secondary intention	Large defect, abundant granulation tissue, significant wound contraction, larger scar
Wound tensile strength	Max 70–80% of normal; never 100%; achieved by 3 months
Keloid vs hypertrophic scar	Keloid extends beyond wound, does not regress; hypertrophic stays within wound, may regress
Fracture healing	Haematoma → soft callus (cartilage) → hard callus (woven bone) → remodelling (lamellar bone)
Thrombospondin-1	Key anti-angiogenic factor; induced by p53; lost in cancer → angiogenic switch
Notch-DLL4	Tip cell (DLL4+) vs stalk cell fate; prevents excessive sprouting
Scarless fetal healing	Hyaluronan-rich ECM, reduced inflammation, Engrailed-1-negative fibroblasts

Diagnostic thinking: excessive collagen + myofibroblasts + contracted scar → keloid/hypertrophic scar (abnormal wound healing)

Diagnostic thinking: foreign body + giant cells + fibrosis → foreign body reaction (check polarised light for birefringent material) (Figure 2.11)

Chapter 4: Haemodynamic Disorders, Thromboembolism, and Shock

THE BIG PICTURE

Haemodynamic disorders reveal how narrow the margin is between normal circulation and catastrophic failure. The same clotting cascade that seals a cut finger can, when dysregulated, occlude a coronary artery or fill the pulmonary trunk with thrombus. Oedema, congestion, thrombosis, embolism, infarction, and shock are not separate diseases but consequences of a small set of failures: Starling forces overwhelmed, endothelium injured, flow made stagnant, blood made hypercoagulable, perfusion lost. The pathologist recognises each stage by its morphology — nutmeg liver of chronic venous congestion, lines of Zahn in an arterial thrombus, saddle embolus at the pulmonary bifurcation, pale wedge of a renal infarct. Reading these patterns correctly tells you not just what happened but what will happen next, because haemodynamic failure drives the clinical trajectory in myocardial infarction, stroke, sepsis, and major trauma alike.

High-yield topics in this chapter: pathogenesis of thrombosis (Virchow's triad); fate of thrombus; pulmonary embolism; types and pathogenesis of shock (especially septic shock with MODS); DIC; pathogenesis of oedema; types of infarction; amniotic fluid embolism; role of endothelium in haemostasis.

Diagnostic thinking: sudden dyspnoea + pleuritic pain + tachycardia + recent immobility → PE

Normal haemostasis maintains blood in a fluid state within intact vessels while enabling rapid clot formation at sites of vascular injury. This balance depends on endothelial anti-thrombotic mechanisms, circulating coagulation factors, platelets, and the fibrinolytic system. Disruption of this balance produces thrombosis and embolism (excessive clotting) or haemorrhage and shock (inadequate clotting). This chapter covers the pathogenesis of oedema, congestion, haemorrhage, thrombosis, embolism, infarction, disseminated intravascular coagulation (DIC), and shock.

Oedema

Oedema is the accumulation of excess interstitial fluid in tissues. When it occurs in body cavities, specific terms are used: hydrothorax (pleural cavity), hydropericardium (pericardial cavity), and hydroperitoneum or ascites (peritoneal cavity). Severe, generalised oedema with diffuse subcutaneous swelling is termed anasarca.

The pathophysiology of oedema is governed by Starling forces: the balance between hydrostatic pressure (which pushes fluid out of capillaries) and oncotic (colloid osmotic) pressure (which retains fluid within capillaries). Oedema results when the net filtration across capillaries exceeds lymphatic drainage.

Table 4.2: Pathophysiological mechanisms and causes of oedema

Mechanism	Pathophysiology	Clinical Examples
↑ Hydrostatic pressure	Increased capillary pressure forces fluid into interstitium	Congestive heart failure, deep vein thrombosis, portal hypertension (ascites), prolonged standing
↓ Oncotic pressure	Reduced plasma albumin decreases osmotic pull	Nephrotic syndrome, liver cirrhosis, protein-losing enteropathy, malnutrition (kwashiorkor)
Lymphatic obstruction	Impaired drainage of interstitial fluid	Filariasis, post-surgical (axillary clearance), malignant infiltration, post-radiation
↑ Vascular permeability	Endothelial injury allows protein-rich fluid leak	Inflammation, burns, anaphylaxis, VEGF-mediated
Sodium and water retention	Renal retention expands plasma volume	Renal failure, excess aldosterone (heart failure, cirrhosis)

Quick Recall: Oedema

Transudate: protein-poor (<3 g/dL), low specific gravity (<1.012); due to hydrostatic or oncotic imbalance.

Exudate: protein-rich (>3 g/dL), high specific gravity (>1.020); due to increased vascular permeability (inflammation).

Most common cause of generalised oedema: congestive heart failure (right-sided or biventricular).

Major cause of lymphoedema (endemic regions): filariasis (Wuchereria bancrofti).

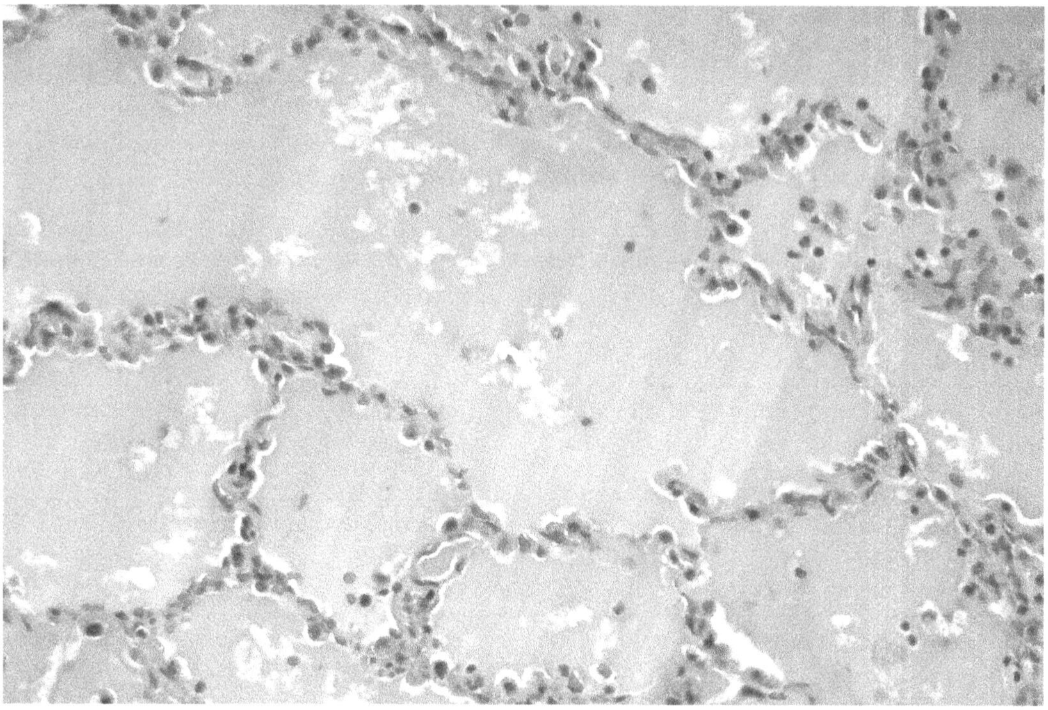

Figure 4.1: Pulmonary oedema. H&E showing alveolar spaces filled with pale eosinophilic transudate and septal congestion. *(Source: Yale Rosen, Wikimedia Commons, CC BY-SA 2.0.)*

Clinical Pearl: Pitting versus non-pitting oedema

A thumb pressed into oedematous tissue either leaves a pit that slowly refills, or it does not — and this simple bedside distinction meaningfully narrows the differential.

Pitting oedema: low-protein transudate that redistributes under pressure and refills over seconds. Causes are the dominant ones: right-sided heart failure, hypoalbuminaemia (nephrotic syndrome, cirrhosis, protein-losing enteropathy, malnutrition), acute and chronic renal failure, and any cause of raised hydrostatic pressure.

Non-pitting oedema: the interstitium is filled with material that does not displace. Two main categories. *Lymphoedema* — high-protein interstitial fluid trapped by lymphatic obstruction; causes include filariasis (Wuchereria bancrofti, endemic in tropical regions), post-mastectomy axillary dissection, and congenital Milroy disease. *Myxoedema* — accumulation of hyaluronic acid and other glycosaminoglycans in hypothyroidism (generalised) and in pretibial myxoedema of Graves disease (localised, paradoxically in a hyperthyroid patient).

Exam cue: proteinuria + pitting oedema → nephrotic syndrome; non-pitting periorbital puffiness + fatigue + bradycardia → hypothyroidism; unilateral non-pitting limb oedema in an endemic region → filariasis.

Hyperaemia and Congestion

Hyperaemia is an active process: arteriolar dilation increases blood inflow to a tissue, producing redness and warmth. It is seen at sites of inflammation and in exercising skeletal muscle. **Congestion** is a passive process: impaired venous outflow leads to the accumulation of deoxygenated blood in a tissue, producing a dusky blue-red (cyanotic) discolouration. Congestion may be localised (e.g., deep vein thrombosis causing limb congestion) or systemic (e.g., right-sided heart failure causing hepatic and splenic congestion).

Chronic hepatic congestion ("nutmeg liver") is the classic morphological consequence of chronic right-sided heart failure. Grossly, the cut surface of the liver shows alternating dark red congested centrilobular zones and tan periportal zones, resembling a cross-section of a nutmeg. Microscopically, there is centrilobular sinusoidal dilation, hepatocyte atrophy, and, in severe cases, centrilobular haemorrhagic necrosis. Longstanding congestion leads to centrilobular fibrosis ("cardiac cirrhosis"), although true cirrhosis with regenerative nodules is uncommon.

Chronic pulmonary congestion results from left-sided heart failure. The alveolar capillaries are engorged, and recurrent microhaemorrhages release erythrocytes into the alveolar spaces. Macrophages phagocytose the red cells and accumulate haemosiderin, becoming **heart failure cells** (haemosiderin-laden macrophages), which are identifiable on Perl's Prussian blue stain. Over time, interstitial fibrosis thickens the alveolar septa, producing the firm, brown lung of chronic passive congestion ("brown induration").

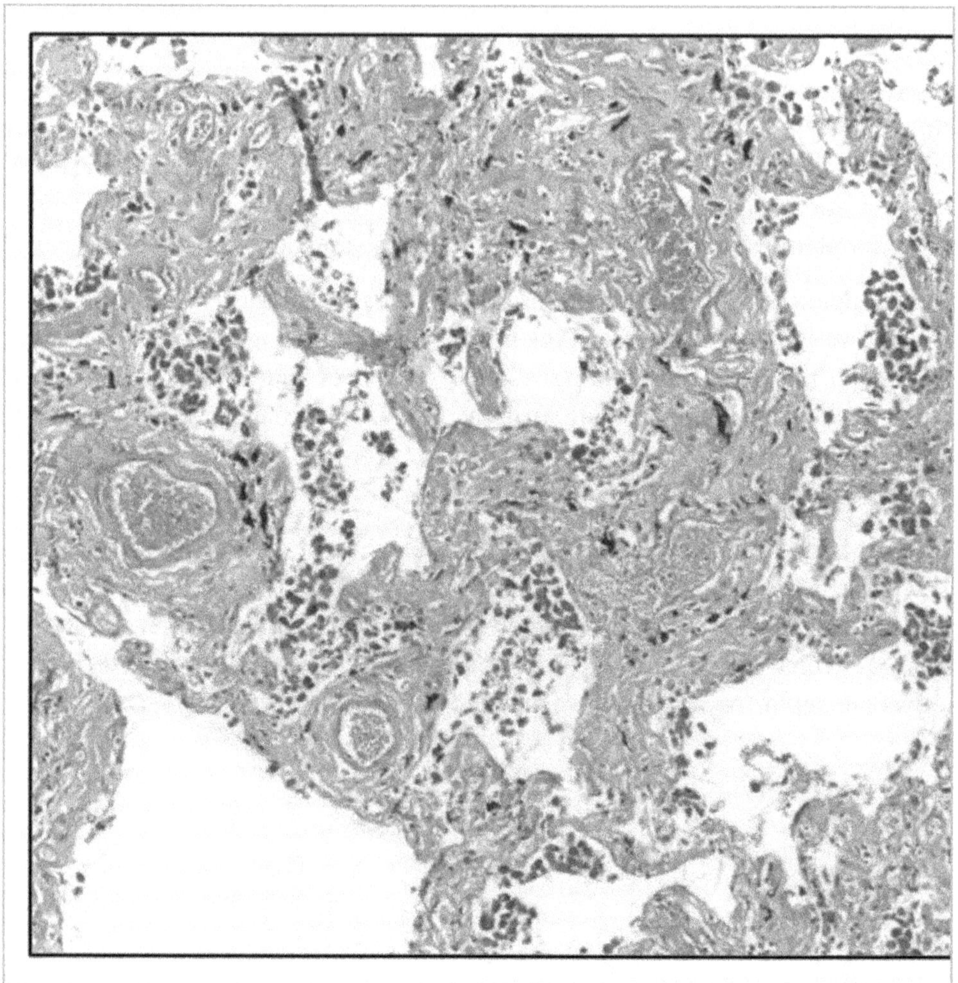

Figure 4.2A: Chronic passive congestion of lung showing thickened alveolar septa, congested capillaries, and haemosiderin-laden macrophages (heart failure cells). H&E, 200×. (Source: Calicut Medical College, Wikimedia Commons, CC BY-SA 4.0.)

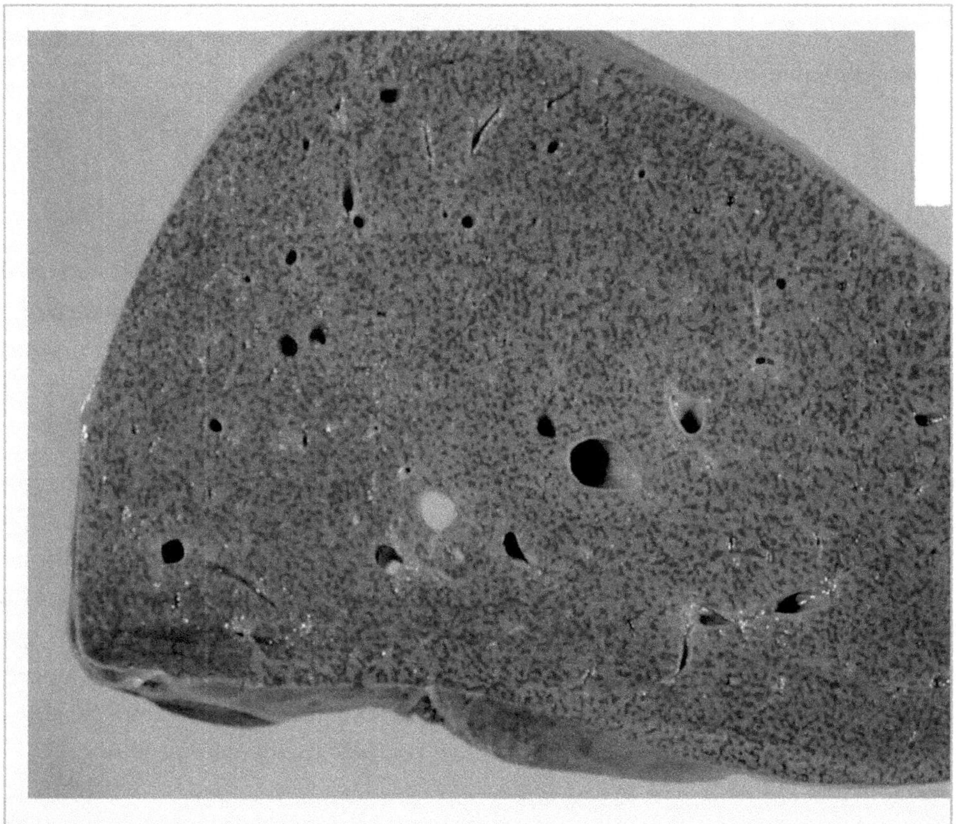

Figure 4.2B: Nutmeg liver: cut surface showing alternating dark red (congested centrilobular) and tan (periportal) zones in chronic right-sided heart failure. Gross photograph, N/A. (Source: Narraburra, Wikimedia Commons, CC0.)

Chronic splenic congestion is the third classic site of chronic passive congestion, and arguably the most common in tropical practice because it accompanies any cause of portal hypertension (cirrhosis, non-cirrhotic portal fibrosis, extrahepatic portal venous obstruction, schistosomiasis) in addition to right-sided heart failure. The spleen is firm, enlarged (typically 500–1000 g against a normal weight of 150 g), and the cut surface is dark red-brown with a thickened, fibrotic capsule and blunted trabeculae. Microscopically, the sinusoids are congested and dilated, the cords of Billroth show progressive reticulin and collagen deposition (the so-called fibrocongestive splenomegaly), and scattered through the red pulp are Gamna-Gandy bodies.

The Pathologist's Eye: Gamna-Gandy bodies

Gamna-Gandy bodies ("tobacco-flecks" of the congested spleen) are a classical viva and SAQ pointer. They are small (1–3 mm) yellow-brown-to-rust-coloured firm nodules formed by organisation of focal parenchymal haemorrhages: fibrous tissue encrusted with haemosiderin and calcium salts, often surrounding residual elastic and collagen fibres from ruptured sinusoidal walls. On H&E they appear as brown-pigmented refractile deposits with a foreign-body giant-cell reaction at the margin; Perl's Prussian blue highlights the iron (blue) and von Kossa the calcium (black). Their presence on a splenectomy specimen is diagnostic of long-standing congestion and strongly suggests portal hypertension until proved otherwise — with non-cirrhotic portal fibrosis (NCPF, endemic in tropical regions and rare in the West) and schistosomiasis prominent on the differential alongside cirrhosis.

Haemorrhage

Haemorrhage is the extravasation of blood from the vascular compartment. It may be external or confined to tissue spaces. Accumulations of blood are designated by location: haematoma (within a tissue), haemothorax (pleural cavity), haemoperitoneum (peritoneal cavity), haemopericardium (pericardial sac, particularly dangerous as even 200–300 mL can cause tamponade), and haemarthrosis (joint space, seen in haemophilia).

Petechiae are minute (1–2 mm) haemorrhages in the skin, mucous membranes, and serosal surfaces, typically due to thrombocytopenia, defective platelet function, or loss of vascular wall support (scurvy, vasculitis). **Purpura** are slightly larger (3–10 mm) haemorrhages, seen in the same conditions as well as in vascular fragility and amyloid infiltration. **Ecchymoses** are larger (>10 mm) subcutaneous haemorrhages (bruises). The characteristic colour change of an ecchymosis (red-blue → blue-green → golden-yellow) reflects the progressive oxidation of haemoglobin to bilirubin and haemosiderin by macrophages. The clinical significance of haemorrhage depends on the volume, rate of blood loss, and the site: rapid loss of 20% of blood volume or slow loss of greater amounts can produce hypovolaemic shock.

Normal Haemostasis

Haemostasis is the process by which blood clots form at sites of vascular injury. It involves a precisely coordinated sequence: (1) arteriolar vasoconstriction (transient, neurogenic and endothelin-mediated), (2) primary haemostasis (platelet adhesion, activation, and aggregation to form a platelet plug), (3) secondary haemostasis (activation of the coagulation cascade to generate thrombin, which converts fibrinogen to fibrin, stabilising the plug), and (4) regulation and termination (antithrombotic mechanisms and fibrinolysis).

Role of Platelets in Haemostasis

Platelets are anucleate cell fragments derived from megakaryocytes in the bone marrow (see Volume 1 for detailed megakaryopoiesis). They circulate for 8-10 days and are normally present at 150,000-400,000/µL. Platelets are the first responders to vascular injury and are essential for primary haemostasis. Their function can be conceptualised in three phases: adhesion, activation/secretion, and aggregation.

Platelet adhesion: When the endothelium is disrupted, subendothelial collagen and von Willebrand factor (vWF) are exposed. Platelets adhere to exposed collagen via glycoprotein Ia/IIa (integrin $\alpha 2\beta 1$) and, critically, via the GPIb-IX-V complex binding to vWF that is itself bound to collagen. The GPIb-vWF interaction is particularly important under conditions of high shear stress (arterial circulation), where the initial tethering of platelets depends on this interaction. Deficiency of GPIb causes Bernard-Soulier syndrome (see Volume 1).

Platelet activation and secretion: Binding to collagen and thrombin triggers platelet activation through intracellular signalling cascades involving phospholipase C, calcium mobilisation, and thromboxane A2 (TXA2) synthesis. Activated platelets undergo a shape change (from discoid to spiny sphere), degranulate their α-granules (releasing fibrinogen, vWF, platelet factor 4, PDGF, P-selectin) and dense granules (releasing ADP, ATP, serotonin, calcium, polyphosphates), and expose phosphatidylserine on their outer membrane (providing a negatively charged surface for assembly of coagulation factor complexes). ADP and TXA2 are potent platelet agonists that recruit additional platelets (the amplification loop). Aspirin irreversibly inhibits cyclooxygenase-1 (COX-1), blocking TXA2 synthesis and providing the basis for antiplatelet therapy. Clopidogrel/prasugrel/ticagrelor block the P2Y12 ADP receptor.

Platelet aggregation: The final step in primary haemostasis is the cross-linking of activated platelets by fibrinogen bridges between GPIIb/IIIa (integrin αIIbβ3) receptors on adjacent platelets, forming the platelet plug. Deficiency of GPIIb/IIIa causes Glanzmann thrombasthenia (see Volume 1). The platelet plug is then stabilised by the fibrin mesh generated by the coagulation cascade (secondary haemostasis).

Vascular injury → Collagen/vWF exposure → Platelet adhesion (GPIb-vWF) → Activation (shape change, degranulation, TXA2) → Aggregation (GPIIb/IIIa-fibrinogen) → Primary platelet plug

Integration: *Platelet biology connects to coagulation cascade and bleeding disorders (Volume 1, Chapters 30-33), DIC (this chapter), thrombotic microangiopathies including TTP and HUS (Volume 1), and antiplatelet therapy in cardiovascular disease (Chapter 13). The dual antiplatelet therapy (aspirin + P2Y12 inhibitor) used after coronary stenting reflects the central role of TXA2 and ADP pathways in platelet activation.*

Role of Endothelium in Haemostasis

The endothelium is the master regulator of haemostasis. Under normal conditions, it maintains an antithrombotic state through multiple mechanisms.

Table 4.3: Antithrombotic and prothrombotic properties of endothelium

Antithrombotic (Normal State)	Prothrombotic (After Injury/Activation)
Prostacyclin (PGI2) and NO: inhibit platelet adhesion and aggregation; cause vasodilation	von Willebrand factor (vWF): mediates platelet adhesion to exposed subendothelium
Heparin-like molecules: activate antithrombin III, which inactivates thrombin and factors Xa, IXa	Tissue factor (TF): activates extrinsic coagulation cascade (factor VII → VIIa)
Thrombomodulin: binds thrombin, activating protein C (which inactivates factors Va and VIIIa)	Plasminogen activator inhibitors (PAI-1): inhibit fibrinolysis

Tissue factor pathway inhibitor (TFPI): inhibits TF-VIIa complex	Downregulation of thrombomodulin expression
Tissue plasminogen activator (tPA): promotes fibrinolysis	Exposure of subendothelial collagen: activates platelets and factor XII
ADPase/CD39: degrades ADP, preventing platelet activation	Release of vWF from Weibel-Palade bodies

The coagulation cascade is covered in detail in Volume 1 (coagulation physiology and bleeding disorders). In brief, the extrinsic pathway is initiated by tissue factor (TF) exposed at sites of endothelial injury, which complexes with factor VIIa. The intrinsic pathway is initiated by contact activation of factor XII. Both converge on factor X, generating the prothrombinase complex (Xa + Va) that converts prothrombin to thrombin. Thrombin cleaves fibrinogen to fibrin monomers, which polymerise and are cross-linked by factor XIIIa to form a stable fibrin mesh. For examination purposes, the cell-based model of coagulation (initiation, amplification, propagation phases occurring on cell surfaces) has largely replaced the classical cascade model, though both are tested (Figures 4.3–4.4).

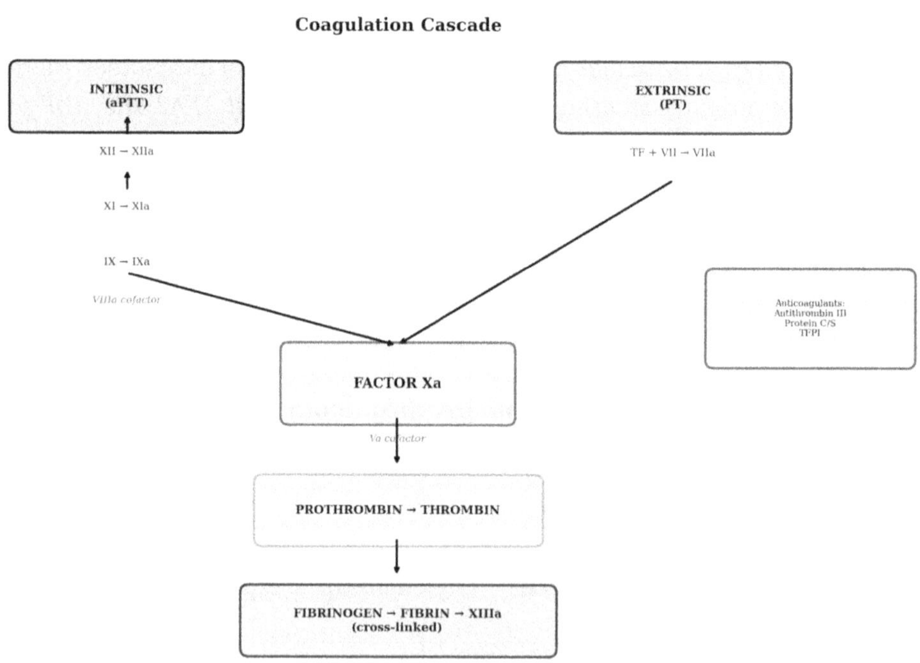

Figure 4.3: Coagulation Cascade. (Source: Author's original.)

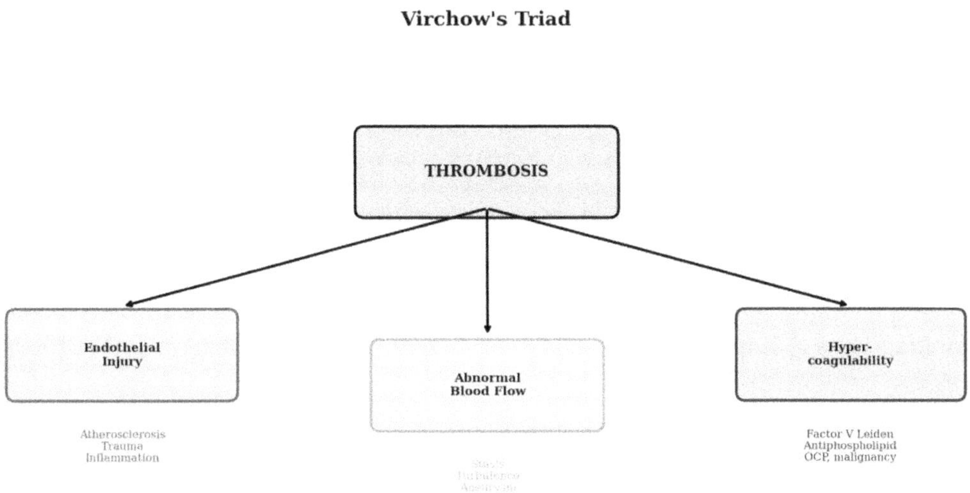

Figure 4.4: Virchow's Triad. *(Source: Author's original.)*

Table 4.4: Virchow's triad

Factor	Mechanism	Clinical Examples
1. Endothelial injury (most important)	Loss of antithrombotic endothelial functions; exposure of subendothelial collagen and tissue factor	Atherosclerosis, vasculitis, endocardial damage (MI, rheumatic fever), indwelling catheters, trauma, turbulent flow over plaques
2. Abnormal blood flow (stasis or turbulence)	Stasis: prevents dilution of activated clotting factors, retards inflow of inhibitors, promotes endothelial activation. Turbulence: causes endothelial injury and creates countercurrents and pockets of stasis	Stasis: atrial fibrillation (left atrial appendage thrombi), immobilisation (DVT), aneurysms. Turbulence: arterial bifurcations, stenotic valves
3. Hypercoagulability	Increased tendency of blood to clot; may be primary (genetic) or secondary (acquired)	Primary: Factor V Leiden, prothrombin G20210A, antithrombin III/protein C/protein S deficiency. Secondary: malignancy, pregnancy, OCP, nephrotic syndrome, HIT, antiphospholipid syndrome, prolonged

		immobilisation

Endothelial injury + Stasis/turbulence + Hypercoagulability → Platelet adhesion and activation → Coagulation cascade → Fibrin deposition → THROMBUS

The key diagnostic clue in distinguishing an ante-mortem thrombus from a post-mortem clot on gross examination is the lines of Zahn: alternating pale (platelet-fibrin) and dark (red cell-rich) laminations seen in thrombi formed in flowing blood. Post-mortem clots are homogeneous, gelatinous, and lack lamination.

Diagnostic thinking: lines of Zahn (alternating pale-dark layers) → antemortem thrombus (not postmortem clot)

Morphology of Thrombi

Arterial thrombi form at sites of endothelial injury or turbulence, typically over atherosclerotic plaques. They are grey-white, friable, and composed predominantly of platelets and fibrin ("white thrombi"). They grow in a retrograde direction (against blood flow). **Venous thrombi (phlebothrombosis)** form in areas of stasis, predominantly in the deep veins of the lower limbs. They are red, soft, and gelatinous, composed predominantly of red cells enmeshed in fibrin ("red thrombi"). They grow in the direction of blood flow (antegrade) and often form long casts of the venous lumen. **Mural thrombi** form on the wall of the heart chambers (typically over areas of myocardial infarction or in dilated, fibrillating atria) or the aorta (over ulcerated atherosclerotic plaques).

Clinical Pearl

Lines of Zahn are the morphological signature of an antemortem thrombus. They are alternating pale layers of platelets and fibrin and dark layers of erythrocytes, formed only when blood is flowing. Post-mortem clots, formed in stagnant blood, lack this lamination and are uniformly dark or have a 'chicken-fat' yellow upper layer with a 'currant-jelly' red lower layer. The medicolegal implication: Lines of Zahn in a pulmonary artery on autopsy confirm pulmonary embolism as a cause of death, while their absence supports a post-mortem clot and excludes thromboembolism. This single histological distinction often determines the cause-of-death certificate in suspected pulmonary embolism.

Fate of Thrombus

A thrombus may undergo one of four outcomes. **Propagation:** the thrombus enlarges by accretion of additional platelets and fibrin. **Embolisation:** the thrombus or a fragment of it dislodges and is carried to a distant site. **Dissolution:** the fibrinolytic system (plasmin) lyses the thrombus, restoring blood flow; this is most effective in the early stages before extensive fibrin cross-linking. **Organisation and recanalisation:** granulation tissue grows into the thrombus, and new channels may form through the organised mass, partially restoring flow. Over time, the organised thrombus is incorporated into the vessel wall.

Thrombus → Propagation / Embolisation / Dissolution (fibrinolysis) / Organisation and recanalisation

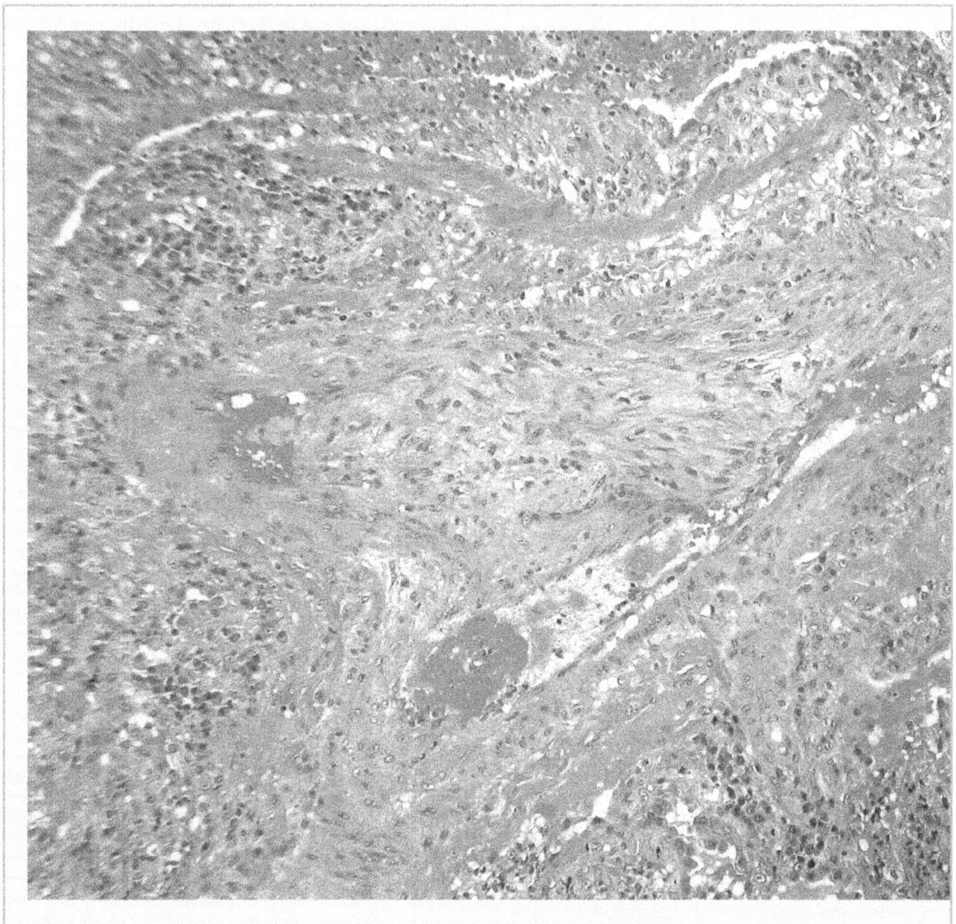

Figure 4.5: Organised thrombus in a vein showing recanalisation channels lined by endothelium, surrounded by fibrous tissue replacing the original thrombus. H&E, 100×. (Source: Yale Rosen, Wikimedia Commons, CC BY-SA 2.0.)

Virchow's Triad: Expanded Molecular Mechanisms

Endothelial injury or dysfunction is the most important element of Virchow's triad and the only element that can independently lead to thrombosis. Normal endothelium maintains an anti-thrombotic surface through multiple mechanisms: production of prostacyclin (PGI2) and nitric oxide (NO), which inhibit platelet adhesion and aggregation; expression of thrombomodulin, which binds thrombin and activates protein C (a natural anticoagulant that inactivates factors Va and VIIIa); expression of heparan sulfate proteoglycans on the cell surface, which potentiate the activity of antithrombin III; expression of tissue factor pathway inhibitor (TFPI); and secretion of tissue plasminogen activator (tPA), which activates fibrinolysis. When the endothelium is damaged or activated (by hypertension, diabetes, cigarette smoke, hyperlipidaemia, bacterial endotoxins, radiation, or cytokines), this anti-thrombotic phenotype shifts to a pro-thrombotic phenotype: tissue factor is expressed on the endothelial surface, thrombomodulin expression is downregulated, von Willebrand factor is released from Weibel-Palade bodies, and plasminogen activator inhibitor-1 (PAI-1) secretion increases, inhibiting fibrinolysis.

Abnormal blood flow encompasses both stasis and turbulence. Stasis disrupts laminar flow, allowing platelets to contact the endothelium (normally, platelets flow in the central axial stream, separated from the vessel wall by a cell-free plasma layer). Stasis also prevents the dilution and clearance of activated coagulation factors by fresh flowing blood and retards the influx of natural anticoagulants (protein C, antithrombin). Turbulence, occurring at arterial bifurcations and aneurysmal dilatations, damages the endothelium and creates pockets of stasis. Clinical scenarios of abnormal flow include atrial fibrillation (stasis in the left atrial appendage, predisposing to mural thrombus and systemic embolism), deep vein thrombosis (stasis in the valve pockets of leg veins during immobilisation), and atherosclerotic plaque-related turbulence (promoting arterial thrombosis superimposed on plaque rupture).

A viva question on thrombosis: 'Why do arterial thrombi form at sites of turbulence while venous thrombi form at sites of stasis?' Arterial thrombi: turbulence at atherosclerotic plaques damages the endothelium and activates platelets under high-shear conditions, producing platelet-rich (white) thrombi that grow retrograde against the direction of flow. Venous thrombi: stasis in valve pockets allows accumulation of activated coagulation factors, producing fibrin-rich (red) thrombi that propagate in the direction of flow. This fundamental difference in pathogenesis explains why arterial thrombosis is treated primarily with antiplatelet agents (aspirin, clopidogrel), while venous thrombosis is treated with anticoagulants (heparin, warfarin, DOACs).

Hypercoagulable States (Thrombophilia)

Hypercoagulability can be primary (inherited) or secondary (acquired). It should be suspected when a patient presents with venous thromboembolism at a young age (under 50), recurrent thrombosis, thrombosis at unusual sites (portal, hepatic, cerebral veins), or a strong family history.

Table 4.3B: Inherited and acquired hypercoagulable states

Category	Condition	Mechanism
Inherited (primary)	Factor V Leiden (most common)	Point mutation (Arg506Gln) renders factor Va resistant to inactivation by activated protein C. Heterozygous in 2–5% of Caucasians; 5-fold increased VTE risk
	Prothrombin gene mutation (G20210A)	Elevated prothrombin levels; 3-fold VTE risk
	Antithrombin III deficiency	Reduced inactivation of thrombin and factor Xa; high VTE risk
	Protein C deficiency	Impaired inactivation of factors Va and VIIIa

	Protein S deficiency	Cofactor for protein C; deficiency impairs APC pathway
Acquired (secondary)	Antiphospholipid syndrome (APLA)	Antibodies against phospholipid-protein complexes (lupus anticoagulant, anticardiolipin, anti-β2GPI); paradoxically: prolonged aPTT in vitro but prothrombotic in vivo
	Heparin-induced thrombocytopenia (HIT)	Antibodies against heparin-PF4 complex activate platelets → thrombosis despite thrombocytopenia
	Malignancy (Trousseau syndrome)	Mucin-secreting adenocarcinomas release tissue factor and procoagulant substances; migratory thrombophlebitis
	Pregnancy / oral contraceptives	Increased hepatic synthesis of coagulation factors; reduced protein S
	Nephrotic syndrome	Urinary loss of antithrombin III; renal vein thrombosis
	Prolonged immobilisation / surgery	Venous stasis

The antiphospholipid syndrome deserves particular emphasis as it is frequently tested. It may be primary or secondary (most commonly associated with SLE). The clinical manifestations include recurrent venous and arterial thromboses, recurrent pregnancy loss (due to placental vessel thrombosis), thrombocytopenia, and cardiac valvular vegetations (Libman-Sacks endocarditis). The laboratory paradox is characteristic: the lupus anticoagulant prolongs the aPTT in vitro (by interfering with phospholipid-dependent clotting assays) but produces a procoagulant state in vivo. Diagnosis requires both clinical criteria (thrombosis or pregnancy morbidity) and laboratory criteria (persistent positivity for lupus anticoagulant, anticardiolipin IgG/IgM, or anti-β2-glycoprotein I antibodies on two occasions at least 12 weeks apart).

When faced with a young patient with unexplained recurrent thrombosis, the first question to ask is whether an inherited or acquired thrombophilia is present. A structured thrombophilia workup should include factor V Leiden mutation analysis, prothrombin gene mutation, antithrombin III, protein C, and protein S levels, and antiphospholipid antibodies. Testing should ideally be performed remote from the acute thrombotic event and off anticoagulation.

Acquired Thrombophilia: Expanded Considerations

While inherited thrombophilias (Factor V Leiden, prothrombin G20210A, protein C/S/antithrombin deficiency) account for a proportion of venous thromboembolism, acquired risk factors are numerically more important in clinical practice. The major acquired thrombophilic conditions include: malignancy-associated thrombosis (Trousseau syndrome), heparin-induced thrombocytopenia (HIT), oral contraceptive/hormone replacement therapy use, pregnancy and the postpartum period, immobilisation and surgery, nephrotic syndrome, myeloproliferative neoplasms (especially polycythaemia vera and essential thrombocythaemia), and paroxysmal nocturnal haemoglobinuria (see Volume 1 for detailed coverage of haematological causes).

Malignancy-associated thrombosis (Trousseau syndrome) deserves particular emphasis. Approximately 10-15% of cancer patients develop clinically apparent VTE, and subclinical thrombosis is even more prevalent. The mechanisms are multifactorial: tumour cells directly activate coagulation through tissue factor expression and cancer procoagulant (a cysteine protease that directly activates factor X), mucin-secreting adenocarcinomas produce circulating mucins that activate platelets and endothelium, chemotherapy causes additional endothelial damage and reduces natural anticoagulant levels, and immobilisation/central venous catheters provide additional risk. Migratory superficial thrombophlebitis (classically affecting unusual sites such as arm or chest wall veins) in a patient without other risk factors should prompt investigation for occult malignancy, particularly pancreatic, gastric, and lung carcinomas.

Heparin-induced thrombocytopenia (HIT) is a prothrombotic disorder (paradoxically, despite thrombocytopenia) caused by IgG antibodies directed against complexes of platelet factor 4 (PF4) and heparin. The PF4-heparin-antibody immune complexes activate platelets via FcγRIIa receptors, leading to intense platelet activation, thrombin generation, and a hypercoagulable state. HIT typically presents 5-10 days after heparin exposure with a 50% or greater drop in platelet count and/or new thrombotic events (both arterial and venous thrombosis are common). The diagnosis is clinical (4Ts score: Thrombocytopenia, Timing, Thrombosis, other causes excluded), confirmed by anti-PF4/heparin ELISA and functional serotonin release assay. All heparin must be discontinued immediately and an alternative non-heparin anticoagulant (argatroban, bivalirudin, fondaparinux) initiated.

The pathogenesis explains the morphology: in HIT, thrombi are characteristically 'white clots' (platelet-rich) rather than the typical red (fibrin/RBC-rich) venous thrombi, reflecting the intense platelet activation that drives the thrombotic process. The pathologist examining arterial thrombectomy specimens in HIT may note an unusually platelet-rich composition. Arterial events (limb ischaemia, stroke, MI) are more common in HIT than in other thrombophilic states, which predominantly cause venous thrombosis.

Quick Recall: Thrombosis

Virchow's triad: endothelial injury (most important), abnormal blood flow, hypercoagulability.

Lines of Zahn: laminated pale/dark layers (Figure 4.10A); present in ante-mortem thrombi, absent in post-mortem clots.

Arterial thrombi: grey-white, platelet-rich, at sites of endothelial injury; grow retrograde.

Venous thrombi: red, RBC-rich, in areas of stasis (deep leg veins); grow antegrade.

Fate: propagation, embolisation, dissolution (fibrinolysis), organisation and recanalisation.
Factor V Leiden: most common inherited hypercoagulable state; point mutation renders factor Va resistant to protein C inactivation.

Embolism

An embolus is an intravascular solid, liquid, or gaseous mass that is carried by the blood to a site distant from its point of origin. The vast majority of emboli (>95%) are fragments of thrombi (thromboembolism). Other types include fat emboli, air emboli, amniotic fluid emboli, atheromatous emboli (cholesterol crystal emboli), and tumour emboli.

Pulmonary Thromboembolism

Pulmonary embolism (PE) is the most important form of thromboembolic disease. In >95% of cases, the emboli originate from deep vein thrombi (DVTs) of the lower extremities, most commonly from the iliofemoral veins. The clinical outcome depends on the size of the embolus. A **saddle embolus** lodges at the bifurcation of the main pulmonary artery and is rapidly fatal because of acute right ventricular failure and cardiovascular collapse. A **large embolus** occluding a major pulmonary artery branch causes acute right heart strain, hypotension, and may be fatal. **Medium-sized emboli** occlude segmental arteries and may cause pulmonary infarction, particularly when the bronchial arterial supply is compromised (as in patients with pre-existing heart failure or lung disease). In individuals with a competent bronchial circulation, the dual blood supply protects against infarction, and the emboli are clinically silent or produce haemorrhage without infarction. **Multiple small recurrent emboli** over time can cause pulmonary hypertension and cor pulmonale (chronic thromboembolic pulmonary hypertension, CTEPH).

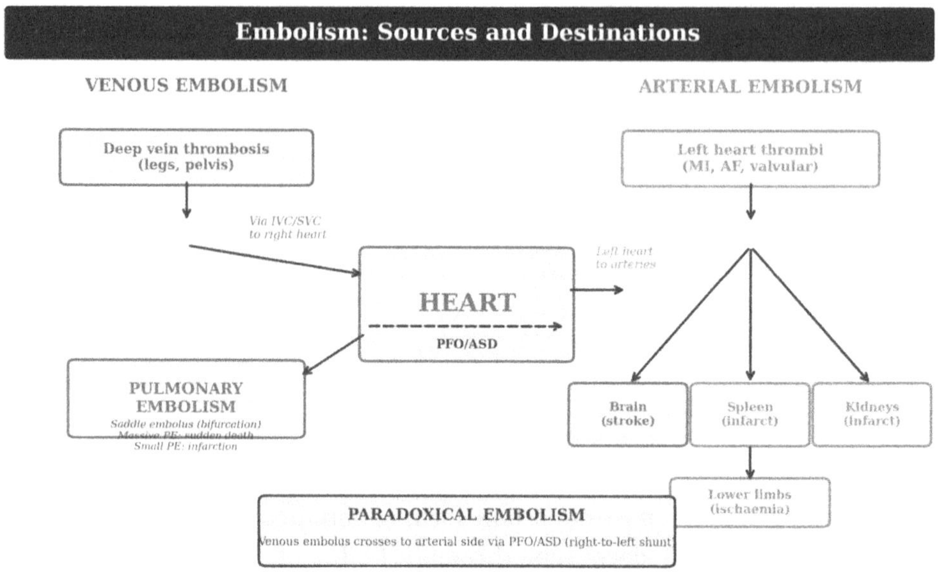

Figure 4.3 : Embolism sources and destinations: venous, arterial, and paradoxical pathways

Figure 4.6: Sources and destinations of emboli. (Source: Author's original.)

Systemic Thromboembolism

Systemic emboli arise from the left heart (mural thrombi over myocardial infarcts, left atrial thrombi in atrial fibrillation, vegetations on heart valves) or from the aorta (ulcerated atheromatous plaques). They travel to the arterial circulation and lodge in end-arteries, causing infarction. The most common sites of systemic embolisation are the lower extremities (most frequent), brain (causing ischaemic stroke), kidneys, spleen, and intestines.

Clinical Pearl

Why some infarcts are red and others pale. Pale (white, anaemic) infarcts occur in solid organs with single (end-) arterial supply: heart, kidney, spleen. Once the artery is occluded, no second source delivers blood, and the infarct is bloodless. Red (haemorrhagic) infarcts occur where dual blood supply or loose tissue architecture allows blood to seep into the infarcted zone: lung (bronchial artery reflow), small bowel (mesenteric collaterals), testis (after torsion-detorsion), and previously congested tissue. The morphological colour is therefore a property of organ vasculature, not of the thrombus or the patient.

Fat Embolism

Fat embolism occurs when marrow fat enters the circulation, most commonly after fractures of long bones (femur, tibia) or orthopaedic surgery. **Fat embolism syndrome** is a clinical triad of respiratory insufficiency (dyspnoea, tachypnoea), neurological symptoms (restlessness, confusion), and a petechial skin rash, typically appearing 1 to 3 days after injury. The pathogenesis involves both mechanical obstruction of pulmonary and cerebral microvasculature by fat globules and biochemical injury from free fatty acids released by lipase action on the fat, which cause endothelial toxicity and activate platelets.

Amniotic Fluid Embolism

Amniotic fluid embolism (AFE) is a rare but catastrophic complication of labour and delivery. It occurs when amniotic fluid containing fetal squamous cells, lanugo hair, mucin, and vernix enters the maternal circulation through tears in the placental membranes or uterine veins. The clinical presentation is dramatic: sudden onset of severe dyspnoea, cyanosis, hypotension, and cardiovascular collapse during or shortly after labour, followed rapidly by DIC. The mortality rate is extremely high (historically 80%, now estimated at 20–40% with modern intensive care). The diagnosis is confirmed by finding fetal squamous cells and mucin in the pulmonary vasculature at autopsy.

Etiopathogenesis and Complications of Amniotic Fluid Embolism

The pathogenesis of AFE is now understood to be more complex than simple mechanical obstruction by amniotic fluid debris. Current evidence supports a two-phase model. In Phase 1 (acute cardiorespiratory collapse), the entry of amniotic fluid into the maternal pulmonary vasculature triggers acute pulmonary vasospasm (mediated by endothelin and leukotrienes in amniotic fluid), leading to acute right ventricular failure, severe hypoxia, and systemic hypotension. This phase lasts 15-30 minutes and is responsible for the sudden cardiovascular collapse. In Phase 2 (haemorrhagic), left ventricular failure develops (possibly due to direct myocardial depressant factors in amniotic fluid), and DIC ensues, driven by tissue factor and phospholipids in amniotic fluid that activate the extrinsic coagulation pathway. Complement activation (anaphylactoid component) and mast cell degranulation contribute to the vasospasm and cardiovascular collapse, leading some authorities to propose the alternative term 'anaphylactoid syndrome of pregnancy.'

Risk factors include advanced maternal age, multiparity, tumultuous/precipitous labour, caesarean section, placental abruption, and uterine rupture. Complications in survivors include hypoxic brain injury (the most devastating long-term consequence), ARDS, acute kidney injury, and Sheehan syndrome (postpartum pituitary necrosis from profound hypotension). The diagnosis remains clinical; there is no specific laboratory test, though the detection of fetal squamous cells in the pulmonary vasculature at autopsy (staining with cytokeratin immunohistochemistry improves detection over H&E alone) or the presence of zinc coproporphyrin (a component of meconium) in maternal serum supports the diagnosis. The mortality rate has decreased from the historical 80% to approximately 20-40% with modern intensive care, but neurological morbidity in survivors remains high.

Quick Recall: Embolism

PE source: >95% from deep vein thrombi of lower limbs (iliofemoral veins).

Saddle embolus: lodges at pulmonary artery bifurcation; rapidly fatal (acute right heart failure).

PE and dual blood supply: competent bronchial circulation protects against infarction; pre-existing heart failure → infarction.

Fat embolism syndrome: triad of respiratory distress + neurological symptoms + petechial rash; 1–3 days after long bone fracture.

Amniotic fluid embolism: sudden collapse during labour; DIC; fetal squames in pulmonary vessels; very high mortality.

Paradoxical embolism: venous embolus crosses to arterial circulation via patent foramen ovale or ASD.

Air Embolism and Decompression Sickness

Air embolism occurs when gas bubbles enter the venous or arterial circulation and obstruct blood flow. Venous air embolism is the more common form and typically results from surgical procedures (particularly neurosurgical operations in the sitting position, laparoscopic surgery, central venous catheter insertion/removal, or haemodialysis circuit disconnection). Approximately 100-300 mL of air entering the venous system rapidly can be fatal, forming an air lock in the right ventricle that prevents effective cardiac output. Smaller volumes may cause symptoms ranging from nothing to chest pain, dyspnoea, and cardiovascular collapse depending on the volume and rate of entry. Arterial air embolism (paradoxical air embolism through a patent foramen ovale, or direct arterial entry during cardiac surgery or vascular procedures) causes cerebral or coronary infarction even with very small volumes. At autopsy, air embolism is demonstrated by submerging the heart under water and puncturing the right ventricle, looking for gas bubbles.

Decompression sickness ('the bends') is a form of gas embolism occurring in divers who ascend too rapidly from depth. At depth, increased ambient pressure dissolves nitrogen in blood and tissues. Rapid decompression causes nitrogen to come out of solution as gas bubbles in the vasculature and tissues. Type I ('pain only') involves bubbles in joints and muscles causing severe pain. Type II involves bubbles in the CNS (causing paraplegia, visual disturbances), pulmonary vasculature ('the chokes'), or inner ear. Chronic decompression sickness in deep-sea divers and caisson workers causes 'caisson disease,' with multiple foci of aseptic (avascular) necrosis of bone, particularly the femoral heads, humeral heads, and tibial condyles. Treatment is emergent recompression in a hyperbaric chamber.

Infarction

An infarct is an area of ischaemic necrosis caused by occlusion of either the arterial supply or the venous drainage of a tissue. Approximately 99% of infarcts result from thrombotic or embolic arterial occlusion. The morphological appearance depends on the nature of the tissue and the type of vascular occlusion.

Table 4.5: Types of infarction

Feature	White (Anaemic) Infarct	Red (Haemorrhagic) Infarct
Mechanism	Arterial occlusion in solid organs with end-arteries	Venous occlusion, or arterial occlusion in loose/dual-supply tissues, or reperfusion

		of ischaemic tissue
Organs affected	Heart, kidney, spleen (solid, single arterial supply)	Lung (dual supply), intestine (collaterals), liver (dual supply), brain (loose tissue), ovary (torsion)
Gross appearance	Pale, wedge-shaped, with apex at occluded vessel; hyperaemic border	Dark red, haemorrhagic; wedge-shaped or diffuse depending on organ
Microscopy	Coagulative necrosis (ghost outlines preserved; except brain: liquefactive)	Coagulative necrosis with extensive haemorrhage into necrotic area

Why is brain infarction liquefactive when other infarcts are coagulative? This is a classic viva question. The brain parenchyma is rich in lipids and has abundant lysosomal enzymes (from microglia) and water content, but relatively little structural protein. The enzymatic digestion therefore predominates over protein denaturation, producing a soft, liquefied necrotic area rather than the firm, ghost-outline pattern of coagulative necrosis seen in protein-rich solid organs such as the heart and kidney.

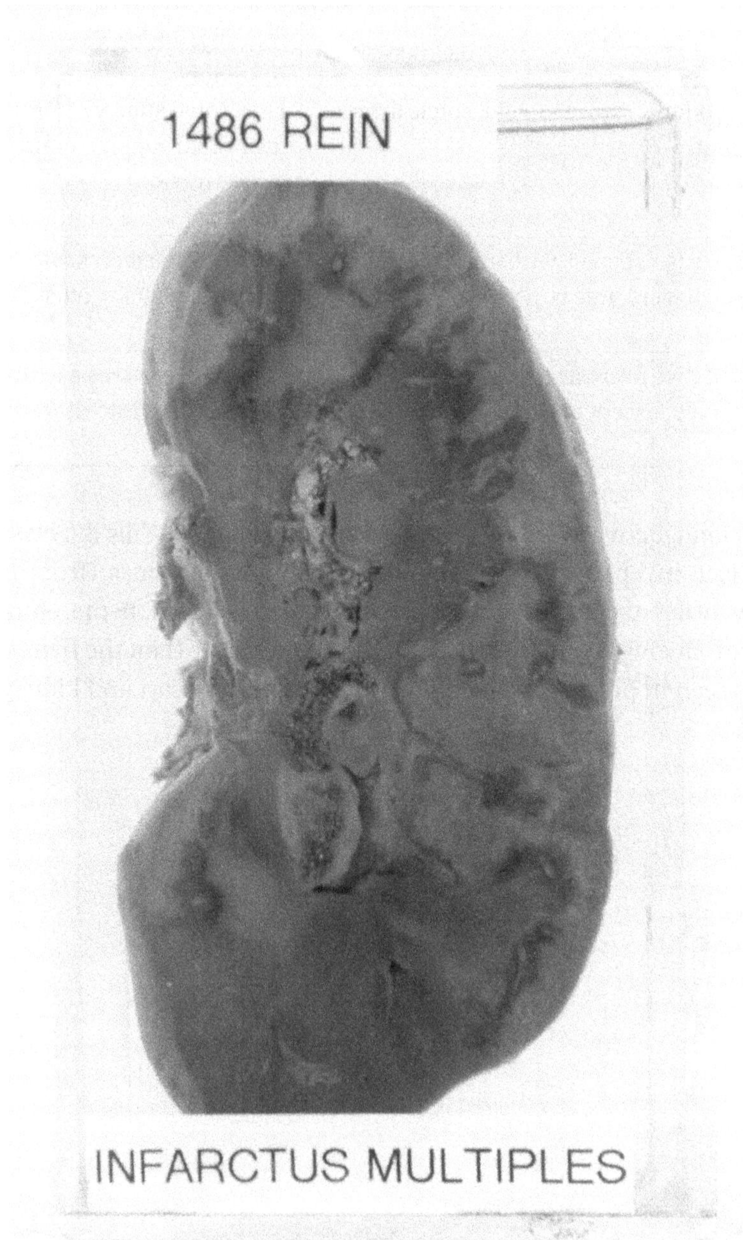

Figure 4.7: Renal infarcts (gross). Multiple wedge-shaped, pale areas of coagulative necrosis on cross-section. *(Source: apatho collection, Wikimedia Commons, CC BY-SA 3.0.)*

[See Figure 3.8 for haemorrhagic infarct of lung (Yale Rosen, CC BY-SA 2.0).]

Disseminated Intravascular Coagulation (DIC)

DIC is not a primary disease but a complication of numerous conditions in which widespread activation of the coagulation cascade leads to the formation of thrombi in the microvasculature, with secondary consumption of platelets and coagulation factors, and activation of fibrinolysis. The paradoxical result is simultaneous thrombosis and bleeding.

Pathogenesis

DIC is triggered by two principal mechanisms. First, release of tissue factor into the circulation (obstetric complications, malignancy, massive tissue injury) directly activates the extrinsic coagulation pathway. Second, widespread endothelial injury (sepsis, especially Gram-negative; vasculitis; severe burns) activates both the intrinsic pathway and exposes tissue factor. The result is thrombin generation throughout the microvasculature, leading to fibrin deposition in small vessels (microthrombi) in multiple organs.

Consumption of platelets and clotting factors (hence the older term "consumption coagulopathy") produces a bleeding diathesis. Simultaneously, the fibrinolytic system is activated, generating fibrin degradation products (FDPs) and D-dimers, which themselves have anticoagulant properties and further impair haemostasis.

Trigger (TF release / endothelial injury) → Widespread thrombin generation → Microvascular fibrin thrombi (organ ischaemia) + Consumption of platelets and factors (bleeding) + Fibrinolysis activation (↑ FDPs, D-dimer)

Table 4.5: Causes of DIC

Category	Examples
Obstetric complications	Abruptio placentae, amniotic fluid embolism, retained dead fetus, eclampsia
Infections (most common cause)	Gram-negative sepsis (endotoxin), Gram-positive sepsis, meningococcaemia, malaria (P. falciparum), rickettsiosis
Malignancy	Acute promyelocytic leukaemia (APL; M3), mucin-secreting adenocarcinomas (pancreas, stomach, ovary)
Massive tissue injury	Trauma, burns, extensive surgery, rhabdomyolysis
Others	Snake envenomation (particularly Echis carinatus, Russell's viper), acute pancreatitis, giant haemangioma (Kasabach-Merritt)

Snake envenomation (saw-scaled viper Echis carinatus, Russell's viper Daboia russelii) is an important cause of DIC in tropical and rural settings. APL (AML-M3) is another critical cause to recognise because specific therapy with all-trans retinoic acid (ATRA) and arsenic trioxide can correct the coagulopathy (see Volume 1).

Laboratory Findings in DIC

The laboratory profile of DIC reflects both consumption and fibrinolysis: thrombocytopenia (platelet count low), prolonged PT and aPTT (factor consumption), elevated D-dimer and FDPs (fibrinolysis), low fibrinogen (consumption, though it may be normal early as an acute-phase reactant), and schistocytes on peripheral blood smear (microangiopathic haemolytic anaemia from RBC fragmentation across fibrin strands in small vessels).

Exam Pitfall

DIC presents with both thrombotic and haemorrhagic manifestations. In examination answers, always describe both sides of the paradox: microvascular thrombosis (causing organ ischaemia) AND consumption coagulopathy (causing bleeding). A common mistake is to describe only the bleeding component.

Quick Recall: DIC

Pathogenesis: widespread thrombin generation → microvascular thrombosis + consumption of platelets/factors + secondary fibrinolysis.

Most common trigger overall: sepsis (especially Gram-negative).

Key lab findings: ↓ platelets, ↑ PT/aPTT, ↑ D-dimer/FDPs, ↓ fibrinogen, schistocytes on smear.

Classic malignancy association: APL (AML-M3); treat with ATRA to correct coagulopathy.

Shock

Shock is a state of systemic hypoperfusion caused by reduction in cardiac output or in effective circulating blood volume. The inadequate tissue perfusion results in cellular hypoxia, metabolic derangement, and, if uncorrected, progressive organ failure and death. Shock is the final common pathway of many lethal clinical events, including massive haemorrhage, severe burns, large myocardial infarction, massive pulmonary embolism, and uncontrolled sepsis (Figures 4.8–4.9).

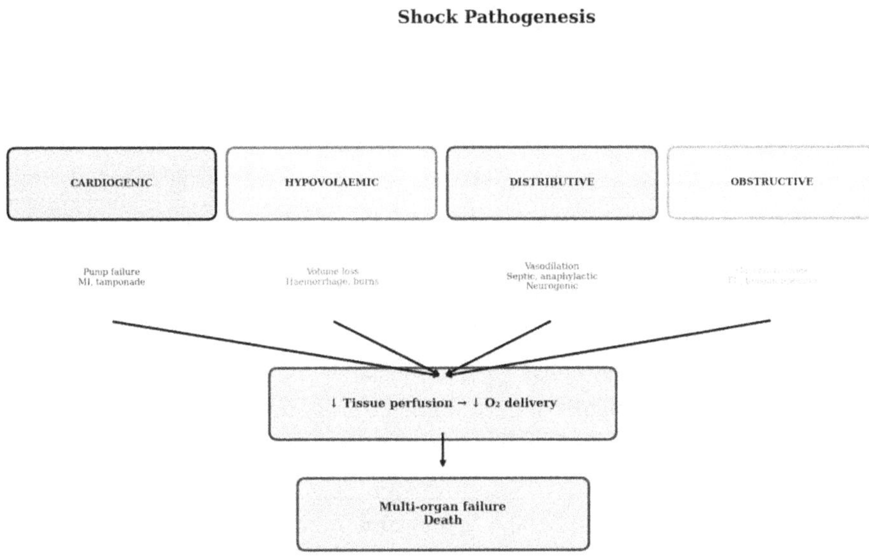

Figure 4.8: Shock Pathogenesis. *(Source: Author's original.)*

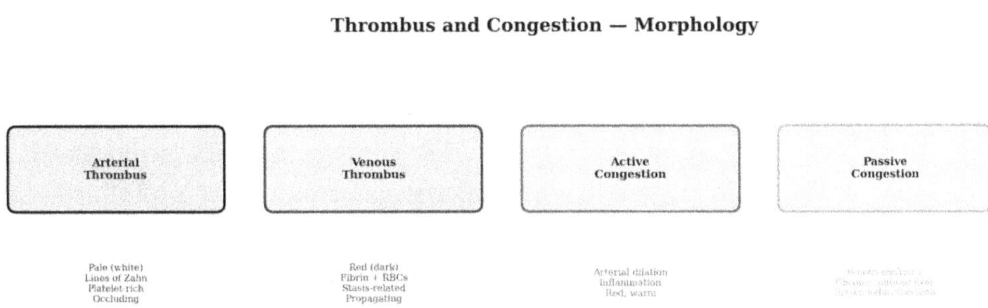

Figure 4.9: Thrombus and Congestion — Morphology. *(Source: Author's original.)*

Types of Shock

Table 4.6: Types and causes of shock

Type	Mechanism	Clinical Causes
Cardiogenic	Failure of the myocardial pump: reduced cardiac output	Large MI (>40% LV mass), myocarditis, arrhythmias, cardiac tamponade, massive PE (obstructive)
Hypovolaemic	Inadequate blood or plasma volume	Haemorrhage (trauma, GI bleed, ruptured aortic aneurysm), fluid loss (severe burns, vomiting, diarrhoea)
Septic	Peripheral vasodilation, endothelial injury, DIC triggered by systemic infection	Gram-negative sepsis (endotoxin/LPS; most common), Gram-positive sepsis (lipoteichoic acid, superantigens), fungal sepsis
Neurogenic	Loss of vascular tone from peripheral vasodilation (sympathetic denervation)	Spinal cord injury, severe head trauma, anaesthetic accident
Anaphylactic	Systemic vasodilation and increased permeability from IgE-mediated mast cell degranulation	Drug reactions (penicillin), insect stings, food allergens (peanut)

Pathogenesis of Septic Shock

Septic shock is the most frequently examined topic in this chapter, and its pathogenesis must be understood in molecular detail. It is triggered when microorganisms or their products (pathogen-associated molecular patterns, PAMPs) activate the innate immune system, producing an overwhelming, dysregulated inflammatory response.

In Gram-negative sepsis, lipopolysaccharide (LPS/endotoxin) is the principal trigger. LPS binds to LPS-binding protein (LBP) in plasma, and this complex interacts with CD14 on monocytes/macrophages. CD14 transfers LPS to TLR4 (Toll-like receptor 4), which, together with the adaptor protein MD2, activates intracellular signalling via the NF-κB and MAP kinase pathways. This triggers the transcription and release of a cascade of pro-inflammatory cytokines: TNF, IL-1, IL-6, IL-12, and IL-18.

In Gram-positive sepsis, lipoteichoic acid and peptidoglycan activate TLR2. Superantigens (TSST-1, streptococcal pyrogenic exotoxins) cross-link MHC II and TCR Vβ, activating up to 20% of T cells and causing massive cytokine release. The downstream effects of this cytokine storm produce the hallmarks of septic shock:

Table 4.8: Pathophysiological effects of septic shock

Effect	Mechanism
Systemic vasodilation and hypotension	TNF, IL-1 induce NO synthase (iNOS) in vascular smooth muscle → massive NO production → vasodilation; impaired myocardial contractility (TNF-mediated)
Endothelial injury and activation	TNF, IL-1 activate endothelium → upregulation of adhesion molecules, tissue factor expression, loss of thrombomodulin → pro-coagulant state
DIC	Tissue factor expression on endothelium and monocytes triggers coagulation; consumption of clotting factors and platelets; impaired anticoagulant mechanisms (protein C, antithrombin)
Metabolic derangement	Insulin resistance, hyperglycaemia, lactic acidosis, mitochondrial dysfunction
Organ dysfunction (MODS)	Combination of hypoperfusion, microvascular thrombosis, and direct cytokine-mediated injury to lungs (ARDS), kidneys (ATN), liver, brain
Immunosuppression (late phase)	Compensatory anti-inflammatory response: IL-10, TGF-β, T-cell apoptosis → immune paralysis → secondary infections

Infection → PAMPs (LPS/lipoteichoic acid) → TLR activation (TLR4/TLR2) → NF-κB → Cytokine storm (TNF, IL-1, IL-6) → Vasodilation (↑NO) + Endothelial injury + DIC + MODS

The Pathologist's Eye

At autopsy, the morphological hallmarks of septic shock include: (1) diffuse alveolar damage in the lungs (hyaline membranes, interstitial oedema, congestion), the morphological substrate of ARDS; (2) renal cortical pallor with tubular epithelial necrosis (acute tubular necrosis, ATN); (3) adrenal haemorrhage (Waterhouse-Friderichsen syndrome, classically in meningococcaemia, but also in other causes of DIC); (4) centrilobular hepatic necrosis ("shock liver"); (5) superficial mucosal haemorrhagic necrosis in the GI tract (stress ulcers). Microthrombi in small vessels (DIC) may be visible on histology, particularly in the glomeruli and pulmonary capillaries.

Sepsis-3 Definitions and the SOFA Score

Sepsis-3 (2016) redefined sepsis as life-threatening organ dysfunction caused by dysregulated host response to infection, replacing the older SIRS-based definition. Organ dysfunction is identified by a ≥2-point increase in the SOFA score.**Suspected infection + ΔSOFA ≥2 = Sepsis → If vasopressors needed for MAP ≥65 + lactate >2 mmol/L = Septic Shock**

Stages of Shock

Regardless of the type, shock progresses through three stages if uncorrected.

Stage 1: Compensated (non-progressive) shock. Baroreceptor reflexes, catecholamine release, activation of the renin-angiotensin-aldosterone system, and ADH secretion maintain blood pressure and vital organ perfusion. Tachycardia, peripheral vasoconstriction (cool, pale extremities), and oliguria are the clinical signs. If the underlying cause is corrected at this stage, full recovery is expected.

Stage 2: Decompensated (progressive) shock. Compensatory mechanisms fail. Widespread tissue hypoxia leads to anaerobic glycolysis, lactic acidosis, and arteriolar vasodilation (loss of vascular tone). Blood pools in the microcirculation, further reducing cardiac output. Endothelial injury triggers DIC. Vital organ function begins to deteriorate: confusion (cerebral hypoperfusion), oliguria progressing to anuria (renal failure), and tachypnoea (metabolic acidosis). Without aggressive intervention, this stage is often irreversible.

Stage 3: Irreversible shock. Cell injury is so severe and widespread that recovery is not possible even with correction of the haemodynamic deficit. Lysosomal enzyme leakage, myocardial depression (myocardial depressant factor), renal shutdown, and bowel necrosis (bacterial translocation and endotoxaemia) create a vicious cycle that leads inexorably to death.

Morphology of Shock (Organ-Specific Changes)

Table 4.9: Organ-specific morphological changes in shock

Organ	Morphological Change
Kidney	Acute tubular necrosis (ATN): ischaemic necrosis of tubular epithelium, particularly proximal tubules and thick ascending limb of Henle; patchy skip lesions; muddy brown casts
Lung	Diffuse alveolar damage (DAD)/ARDS: congestion, interstitial oedema, hyaline membranes, type II pneumocyte hyperplasia (proliferative phase)
Liver	Centrilobular haemorrhagic necrosis ("shock liver"); hepatocyte dropout around central veins
GI tract	Superficial mucosal haemorrhagic necrosis; stress ulcers (Curling ulcers in burns, Cushing ulcers in CNS injury)
Adrenals	Adrenal haemorrhage (Waterhouse-Friderichsen syndrome in meningococcal sepsis); cortical lipid depletion
Brain	Ischaemic encephalopathy; laminar necrosis of cortex; selective neuronal necrosis

	(Purkinje cells, hippocampal CA1)
Heart	Contraction band necrosis (coagulative myocytolysis); subendocardial haemorrhage

Quick Recall: Shock

Most common cause of septic shock: Gram-negative sepsis (LPS → LBP → CD14 → TLR4/MD2 → NF-κB → TNF, IL-1, IL-6).

Superantigens: S. aureus TSST-1, streptococcal pyrogenic exotoxins; activate up to 20% T cells via Vβ-MHC II cross-linking.

iNOS and NO: TNF/IL-1 induce iNOS → massive NO → vasodilation → refractory hypotension.

Waterhouse-Friderichsen: bilateral adrenal haemorrhage in meningococcal sepsis (DIC-mediated).

Three stages: compensated (reversible) → decompensated (progressive, potentially reversible) → irreversible.

Key autopsy finding: ATN (kidney), DAD/hyaline membranes (lung), centrilobular necrosis (liver), stress ulcers (GI).

Integration: *Haemodynamic disorders connect to cardiovascular pathology (atherosclerosis and MI, Chapter 13 and 14), respiratory pathology (ARDS/DAD in shock, PE infarction, Chapter 15), renal pathology (ATN, renal vein thrombosis, Chapter 23), hepatobiliary pathology (Budd-Chiari syndrome, shock liver, Chapter 20), and haematopathology (DIC, thrombophilia, HIT, see Volume 1).*

Recent Advances

Immunothrombosis and COVID-19. The COVID-19 pandemic highlighted the concept of immunothrombosis, the pathological interplay between innate immunity and coagulation in which neutrophil extracellular traps (NETs), complement activation, and endothelial injury drive microvascular thrombosis. SARS-CoV-2 directly infects endothelial cells via ACE2 receptors, causing endotheliitis and a procoagulant state. Elevated D-dimer emerged as a major predictor of mortality in severe COVID-19. The term "COVID-19-associated coagulopathy" (CAC) describes a distinct thrombotic phenotype characterised by pulmonary microvascular thrombosis, elevated D-dimer with relatively preserved PT/aPTT (unlike classic DIC), and venous thromboembolism rates of 20–30% in ICU patients.

Sepsis-3 definition and the role of biomarkers. The Third International Consensus Definitions for Sepsis (Sepsis-3, 2016) redefined sepsis as "life-threatening organ dysfunction caused by a dysregulated host response to infection," operationalised by an increase of 2 or more points in the Sequential Organ Failure Assessment (SOFA) score. Septic shock is defined as sepsis with persistent hypotension requiring vasopressors and a serum lactate >2 mmol/L despite adequate fluid resuscitation. Procalcitonin-guided antibiotic de-escalation and the use of presepsin (sCD14-ST) as a diagnostic biomarker are gaining wider clinical adoption.

Direct oral anticoagulants (DOACs) and VTE management. DOACs (rivaroxaban, apixaban, dabigatran, edoxaban) have largely replaced warfarin for treatment and secondary prevention of venous thromboembolism in international guidelines. These agents directly inhibit factor Xa (rivaroxaban, apixaban, edoxaban) or thrombin (dabigatran) without requiring INR monitoring. Specific reversal agents are now available: idarucizumab for dabigatran and andexanet alfa for factor Xa inhibitors.

International Frameworks

ISTH overt-DIC scoring. The International Society on Thrombosis and Haemostasis (ISTH) overt-DIC scoring system stratifies disseminated intravascular coagulation using four routinely available laboratory parameters: platelet count, fibrin-related markers (D-dimer or fibrin degradation products), prothrombin time prolongation, and fibrinogen level. A composite score of ≥5 in a patient with an underlying disorder known to be associated with DIC (sepsis, malignancy, obstetric complications, trauma, vascular abnormalities) is compatible with overt DIC; serial scoring is recommended to track trajectory. The ISTH framework is the international reference standard for DIC diagnosis in clinical trials and audit. Citation: Taylor FB Jr, et al. Thromb Haemost 2001;86(5):1327–1330. PMID 11816725.

Ultra High-Yield Chapter Summary

Topic	Must Remember
Oedema mechanisms	↑ hydrostatic, ↓ oncotic, lymphatic obstruction, ↑ permeability, Na/H2O retention
Transudate vs exudate	Transudate: protein-poor, <1.012 SG; Exudate: protein-rich, >1.020 SG, due to inflammation
Nutmeg liver	Chronic hepatic congestion (right heart failure); centrilobular sinusoidal dilation and hepatocyte atrophy
Heart failure cells	Haemosiderin-laden macrophages in alveoli; Perl's stain positive; chronic left heart failure
Virchow's triad	Endothelial injury (most important) + abnormal blood flow + hypercoagulability
Lines of Zahn	Laminated pale/dark layers in ante-mortem thrombi; absent in post-mortem clots
Arterial vs venous thrombi	Arterial: white, platelet-rich, retrograde.
Fate of thrombus	Propagation, embolisation, dissolution (fibrinolysis), organisation and recanalisation
Factor V Leiden	Most common inherited hypercoagulable state; mutation renders Va resistant to protein C

Pulmonary embolism	>95% from lower limb DVT; saddle embolus = rapidly fatal; medium emboli → infarction if dual supply compromised
Fat embolism syndrome	Long bone fractures; triad: respiratory distress + neuro symptoms + petechial rash; 1–3 days post-injury
Amniotic fluid embolism	Labour/delivery; sudden collapse, DIC; fetal squames in pulmonary vessels; very high mortality
White vs red infarct	White: solid organs, end-arteries (heart, kidney, spleen).
Brain infarction	Liquefactive (not coagulative); lipid-rich, abundant lysosomes, high water content
DIC	Widespread thrombin generation → microvascular thrombosis + consumption coagulopathy + secondary fibrinolysis
DIC labs	↓ platelets, ↑ PT/aPTT, ↑ D-dimer, ↓ fibrinogen, schistocytes
Septic shock: TLR4 pathway	LPS → LBP → CD14 → TLR4/MD2 → NF-κB → TNF, IL-1, IL-6 → vasodilation, DIC, MODS
Superantigens	S. aureus TSST-1, streptococcal exotoxins; cross-link MHC II with TCR Vβ; activate 20% T cells
Stages of shock	Compensated → decompensated → irreversible
Waterhouse-Friderichsen	Bilateral adrenal haemorrhage in meningococcal DIC; acute adrenal insufficiency
Shock kidney	ATN: ischaemic necrosis of proximal tubules; muddy brown casts
Shock lung	DAD: hyaline membranes, interstitial oedema; ARDS (Figure 4.1)

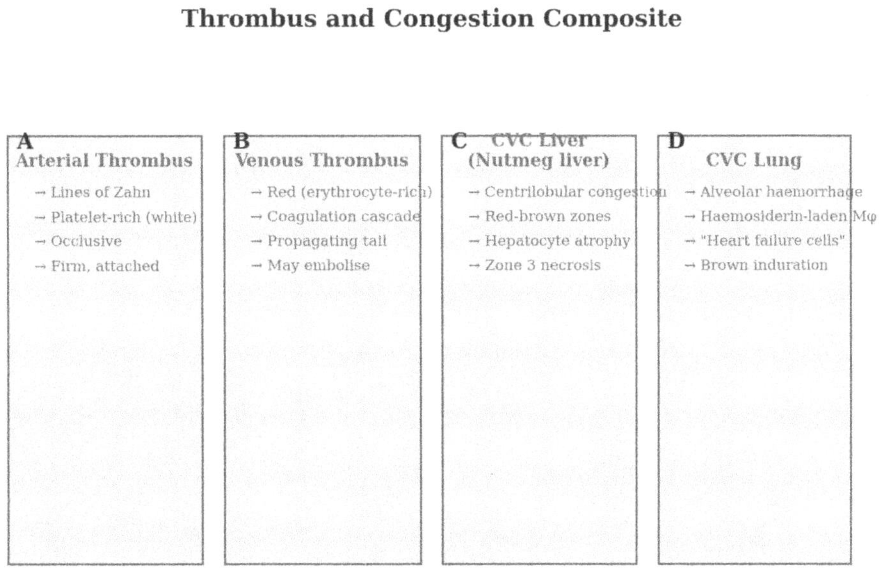

Figure 4.10: Thrombus and Congestion Composite. (Source: Author's original.)

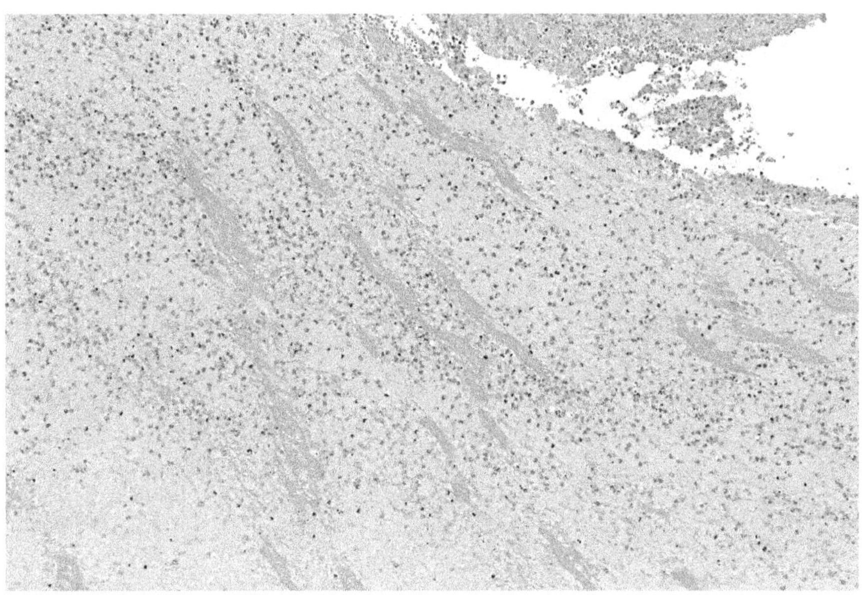

Figure 4.10A: Arterial thrombus (Lines of Zahn): Laminations of alternating platelets/fibrin and erythrocytes (H&E, intermed mag). (Source: Nephron, Wikimedia Commons, CC BY-SA 3.0.)

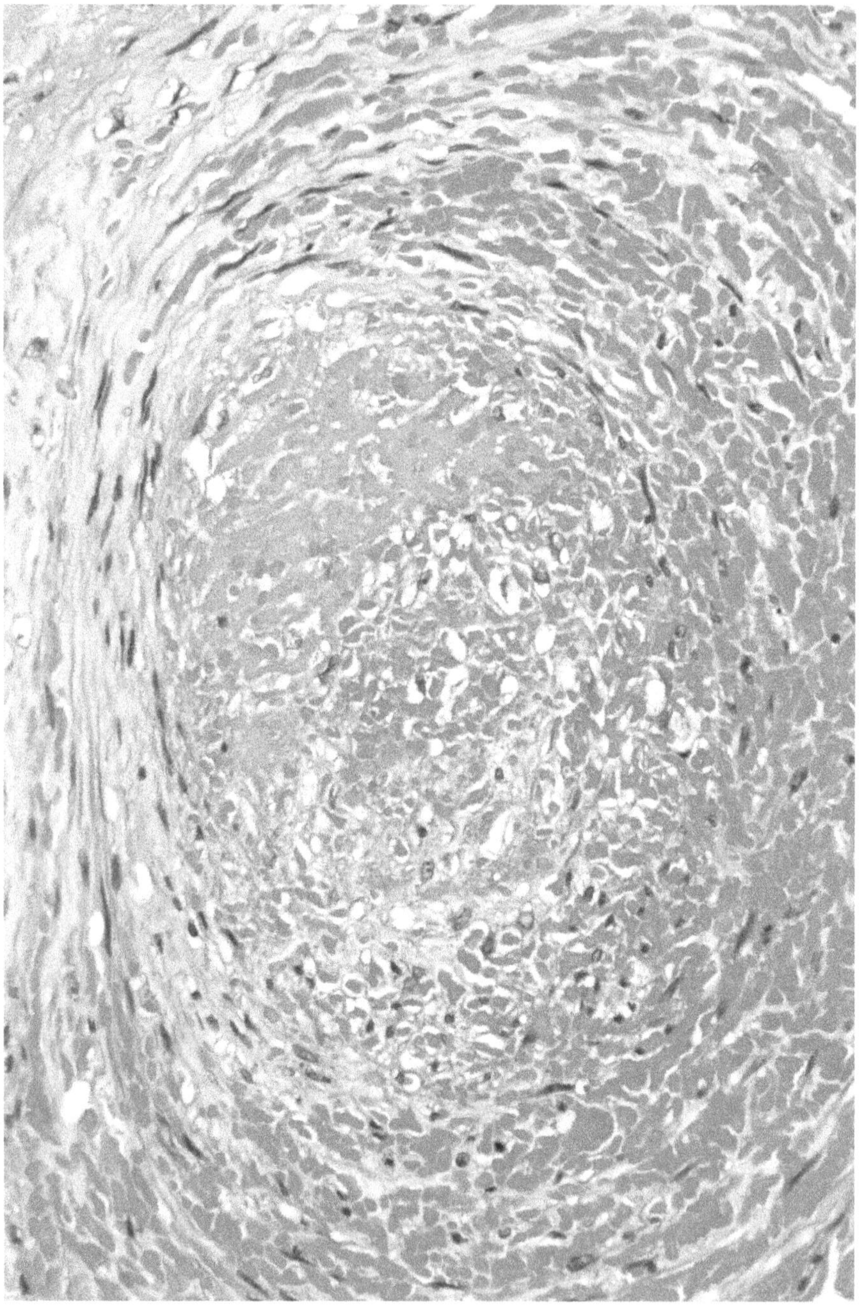

Figure 4.10B: Venous thrombus: Fetal thrombotic vasculopathy showing thrombi in small vessels (H&E, very high mag). (Source: Nephron, Wikimedia Commons, CC BY-SA 3.0.)

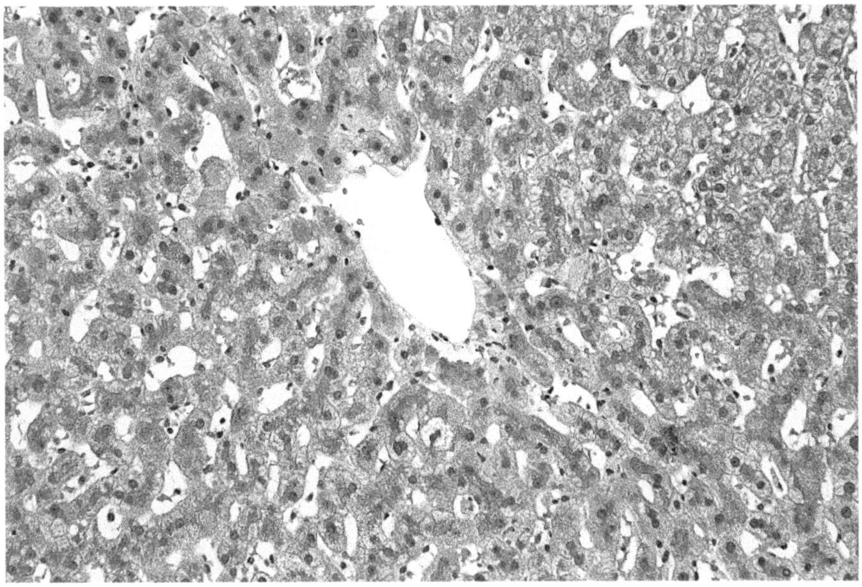

Figure 4.10C: Chronic venous congestion of liver (Nutmeg liver): Dilated sinusoids in Zone III with early perisinusoidal fibrosis (H&E, high mag). (Source: Nephron, Wikimedia Commons, CC BY-SA 3.0.)

Chapter 5: Diseases of the Immune System

THE BIG PICTURE

The immune system protects against infection and surveils for neoplasia. Dysregulation produces immune-mediated disease: hypersensitivity reactions damage host tissues through excessive or misdirected immune responses; autoimmune diseases arise when tolerance to self-antigens breaks down; immunodeficiency states leave the host vulnerable to opportunistic pathogens; and amyloidosis results when misfolded proteins, many derived from immunoglobulin light chains or inflammatory mediators, accumulate in tissues and destroy organ architecture. This chapter covers the full spectrum of immune-mediated disease.

High-yield topics in this chapter: hypersensitivity reactions (types I–IV); mechanisms of autoimmunity and immunological tolerance; SLE (pathogenesis, ANA patterns, lupus nephritis); amyloidosis (classification, pathogenesis, diagnosis); HIV/AIDS (pathogenesis, CD4 lifecycle, opportunistic infections); transplant rejection and graft-versus-host disease; primary immunodeficiency diseases; MHC molecules and antigen presentation.

The immune system distinguishes dangerous from non-dangerous signals. Failure of this discrimination results in immune-mediated disease affecting virtually every organ system. SLE destroys kidneys, type 1 diabetes destroys islets, Graves disease drives thyrotoxicosis, and rheumatoid arthritis erodes joints. For the pathologist, immune-mediated disease is encountered on every slide and in every laboratory: from the IF pattern on a renal biopsy to the CD4 count in an HIV patient to the Congo red stain on an amyloid deposit. Mastery of immunopathology is not optional; it is foundational.

The Major Histocompatibility Complex (MHC)

The MHC (HLA system, chromosome 6p21) is the most polymorphic genetic region. Class I (HLA-A, B, C) presents intracellular peptides to CD8+ T cells; Class II (HLA-DR, DQ, DP) presents extracellular peptides to CD4+ T cells. Key disease associations: HLA-B27 (ankylosing spondylitis), HLA-DR3/DR4 (type 1 diabetes), HLA-DQ2/DQ8 (coeliac disease). See table.**MHC class I molecules (HLA-A, HLA-B, HLA-C)** are expressed on virtually all nucleated cells. They present intracellular (endogenous) peptides (derived from cytoplasmic proteins, including viral and tumour antigens, degraded by the proteasome) to CD8+ cytotoxic T lymphocytes. The molecule consists of a polymorphic α chain (heavy chain) non-covalently associated with β2-microglobulin. The peptide-binding groove accommodates peptides of 8–10 amino acids.

MHC class II molecules (HLA-DP, HLA-DQ, HLA-DR) are expressed constitutively only on antigen-presenting cells (dendritic cells, macrophages, B lymphocytes) and thymic epithelium, but can be induced on other cells by IFN-γ. They present extracellular (exogenous) peptides (derived from endocytosed proteins, degraded in lysosomes) to CD4+ helper T lymphocytes. The molecule is a heterodimer of α and β chains, both transmembrane. The peptide-binding groove accommodates longer peptides (13–25 amino acids). The invariant chain (Ii) and HLA-DM regulate peptide loading.

Table 5.0: Comparison of MHC class I and class II

Feature	MHC Class I	MHC Class II
Loci	HLA-A, -B, -C	HLA-DP, -DQ, -DR
Structure	α chain + β2-microglobulin	α chain + β chain (heterodimer)
Expression	All nucleated cells	APCs (dendritic cells, macrophages, B cells); inducible by IFN-γ
Peptide source	Endogenous (cytoplasmic; proteasome)	Exogenous (endocytosed; lysosomal)
Peptide length	8–10 amino acids	13–25 amino acids
Recognised by	CD8+ CTLs	CD4+ helper T cells
Disease associations	HLA-B27: ankylosing spondylitis; HLA-B51: Behçet disease	HLA-DR4: RA, type 1 DM; HLA-DR3: SLE; HLA-DQ2/DQ8: coeliac disease

Quick Recall: MHC/HLA

Class I: HLA-A/B/C; all nucleated cells; endogenous peptides → CD8+ CTLs.

Class II: HLA-DP/DQ/DR; APCs; exogenous peptides → CD4+ T helpers.

Strongest disease association: HLA-B27 with ankylosing spondylitis (>90% of patients are B27+).

HLA matching: critical for transplant outcome; mismatch → allorecognition → rejection.

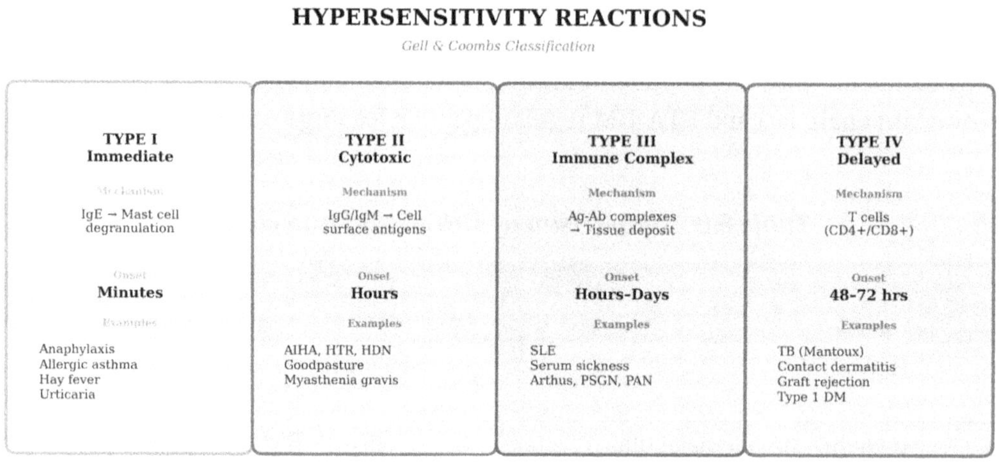

Figure 5.1: Hypersensitivity Reactions: Gell and Coombs Classification. (Source: Author's original.)

Hypersensitivity Reactions

Hypersensitivity refers to immune responses that are excessive, misdirected, or poorly controlled and result in tissue injury. Gell and Coombs classified these into four types based on the immunological mechanism involved. In clinical practice, hypersensitivity reactions are rarely pure; many diseases involve a combination of mechanisms. However, the classification remains essential for examination purposes and for understanding the pathogenesis of specific diseases.

Table 5.1: Gell and Coombs classification of hypersensitivity reactions

Type	Mechanism	Mediators	Time Course	Clinical Examples
I: Immediate (anaphylactic)	IgE-mediated mast cell/basophil degranulation	Histamine, leukotrienes (LTC4/D4/E4), prostaglandins, PAF, cytokines (TNF, IL-4, IL-5, IL-13)	Minutes (immediate phase); 2–24 hrs (late phase)	Anaphylaxis, allergic asthma, allergic rhinitis (hay fever), urticaria, food allergy
II: Antibody-mediated (cytotoxic)	IgG/IgM antibodies against cell surface or ECM antigens → complement activation, ADCC, opsonisation, or	Complement (MAC, C3b), Fc receptor-bearing cells (NK, macrophages)	Hours	Autoimmune haemolytic anaemia, Rh haemolytic disease, Goodpasture syndrome, myasthenia gravis, Graves disease, acute rheumatic fever

	functional alteration			
III: Immune complex	Antigen-antibody (IgG) complexes deposit in tissues → complement activation → neutrophil recruitment → tissue damage	Complement (C3a, C5a), neutrophil enzymes, ROS	Hours to days	SLE, post-streptococcal GN, serum sickness, Arthus reaction, polyarteritis nodosa (HBV-associated)
IV: Cell-mediated (delayed)	T cell-mediated: (a) CD4+ Th1/Th17 → macrophage activation; (b) CD8+ CTL → direct cytotoxicity	Cytokines (IFN-γ, TNF, IL-17), activated macrophages, cytotoxic T cells	24–72 hrs (delayed)	Contact dermatitis, tuberculin reaction, granulomatous inflammation (TB, sarcoidosis), transplant rejection, type 1 diabetes, MS

Type I Hypersensitivity: Immediate (Figure 5.1)

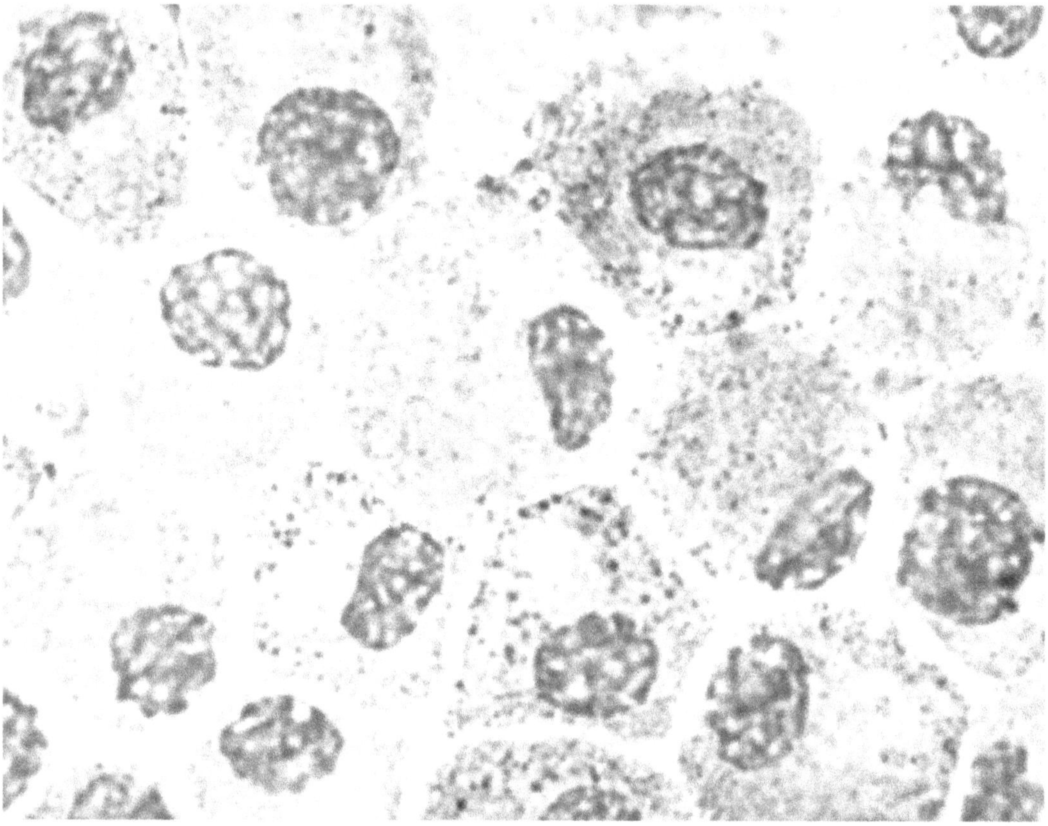

Figure 5.2: Type I hypersensitivity — mast cell with metachromatic granules (toluidine blue). Arrow indicates mast cell with characteristic purple granules (Source: Rubber, Wikimedia Commons, Copyrighted free use.)

Type I reactions are mediated by IgE antibodies bound to FcεRI receptors on mast cells and basophils. On first exposure to an allergen, susceptible individuals mount a Th2 response (IL-4, IL-5, IL-13) that drives B-cell class switching to IgE. The IgE binds to mast cells (sensitisation). On subsequent exposure, the allergen cross-links cell-bound IgE, triggering mast cell degranulation and release of preformed mediators (histamine, tryptase, proteases) within minutes (the immediate phase). This is followed by synthesis of lipid mediators (leukotrienes, prostaglandins) and cytokines that recruit eosinophils and produce the late phase response (2–24 hours later), which is responsible for the chronic tissue damage in conditions like asthma.

Allergen exposure → Th2 response (IL-4) → IgE class switch → IgE binds FcεRI on mast cells (sensitisation) → Re-exposure → Cross-linking → Degranulation → Immediate phase (histamine) + Late phase (leukotrienes, eosinophils)

Table 5.1B: Mediators of type I hypersensitivity

Mediator	Source	Actions
Histamine	Preformed; mast cell granules	Vasodilation, ↑ vascular permeability, bronchospasm, mucus secretion
Tryptase	Preformed; mast cell granules	Serum tryptase is a marker of mast cell activation (elevated in anaphylaxis and mastocytosis)
Leukotrienes (LTC4, LTD4, LTE4)	Newly synthesised; arachidonic acid/5-LOX pathway	Prolonged bronchospasm (1000× more potent than histamine), ↑ vascular permeability, mucus secretion
Prostaglandin D2	Newly synthesised; COX pathway	Bronchospasm, vasodilation
PAF (platelet-activating factor)	Newly synthesised	Platelet aggregation, bronchospasm, vasodilation, chemotaxis
Cytokines (TNF, IL-4, IL-5, IL-13)	Synthesised de novo	Late phase: eosinophil recruitment (IL-5), IgE production (IL-4), mucus secretion (IL-13)

Anaphylaxis is the most severe manifestation of type I hypersensitivity, characterised by systemic vasodilation, increased vascular permeability, bronchospasm, and laryngeal oedema. It can be rapidly fatal if untreated. The immediate treatment is intramuscular adrenaline (epinephrine), which acts via α1 receptors (vasoconstriction, reverses hypotension) and β2 receptors (bronchodilation). Post-mortem findings in fatal anaphylaxis include pulmonary hyperinflation, laryngeal oedema, and visceral congestion; however, the pathological findings may be minimal, making the diagnosis predominantly clinical and supported by elevated post-mortem serum tryptase.

Type II Hypersensitivity: Antibody-Mediated

Table 5.1C: Subtypes of type II hypersensitivity with examples

Mechanism	Antibody Target	Disease
Opsonisation and phagocytosis	RBC surface antigens	Autoimmune haemolytic anaemia, Rh haemolytic disease of newborn
	Platelet antigens	Immune thrombocytopenic purpura (ITP)

Complement/ADCC-mediated cytotoxicity	GBM (type IV collagen)	Goodpasture syndrome (linear IF along GBM)
	Donor HLA antigens	Hyperacute transplant rejection
Antibody-mediated dysfunction (stimulatory)	TSH receptor	Graves disease (thyroid-stimulating antibody)
Antibody-mediated dysfunction (blocking)	AChR	Myasthenia gravis (blocks neuromuscular transmission)
Antibody-mediated dysfunction (blocking)	Intrinsic factor / parietal cell	Pernicious anaemia

In type II reactions, IgG or IgM antibodies are directed against antigens on cell surfaces or in the extracellular matrix. Three mechanisms of tissue injury operate. **Opsonisation and phagocytosis:** antibodies coat cells, promoting complement fixation (C3b opsonisation) and Fc receptor-mediated phagocytosis (autoimmune haemolytic anaemia, ITP). **Complement-dependent and antibody-dependent cytotoxicity:** the membrane attack complex (C5b-9) lyses target cells; NK cells and macrophages kill via ADCC (transfusion reactions, hyperacute transplant rejection, Goodpasture syndrome where anti-GBM antibodies destroy the glomerular basement membrane). **Antibody-mediated cellular dysfunction:** antibodies bind to receptors and either stimulate or block function without causing cell destruction. This mechanism underlies Graves disease (stimulatory anti-TSH receptor antibodies) and myasthenia gravis (blocking anti-acetylcholine receptor antibodies).

Type III Hypersensitivity: Immune Complex

Type III reactions result from the deposition of antigen-antibody (immune) complexes in tissues, with subsequent complement activation and neutrophil-mediated tissue damage. The key determinants of pathogenicity are the size of the complex (intermediate-sized complexes are most pathogenic because they are not efficiently cleared), the antigen-to-antibody ratio (slight antigen excess favours intermediate complex formation), and the haemodynamic characteristics of the deposition site (complexes preferentially deposit where blood is filtered or where there is turbulence: glomeruli, joints, skin, small vessels). SLE is the prototype systemic immune complex disease. The **Arthus reaction** is the localised form: intradermal injection of antigen in a previously sensitised individual produces localised vasculitis within 4–8 hours. **Serum sickness** is the systemic form: administration of a large dose of foreign protein (historically horse anti-tetanus serum) produces fever, urticaria, arthralgia, and glomerulonephritis 7–10 days later as immune complexes form and deposit.

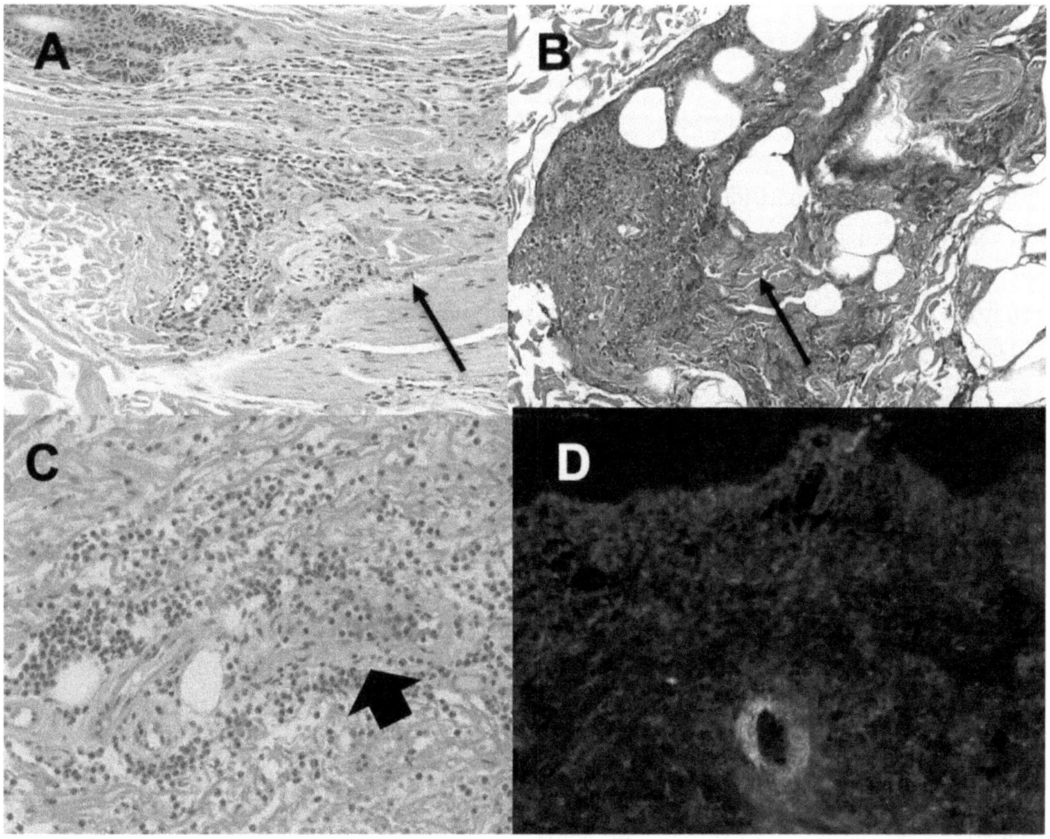

Figure 5.3: Type III hypersensitivity — immune complex vasculitis. (A) Fibrinoid necrosis of vessel wall, H&E. (B) Fibrinoid necrosis, PAS. (C) Leukocytoclastic vasculitis with nuclear dust, H&E. (D) Vascular IgG deposits, IF. (Source: Fraticelli P et al., Intern Emerg Med, CC BY 4.0. DOI: 10.1007/s11739-021-02688-x.)

Type IV Hypersensitivity: Cell-Mediated

Type IV reactions are mediated by T lymphocytes rather than antibodies. Two subtypes are recognised. **CD4+ T cell-mediated inflammation (delayed-type hypersensitivity, DTH):** CD4+ Th1 cells recognise antigen presented by macrophages, secrete IFN-γ and TNF, and activate macrophages, which become the principal effector cells. The classic example is the tuberculin (Mantoux) reaction: a zone of induration appears 24–72 hours after intradermal injection of PPD in a sensitised individual, composed of perivascular CD4+ T cells and activated macrophages. Granulomatous inflammation (TB, sarcoidosis, leprosy) is a variant in which persistent, poorly degradable antigens drive chronic macrophage activation, epithelioid cell transformation, and giant cell formation (see Chapter 2). CD4+ Th17 cells contribute to neutrophilic inflammation in contact dermatitis and certain autoimmune diseases. **CD8+ cytotoxic T lymphocyte (CTL)-mediated cytotoxicity:** CTLs recognise peptides presented on MHC class I and kill target cells via perforin-granzyme and Fas-FasL pathways. This mechanism is central to transplant rejection, viral hepatitis, and type 1 diabetes (destruction of beta cells).

Quick Recall: Hypersensitivity Reactions

Type I: IgE + mast cells; minutes; anaphylaxis, asthma, hay fever. Mediators: histamine, leukotrienes.

Type II: IgG/IgM vs cell surface antigens; complement, ADCC, receptor dysfunction. Graves (stimulatory), MG (blocking), Goodpasture (anti-GBM).

Type III: immune complex deposition; complement + neutrophils; SLE, PSGN, serum sickness.

Type IV: T cell-mediated; delayed (24–72 hrs); DTH (CD4+Th1, tuberculin), CTL (CD8+, transplant rejection).

Granulomatous inflammation: variant of type IV; persistent antigen → macrophage activation → epithelioid cells + giant cells.

Autoimmunity

Autoimmune diseases arise when the immune system mounts a sustained response against self-antigens. They affect 3–5% of the population and are a major cause of chronic morbidity. Two broad categories are recognised: **organ-specific** autoimmune diseases (immune response directed against a single organ, e.g., Hashimoto thyroiditis, type 1 diabetes, myasthenia gravis) and **systemic** autoimmune diseases (immune complexes or autoantibodies affect multiple organs, e.g., SLE, rheumatoid arthritis, systemic sclerosis).

Immunological Tolerance and Its Breakdown

Immunological tolerance is maintained by central mechanisms (clonal deletion; AIRE gene) and peripheral mechanisms (anergy, Tregs, Fas-FasL deletion, immune privilege), as summarised below.

Mechanisms of Autoimmunity

Autoimmunity results from failure of tolerance (defective AIRE→APECED; FOXP3 mutations→IPEX), molecular mimicry, release of sequestered antigens, epitope spreading, bystander activation, and HLA-linked genetic susceptibility (see Quick Recall box).

Quick Recall: Autoimmunity

Central tolerance: clonal deletion in thymus/marrow; AIRE gene drives ectopic self-antigen expression.

Peripheral tolerance: anergy, Tregs (FOXP3+), Fas-FasL deletion, immune privilege.

Molecular mimicry: strep M protein vs cardiac myosin (rheumatic fever); C. jejuni vs GM1 ganglioside (Guillain-Barré).

AIRE mutation: APECED (APS-1); FOXP3 mutation: IPEX syndrome (neonatal autoimmunity).

Strongest HLA associations: HLA-B27 (ankylosing spondylitis), HLA-DR4 (RA, type 1 DM), HLA-DQ2/DQ8 (coeliac disease).

Systemic Lupus Erythematosus (SLE)

SLE is the prototype systemic autoimmune disease, characterised by the production of autoantibodies against nuclear antigens and the deposition of immune complexes in multiple organs. It predominantly affects women of childbearing age (female-to-male ratio 9:1) with a peak incidence between 15 and 45 years.

SLE Pathogenesis

The pathogenesis of SLE involves genetic susceptibility (HLA-DR2/DR3, complement deficiencies C1q/C2/C4, polymorphisms in FcR genes, IRF5, STAT4, ITGAM), hormonal factors (oestrogen enhances and testosterone suppresses immune responses), environmental triggers (UV light induces apoptosis and DNA damage; EBV; drugs such as hydralazine, procainamide, isoniazid produce drug-induced lupus), and defective clearance of apoptotic cells (deficiency of C1q or DNase I impairs clearance of nuclear debris, exposing nuclear antigens to the immune system). The central immunological defect is a failure of tolerance to nuclear antigens, particularly double-stranded DNA (dsDNA), histones, and ribonucleoprotein complexes (Sm, RNP, Ro/SSA, La/SSB). Anti-dsDNA antibodies form immune complexes that deposit in the glomeruli, skin, joints, and serosal surfaces, causing type III hypersensitivity-mediated injury.

Antinuclear Antibodies (ANA) and Their Patterns

ANA testing by indirect immunofluorescence on HEp-2 cells is the screening test for SLE (sensitivity >95%). However, ANA positivity is not specific; it occurs in many autoimmune diseases, infections, and even in healthy individuals (low titres). The pattern of nuclear staining and the specificity of the antibody provide diagnostic and prognostic information.

Table 5.6: ANA patterns and associated antibodies in SLE and related diseases

IF Pattern	Target Antigen	Disease Association
Homogeneous (diffuse)	dsDNA, histones	SLE (active disease; anti-dsDNA correlates with nephritis), drug-induced lupus (anti-histone) **Clinical Pearl** SLE serology is a diagnostic ladder. Step one: ANA (homogeneous, speckled, rim, nucleolar). Sensitive but not specific; positive in scleroderma, MCTD, drug-induced lupus, Sjogren, even some healthy elderly. Step two: anti-dsDNA and anti-Smith are SLE-specific; anti-dsDNA correlates with disease activity and lupus nephritis; anti-Sm is specific but less sensitive. Step three: anti-Ro (SSA) and anti-La (SSB) point to Sjogren overlap, neonatal lupus risk, and subacute cutaneous lupus; anti-

		histone points to drug-induced lupus; anti-ribosomal P points to neuropsychiatric lupus. Read the ladder, not just the rung.
Rim (peripheral)	dsDNA, nuclear envelope (lamins)	SLE (highly specific for lupus nephritis; anti-dsDNA)
Speckled	Sm (Smith), U1-RNP, Ro/SSA, La/SSB	Anti-Sm: highly specific for SLE (low sensitivity). Anti-RNP: MCTD. Anti-Ro: Sjögren, neonatal lupus. Anti-La: Sjögren
Nucleolar	RNA polymerase I/III, fibrillarin, Scl-70 (topoisomerase I)	Systemic sclerosis (scleroderma); anti-Scl-70: diffuse SSc
Centromere	CENP-A/B/C	Limited cutaneous systemic sclerosis (CREST syndrome)

The key diagnostic clue: anti-dsDNA antibodies (detected by Farr assay or CLIF on Crithidia luciliae) are both highly specific for SLE and correlate with disease activity, particularly nephritis. Rising anti-dsDNA titres with falling complement levels (C3, C4) herald a lupus flare. Anti-Sm antibodies are the most specific for SLE but are present in only 25–30% of patients.

Diagnostic thinking: ANA + anti-dsDNA + wire-loop GN + full-house IF → SLE

Lupus Nephritis

Renal involvement occurs in 50–70% of SLE patients and is a major determinant of morbidity and mortality. The ISN/RPS classification (2003, revised 2018) divides lupus nephritis into six classes based on the renal biopsy (see Chapter 22 for detailed renal pathology).

Table 5.7: ISN/RPS classification of lupus nephritis (summary)

Class	Pattern	Key Features	Prognosis
I	Minimal mesangial	Normal LM; mesangial immune deposits on IF/EM only	Excellent
II	Mesangial proliferative	Mesangial hypercellularity on LM; mesangial deposits	Good
III	Focal lupus	<50% glomeruli affected; segmental	Variable; may progress

	nephritis	endocapillary ± extracapillary proliferation; subendothelial deposits	
IV	Diffuse lupus nephritis	≥50% glomeruli; diffuse endocapillary proliferation; "wire-loop" lesions (massive subendothelial deposits); most severe form	Poor without treatment
V	Membranous lupus nephritis	Diffuse thickening of GBM; subepithelial deposits; resembles primary membranous nephropathy	Nephrotic syndrome; moderate
VI	Advanced sclerotic	>90% globally sclerosed glomeruli	End-stage; irreversible

On IF microscopy, lupus nephritis shows the characteristic "full house" pattern: granular deposits of IgG, IgA, IgM, C3, and C1q along the GBM and in the mesangium. This pattern is virtually diagnostic of lupus nephritis. On EM, electron-dense deposits are seen in subendothelial (class III/IV), subepithelial (class V), and mesangial locations. Tubuloreticular inclusions ("interferon footprints") in endothelial cells are another EM hallmark.

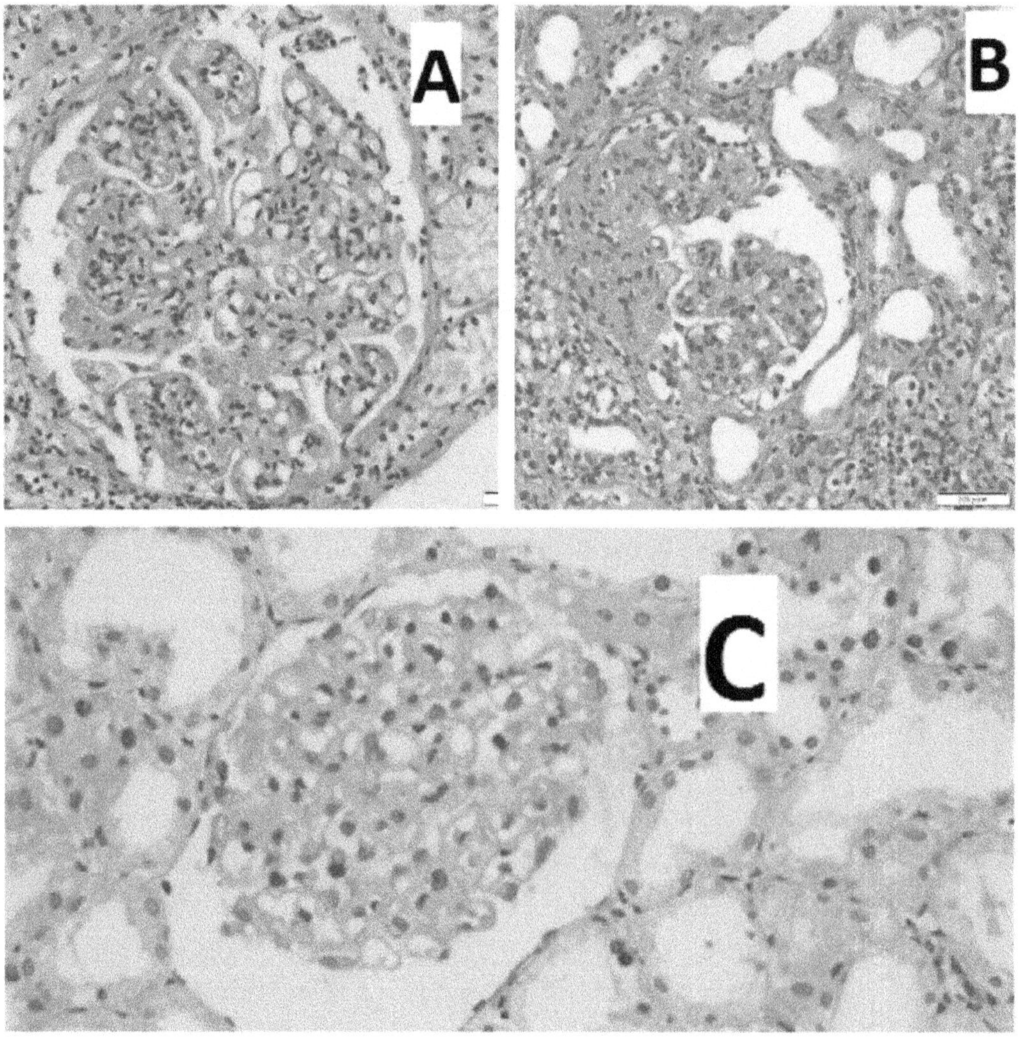

Figure 5.4: Lupus nephritis — wire loop lesion. H&E. (A) Diffuse proliferative GN with thickened capillary walls, (B) mesangial proliferation, (C) wire loop lesions at high power. (Source: Javeed S et al., Cureus 2022, CC BY 3.0. DOI: 10.7759/cureus.28363.)

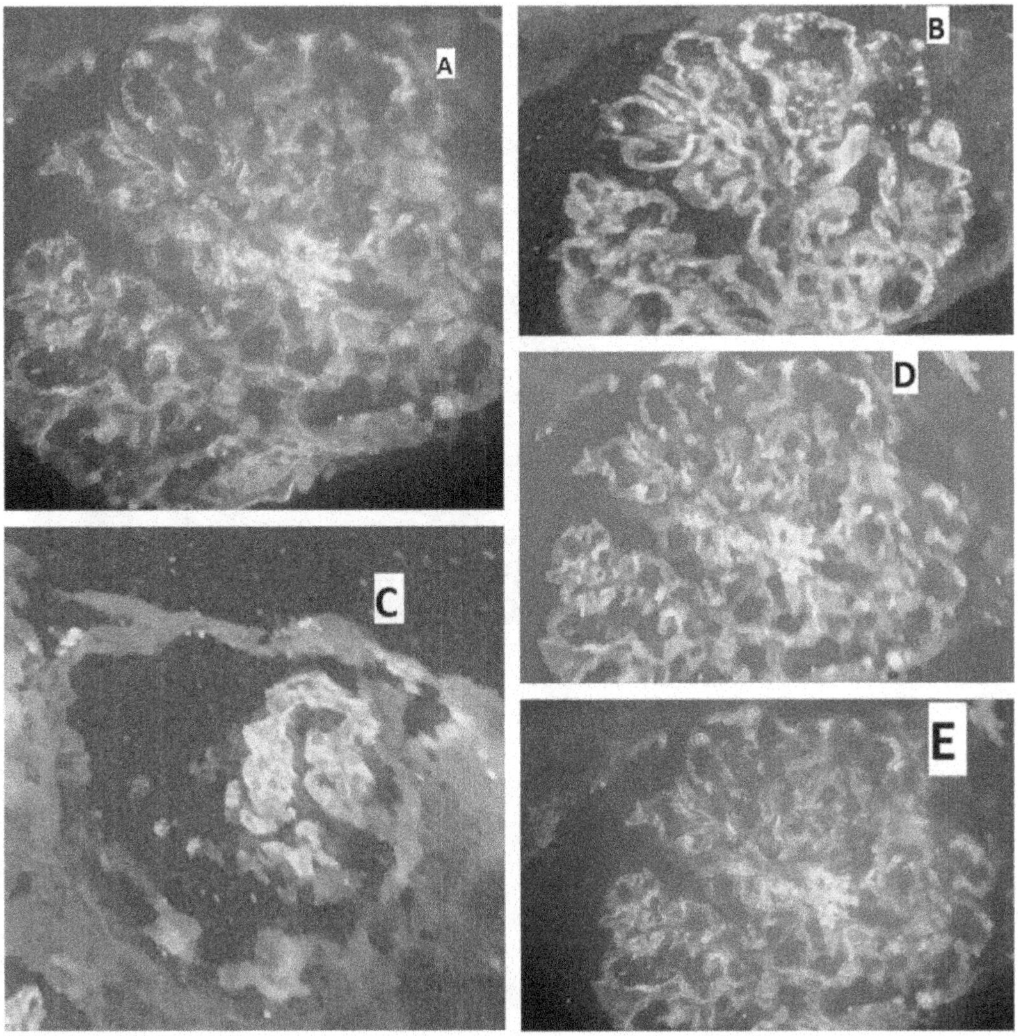

Figure 5.5: Lupus nephritis — full house immunofluorescence. Granular capillary wall staining for (A) IgG, (B) IgM, (C) C1q, (D) C3, (E) IgA. (Source: Javeed S et al., Cureus 2022, CC BY 3.0. DOI: 10.7759/cureus.28363.)

Integration: *Lupus nephritis is covered in detail in Chapter 22 (Renal Pathology Part 1). The IF and EM findings of SLE nephritis are among the most frequently tested topics across both general pathology and systemic pathology papers.*

Exam Pitfall

Drug-induced lupus (hydralazine, procainamide, isoniazid) presents with anti-histone antibodies (homogeneous ANA pattern), arthralgia, serositis, and rash, but does NOT cause renal or CNS disease. Anti-dsDNA is characteristically absent. Symptoms resolve on drug withdrawal (Figure 5.6).

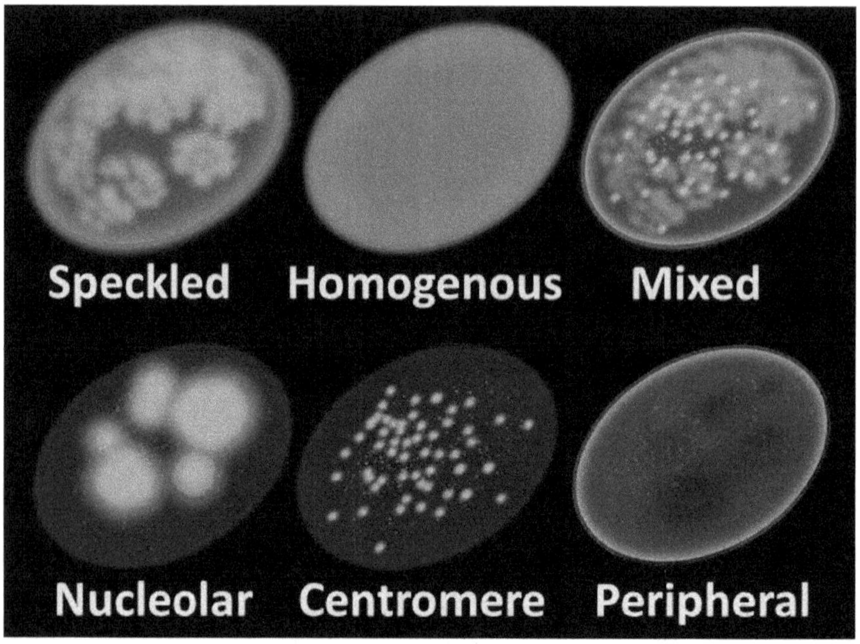

Figure 5.6: Antinuclear antibody (ANA) immunofluorescence patterns on HEp-2 cells. Top row: speckled, homogeneous, mixed. Bottom row: nucleolar, centromere, peripheral. Each pattern correlates with specific autoantibodies (see Table 5.6). (Source: Al-Mughales JA. Minor edits by Mikael Häggström, Wikimedia Commons, CC BY 2.0.)

Quick Recall: SLE

F:M ratio: 9:1; peak 15–45 years; South Asian prevalence likely underestimated.

Pathogenesis: defective clearance of apoptotic debris → nuclear antigen exposure → anti-dsDNA/anti-Sm → immune complex deposition (Figure 5.7).

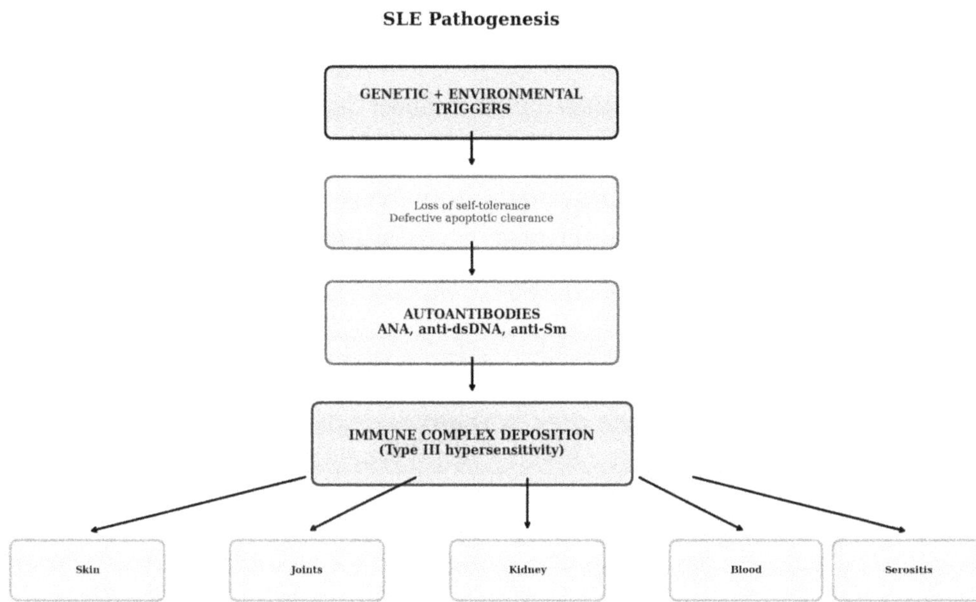

Figure 5.7: SLE Pathogenesis. *(Source: Author's original.)*

Anti-dsDNA: specific for SLE; correlates with nephritis and disease activity.
Anti-Sm: most specific for SLE (but low sensitivity, ~25–30%).
Full house IF: IgG + IgA + IgM + C3 + C1q; diagnostic of lupus nephritis.
Wire-loop lesion: class IV (diffuse) lupus nephritis; massive subendothelial immune deposits.
Drug-induced lupus: anti-histone antibodies; no renal/CNS disease; resolves on drug withdrawal.

Organ Manifestations of SLE Beyond the Kidney

Skin: The classic butterfly (malar) rash is a photosensitive erythema over the cheeks and nasal bridge, sparing the nasolabial folds. Discoid lupus produces well-defined erythematous plaques with adherent keratotic scaling, follicular plugging, and atrophic scarring. Histologically, skin lesions show interface dermatitis with basal vacuolar change, perivascular lymphocytic infiltrate, thickening of the basement membrane zone ("lupus band" on direct IF showing granular IgG/IgM/C3 deposits at the dermal-epidermal junction), and mucin deposition in the dermis.

Joints: Non-erosive arthritis affecting small joints is one of the most common presenting features. Unlike rheumatoid arthritis, lupus arthropathy does not typically produce joint destruction (Jaccoud arthropathy is a deforming but non-erosive pattern).

Serosal surfaces: Pleuritis and pericarditis (serositis) occur in >50% of patients and may produce effusions.

Cardiovascular: Libman-Sacks endocarditis (sterile verrucous vegetations on both surfaces of the mitral and aortic valves) is characteristic. Accelerated atherosclerosis is a major cause of late morbidity and mortality in SLE, driven by chronic inflammation and corticosteroid therapy.

Haematological: autoimmune haemolytic anaemia, thrombocytopenia, leucopenia, and lymphopenia are common. Anti-phospholipid antibodies (present in 30–40% of SLE patients) predispose to thrombosis and pregnancy loss (see Chapter 4).

CNS: Neuropsychiatric lupus manifests as seizures, psychosis, cerebrovascular disease, and cognitive dysfunction, resulting from vasculopathy, autoantibody-mediated neuronal injury, and complement-mediated damage (Figure 5.8).

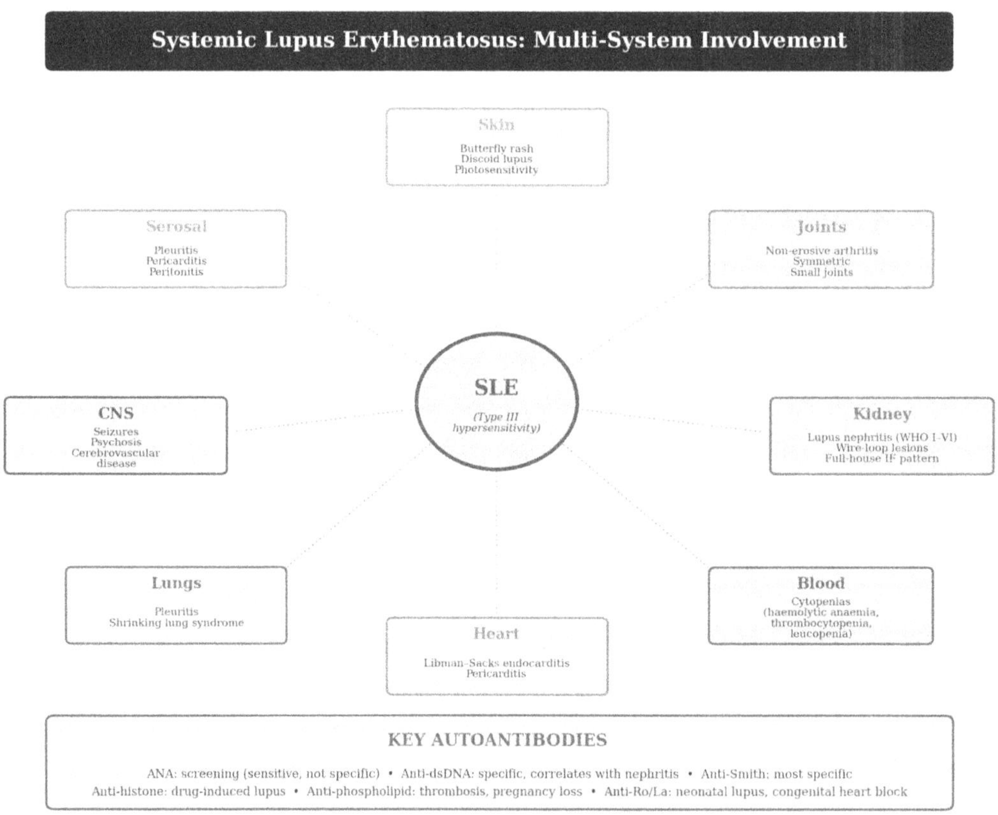

Figure 5.8: Multi-system involvement in systemic lupus erythematosus (SLE). (Source: Author's original.)

Other Selected Autoimmune Diseases

Sjögren Syndrome

Sjögren syndrome is a chronic autoimmune disorder characterised by immune-mediated destruction of the lacrimal and salivary glands, producing keratoconjunctivitis sicca (dry eyes) and xerostomia (dry mouth). It may be primary or secondary (associated with another autoimmune disease, most commonly RA or SLE). Histologically, the salivary glands show a dense lymphoplasmacytic infiltrate (predominantly CD4+ T cells) surrounding and replacing acinar tissue, with formation of epimyoepithelial islands (lymphoepithelial lesions). Autoantibodies include anti-Ro/SSA and anti-La/SSB (anti-Ro is associated with neonatal lupus and congenital heart block when present in pregnant women). Patients with Sjögren syndrome have a 40-fold increased risk of developing mucosa-associated lymphoid tissue (MALT) lymphoma of the parotid gland.

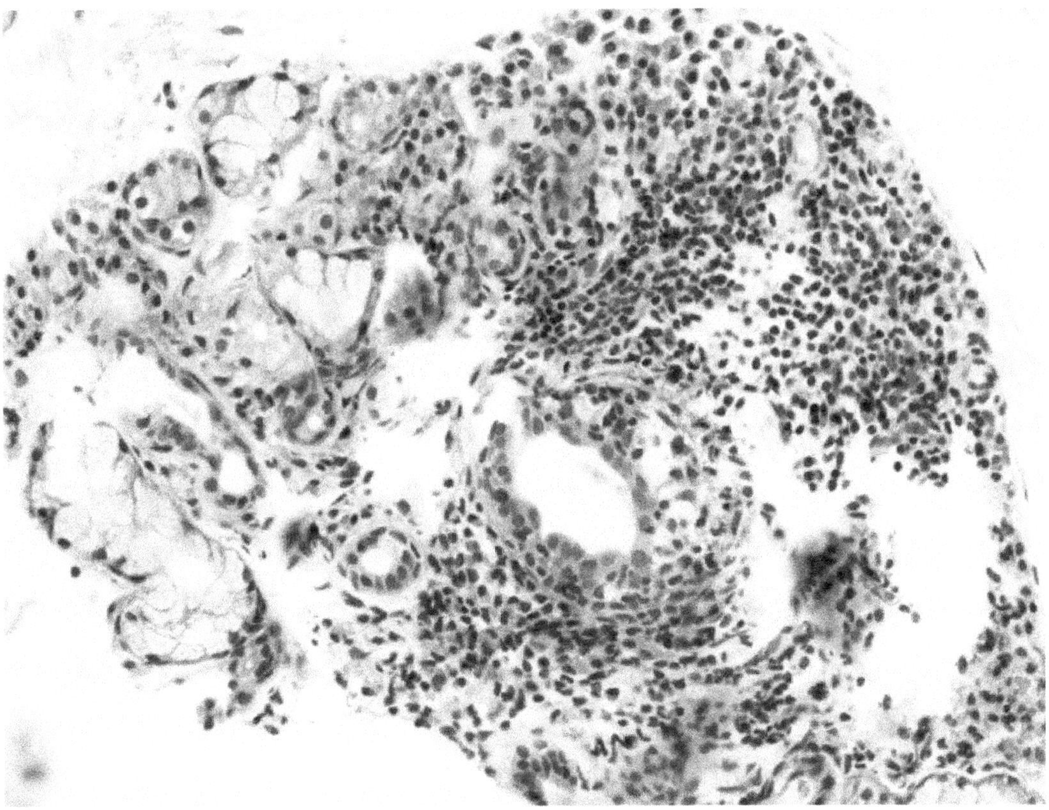

Figure 5.9: Sjögren syndrome — lymphocytic sialadenitis. Salivary gland biopsy showing dense lymphocytic infiltrate with periductal aggregates and acinar destruction. H&E. (Source: Nephron, Wikimedia Commons, CC BY-SA 3.0.)

Systemic Sclerosis (Scleroderma)

Systemic sclerosis is characterised by excessive fibrosis in the skin and visceral organs, obliterative vascular disease, and autoimmunity. Two clinical subtypes are recognised. **Diffuse cutaneous SSc** involves widespread skin thickening (proximal and distal) and early visceral involvement (lung, kidney, GI, heart). It is associated with anti-Scl-70 (anti-topoisomerase I) antibodies and a nucleolar ANA pattern. **Limited cutaneous SSc (CREST syndrome)** features calcinosis, Raynaud phenomenon, oesophageal dysmotility, sclerodactyly, and telangiectasia. It is associated with anti-centromere antibodies. Pulmonary arterial hypertension is a major cause of death in limited SSc.

The pathogenesis involves three interconnected processes: vascular injury (endothelial damage, intimal fibrosis of small arteries), immune activation (CD4+ T cells, macrophages, fibrogenic cytokines including TGF-β, PDGF, and IL-13), and progressive fibrosis (myofibroblast activation and excessive collagen deposition). Histologically, the skin shows progressive dermal fibrosis with loss of adnexa, thinning of the epidermis, and perivascular lymphocytic infiltrate in early lesions.

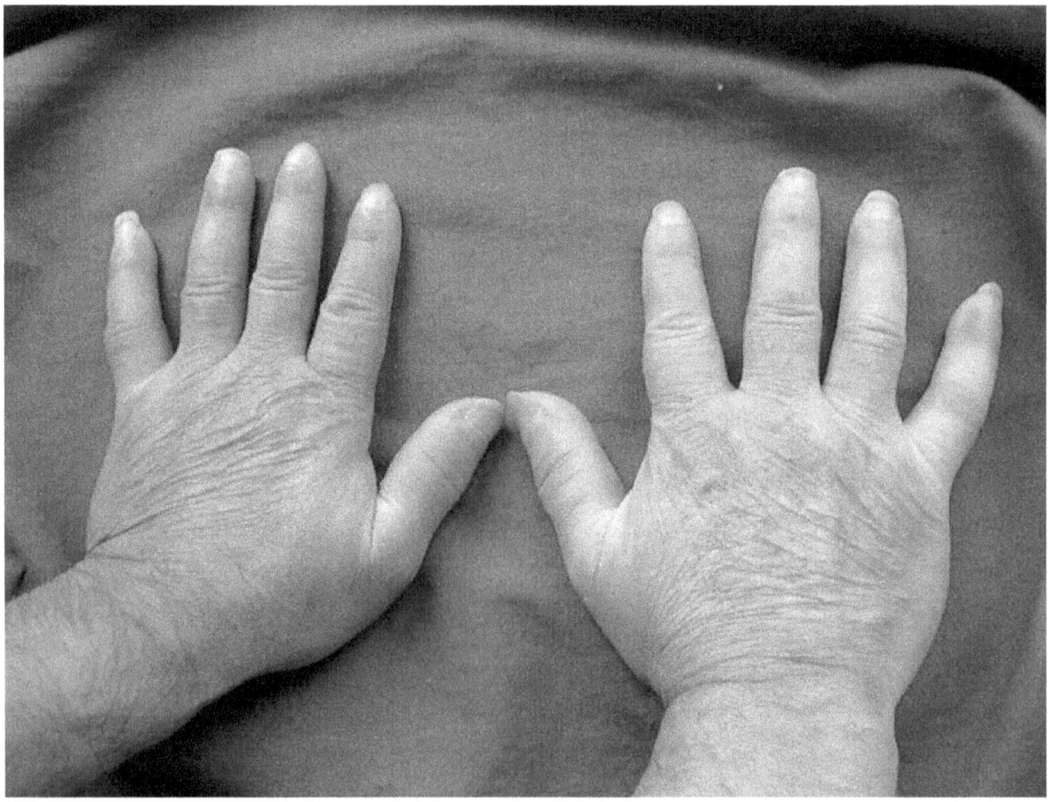

Figure 5.10: Systemic sclerosis — bilateral hand involvement showing sclerodactyly with taut, shiny skin and flexion contractures (Clinical photograph) (Source: Maria Sieglinda von Nudeldorf, Wikimedia Commons, CC BY-SA 4.0.)

IgG4-Related Disease

IgG4-related disease (IgG4-RD) is a recently recognised fibroinflammatory condition characterised by tumour-like swelling of affected organs, a dense lymphoplasmacytic infiltrate rich in IgG4-positive plasma cells, storiform fibrosis (a characteristic "cartwheel" pattern), obliterative phlebitis, and elevated serum IgG4 levels (though not universally present). It can affect virtually any organ, but the most commonly involved sites are the pancreas (autoimmune pancreatitis type 1, previously called lymphoplasmacytic sclerosing pancreatitis), salivary glands (Mikulicz disease), lacrimal glands, retroperitoneum (retroperitoneal fibrosis), aorta, kidneys (tubulointerstitial nephritis), and thyroid (Riedel thyroiditis). The histological triad of storiform fibrosis, >10 IgG4+ plasma cells per HPF (or IgG4/IgG ratio >40%), and obliterative phlebitis is diagnostic. IgG4-RD responds dramatically to corticosteroids and rituximab (anti-CD20).

Disease	Key Antibody	Key Features
Sjögren syndrome	Anti-Ro/SSA, Anti-La/SSB	Dry eyes + dry mouth; lymphocytic sialadenitis; 40× MALT lymphoma risk
Diffuse SSc	Anti-Scl-70 (topoisomerase I)	Widespread skin + visceral fibrosis; scleroderma renal crisis
Limited SSc (CREST)	Anti-centromere	Calcinosis, Raynaud, oesophageal dysmotility, sclerodactyly, telangiectasia; PAH
IgG4-RD	Elevated serum IgG4 (variable)	Storiform fibrosis + IgG4+ plasma cells + obliterative phlebitis; responds to steroids/rituximab
Rheumatoid arthritis	RF (IgM anti-IgG), Anti-CCP (most specific)	Symmetric erosive polyarthritis; pannus formation; rheumatoid nodules; see Chapter 29
Dermatomyositis	Anti-Mi-2, Anti-MDA5	Proximal muscle weakness + heliotrope rash + Gottron papules; malignancy screen mandatory

The Complement System in Disease

The complement system consists of over 30 proteins activated sequentially via three pathways (classical, alternative, lectin) that converge on C3 convertase formation, leading to opsonisation (C3b), chemotaxis/anaphylatoxins (C3a, C5a), and cell lysis (C5b-9 MAC). See table for pathway details and regulatory proteins. Complement deficiencies: C1q/C2/C4 deficiency predisposes to SLE (impaired immune complex clearance); C3 deficiency causes severe pyogenic infections; C5-9 (MAC) deficiency predisposes to Neisseria infections; C1-INH deficiency causes hereditary angioedema. See table.

Quick Recall: Complement in Disease

C1q/C2/C4 deficiency: SLE-like immune complex disease (impaired clearance).

C3 deficiency: severe recurrent pyogenic infections (loss of opsonisation).

C5–C9 deficiency: recurrent Neisseria infections (meningococcal, gonococcal).

C1-INH deficiency: hereditary angioedema (bradykinin-mediated; NOT histamine-mediated → does not respond to antihistamines/adrenaline).

PNH: PIG-A mutation → loss of CD55/CD59 → unregulated MAC → complement-mediated haemolysis; eculizumab (anti-C5) is therapeutic.

Transplant Rejection and Graft-versus-Host Disease (Figure 5.11)

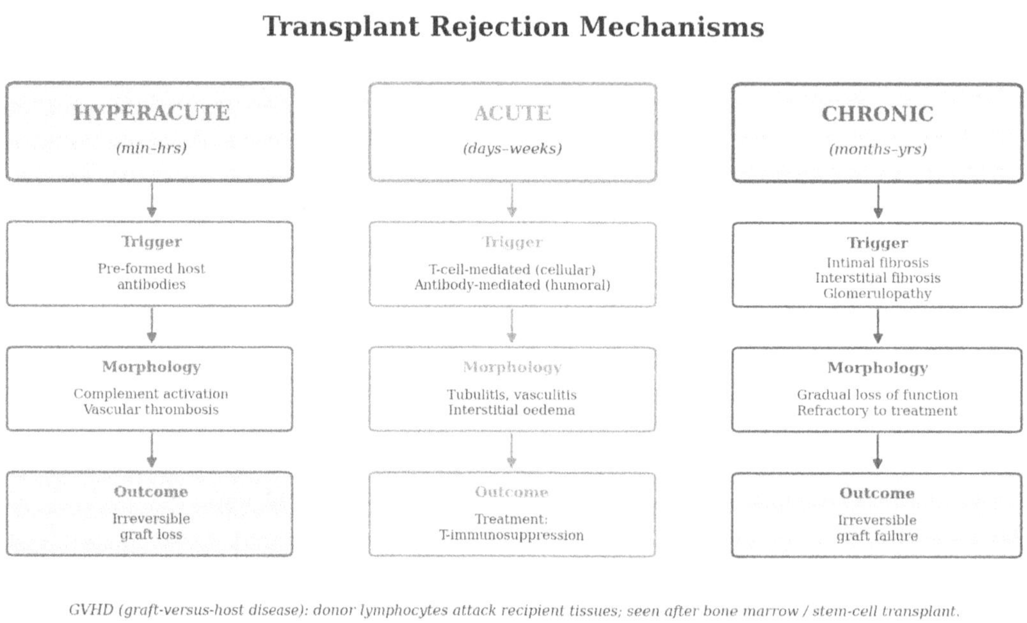

Figure 5.11: Transplant Rejection Mechanisms. *(Source: Author's original.)*

Transplant rejection is an immune response directed against foreign HLA antigens on the graft. Three temporal patterns are recognised based on the mechanism and time course.

Table 5.8: Mechanisms of transplant rejection

Type	Time Course	Mechanism	Morphology
Hyperacute	Minutes to hours	Preformed antibodies against donor HLA or ABO antigens; complement activation; endothelial injury	Widespread thrombosis, fibrinoid necrosis of graft vessels; graft becomes

			cyanotic and infarcted
Acute	Days to weeks (cellular) or weeks to months (humoral)	Cellular: CD8+ CTL kill graft cells (tubulitis, endotheliitis). Humoral: donor-specific antibodies against HLA; complement (C4d deposition)	Cellular: interstitial lymphocytic infiltrate, tubulitis. Humoral: vasculitis, C4d+ on peritubular capillaries
Chronic	Months to years	Combination of T cell and antibody-mediated injury; vascular intimal fibrosis (graft arteriosclerosis)	Intimal fibrosis of graft vessels ("transplant vasculopathy"); interstitial fibrosis and tubular atrophy (IFTA)

Graft-versus-Host Disease (GVHD)

GVHD occurs when immunocompetent donor T cells in the graft recognise and attack host tissues. It is the principal complication of allogeneic haematopoietic stem cell transplantation (see Volume 1) and may also occur after transfusion of non-irradiated blood products to immunocompromised patients. GVHD is classified as acute (typically within 100 days of transplant, though the modern definition is based on clinical features rather than time) or chronic (after 100 days).

Acute GVHD targets three organs: skin (maculopapular rash, may progress to erythroderma and epidermal necrolysis), liver (jaundice from bile duct destruction), and GI tract (diarrhoea, mucosal ulceration, crypt apoptosis). The histological hallmark is apoptosis of epithelial cells (satellite cell necrosis: apoptotic cell with adjacent lymphocyte) in the affected organs.

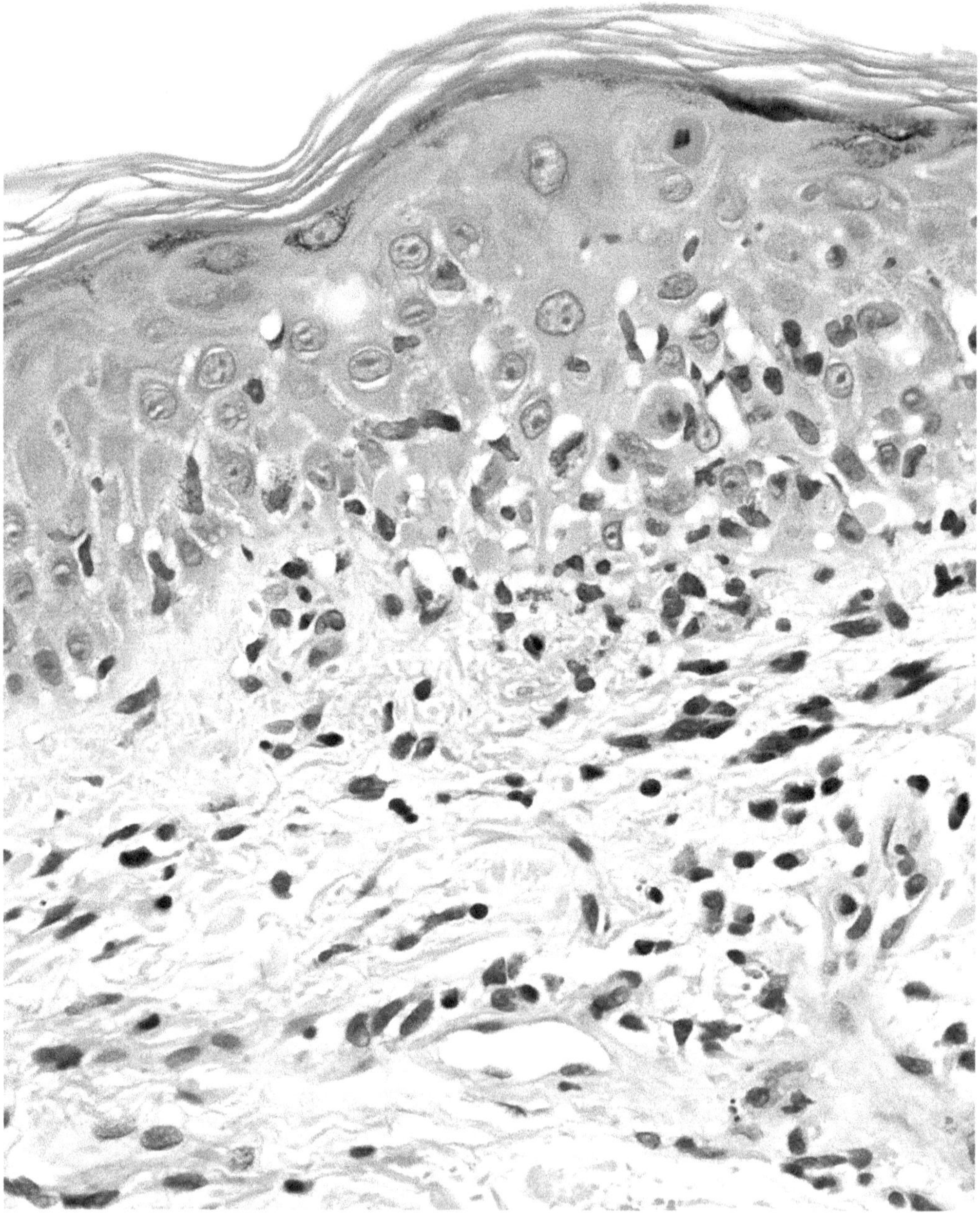

Figure 5.12: Graft-versus-host disease — skin. H&E, high magnification. Interface dermatitis with basal vacuolization, dyskeratotic keratinocytes (apoptotic bodies), dermal lymphocytic infiltrate, and melanin incontinence. (Source: Nephron, Wikimedia Commons, CC BY-SA 3.0.)

Chronic GVHD resembles a systemic autoimmune disease, with features of scleroderma (skin fibrosis), Sjögren syndrome (sicca), bronchiolitis obliterans (lung), and chronic liver disease. It may follow acute GVHD or arise de novo.

Integration: Transplant rejection connects to renal transplant pathology (Chapter 23, antibody-mediated rejection and C4d staining), autoimmune hepatitis and recurrent disease in liver allografts (Chapter 20), cardiac allograft vasculopathy (Chapter 14), and GVHD in allogeneic HSCT (Volume 1, Chapters 35–36). The HLA matching principles discussed here underpin organ allocation algorithms and post-transplant immunosuppressive protocols across all solid organ and haematopoietic stem cell transplantation settings.

HIV Infection and AIDS

HIV (human immunodeficiency virus) is a retrovirus of the lentivirus family. HIV-1 is responsible for the vast majority of infections worldwide; HIV-2 is largely confined to West Africa and is less virulent.

HIV Pathogenesis

HIV targets CD4+ T lymphocytes. The viral envelope glycoprotein gp120 binds to CD4 on the T cell surface, then undergoes conformational change to bind a co-receptor: CCR5 (on macrophages and memory T cells; used by R5/macrophage-tropic strains in early disease) or CXCR4 (on T cells; used by X4/T-tropic strains in late disease). The transmembrane glycoprotein gp41 mediates fusion of the viral and cell membranes. After entry, reverse transcriptase converts viral RNA to DNA, which integrase inserts into the host genome (provirus). The provirus may remain latent in resting memory CD4+ T cells (the latent reservoir, the major barrier to cure) or, upon T-cell activation, is transcribed, assembled, and released by budding.

gp120 binds CD4 → gp120 binds CCR5/CXCR4 (co-receptor) → gp41-mediated fusion → Reverse transcriptase (RNA → DNA) → Integrase (provirus) → Latent reservoir OR Transcription → Assembly → Budding (protease)

CD4+ T-cell depletion occurs through multiple mechanisms: direct viral cytopathic effect, activation-induced apoptosis of uninfected bystander cells, CTL killing of infected cells, and impaired thymic output. The clinical consequence is progressive immunodeficiency, with susceptibility to opportunistic infections and certain neoplasms once the CD4 count falls below 200 cells/µL (the WHO/CDC threshold for AIDS).

Table 5.11: AIDS-defining opportunistic infections and neoplasms

CD4 Count	Opportunistic Infections	AIDS-Defining Neoplasms
<200/µL	Pneumocystis jirovecii pneumonia (PCP), oesophageal candidiasis, disseminated histoplasmosis	Kaposi sarcoma (HHV-8), primary CNS lymphoma (EBV)

<100/µL	Toxoplasma encephalitis, cryptosporidiosis (chronic diarrhoea), microsporidiosis	Non-Hodgkin lymphoma (diffuse large B-cell, Burkitt)
<50/µL	Disseminated Mycobacterium avium complex (MAC), CMV retinitis, progressive multifocal leukoencephalopathy (JC virus)	Invasive cervical carcinoma (HPV)

Natural History of HIV Infection

The clinical course of untreated HIV infection follows three phases. The **acute (primary) phase** occurs 2–4 weeks after exposure: high viraemia, widespread viral dissemination to lymphoid tissue, a sharp drop in CD4 count, and a transient mononucleosis-like illness (fever, pharyngitis, lymphadenopathy, rash) in 50–70% of patients. The immune response (HIV-specific CTLs) partially controls viraemia, establishing a viral set point. The **chronic (clinical latency) phase** lasts years (median 8–10 years without ART): the patient is often asymptomatic or has persistent generalised lymphadenopathy, but the virus is actively replicating in lymphoid tissue, and CD4 counts decline progressively at a rate of approximately 50–65 cells/µL per year. Minor opportunistic infections (oral candidiasis, herpes zoster, oral hairy leukoplakia) may appear as CD4 counts fall below 500. **AIDS** is the final phase, defined by CD4 <200/µL or an AIDS-defining illness. Without treatment, survival after an AIDS diagnosis was historically 1–3 years. ART has transformed this; with adherence, near-normal life expectancy is achievable.

Acute infection (high viraemia, ↓CD4) → Immune response (CTL, set point) → Clinical latency (years, progressive CD4 decline) → AIDS (CD4 <200, OIs, neoplasms)

Laboratory Diagnosis of HIV

The WHO-recommended testing strategy uses a sequential rapid-test algorithm: three rapid tests ("tridot" or immunochromatographic assays using different antigen preparations) are performed sequentially; if the first is reactive, a second test with a different assay principle is performed, and if discordant, a third test decides. Fourth-generation assays detect both anti-HIV antibodies and p24 antigen simultaneously, narrowing the window period to approximately 2 weeks. **Viral load (HIV RNA by RT-PCR)** is the gold standard for monitoring treatment response and is the earliest marker of infection (detectable within 10 days of exposure, during the window period before antibody seroconversion). **CD4 count** is used for staging and for determining when to initiate or modify prophylaxis against opportunistic infections. Western blot, once used as a confirmatory test, has been replaced by fourth-generation assays and nucleic acid testing in most guidelines.

Morphology of HIV Lymphadenopathy

Lymph node biopsy in HIV shows a progression of histological changes that mirrors the clinical phases. In early disease, there is follicular hyperplasia with large, irregular germinal centres showing follicle lysis (disruption of the follicular dendritic cell network by HIV, with "naked" germinal centres devoid of mantle zones). As disease progresses, there is involution of follicles, depletion of lymphocytes, increased vascularity, and fibrosis ("burnt-out" lymphadenopathy). In advanced AIDS, the lymph node architecture is effaced, with marked lymphocyte depletion. The pathologist must also consider opportunistic infections (mycobacterial, fungal) and lymphomas (DLBCL, Burkitt, primary effusion lymphoma) in the differential of lymphadenopathy in HIV-positive patients (Figure 5.13).

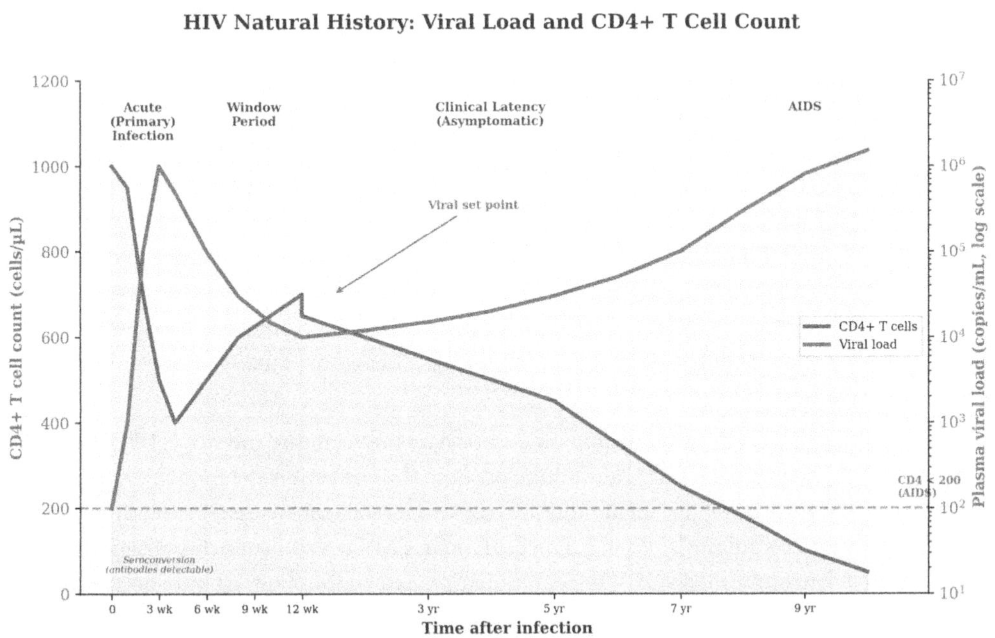

Figure 5.13: Natural history of HIV infection: viral load and CD4 count over time. (Source: Author's original.)

Quick Recall: HIV/AIDS

HIV entry: gp120 → CD4 → CCR5/CXCR4 co-receptor → gp41 fusion. CCR5Δ32 homozygosity confers near-complete resistance.

Latent reservoir: resting memory CD4+ T cells harbour integrated provirus; major barrier to cure.

AIDS definition: CD4 <200/µL or AIDS-defining illness.

Most common OI in TB-endemic settings: tuberculosis (pulmonary and extrapulmonary).

AIDS-defining neoplasms: Kaposi sarcoma (HHV-8), NHL (EBV-driven), invasive cervical carcinoma (HPV).

WHO Clinical Staging of HIV/AIDS (Adults and Adolescents)

WHO clinical staging classifies HIV disease by clinical events that predict prognosis and guide ART initiation decisions, particularly where CD4 testing is not routine. Stage 4 conditions are AIDS-defining.

Table 9.3a: WHO Clinical Stages of HIV/AIDS

Stage	Clinical features (representative)
Stage 1 — Asymptomatic	Asymptomatic HIV infection; persistent generalised lymphadenopathy. Performance scale 1 (normal activity).
Stage 2 — Mild symptoms	Moderate unexplained weight loss (<10%); recurrent respiratory tract infections (sinusitis, otitis, pharyngitis); herpes zoster; angular cheilitis; recurrent oral ulcers; papular pruritic eruptions; seborrhoeic dermatitis; fungal nail infections.
Stage 3 — Advanced symptoms	Unexplained severe weight loss (>10%); unexplained chronic diarrhoea >1 month; unexplained persistent fever >1 month; persistent oral candidiasis; oral hairy leukoplakia; pulmonary tuberculosis; severe bacterial infections (pneumonia, pyomyositis, empyema); acute necrotising ulcerative stomatitis/gingivitis/periodontitis; unexplained anaemia (<8 g/dL), neutropenia ($<0.5\times10^9$/L), or chronic thrombocytopenia ($<50\times10^9$/L).
Stage 4 — Severe symptoms (AIDS)	HIV wasting syndrome; Pneumocystis jirovecii pneumonia (PCP); recurrent severe bacterial pneumonia; chronic HSV infection (>1 month) or visceral HSV; oesophageal candidiasis (or candidiasis of trachea/bronchi/lungs); extrapulmonary TB; Kaposi sarcoma; CMV retinitis or other organ CMV; CNS toxoplasmosis; HIV encephalopathy; extrapulmonary cryptococcosis (including meningitis); disseminated NTM infection; progressive multifocal leukoencephalopathy (PML); chronic cryptosporidiosis/isosporiasis; disseminated mycosis (histoplasmosis, coccidioidomycosis); non-typhoidal Salmonella septicaemia; lymphoma (Burkitt, DLBCL, primary CNS); invasive cervical carcinoma; atypical disseminated leishmaniasis; symptomatic HIV-associated nephropathy or cardiomyopathy.

Under the current WHO "treat-all" policy (2016 onwards), antiretroviral therapy is initiated at diagnosis regardless of CD4 count or clinical stage. Staging remains useful for prognosis and for opportunistic-infection prophylaxis decisions (e.g., PCP prophylaxis at CD4 <200 or WHO Stage 3/4).

Primary Immunodeficiency Diseases

Primary (congenital) immunodeficiencies are genetically determined defects in the immune system. Though individually rare, they are important for understanding immune function and are frequently tested. They are classified by the component of the immune system that is defective.

Table 5.13: Selected primary immunodeficiency diseases

Defect	Disease	Gene/Mechanism	Key Features

B-cell (humoral)	X-linked agammaglobulinaemia (Bruton)	BTK gene mutation; block in pre-B to B-cell maturation	Males; absent B cells and Ig; recurrent bacterial infections after 6 months (maternal IgG wanes)
	Common variable immunodeficiency (CVID)	Heterogeneous; defective B-cell differentiation	Adults; low IgG/IgA; recurrent sinopulmonary infections; increased lymphoma and autoimmune risk
	Selective IgA deficiency	Most common primary immunodeficiency	Usually asymptomatic; mucosal infections; anaphylaxis to blood products containing IgA
	Hyper-IgM syndrome	CD40L (X-linked) or AID mutation; defective class switching	Elevated IgM, absent IgG/IgA/IgE; susceptible to Pneumocystis, Cryptosporidium
T-cell (cellular)	DiGeorge syndrome	22q11.2 deletion (TBX1); thymic hypoplasia	T-cell deficiency, hypoparathyroidism (hypocalcaemia), cardiac defects, facial dysmorphism
Combined B+T	Severe combined immunodeficiency (SCID)	Multiple genes (IL-2Rγc most common X-linked; ADA deficiency autosomal recessive)	Absent T cells ± B cells ± NK cells; fatal in infancy without HSCT; "bubble boy" disease
Phagocyte	Chronic granulomatous disease (CGD)	NADPH oxidase deficiency (CYBB, X-linked most common)	Cannot generate respiratory burst; recurrent catalase-positive infections (S. aureus, Aspergillus); granuloma formation; negative NBT/DHR test
	Chédiak-Higashi syndrome	LYST gene; defective lysosomal trafficking	Giant granules in neutrophils; oculocutaneous albinism; recurrent pyogenic infections
Combined (with syndromic features)	Wiskott-Aldrich syndrome	WAS gene (WASP protein); X-linked	Triad: thrombocytopenia (small platelets), eczema, recurrent infections; increased risk of lymphoma; IgM low, IgA/IgE elevated

Complement	C2/C4 deficiency		Increased susceptibility to immune complex disease (SLE-like)
	C5–C9 (MAC) deficiency		Recurrent Neisseria (meningococcal/gonococcal) infections

Why does a patient with SCID present with absent T cells but variable B and NK cell numbers? The answer lies in the specific genetic defect. X-linked SCID (IL-2Rγc mutation) affects the common gamma chain shared by receptors for IL-2, IL-4, IL-7, IL-9, IL-15, and IL-21. IL-7 is essential for T-cell development, and IL-15 for NK-cell development; hence this form produces T−B+NK− SCID. ADA deficiency, by contrast, causes accumulation of toxic purine metabolites in all lymphocyte lineages, producing T−B−NK− SCID.

The distinction between humoral and cellular immunodeficiency is clinically important: humoral (B-cell) deficiencies present with recurrent sinopulmonary and GI tract bacterial infections (encapsulated organisms: pneumococcus, Haemophilus) because antibody-mediated opsonisation is impaired. Cellular (T-cell) deficiencies present with severe viral, fungal, and intracellular bacterial infections (CMV, PCP, mycobacteria) because cell-mediated immunity is impaired. Combined deficiencies present with both spectra.

Quick Recall: Primary Immunodeficiency

Bruton (XLA): BTK mutation; no B cells/Ig; recurrent bacterial infections after 6 months.

SCID: most severe; IL-2Rγc (T−B+NK−) or ADA (T−B−NK−); fatal without HSCT.

DiGeorge: 22q11.2 deletion; thymic hypoplasia; T-cell deficiency + hypoparathyroidism + cardiac defects.

CGD: NADPH oxidase defect; catalase-positive organisms; NBT/DHR test diagnostic.

Wiskott-Aldrich: WAS gene; triad of thrombocytopenia (small platelets) + eczema + infections.

IgA deficiency: most common PID; usually asymptomatic; anaphylaxis risk with IgA-containing blood products.

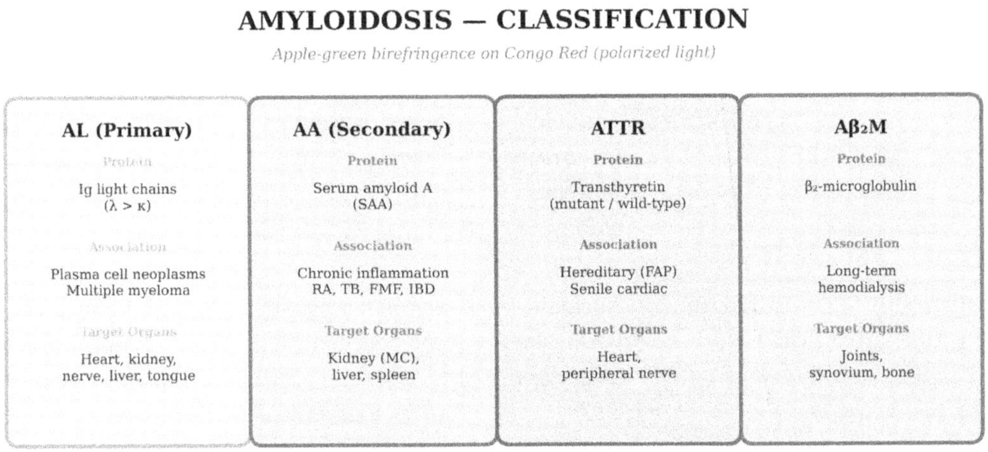

Figure 5.14: Amyloidosis Classification. (Source: Author's original.)

Amyloidosis

Amyloidosis is a group of disorders characterised by the extracellular deposition of abnormally folded proteins (amyloid) that aggregate into insoluble fibrils with a characteristic beta-pleated sheet configuration. Regardless of the precursor protein, all forms of amyloid share three defining properties: (1) Congo red staining with apple-green birefringence under polarised light; (2) fibrillar ultrastructure (7.10–10 nm non-branching fibrils on EM); and (3) a rigid, non-branching, cross-beta-pleated sheet conformation detectable by X-ray diffraction.

Diagnostic thinking: apple-green birefringence under polarised light on Congo red → amyloid

Classification and Pathogenesis

Table 5.14: Classification of amyloidosis

Type	Fibril Protein	Precursor	Clinical Setting	Organ Involvement
AL (primary; most common systemic form in the West)	Immunoglobulin light chains (κ or λ)	Monoclonal Ig from plasma cell neoplasm	Plasma cell myeloma, MGUS, Waldenström macroglobulinaemia	Heart (restrictive CMP), kidney (nephrotic), liver, tongue (macroglossia), peripheral nerves
AA (secondary/reactive)	Serum amyloid A (SAA)	Hepatic acute-phase reactant	Chronic inflammatory conditions: RA, IBD, TB, FMF,	Kidney (most common and earliest), liver, spleen; does NOT involve heart

			bronchiectasis, chronic osteomyelitis	
Aβ (cerebral)	Aβ peptide (from APP)	Amyloid precursor protein (APP)	Alzheimer disease, Down syndrome (trisomy 21)	Brain: senile plaques, cerebral amyloid angiopathy
ATTR (transthyretin)	Transthyretin (TTR)	Normal (wild-type) or mutant TTR	Familial amyloid polyneuropathy (FAP); senile cardiac amyloidosis (wild-type ATTR)	Peripheral nerves (mutant); heart (wild-type, elderly males)
Aβ2M (dialysis-associated)	Beta-2 microglobulin	Not cleared by dialysis membranes	Long-term haemodialysis	Carpal tunnel, joints, bones

In TB-endemic regions, AA amyloidosis secondary to tuberculosis and chronic suppurative infections remains the most commonly encountered form, though AL amyloidosis is increasingly recognised with improved diagnostic facilities. Renal amyloidosis is the most common presentation of AA amyloidosis, typically manifesting as nephrotic syndrome.

Clinical Pearl

Reading amyloid type from clinical context. AL amyloid (light chain) is the disease of plasma cell dyscrasias: multiple myeloma, MGUS with progression, Waldenstrom macroglobulinaemia. AA amyloid (serum amyloid A) is the disease of chronic inflammation: tuberculosis, bronchiectasis, rheumatoid arthritis, leprosy, Crohn disease, familial Mediterranean fever. ATTR amyloid (transthyretin) is the disease of familial cardiomyopathy and senile cardiac involvement. In TB-endemic settings, AA dominates because chronic infectious disease dominates; a renal biopsy showing amyloid in a young patient from such a setting should prompt a TB workup before serum free light chains.

Diagnosis of Amyloidosis

The gold standard for diagnosis is tissue biopsy with Congo red staining. Under polarised light, amyloid deposits show characteristic apple-green birefringence. Common biopsy sites include the abdominal fat pad aspirate (sensitivity ~80%), rectal mucosa, gingival biopsy, and the affected organ (kidney, liver, heart). Once amyloid is confirmed, typing is essential for treatment: AL requires chemotherapy targeting the plasma cell clone; AA requires treatment of the underlying inflammatory condition; ATTR may respond to tafamidis (a TTR stabiliser) or patisiran/inotersen (RNA interference therapies targeting hepatic TTR production). Immunohistochemistry, mass spectrometry (the most accurate method for typing), and serum free light chain assays are used for classification.

Amyloid deposition in the spleen produces two patterns: the sago spleen (small, firm, translucent deposits within splenic follicles, resembling sago granules) and the lardaceous spleen (diffuse deposition throughout the red pulp, producing a pale, waxy, enlarged organ). These are classic gross pathology descriptions tested in examinations.

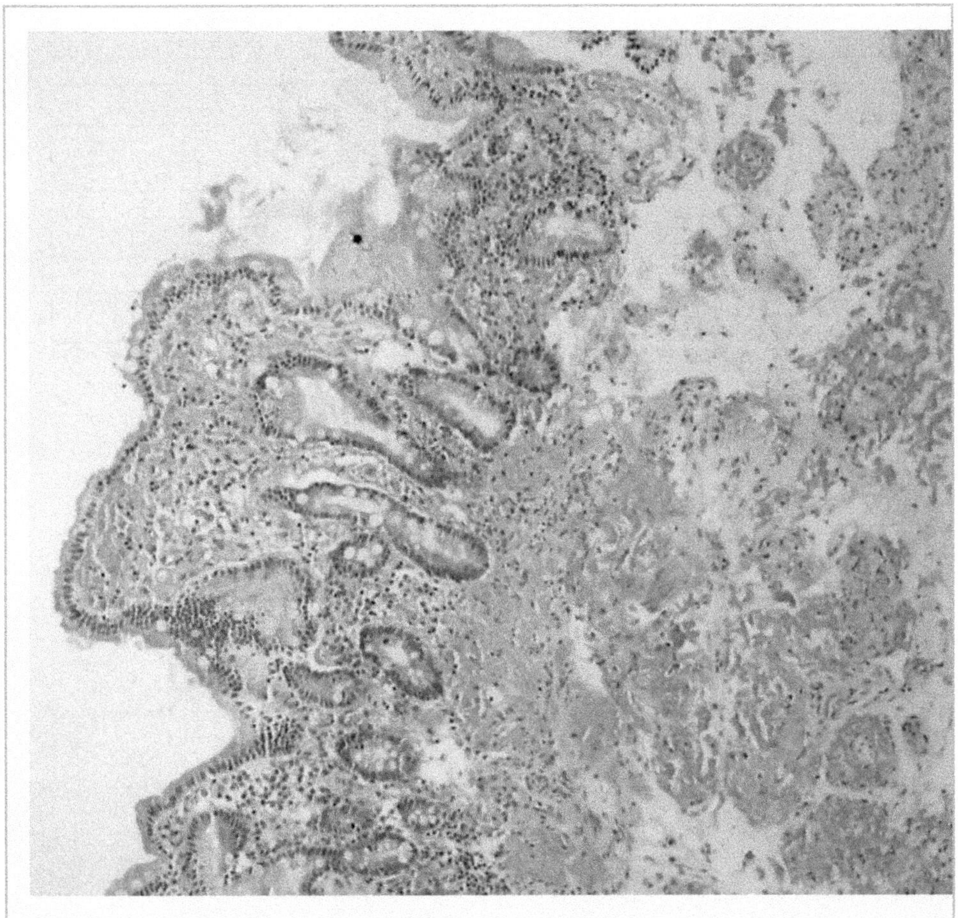

Figure 5.15: Amyloid deposit in small bowel duodenum mucosa — Congo red staining highlighting characteristic salmon-pink amyloid deposits in the lamina propria. Congo red, ×10. (Source: Michael Feldman, Wikimedia Commons, CC BY 2.0.)

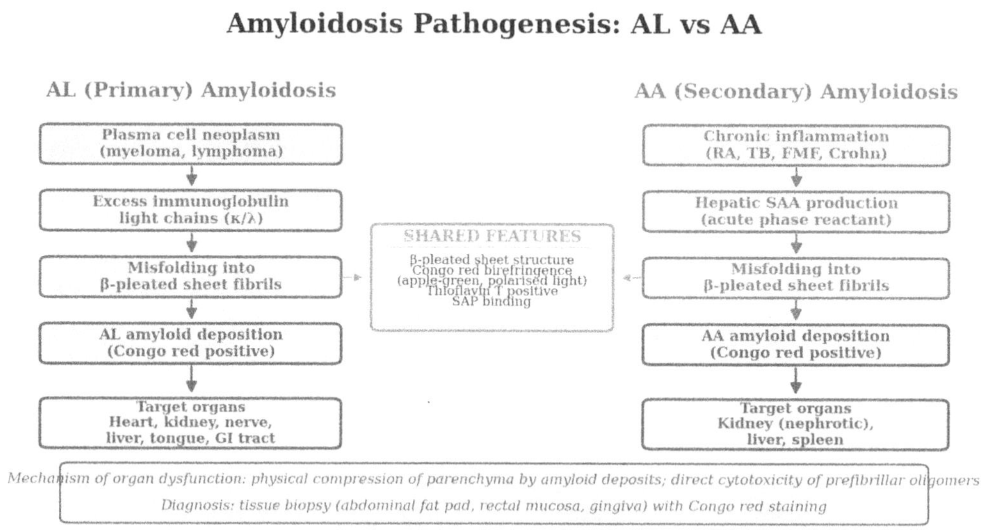

Figure 5.16: Pathogenesis of AL and AA amyloidosis. (Source: Author's original.)

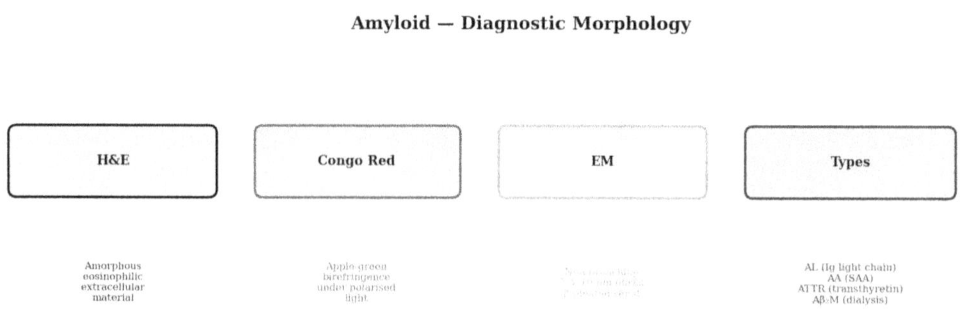

Figure 5.17: Amyloid — Diagnostic Morphology. *(Source: Author's original.)*

The Pathologist's Eye

When evaluating a Congo red-stained section for amyloid, always confirm with polarised light. False positives on Congo red (non-specific staining of collagen and fibrin) are common; only true amyloid shows the pathognomonic apple-green birefringence. In renal biopsies, amyloid deposits are mesangial and along the GBM; they are Congo red-positive and negative for PAS staining (unlike diabetic nodular glomerulosclerosis, which is PAS-positive). Electron microscopy shows randomly arranged, non-branching fibrils of 7.10–10 nm diameter, distinct from the organised fibrils of fibrillar glomerulonephritis (20 nm) and immunotactoid glomerulopathy (30–50 nm microtubules).

Quick Recall: Amyloidosis

Congo red: apple-green birefringence under polarised light; gold standard for diagnosis.

AL: light chains; plasma cell neoplasm; involves heart (restrictive CMP), kidney, tongue.

AA: SAA; chronic inflammation (TB, RA, FMF); involves kidney (most common), liver, spleen; spares heart.

Aβ: Alzheimer disease; senile plaques and cerebral amyloid angiopathy.

ATTR: transthyretin; mutant (FAP) or wild-type (senile cardiac); tafamidis is a disease-modifying therapy.

Sago spleen: follicular amyloid deposits. Lardaceous spleen: diffuse red pulp deposits.

Typing: mass spectrometry (most accurate), IHC, serum free light chains.

Reactive Lymph Node Patterns

Reactive lymphadenopathy is far more common than neoplastic lymphadenopathy, and the pattern of reactive change on biopsy narrows the differential diagnosis.

Pattern	Key Features	Causes
Follicular hyperplasia	Reactive germinal centres with polarity (dark/light zones), tingible body macrophages, mixed centroblasts/centrocytes, preserved mantle zones	Rheumatoid arthritis, HIV (early), toxoplasmosis, syphilis
Paracortical hyperplasia	Expanded T-zone (paracortex), immunoblasts, high endothelial venules prominent	Viral infections (EBV, CMV), drug reactions, dermatopathic lymphadenopathy
Sinus histiocytosis	Expanded sinuses filled with histiocytes; Rosai-Dorfman disease if emperipolesis + S100+	Draining LN of carcinoma, Rosai-Dorfman disease
Granulomatous	Epithelioid granulomas +/- necrosis; caseating vs non-caseating is key branch point	TB, sarcoidosis, fungal infections, cat-scratch disease (stellate microabscesses)

Necrotising (Kikuchi-Fujimoto)	Karyorrhexis, crescentic histiocytes, CD123+ plasmacytoid DCs, absence of neutrophils; self-limiting	Kikuchi-Fujimoto disease (young Asian women); exclude SLE (check ANA)

Spleen Pathology

The spleen functions as a filter for senescent red cells, a site of immune surveillance, and a reservoir of monocytes and platelets. Splenomegaly results from four broad mechanisms: congestive (portal hypertension, right heart failure), infiltrative (leukaemia, lymphoma, Gaucher disease), hyperplastic/work hypertrophy (immune thrombocytopenia, autoimmune haemolytic anaemia), and infective (malaria, kala-azar, infectious mononucleosis).

Hypersplenism is defined as splenomegaly accompanied by one or more cytopenias (anaemia, leucopenia, thrombocytopenia) and compensatory bone marrow hyperplasia, with correction after splenectomy. The mechanism is sequestration and accelerated destruction of blood cells within the expanded splenic cords.

Gamna-Gandy bodies (siderotic nodules) are small, brown-yellow foci of organised focal haemorrhage in the spleen, composed of haemosiderin and calcium encrusted on connective tissue and elastic fibres. They occur in congestive splenomegaly (portal hypertension) and sickle cell disease. On histology, they appear as iron- and calcium-positive nodules; on MRI, they produce characteristic punctate low-signal foci.

Recent Advances

IUIS 2022 — inborn errors of immunity classification update. The International Union of Immunological Societies Expert Committee released its 2022 update on the classification of human inborn errors of immunity (Tangye et al. Journal of Clinical Immunology 2022; 42: 1473–1507; PMID 35748970). Building on the January 2020 iteration, the committee incorporated 55 newly described monogenic gene defects together with one phenocopy due to autoantibodies, taking the total recognised inborn errors of immunity to 485 entries. The committee retained the customary ten-table organisation: combined immunodeficiencies; combined immunodeficiencies with associated or syndromic features; predominantly antibody deficiencies; diseases of immune dysregulation; congenital defects of phagocyte number or function; defects in intrinsic and innate immunity; autoinflammatory disorders; complement deficiencies; bone marrow failure; and phenocopies of inborn errors of immunity. The classification is the operational reference for clinical immunology, for laboratory genetic-test panel design, and for curated databases used in variant interpretation; the expansion in entry numbers reflects the diagnostic yield of next-generation sequencing in undiagnosed-disease programmes.

Checkpoint immunotherapy and autoimmune adverse events. Immune checkpoint inhibitors (anti-PD-1: pembrolizumab, nivolumab; anti-CTLA-4: ipilimumab; anti-PD-L1: atezolizumab) have transformed oncology but produce immune-related adverse events (irAEs) in 30–60% of patients, essentially iatrogenic autoimmune diseases. These include colitis, hepatitis, thyroiditis, pneumonitis, myocarditis, and hypophysitis. The pathologist increasingly encounters biopsies of irAE-affected organs, which show patterns resembling classical autoimmune diseases (e.g., checkpoint colitis mimics IBD on biopsy).

Recognition of irAEs is critical because they require immunosuppression, not more immune activation (see Chapter 6 for checkpoint biology in neoplasia).

CAR-T cell therapy and cytokine release syndrome. Chimeric antigen receptor T-cell (CAR-T) therapy, in which the patient's T cells are engineered to express a receptor targeting a tumour antigen (most commonly CD19 for B-cell lymphomas and ALL), has produced remarkable responses in haematological malignancies. The major complication is cytokine release syndrome (CRS), a systemic inflammatory response driven by massive release of IL-6, IFN-γ, and TNF from activated CAR-T cells and macrophages. CRS is managed with tocilizumab (anti-IL-6R antibody). CAR-T programmes are now operational at major centres internationally (see Volume 1).

Advances in amyloid typing and therapy. Laser microdissection and mass spectrometry (LMD/MS) has become the gold standard for amyloid typing, replacing immunohistochemistry in reference centres. For ATTR amyloidosis, RNA interference therapies (patisiran, vutrisiran) and antisense oligonucleotides (inotersen) that suppress hepatic TTR production have shown dramatic efficacy in clinical trials. For AL amyloidosis, daratumumab (anti-CD38) combined with bortezomib-based regimens has improved haematological response rates substantially.

International Frameworks

2019 EULAR/ACR SLE classification. The 2019 European Alliance of Associations for Rheumatology and American College of Rheumatology criteria for systemic lupus erythematosus require a positive antinuclear antibody titre ≥1:80 on HEp-2 cells as an obligatory entry criterion. Beyond entry, additive weighted criteria are scored across seven clinical domains (constitutional, haematological, neuropsychiatric, mucocutaneous, serosal, musculoskeletal, renal) and three immunological domains (antiphospholipid antibodies, complement proteins, SLE-specific antibodies). Each criterion carries a weight from 2 to 10, and a cumulative score of ≥10 with at least one clinical criterion classifies the patient as SLE. Validation reported sensitivity 96.1% and specificity 93.4%, outperforming both ACR 1997 and SLICC 2012 criteria. Renal biopsy interpretation continues to use the ISN/RPS class I–VI scheme with separate activity and chronicity indices. Citation: Aringer M, et al. Arthritis Rheumatol 2019;71(9):1400–1412. PMID 31385462.

Chapel Hill 2012 vasculitis nomenclature. The 2012 revised International Chapel Hill Consensus Conference (CHCC) nomenclature classifies vasculitides by predominant vessel size and pathogenic mechanism. Large-vessel vasculitis includes giant cell arteritis and Takayasu arteritis. Medium-vessel vasculitis includes polyarteritis nodosa and Kawasaki disease. Small-vessel vasculitis is subdivided into ANCA-associated (microscopic polyangiitis, granulomatosis with polyangiitis, eosinophilic granulomatosis with polyangiitis) and immune-complex (anti-GBM disease, IgA vasculitis, cryoglobulinaemic vasculitis, hypocomplementaemic urticarial vasculitis). Variable-vessel vasculitis includes Behçet disease and Cogan syndrome. Single-organ, vasculitis-associated-with-systemic-disease, and vasculitis-with-probable-aetiology categories complete the framework. The 2012 update retired eponymous names where descriptive alternatives exist and is the international reference for histopathological reporting. Citation: Jennette JC, et al. Arthritis Rheum 2013;65(1):1–11. PMID 23045170.

Ultra High-Yield Chapter Summary

Topic	Must Remember
Type I hypersensitivity	IgE + mast cell degranulation; histamine, leukotrienes; anaphylaxis, asthma, allergic rhinitis
Type II hypersensitivity	IgG/IgM vs cell surface; opsonisation, ADCC, receptor dysfunction; Graves (stimulatory), MG (blocking), Goodpasture (anti-GBM)
Type III hypersensitivity	Immune complex deposition; complement + neutrophils; SLE, PSGN, serum sickness, Arthus
Type IV hypersensitivity	T cell-mediated; DTH (CD4+Th1, tuberculin), CTL (CD8+, rejection); granulomatous = variant

Central tolerance	Clonal deletion in thymus/marrow; AIRE gene (APECED if mutant)
Peripheral tolerance	Anergy, Tregs (FOXP3+; IPEX if mutant), Fas-FasL deletion, immune privilege
Molecular mimicry	Strep M protein vs cardiac myosin (rheumatic fever)
SLE pathogenesis	Defective clearance of apoptotic debris → anti-nuclear antibodies → immune complex deposition
Anti-dsDNA	Specific for SLE; correlates with nephritis and disease activity
Anti-Sm	Most specific for SLE (low sensitivity ~25–30%)
Full house IF	IgG+IgA+IgM+C3+C1q in lupus nephritis
Wire-loop lesion	Class IV diffuse lupus nephritis; massive subendothelial deposits
Drug-induced lupus	Anti-histone Ab; no renal/CNS disease; hydralazine, procainamide, isoniazid
Hyperacute rejection	Preformed antibodies; minutes; complement → thrombosis → infarction
Acute rejection	Cellular (CTL, tubulitis) + humoral (DSA, C4d+); days to weeks
GVHD targets	Skin + liver + GI tract; satellite cell necrosis (apoptosis + adjacent lymphocyte)
HIV entry	gp120 → CD4 → CCR5/CXCR4 → gp41 fusion
Latent reservoir	Resting memory CD4+ T cells; barrier to cure
CCR5Δ32	Homozygous = near-complete HIV resistance
AL amyloidosis	Light chains; plasma cell neoplasm; heart, kidney, tongue, nerves
AA amyloidosis	SAA; chronic inflammation (TB, RA); kidney, liver, spleen; spares heart
Congo red	Apple-green birefringence under polarised light; gold standard for amyloid diagnosis

SCID	Absent T cells; IL-2Rγc (X-linked: T−B+NK−) or ADA (T−B−NK−); fatal without HSCT
CGD	NADPH oxidase defect; catalase-positive organisms; NBT/DHR test negative
MHC class I	HLA-A/B/C; all nucleated cells; endogenous peptides to CD8+ CTLs; HLA-B27 → ankylosing spondylitis
MHC class II	HLA-DP/DQ/DR; APCs only; exogenous peptides to CD4+ T helpers; HLA-DR4 → RA, type 1 DM
Sjögren syndrome	Anti-Ro/SSA + Anti-La/SSB; dry eyes + dry mouth; 40× MALT lymphoma risk
Diffuse SSc	Anti-Scl-70 (topoisomerase I); widespread skin + visceral fibrosis; scleroderma renal crisis
Limited SSc (CREST)	Anti-centromere; calcinosis, Raynaud, oesophageal dysmotility, sclerodactyly, telangiectasia; PAH
IgG4-RD	Storiform fibrosis + IgG4+ plasma cells + obliterative phlebitis; responds to steroids/rituximab
Complement C1q/C2/C4 deficiency	SLE-like immune complex disease (impaired clearance of apoptotic debris)
Complement C5–9 deficiency	Recurrent Neisseria infections (meningococcal, gonococcal)
Hereditary angioedema	C1-INH deficiency; bradykinin-mediated (NOT histamine); does not respond to antihistamines
Wiskott-Aldrich	WAS gene; thrombocytopenia (small platelets) + eczema + infections; lymphoma risk
Bruton (XLA)	BTK mutation; no B cells; recurrent bacterial infections after 6 months when maternal IgG wanes
DiGeorge	22q11.2 deletion; thymic hypoplasia; T-cell deficiency + hypoparathyroidism + cardiac defects
Libman-Sacks endocarditis	SLE; sterile verrucous vegetations on both surfaces of mitral/aortic valves

Checkpoint irAEs	Anti-PD-1/CTLA-4 therapy → iatrogenic autoimmune colitis, hepatitis, thyroiditis, myocarditis

Chapter 6: Neoplasia Part 1: Biology and Behaviour

THE BIG PICTURE

Cancer is fundamentally a disease of disordered gene regulation. A neoplasm arises when a cell acquires a series of genetic and epigenetic alterations that confer growth advantages, enabling it to proliferate autonomously, evade cell death, and ultimately invade and metastasise. These alterations converge on a finite number of molecular pathways, codified as the "hallmarks of cancer" by Hanahan and Weinberg. This chapter builds the molecular framework: the oncogenes that accelerate growth, the tumour suppressor genes whose loss removes the brakes, the mechanisms of carcinogenesis (chemical, radiation, biological), and the multistep process by which a normal cell transforms into an invasive, metastatic cancer. Understanding these principles is the foundation for interpreting every systemic pathology chapter that follows.

High-yield topics in this chapter: hallmarks of cancer; oncogenes and mechanisms of activation (RAS, MYC, ABL, HER2, EGFR); tumour suppressor genes (p53, RB, APC, BRCA1/2, VHL); cell cycle regulation and checkpoints; chemical carcinogenesis (initiation, promotion, progression); radiation carcinogenesis; viral and biological carcinogenesis (HPV, EBV, HBV, HHV-8, H. pylori); molecular basis of invasion and metastasis (EMT, metastatic cascade); epigenetics in cancer.

Cancer kills more than 10 million people worldwide each year, with regional registries documenting that tobacco-related cancers (oral cavity, lung, oesophagus) and cervical cancer dominate in many low- and middle-income settings. Yet despite this diversity, all cancers share a common molecular logic. A lung adenocarcinoma driven by an EGFR mutation and a colon carcinoma driven by APC loss both deploy the same fundamental strategies: self-sufficiency in growth signals, evasion of apoptosis, limitless replication, sustained angiogenesis, and the capacity to invade and metastasise. The pathologist who understands these strategies can decode the biology behind the microscopic pattern, predict behaviour, and guide targeted therapy.

Nomenclature and Classification of Neoplasms

A **neoplasm** ("new growth") is an abnormal mass of tissue whose growth exceeds and is uncoordinated with that of normal tissues and persists after cessation of the stimulus that evoked the change. Neoplasms are classified as **benign** or **malignant** based on their biological behaviour.

Table 6.4: Benign vs malignant neoplasms

Feature	Benign	Malignant
Differentiation	Well differentiated; resembles tissue of origin	Variable; ranges from well differentiated to anaplastic

Growth rate	Usually slow	Variable; often rapid
Growth pattern	Expansile, encapsulated, well-circumscribed	Infiltrative, invasive; poorly circumscribed
Mitoses	Rare, normal	Frequent, may be abnormal (atypical mitoses)
Necrosis/haemorrhage	Rare	Common (outgrows blood supply)
Metastasis	Absent (by definition)	Defines malignancy; present in advanced disease
Local recurrence	Rare if completely excised	Common; depends on completeness of excision
Nuclear features	Uniform, normal N:C ratio	Pleomorphism, hyperchromasia, high N:C ratio, prominent nucleoli

Nomenclature conventions: Benign tumours of epithelial origin are named by adding "-oma" to the tissue type: adenoma (glandular), papilloma (surface epithelium with finger-like projections), cystadenoma (cystic). Malignant epithelial tumours are carcinomas (adenocarcinoma, squamous cell carcinoma). Benign mesenchymal tumours follow the pattern: lipoma, fibroma, chondroma, osteoma, leiomyoma, haemangioma. Malignant mesenchymal tumours are sarcomas: liposarcoma, fibrosarcoma, osteosarcoma, leiomyosarcoma, angiosarcoma. Important exceptions include: lymphoma (malignant, not benign), melanoma (malignant), seminoma and hepatoblastoma (malignant), mesothelioma (malignant), and teratoma (variable behaviour depending on tissue maturity and components).

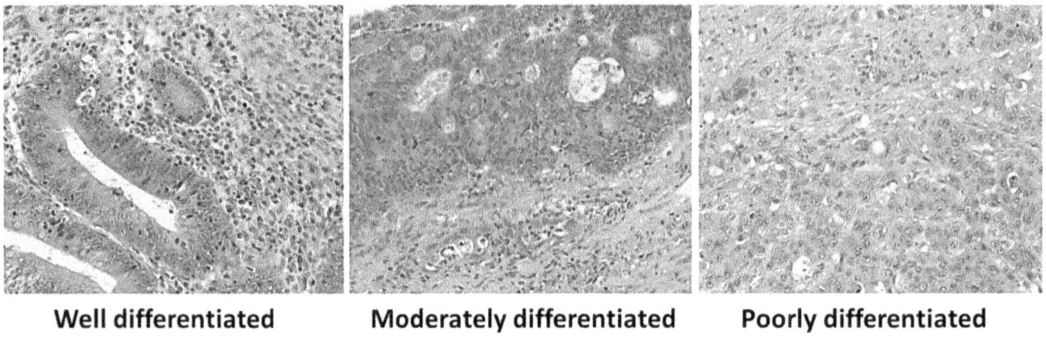

Figure 6.1: Well, moderately, and poorly differentiated colorectal adenocarcinoma. H&E. Left: well-differentiated with gland formation. Centre: moderately differentiated. Right: poorly differentiated with solid sheets, loss of glandular architecture. (Source: Mikael Häggström/Nephron, Wikimedia Commons, CC0 1.0/Public Domain.)

> **Exam Pitfall**
>
> The suffix "-oma" does not always mean benign. Lymphoma, melanoma, mesothelioma, seminoma, and hepatoblastoma are all malignant. Conversely, a hamartoma is not a true neoplasm but a disorganised mass of tissue indigenous to the site. A choristoma is normal tissue in an abnormal location.

Dysplasia and the Dysplasia-Carcinoma Continuum

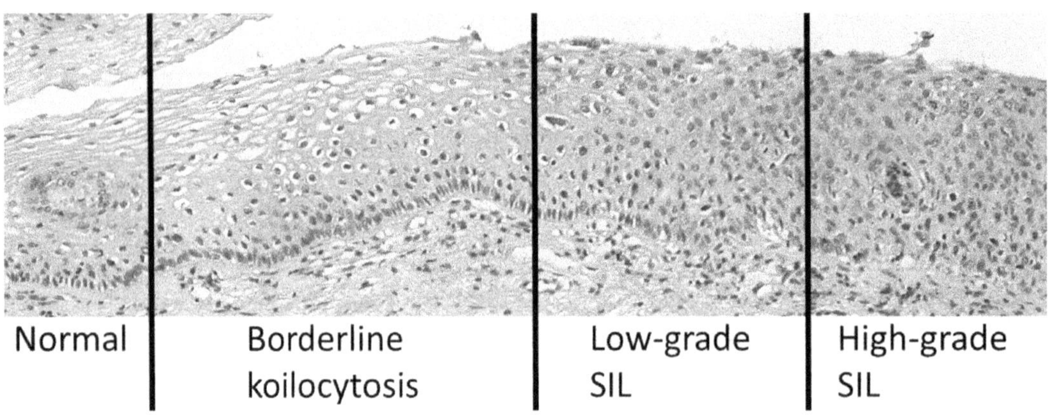

Figure 6.2: Spectrum of squamous intraepithelial lesions (cervical dysplasia). Normal → borderline koilocytosis → low-grade SIL → high-grade SIL. H&E. Note progressive loss of maturation and full-thickness atypia in HSIL. (Source: Mikael Häggström, Wikimedia Commons, CC0 1.0/Public Domain.)

Dysplasia refers to disordered epithelial growth characterised by loss of uniformity of individual cells and loss of architectural orientation. Dysplastic cells exhibit nuclear pleomorphism, hyperchromasia, increased nuclear-to-cytoplasmic ratio, increased mitotic activity (including abnormal mitoses), and disordered maturation. Dysplasia is graded as mild (low-grade), moderate, or severe (high-grade). When dysplastic changes involve the full thickness of the epithelium without breaching the basement membrane, the lesion is termed **carcinoma in situ (CIS)**. CIS is a pre-invasive malignancy: it has the cytological features of malignancy but has not yet acquired the ability to invade. Once the dysplastic cells penetrate the basement membrane, the lesion becomes an invasive carcinoma.

The dysplasia-carcinoma sequence is best documented in the cervix (CIN 1–3 to SCC), the colorectum (adenoma with dysplasia to carcinoma), and the oesophagus (Barrett oesophagus with dysplasia to adenocarcinoma). Not all dysplasias progress to cancer: low-grade dysplasia may regress, remain stable, or progress, whereas high-grade dysplasia/CIS has a much higher probability of progressing to invasive carcinoma if untreated.

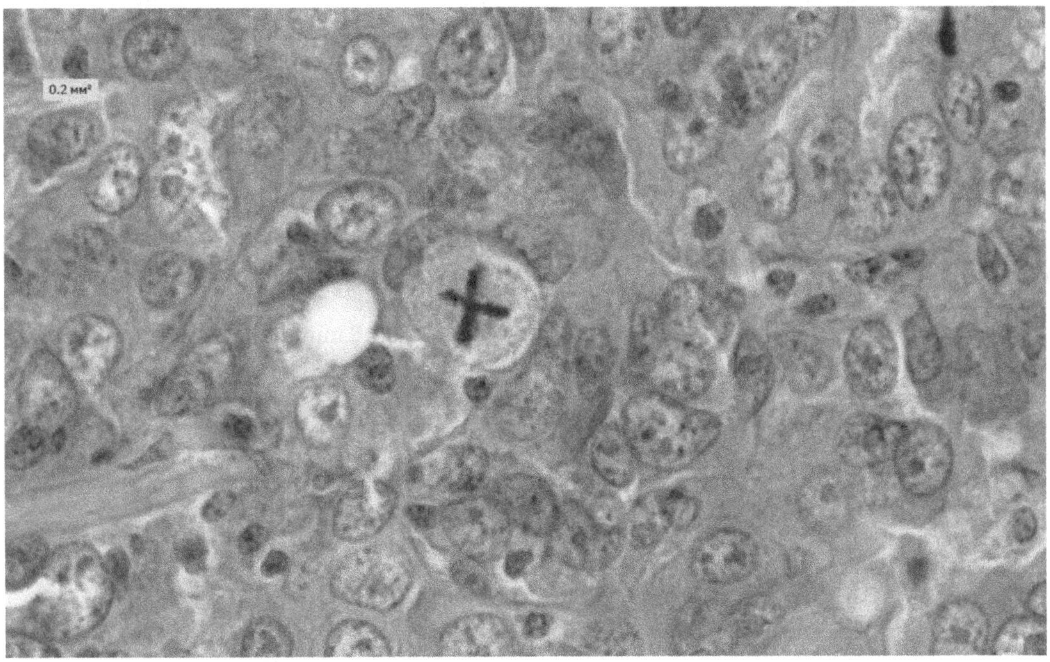

Figure 6.3: Anaplasia — pathologic (tetrapolar) mitotic figure. H&E, high power. Marked nuclear pleomorphism with abnormal mitotic spindle formation. (Source: KGH, Wikimedia Commons, CC BY-SA 3.0.)

The distinction between dysplasia and reactive atypia is a common diagnostic challenge. Reactive atypia (seen in inflammation, ulceration, radiation) shows nuclear enlargement and prominent nucleoli but retains an orderly maturation pattern, normal polarity, and lacks the architectural disorder of dysplasia. This distinction has direct clinical implications: dysplasia requires follow-up or treatment, while reactive atypia requires treatment of the underlying cause.

Cancer Epidemiology: A Global Perspective

Hallmarks of Cancer

In their landmark papers (2000, updated 2011 and 2022), Douglas Hanahan and Robert Weinberg proposed that the complexity of cancer can be reduced to a set of acquired functional capabilities, the "hallmarks of cancer." These hallmarks provide the organising framework for understanding cancer biology and are the backbone of examination answers on neoplasia.

Clinical Pearl

Each hallmark of cancer maps to a class of targeted therapy. Sustained proliferative signalling: BRAF inhibitors (vemurafenib, dabrafenib), EGFR inhibitors (gefitinib, osimertinib), HER2 antibodies (trastuzumab). Evading apoptosis: BCL-2 inhibitors (venetoclax). Limitless replicative potential: telomerase inhibitors (under trial). Sustained angiogenesis: VEGF antibodies (bevacizumab) and VEGFR TKIs (sunitinib, pazopanib). Genome instability: PARP inhibitors (olaparib, niraparib) in BRCA-mutated tumours. Avoiding immune destruction: PD-1, PD-L1, and CTLA-4 antibodies (pembrolizumab, nivolumab, ipilimumab). The hallmarks framework is not just teaching scaffolding; it is the architecture of modern oncological pharmacology.

Table 6.5: Hallmarks of cancer

Hallmark	Mechanism	Examples
1. Self-sufficiency in growth signals	Oncogene activation provides constitutive growth signalling	RAS mutations, HER2 amplification, BCR-ABL fusion, EGFR mutations
2. Insensitivity to growth inhibitors	Loss of tumour suppressors removes cell cycle checkpoints	RB loss (loss of G1/S checkpoint), APC loss (Wnt pathway activation), TGF-β receptor inactivation
3. Evasion of apoptosis	Disabled apoptotic pathways allow survival of damaged cells	p53 mutation (loss of guardian), BCL2 overexpression (follicular lymphoma), loss of Fas/FasL pathway
4. Limitless replicative potential	Telomerase reactivation prevents telomere shortening	Telomerase (hTERT) expressed in >90% of cancers; alternative lengthening of telomeres (ALT) in sarcomas
5. Sustained angiogenesis	Tumour secretes pro-angiogenic factors; anti-angiogenic factors are lost	VEGF overexpression; loss of TSP-1 (p53-dependent); angiogenic switch (see Chapter 3)
6. Invasion and metastasis	EMT, loss of E-cadherin, MMP activity, motility	E-cadherin downregulation, Snail/Slug/Twist transcription factors, MMP-2/9, chemokine-guided homing

7. Reprogramming energy metabolism	Warburg effect: aerobic glycolysis even in presence of oxygen	Increased glucose uptake (↑GLUT1); basis of FDG-PET imaging
8. Evading immune destruction	Tumour evades immune surveillance	PD-L1 expression (inhibits T cells); loss of MHC class I; Treg recruitment; basis of checkpoint immunotherapy
Enabling characteristics:		
Genome instability and mutation	Defective DNA repair accelerates acquisition of hallmark mutations	MSI (MLH1, MSH2), BRCA1/2, p53 mutation (guardian of the genome)
Tumour-promoting inflammation	Chronic inflammation provides growth factors, survival signals, and mutagenic ROS	Colitis-associated CRC, HBV/HCV-associated HCC, H. pylori-associated gastric cancer (Figure 6.4)

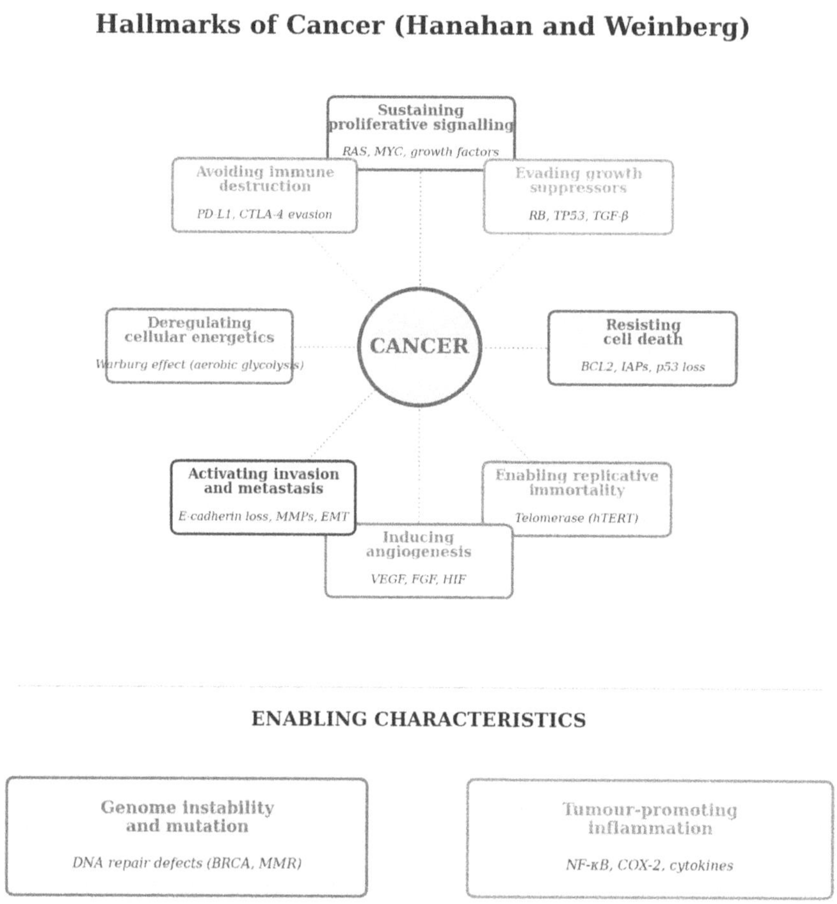

Figure 6.4: The Hallmarks of Cancer (Hanahan and Weinberg). (Source: Author's original.)

In 2022, Hanahan proposed four additional dimensions: phenotypic plasticity (lineage switching), non-mutational epigenetic reprogramming (chromatin/DNA methylation changes driving hallmark capabilities), polymorphic microbiomes (tumour-associated microbial communities influencing immunity and metabolism), and senescent cells (SASP providing growth factors and inflammatory mediators to the tumour microenvironment).

Clinical Pearl

Phenotypic plasticity is the morphology behind targeted-therapy escape. Adenocarcinoma of lung treated with EGFR inhibitors can transform into small cell carcinoma; prostate adenocarcinoma treated with androgen receptor targeting can transform into neuroendocrine carcinoma. The underlying biology is lineage switching, not new mutation. The diagnostic implication: every progression biopsy after targeted therapy must be re-examined for histological transformation, even when the clinical course suggests simple resistance. A small-cell phenotype in a patient previously diagnosed with lung adenocarcinoma is not a new diagnosis; it is the same tumour wearing different clothes.

Oncogenes

Proto-oncogenes are normal cellular genes that encode proteins involved in growth signalling, cell cycle progression, or inhibition of apoptosis. When mutated, amplified, or translocated, they become oncogenes, which produce proteins with enhanced or constitutive activity that drives unregulated cell proliferation. Oncogenes act in a **dominant** fashion: mutation of a single allele is sufficient to confer a growth advantage (gain-of-function).

Mechanisms of Oncogene Activation

Mechanism	Molecular Event	Example
Point mutation	Single nucleotide change creates constitutively active protein	RAS (KRAS, NRAS, HRAS): most commonly mutated oncogene in human cancers (~30%); constitutive GTPase activity → sustained MAP kinase signalling; BRAF V600E: constitutive serine/threonine kinase activity (melanoma, PTC, hairy cell leukaemia)
Gene amplification	Increased copy number → overexpression of normal protein	HER2/ERBB2 amplification (breast cancer; target of trastuzumab); NMYC amplification (neuroblastoma; poor prognosis); MYC amplification (breast, ovary)
Chromosomal translocation (fusion gene)	Juxtaposition of coding sequences creates a chimeric oncoprotein	BCR-ABL t(9;22): CML (constitutive tyrosine kinase; imatinib target); EWS-FLI1 t(11;22): Ewing sarcoma; PML-RARA t(15;17): APL; PAX3-FOXO1 t(2;13): alveolar RMS; ALK rearrangements: ALCL, NSCLC
Chromosomal translocation (promoter swap)	Proto-oncogene placed under control of a strong promoter	MYC-IGH t(8;14): Burkitt lymphoma (MYC under Ig heavy chain enhancer); BCL2-IGH t(14;18): follicular lymphoma; CCND1-IGH t(11;14): mantle cell lymphoma
Insertional mutagenesis	Viral integration near a proto-oncogene	Retroviral insertion near MYC (avian leukosis); HBV integration near cellular genes

Key Oncogene Pathways

The RAS-MAP kinase pathway is the most frequently mutated signalling pathway in cancer. RAS proteins (KRAS, NRAS, HRAS) are small GTPases that cycle between an active GTP-bound state and an inactive GDP-bound state. Growth factor binding to a receptor tyrosine kinase (e.g., EGFR) activates RAS via the adaptor proteins GRB2 and SOS. Oncogenic RAS mutations (most commonly at codons 12, 13, or 61) lock the protein in the GTP-bound (active) state, resulting in constitutive signalling through RAF → MEK → ERK (MAP kinase cascade), driving proliferation. KRAS mutations are found in ~90% of pancreatic cancers, ~50% of colon cancers, and ~30% of lung adenocarcinomas. The development of direct KRAS G12C inhibitors (sotorasib, adagrasib) has been a major breakthrough in targeted therapy (see Recent Advances).

Growth factor → RTK → GRB2/SOS → RAS (GDP→GTP) → RAF → MEK → ERK → Transcription factors (MYC, FOS, JUN) → Cell proliferation

MYC is a transcription factor that regulates expression of genes controlling cell growth, proliferation, metabolism, and apoptosis. It is activated by translocation (Burkitt lymphoma), amplification (neuroblastoma, breast cancer), or increased protein stability. MYC activates expression of cyclins and CDKs (promoting cell cycle entry), hTERT (telomerase), and genes involved in ribosome biogenesis and metabolism. Paradoxically, MYC also activates p53-dependent apoptosis, which acts as a safety brake; this explains why MYC-driven cancers often require concomitant loss of p53 for full malignant transformation.

> **Quick Recall: Oncogenes**
>
> **RAS:** most commonly mutated oncogene (~30% of all cancers); constitutive GTPase; codons 12/13/61; KRAS G12C inhibitors (sotorasib).
>
> **MYC:** transcription factor; Burkitt t(8;14); amplification in neuroblastoma (NMYC), breast.
>
> **BCR-ABL:** t(9;22) Philadelphia chromosome; CML; constitutive tyrosine kinase; imatinib.
>
> **HER2:** amplification in 20% breast cancers; trastuzumab; also amplified in gastric cancer.
>
> **BRAF V600E:** melanoma, PTC, hairy cell leukaemia; vemurafenib, dabrafenib.
>
> **Dominant:** single allele mutation sufficient (gain-of-function).

Tumour Suppressor Genes

Tumour suppressor genes encode proteins that restrain cell growth, promote apoptosis, or maintain genomic integrity. Unlike oncogenes, tumour suppressors act **recessively**: both alleles must be inactivated for loss of function (Knudson's two-hit hypothesis). The first hit may be inherited (germline mutation, conferring cancer predisposition) or acquired (somatic mutation); the second hit is typically a somatic event (deletion, mutation, or epigenetic silencing of the remaining allele, termed loss of heterozygosity, LOH).

The p53 Tumour Suppressor: Guardian of the Genome

TP53 is the most frequently mutated gene in human cancers (mutated in >50% of all cancers). The p53 protein is a transcription factor that integrates stress signals (DNA damage, hypoxia, oncogene activation) and mediates cellular responses: cell cycle arrest (via p21/WAF1, which inhibits CDK4/cyclin D and CDK2/cyclin E complexes), DNA repair, apoptosis (via BAX, PUMA, NOXA), and senescence. Under normal conditions, p53 levels are kept low by MDM2, an E3 ubiquitin ligase that targets p53 for proteasomal degradation. Upon DNA damage, kinases such as ATM and CHK2 phosphorylate both p53 (stabilising it) and MDM2 (inhibiting its activity), allowing p53 to accumulate and activate its target genes.

DNA damage → ATM/CHK2 phosphorylation → p53 stabilisation (MDM2 inhibited) → p21 (cell cycle arrest at G1/S) / BAX, PUMA (apoptosis) / DNA repair genes

Li-Fraumeni syndrome results from germline TP53 mutations (autosomal dominant). Affected individuals develop multiple cancers at a young age, including sarcomas, breast cancer, brain tumours, leukaemias, and adrenocortical carcinomas (the classic "SBLA" spectrum). The syndrome dramatically illustrates the guardian role of p53: with one allele already mutated, loss of the second allele (somatic) occurs frequently in different tissues, producing diverse malignancies.

HPV and p53: High-risk HPV types (16, 18) express the E6 oncoprotein, which recruits the E6AP ubiquitin ligase to degrade p53, effectively removing the guardian without a mutation in TP53 itself. This is a key mechanism in cervical carcinogenesis and is also relevant in HPV-associated oropharyngeal squamous cell carcinoma.

The Retinoblastoma Gene (RB1)

RB is the prototypic tumour suppressor and the first to be discovered. The RB protein governs the G1/S transition by binding and sequestering E2F transcription factors. In its hypophosphorylated (active) state, RB blocks E2F-mediated transcription of genes required for S-phase entry (cyclins A and E, DNA polymerase). Mitogenic signals activate CDK4/6-cyclin D complexes, which phosphorylate RB, releasing E2F and allowing cell cycle progression. Loss of RB function (by mutation, deletion, or HPV E7-mediated degradation) removes the G1/S checkpoint, permitting unregulated proliferation.

Growth signals → CDK4/6-Cyclin D → RB phosphorylation → E2F release → S-phase entry genes. Loss of RB → constitutive E2F activity → uncontrolled proliferation

Knudson's two-hit hypothesis was formulated from the study of retinoblastoma. In the familial (hereditary) form, one RB allele is mutated in the germline (first hit, inherited); somatic loss of the second allele (second hit) occurs in retinal cells, producing bilateral, multifocal retinoblastomas at an early age. In the sporadic form, both hits are somatic and occur in the same retinal cell, producing unilateral, unifocal retinoblastoma at a later age. This model applies broadly to other tumour suppressor genes.

Other Major Tumour Suppressors

Gene	Protein / Function	Cancer Syndrome	Sporadic Cancers

		(Germline)	
APC	Component of β-catenin destruction complex; regulates Wnt signalling. Loss → β-catenin accumulation → nuclear translocation → MYC and cyclin D1 transcription	Familial adenomatous polyposis (FAP): hundreds of colonic polyps by adolescence; near-100% CRC risk	Sporadic CRC (APC mutation is the initiating event in the adenoma-carcinoma sequence)
BRCA1/BRCA2	DNA double-strand break repair by homologous recombination	Hereditary breast-ovarian cancer syndrome: 60–80% lifetime breast cancer risk, 20–40% ovarian cancer risk	Sporadic breast and ovarian cancer (BRCA1 promoter methylation)
VHL	E3 ubiquitin ligase component targeting HIF-1α for degradation under normoxic conditions. Loss → HIF-1α accumulation → VEGF, PDGF overexpression	von Hippel-Lindau syndrome: clear cell RCC, cerebellar haemangioblastoma, phaeochromocytoma	Sporadic clear cell RCC (VHL inactivation in >70%)
WT1	Transcription factor; Wilms tumour suppressor	WAGR syndrome (WT1 deletion + aniridia + genitourinary anomalies + intellectual disability); Denys-Drash	Wilms tumour (nephroblastoma)
NF1	Neurofibromin: RAS-GAP (converts RAS-GTP to RAS-GDP). Loss → sustained RAS activation	Neurofibromatosis type 1: neurofibromas, café-au-lait spots, optic glioma, MPNST risk	Sporadic MPNST, juvenile myelomonocytic leukaemia (JMML)
NF2	Merlin: cytoskeletal-membrane linker	Neurofibromatosis type 2: bilateral acoustic schwannomas, meningiomas	Sporadic schwannomas, meningiomas
PTEN	Lipid phosphatase; opposes PI3K/AKT pathway. Loss → constitutive AKT activation → survival and proliferation	Cowden syndrome: hamartomas, breast/thyroid/endometrial cancer risk	Endometrial, prostate, glioblastoma

Quick Recall: Tumour Suppressors

p53: guardian of the genome; most commonly mutated gene in cancer; Li-Fraumeni syndrome; degraded by HPV E6.

RB: G1/S checkpoint; Knudson two-hit; phosphorylated by CDK4/6-Cyclin D; degraded by HPV E7.

APC: Wnt/β-catenin pathway; FAP; initiating mutation in CRC adenoma-carcinoma sequence.

BRCA1/2: homologous recombination DNA repair; hereditary breast-ovarian cancer; PARP inhibitor sensitivity.

VHL: HIF-1α degradation; VHL syndrome (clear cell RCC, haemangioblastoma, phaeo).

Two-hit: both alleles must be lost (recessive); first hit germline or somatic, second hit always somatic (LOH, methylation).

Hereditary Cancer Syndromes

Inherited cancer predisposition syndromes dramatically illustrate the role of tumour suppressors and DNA repair genes. These account for approximately 5–10% of all cancers and are characterised by early-onset disease, bilateral or multifocal tumours, and a family history across generations (autosomal dominant inheritance with variable penetrance). Recognition is essential for genetic counselling and cancer surveillance.

Table 6.6: Major hereditary cancer syndromes

Syndrome	Gene	Cancers
FAP (familial adenomatous polyposis)	APC (5q21)	Colorectal (near-100% risk); duodenal, desmoid tumours, hepatoblastoma (Gardner variant: osteomas, fibromatosis, epidermoid cysts)
Lynch syndrome (HNPCC)	MLH1, MSH2, MSH6, PMS2 (MMR genes)	Colorectal (right-sided), endometrial, ovarian, gastric, urothelial (Amsterdam/Bethesda criteria for testing)
Hereditary breast-ovarian cancer	BRCA1 (17q21), BRCA2 (13q12)	Breast (60–80%), ovarian (20–40%), prostate, pancreas; BRCA1: triple-negative breast cancer; PARP inhibitor sensitivity
Li-Fraumeni	TP53	Sarcomas, breast cancer, brain tumours, leukaemia, adrenocortical carcinoma (childhood)
Retinoblastoma (hereditary)	RB1 (13q14)	Bilateral retinoblastoma; osteosarcoma in survivors

von Hippel-Lindau	VHL (3p25)	Clear cell RCC, cerebellar haemangioblastoma, phaeochromocytoma, retinal angioma
MEN1	MEN1 (menin)	Pituitary adenoma, parathyroid hyperplasia/adenoma, pancreatic islet tumours (3 Ps)
MEN2A/2B	RET proto-oncogene (gain-of-function)	Medullary thyroid carcinoma, phaeochromocytoma, parathyroid hyperplasia (2A); mucosal neuromas, marfanoid habitus (2B)
Cowden syndrome	PTEN	Breast, thyroid, endometrial cancer; hamartomatous polyps; trichilemmomas
Neurofibromatosis type 1	NF1	Neurofibromas, MPNST (5–10% risk), optic glioma, JMML, café-au-lait spots
Xeroderma pigmentosum	NER genes (XPA–XPG)	BCC, SCC, melanoma (UV-induced; extreme photosensitivity)

When faced with a young patient with cancer, the first question to ask is whether the presentation fits a hereditary cancer syndrome. Red flags include: age of onset younger than expected for that tumour type, bilateral or multifocal disease, multiple primary cancers, family history of the same or related cancers across generations, and unusual tumour types (e.g., medullary thyroid carcinoma → always test for RET germline mutation; adrenocortical carcinoma in a child → suspect Li-Fraumeni).

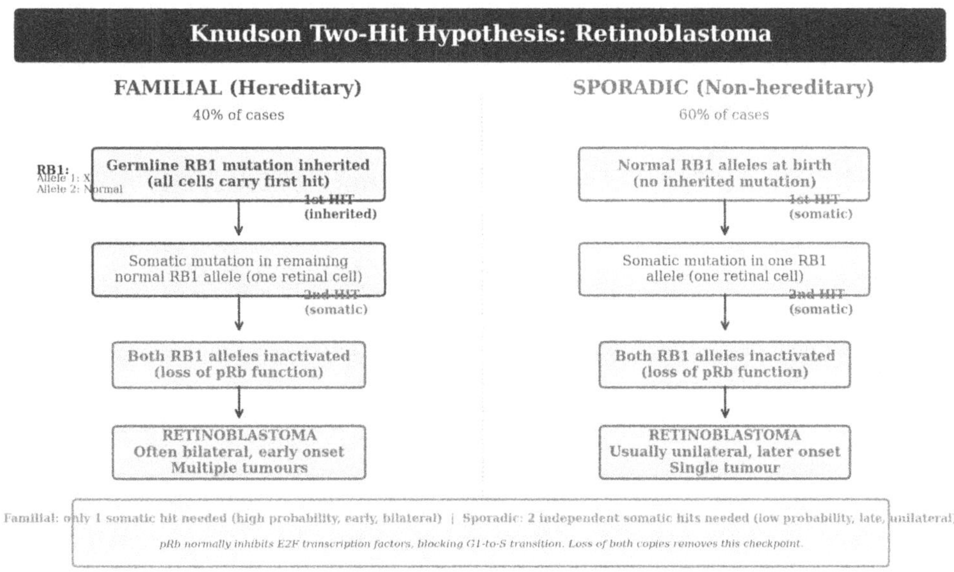

Figure 6.5: Knudson's two-hit hypothesis in retinoblastoma. (Source: Author's original.)

The Multistep Model: Adenoma-Carcinoma Sequence

The colorectal adenoma-carcinoma sequence (Vogelstein/Fearon model) exemplifies multistep carcinogenesis: APC loss (initiation) → KRAS activation → SMAD4 loss → TP53 loss → carcinoma, spanning 10–15 years (the rationale for screening colonoscopy). The full molecular detail of CIN and serrated/MSI pathways is covered in Chapter 19.**APC loss** (5q21) is the initiating event, producing a small adenomatous polyp. **KRAS activation** drives adenoma growth (intermediate adenoma). **SMAD4 loss** (18q21; loss of TGF-β signalling) promotes progression to a large adenoma with high-grade dysplasia. **TP53 loss** (17p) is the final gatekeeping event that permits the transition from adenoma to invasive carcinoma. Additional mutations (e.g., activation of telomerase, loss of DCC) accumulate during tumour progression. The entire sequence spans 10–15 years, which is the rationale for colonoscopic screening and polypectomy as a cancer prevention strategy.

Normal epithelium → APC loss → Early adenoma → KRAS mutation → Intermediate adenoma → SMAD4/18q loss → Late adenoma → p53 loss → Carcinoma → Additional mutations → Metastasis

Integration: *The adenoma-carcinoma sequence is covered in detail in Chapter 19 (Lower GI Pathology). The alternative pathway through MSI (Lynch syndrome and sporadic MLH1 methylation) is discussed in the Genomic Instability section of this chapter and in Chapter 19.*

The serrated neoplasia pathway accounts for 20–30% of CRC and is molecularly distinct from the CIN (adenoma-carcinoma) pathway. It proceeds: BRAF V600E mutation → sessile serrated lesion (SSL) → progressive CpG island methylation (CIMP-high) → MLH1 promoter methylation → mismatch repair deficiency → MSI-H carcinoma. Unlike Lynch syndrome (germline MMR mutation), serrated pathway MSI-H cancers are sporadic. The IHC–molecular algorithm distinguishes these: loss of MLH1+PMS2 on IHC triggers reflex BRAF V600E testing. If BRAF-mutant, the cause is sporadic MLH1 methylation. If BRAF wild-type, suspect Lynch syndrome and proceed to germline testing (see Chapter 19) (Figure 6.6).

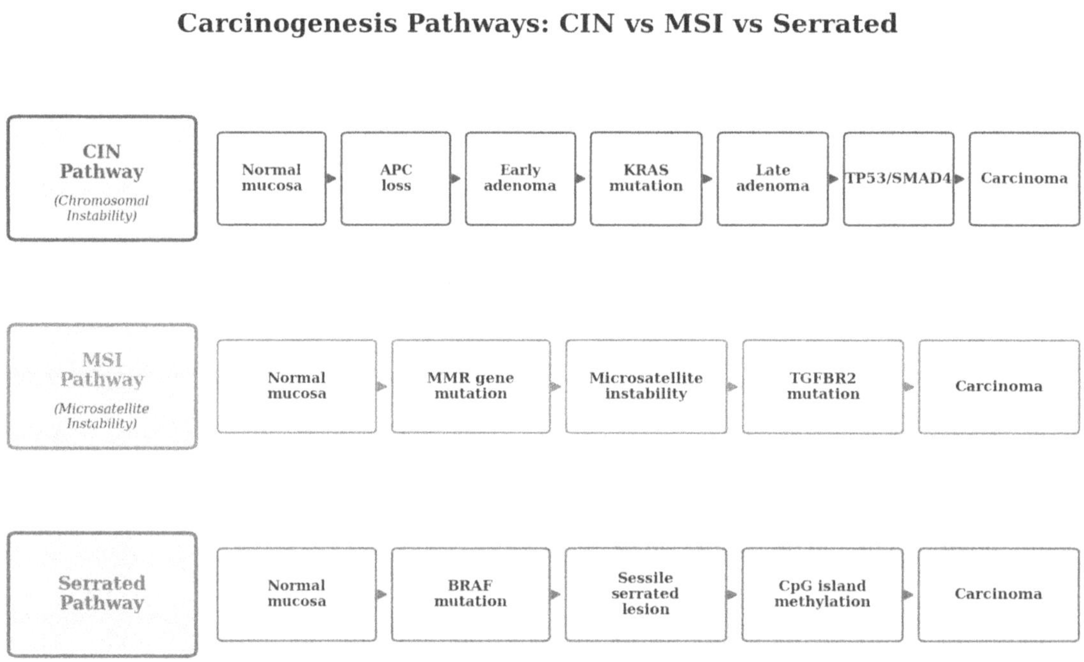

Figure 6.6: Carcinogenesis Pathways: CIN vs MSI vs Serrated. *(Source: Author's original.)*

Cell Cycle Regulation and Cancer

The cell cycle is regulated by the sequential activation of cyclin-dependent kinases (CDKs) complexed with their cyclin partners. CDK inhibitors (CKIs) act as brakes. In cancer, this system is subverted at multiple levels.

Phase	CDK-Cyclin Complex	Checkpoint / Key Events	Cancer Relevance
G1	CDK4/6-Cyclin D	Restriction point; RB	CDK4/6 inhibitors (palbociclib,

		phosphorylation	ribociclib) in HR+ breast cancer; Cyclin D1 overexpression in mantle cell lymphoma t(11;14)
G1/S transition	CDK2-Cyclin E	RB fully phosphorylated; E2F released; S-phase gene transcription	p21 (CDK inhibitor induced by p53) arrests cell here after DNA damage
S	CDK2-Cyclin A	DNA replication	BRCA1/2 repair DSBs during replication; ATR-CHK1 checkpoint
G2/M	CDK1(CDC2)-Cyclin B	DNA damage checkpoint before mitosis	ATM-CHK2-p53 pathway; DNA damage → G2 arrest
M	CDK1-Cyclin B	Spindle assembly checkpoint (SAC)	BUB1, MAD2 mutations → aneuploidy; taxanes target spindle

CDK inhibitors are divided into two families. The INK4 family (p15/INK4b, **p16/INK4a**, p18, p19) specifically inhibits CDK4/6, preventing cyclin D binding. The CIP/KIP family (**p21/WAF1**, p27, p57) broadly inhibits CDK2 and CDK1 complexes. p16 is frequently inactivated in cancers (deletion, promoter hypermethylation) and is used as a surrogate marker for HPV-driven oropharyngeal carcinoma (HPV E7 degrades RB → compensatory p16 overexpression; strong diffuse nuclear and cytoplasmic p16 staining by IHC).

Integration: *Cell cycle checkpoints connect to DNA repair (BRCA, ATM), apoptosis (p53-mediated), and telomere biology (see Chapter 1). CDK4/6 inhibitors are transforming the treatment of HR-positive breast cancer (see Chapter 26).*

Carcinogenesis

Carcinogenesis is a multistep process in which normal cells acquire the hallmark capabilities through the accumulation of genetic and epigenetic alterations. Three major categories of carcinogens are recognised: chemical, radiation, and biological (microbial). The IARC classification of chemical agents (Groups 1, 2A, 2B) and the clinical/occupational perspective on specific carcinogens are consolidated in Chapter 7.

Chemical Carcinogenesis

Chemical carcinogenesis proceeds through three stages. **Initiation** is an irreversible genetic alteration caused by a chemical mutagen (the initiator). Most chemical carcinogens are procarcinogens that require metabolic activation (typically by cytochrome P-450 mixed-function oxidases in the liver) to form ultimate carcinogens, which are reactive electrophiles that bind to and damage DNA. **Promotion** is a reversible process in which promoters (non-mutagenic agents) stimulate proliferation of initiated cells, expanding the clone and increasing the probability of additional mutations. Promoters include oestrogens (endometrial and breast cancer), phorbol esters, and chronic inflammation. **Progression** is the acquisition of additional mutations that confer malignant properties (invasion, metastasis, drug resistance) to the growing tumour. This stage is characterised by increasing genetic instability and clonal heterogeneity.

Procarcinogen → P-450 activation → Ultimate carcinogen (electrophile) → DNA damage (INITIATION) → Promoter-driven proliferation (PROMOTION) → Additional mutations (PROGRESSION) → Malignant neoplasm

Chemical Carcinogen	Activated Form / Mechanism	Associated Cancer
Polycyclic aromatic hydrocarbons (benzo[a]pyrene)	Epoxide intermediates (P-450); tobacco smoke, smoked foods	Lung, larynx, oral cavity, oesophagus, bladder
Aromatic amines (β-naphthylamine, benzidine)	N-hydroxylation in liver; excreted in urine	Bladder (occupational: dye workers, rubber industry)
Nitrosamines	Formed from nitrites in GI tract	Stomach, oesophagus (dietary nitrites in preserved food)
Aflatoxin B1 (Aspergillus flavus/parasiticus)	Epoxide; p53 codon 249 hotspot mutation (Arg→Ser)	Hepatocellular carcinoma (synergistic with HBV); grain contamination in tropical regions
Alkylating agents (cyclophosphamide)	Direct-acting; DNA cross-linking	Treatment-related AML, bladder cancer
Benzene	Metabolised to epoxides and aldehydes	AML, MDS
Asbestos	Chronic irritation, ROS generation, mesothelial injury	Mesothelioma (crocidolite > amosite > chrysotile); bronchogenic carcinoma (synergistic with smoking)
Vinyl chloride	Chloroethylene oxide	Angiosarcoma of the liver (occupational)

Betel nut / areca nut	Arecoline and nitrosamines	Oral submucous fibrosis → oral SCC (major cause in South Asia)

Radiation Carcinogenesis

Both ionising radiation (X-rays, gamma rays, neutrons) and ultraviolet radiation are established carcinogens. Ionising radiation causes DNA damage through direct double-strand breaks and indirect damage via free radical generation. The cancers most associated with ionising radiation include leukaemia (especially AML and CML, as seen in atomic bomb survivors), thyroid cancer (Chernobyl), breast cancer, lung cancer, and sarcomas. There is no safe threshold dose; risk increases linearly with dose (linear no-threshold model). UV radiation (UVB, 280–320 nm) causes pyrimidine dimer formation in DNA. If not repaired by the nucleotide excision repair (NER) pathway, these dimers cause CC→TT signature mutations. Xeroderma pigmentosum (XP), caused by inherited defects in NER genes, results in extreme UV sensitivity and a several-thousand-fold increase in skin cancer risk. UV-associated cancers include basal cell carcinoma, squamous cell carcinoma, and melanoma of the skin.

Biological (Microbial) Carcinogenesis

Approximately 15–20% of all cancers worldwide are caused by infectious agents. This proportion is higher in developing countries, including India, where HPV, H. pylori, HBV, and HCV together contribute to a substantial fraction of the cancer burden.

Agent	Mechanism	Associated Cancer
HPV (types 16, 18)	E6 degrades p53; E7 degrades RB; integration disrupts E2 (negative regulator)	Cervical SCC and adenocarcinoma, oropharyngeal SCC, vulvar, vaginal, penile, anal SCC
EBV	Latent membrane protein 1 (LMP1) mimics CD40 signalling; EBNA2 activates MYC; episomal maintenance	Burkitt lymphoma (endemic), nasopharyngeal carcinoma, Hodgkin lymphoma (mixed cellularity/lymphocyte-depleted), post-transplant lymphoma (PTLD), NK/T-cell lymphoma (nasal type)
HBV	Insertional mutagenesis; HBx protein activates NF-κB, inactivates p53; chronic inflammation and regeneration	Hepatocellular carcinoma
HCV	Chronic inflammation and cirrhosis (no DNA integration); core protein may directly	Hepatocellular carcinoma

	modulate signalling	
HHV-8 (KSHV)	LANA inhibits p53 and RB; viral IL-6, viral cyclin D; angiogenic factors	Kaposi sarcoma, primary effusion lymphoma, multicentric Castleman disease
HTLV-1	Tax protein activates NF-κB, cyclin D, inactivates p53	Adult T-cell leukaemia/lymphoma (ATLL)
H. pylori	CagA oncoprotein injected via type IV secretion system; activates SHP2 phosphatase, β-catenin signalling; chronic gastritis → intestinal metaplasia → dysplasia → carcinoma	Gastric adenocarcinoma, gastric MALT lymphoma
Opisthorchis / Clonorchis (liver flukes)	Chronic biliary inflammation	Cholangiocarcinoma (SE Asia)
Schistosoma haematobium	Chronic cystitis; urothelial hyperplasia	Squamous cell carcinoma of bladder (Egypt, sub-Saharan Africa)

Quick Recall: Carcinogenesis

Initiation-promotion-progression: initiation = irreversible DNA damage; promotion = clonal expansion (reversible); progression = malignant evolution.

Aflatoxin B1: p53 codon 249 (Arg→Ser); HCC; synergistic with HBV.

Asbestos: mesothelioma (crocidolite worst) + bronchogenic carcinoma (synergistic with smoking).

HPV: E6 → p53 degradation; E7 → RB degradation; cervical, oropharyngeal, anal SCC.

EBV: Burkitt, NPC, HL (MC/LD), PTLD, NK/T-cell lymphoma.

H. pylori: gastric adenocarcinoma (CagA+), MALT lymphoma.

Epigenetics in Cancer

Cancer Metabolism: The Warburg Effect

Normal cells generate ATP primarily through oxidative phosphorylation in the mitochondria. Cancer cells, even in the presence of abundant oxygen, preferentially use aerobic glycolysis, converting glucose to lactate rather than feeding pyruvate into the TCA cycle. This metabolic shift, described by Otto Warburg in the 1920s, is termed the **Warburg effect**. Although glycolysis is far less efficient than oxidative phosphorylation (2 ATP vs 36 ATP per glucose molecule), it provides rapidly dividing cancer cells with two advantages: (1) fast ATP generation (glycolysis is rapid, supporting high proliferation rates), and (2) biosynthetic intermediates (glycolytic intermediates are shunted into anabolic pathways producing nucleotides, amino acids, and lipids needed for new cell assembly).

Cancer cells upregulate glucose transporters (GLUT1) and glycolytic enzymes (hexokinase, pyruvate kinase M2/PKM2). The increased glucose uptake is exploited clinically in **FDG-PET imaging**: fluorodeoxyglucose (FDG), a glucose analogue, is preferentially taken up by metabolically active tumour cells and detected by positron emission tomography. FDG-PET is used for staging, response assessment, and detection of recurrence in lymphomas, lung cancers, and many other malignancies.

Beyond the Warburg effect, cancer metabolism is now recognised to be highly context-dependent. Some tumour cells rely on glutamine (glutaminolysis), fatty acid oxidation, or mitochondrial oxidative phosphorylation depending on the tissue of origin, genetic drivers (e.g., MYC drives glutaminolysis; VHL loss drives HIF-mediated glycolysis), and microenvironmental conditions. Metabolic heterogeneity within a single tumour is common, with glycolytic cells and oxidative cells cooperating in a metabolic symbiosis.

Limitless Replicative Potential: Telomerase in Cancer

Normal somatic cells have a finite replicative lifespan (the Hayflick limit, approximately 60–70 doublings for human fibroblasts). With each cell division, the telomeres (repetitive TTAGGG sequences at chromosome ends) shorten because DNA polymerase cannot fully replicate the 3' ends of linear chromosomes (the end-replication problem). When telomeres shorten to a critical length, the exposed chromosome ends activate the DNA damage response (p53 and RB pathways), triggering replicative senescence or apoptosis. This acts as a tumour suppressor mechanism, a "molecular clock" that limits proliferative capacity.

Cancer cells bypass this barrier by reactivating **telomerase**, a ribonucleoprotein enzyme (reverse transcriptase) that adds TTAGGG repeats to telomere ends, maintaining telomere length and conferring unlimited replicative potential. The catalytic subunit of telomerase is **hTERT (human telomerase reverse transcriptase)**. Telomerase is expressed in >90% of human cancers but is absent in most normal somatic cells (it is normally active only in germ cells, stem cells, and activated lymphocytes). **TERT promoter mutations** (C228T and C250T) create new binding sites for ETS transcription factors, upregulating hTERT expression. These mutations are common in melanoma, glioblastoma, urothelial carcinoma, hepatocellular carcinoma, and thyroid carcinoma, and are emerging as diagnostically useful biomarkers.

A minority of cancers (approximately 10–15%, predominantly sarcomas and gliomas) maintain telomere length through the alternative lengthening of telomeres (ALT) mechanism, a recombination-based pathway independent of telomerase.

Normal cell: telomere shortening with each division → critical length → p53/RB activation → senescence/apoptosis. Cancer cell: telomerase reactivation (hTERT) → telomere maintenance → unlimited replication

The Tumour Microenvironment

The tumour microenvironment (TME) comprises cancer-associated fibroblasts (CAFs), immune cells (tumour-infiltrating lymphocytes, tumour-associated macrophages, MDSCs, Tregs), endothelial cells, pericytes, and the extracellular matrix. These components are not passive bystanders; they actively support tumour growth and may also restrain it.

Cancer-associated fibroblasts (CAFs) are the most abundant stromal cell in many carcinomas. They secrete growth factors (HGF, EGF, IGF), cytokines, and chemokines that promote tumour cell proliferation, survival, and invasion. They produce the desmoplastic stroma (dense collagen-rich matrix) characteristic of pancreatic ductal adenocarcinoma, which acts as a physical barrier to drug delivery and immune cell infiltration. CAFs also remodel the ECM by secreting MMPs and lysyl oxidase, facilitating invasion.

Tumour-associated macrophages (TAMs) are often polarised toward an M2 (anti-inflammatory, pro-tumour) phenotype by tumour-derived signals (IL-4, IL-10, CSF1). M2 TAMs promote angiogenesis (VEGF), suppress anti-tumour immunity (IL-10, TGF-β, arginase), and facilitate invasion and metastasis (MMP secretion, cathepsin expression). High TAM density in the tumour stroma correlates with poor prognosis in most solid tumours. Targeting TAMs (CSF1R inhibitors, CD47-SIRPα checkpoint blockade) is an active area of therapeutic investigation.

The concept of "hot" versus "cold" tumours describes the degree of immune cell infiltration in the TME. "Hot" tumours (abundant TILs, inflamed stroma) are more likely to respond to immune checkpoint inhibitors. "Cold" tumours (immune-desert or immune-excluded) lack T-cell infiltration and are resistant to immunotherapy. Strategies to convert cold tumours to hot (radiation, oncolytic viruses, STING agonists) are in clinical development.

Evasion of Immune Destruction

The immune system constantly surveys for and eliminates nascent tumours, a process termed immune surveillance. Successful cancers are those that have evolved mechanisms to evade this surveillance. The concept of "cancer immunoediting" describes three phases: elimination (immune system destroys most tumour cells), equilibrium (immune system contains but does not eradicate residual tumour cells, which may persist for years), and escape (tumour cells acquire mutations or express molecules that allow them to evade immune attack).

The major mechanisms of immune evasion include: (1) **loss of MHC class I expression** (tumour cells become invisible to CTLs); (2) **expression of immune checkpoint ligands**, most importantly PD-L1 (programmed death-ligand 1), which binds PD-1 on activated T cells and delivers an inhibitory signal, inducing T-cell exhaustion and anergy; (3) secretion of immunosuppressive cytokines (TGF-β, IL-10); (4) recruitment of regulatory T cells (Tregs) and myeloid-derived suppressor cells (MDSCs) to the tumour microenvironment; and (5) loss of tumour antigens through immunoediting.

Immune checkpoint inhibitors have revolutionised cancer therapy by blocking these inhibitory signals. Anti-PD-1 antibodies (pembrolizumab, nivolumab) and anti-PD-L1 antibodies (atezolizumab, durvalumab) restore T-cell activity against tumour cells. Anti-CTLA-4 antibodies (ipilimumab) enhance T-cell activation by blocking a co-inhibitory receptor on T cells. These agents have produced durable responses in melanoma, NSCLC, RCC, Hodgkin lymphoma, and MSI-high cancers. Predictive biomarkers for checkpoint inhibitor response include PD-L1 expression by IHC, tumour mutational burden (TMB), and MSI/dMMR status.

Tumour antigen → T-cell recognition via TCR/MHC I → PD-L1 (tumour) binds PD-1 (T cell) → T-cell exhaustion. Anti-PD-1/PD-L1 antibody blocks this interaction → T-cell reactivation → Tumour killing

Cancer Stem Cells

The cancer stem cell (CSC) hypothesis proposes that tumours are hierarchically organised, with a small subpopulation of cells (cancer stem cells or tumour-initiating cells) that possess the capacity for self-renewal, differentiation, and tumour regeneration. The bulk of the tumour consists of rapidly dividing transit-amplifying cells that have limited replicative potential. CSCs are relatively resistant to chemotherapy and radiation (due to quiescence, enhanced DNA repair, and drug efflux pumps such as ABC transporters), which may explain tumour recurrence after apparently successful therapy. CSCs have been identified in AML (CD34+CD38−), breast cancer (CD44+CD24−), glioblastoma (CD133+), and colon cancer (Lgr5+). The CSC model has therapeutic implications: to eradicate a tumour, the CSC population must be eliminated, not just the bulk tumour cells.

Genomic Instability and DNA Repair Defects

Lynch syndrome (HNPCC) results from germline MMR gene mutations (MLH1, MSH2, MSH6, PMS2), accounting for 3–5% of CRC. Tumours are characteristically right-sided, mucinous/medullary, with TILs and accelerated adenoma–carcinoma progression. Universal MMR IHC on all new CRC is standard; MLH1/PMS2 loss triggers BRAF V600E and MLH1 methylation testing to distinguish sporadic from Lynch (see Chapter 25 for gynaecological Lynch cancers).

Other DNA repair pathway defects in cancer include: BRCA1/2 deficiency (homologous recombination repair; breast, ovarian, pancreatic, prostate cancers; sensitivity to PARP inhibitors, which exploit synthetic lethality); XP (nucleotide excision repair; skin cancers); and ATM deficiency (DNA damage signalling; lymphomas, breast cancer).

> **Quick Recall: Genomic Instability**
>
> **CIN:** chromosomal instability; aneuploidy; most common in solid tumours.
>
> **MSI:** microsatellite instability; dMMR (MLH1, MSH2, MSH6, PMS2); Lynch syndrome (germline) or MLH1 methylation (sporadic).
>
> **MSI-H tumours:** right-sided CRC, lymphocytic infiltrate, high neoantigen load, checkpoint inhibitor responsive.
>
> **BRCA1/2 deficiency:** HRR defect; breast-ovarian-pancreas-prostate; PARP inhibitor sensitivity (synthetic lethality).
>
> **Synthetic lethality:** PARP inhibition + BRCA loss = cell death; neither alone is lethal.

Routes of Spread and Organ Tropism

Malignant tumours spread by four routes. **Direct (local) extension:** invasion through tissue planes into adjacent structures. **Lymphatic spread:** the most common initial route for carcinomas. Tumour cells enter lymphatics and are carried to regional lymph nodes ("sentinel node" concept). Involvement of lymph nodes is a major prognostic factor and the basis of the N component in TNM staging. **Haematogenous spread:** the typical route for sarcomas, renal cell carcinoma, hepatocellular carcinoma, and choriocarcinoma. Tumour cells enter veins, and the pattern of organ metastasis follows venous drainage: GI tract tumours → liver (portal system); all other tumours → lungs (systemic veins → pulmonary capillary bed); lung tumours → brain, bone, adrenals (systemic arterial spread). Exceptions to the expected drainage pattern suggest involvement of the vertebral venous plexus (Batson plexus: valveless; allows prostate, breast, thyroid, kidney, and lung cancers to metastasise to the vertebral bodies). **Transcoelomic (seeding):** tumour cells shed into body cavities (peritoneum, pleura) and implant on serosal surfaces. Classic examples include ovarian carcinoma (peritoneal carcinomatosis) and gastric carcinoma (Krukenberg tumour: bilateral ovarian metastasis via transcoelomic spread of signet-ring cell carcinoma).

Primary Cancer	Common Metastatic Sites	Route
Lung carcinoma	Brain, bone, adrenal, liver, contralateral lung	Haematogenous
Breast carcinoma	Bone (most common), lung, liver, brain	Haematogenous + lymphatic (axillary nodes)
Colorectal carcinoma	Liver (portal venous drainage), lung, peritoneum	Haematogenous + transcoelomic

Prostate carcinoma	Bone (osteoblastic; vertebral bodies via Batson plexus), lymph nodes	Haematogenous
Renal cell carcinoma	Lung, bone, brain; invades renal vein/IVC	Haematogenous
Ovarian carcinoma	Peritoneum (carcinomatosis), omentum, contralateral ovary	Transcoelomic
Melanoma	Widespread: lung, liver, brain, skin, small bowel	Haematogenous + lymphatic
Gastric carcinoma (signet ring)	Ovaries (Krukenberg tumour), peritoneum, Virchow node (left supraclavicular)	Transcoelomic + lymphatic (Figure 6.7)

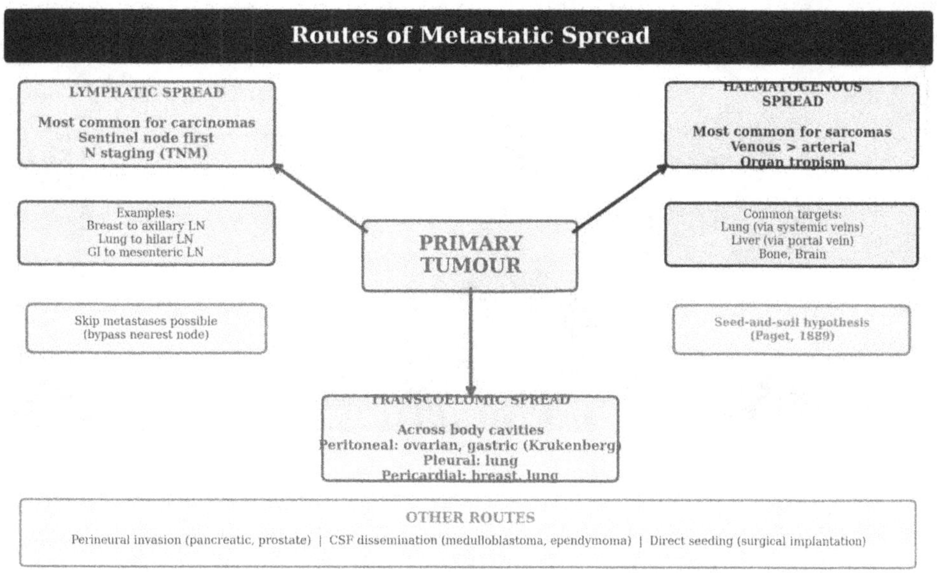

Figure 6.7: Routes of metastatic spread. (Source: Author's original.)

Molecular Basis of Invasion and Metastasis

The ability to invade surrounding tissues and metastasise to distant sites is the defining feature of malignancy and the cause of the vast majority of cancer deaths. The metastatic cascade is a complex, multistep process with multiple rate-limiting steps.

The Metastatic Cascade

Step 1: Local invasion. Tumour cells must detach from neighbours and penetrate the basement membrane and surrounding interstitial matrix. Key molecular events include downregulation of E-cadherin (loss of cell-cell adhesion), secretion of matrix metalloproteinases (MMP-2, MMP-9) that degrade type IV collagen in the basement membrane, and acquisition of motility through the epithelial-to-mesenchymal transition (EMT).

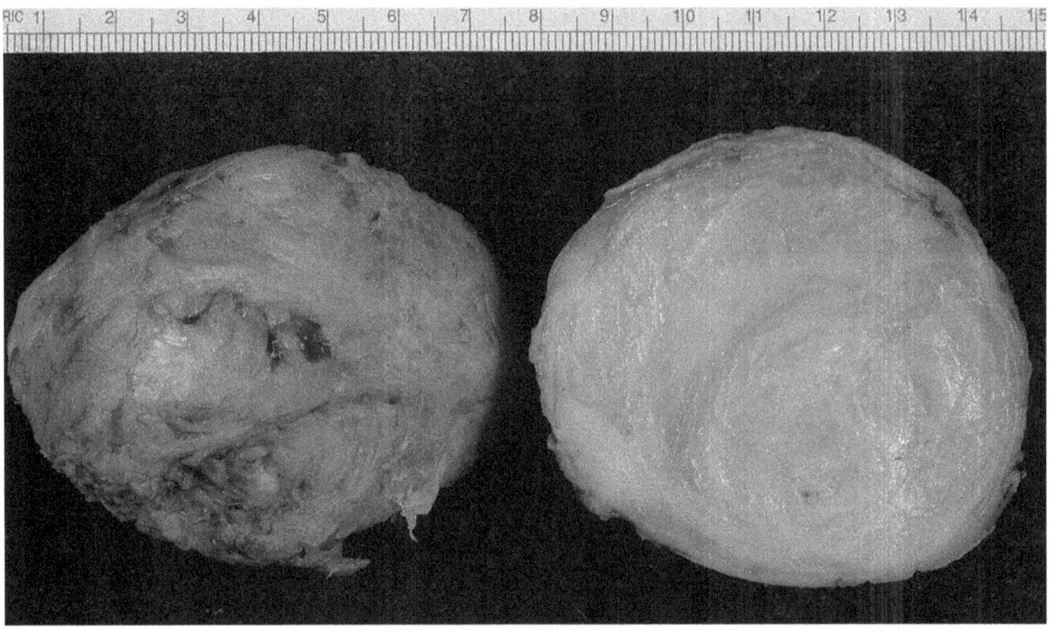

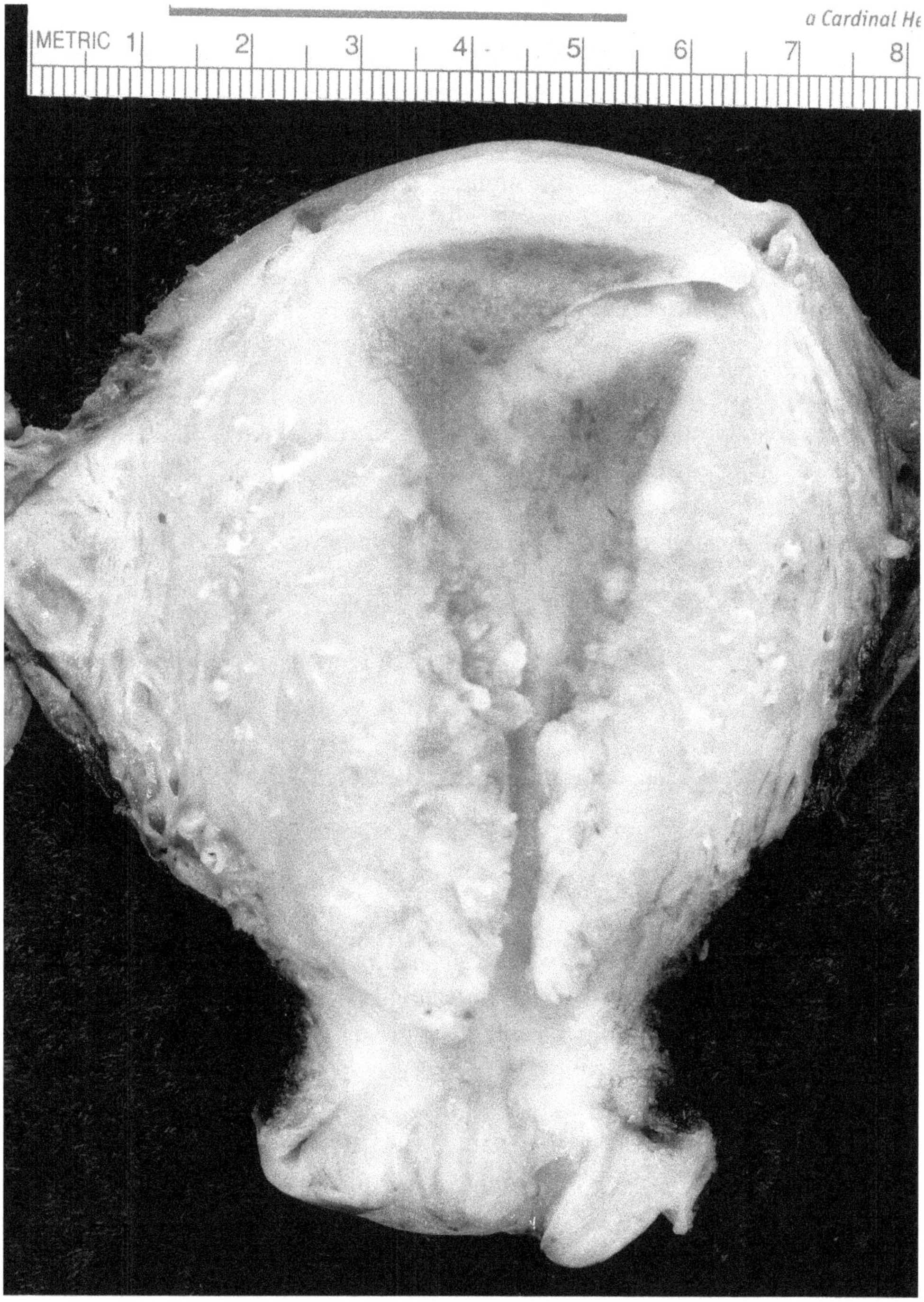

Figure 6.8: Benign versus malignant tumour — gross comparison. Top: Leiomyoma — well-circumscribed, encapsulated, whorled cut surface (benign). Bottom: Endometrioid adenocarcinoma, FIGO grade III — irregular infiltrative tumour invading myometrium (malignant) (Source: Ed Uthman, Wikimedia Commons, CC BY 2.0.)

Step 2: Intravasation. Tumour cells enter blood vessels (haematogenous spread) or lymphatics (lymphatic spread). This requires traversal of the vascular basement membrane, aided by tumour-associated macrophages and VEGF-mediated vascular permeability.

Step 3: Survival in the circulation. Circulating tumour cells (CTCs) are vulnerable to shear stress, anoikis (detachment-induced apoptosis), and immune attack. Survival strategies include coating with platelets (platelet cloaking, which shields from NK cells), travelling as tumour cell clusters, and expression of anti-apoptotic proteins.

Step 4: Extravasation. Tumour cells arrest in the microvasculature of distant organs, adhere to endothelium (via selectins, integrins), and migrate through the vessel wall into the parenchyma.

Step 5: Colonisation (metastatic growth). This is the most rate-limiting step. The tumour cell must adapt to the foreign microenvironment of the distant organ, recruit blood supply, and evade local immune defences. Many tumour cells remain dormant as micrometastases for years before emerging as clinically detectable metastases. The "seed and soil" hypothesis (Paget, 1889) explains organ tropism: certain cancers preferentially metastasise to specific organs because the tumour cells ("seed") are compatible with the microenvironment ("soil") of those organs. Chemokine-receptor interactions (e.g., CXCR4 on breast cancer cells homing to CXCL12-rich organs: bone, lung, liver) and pre-metastatic niche formation (tumour-derived exosomes and cytokines prepare distant sites for colonisation) are the molecular basis of organ tropism (Figure 6.1).

Local invasion (E-cadherin loss, MMP, EMT) → Intravasation → Survival in circulation (platelet cloaking) → Extravasation (selectins, integrins) → Colonisation (seed and soil, pre-metastatic niche, dormancy) (Figure 6.2)

Epithelial-to-Mesenchymal Transition (EMT)

EMT is a developmental programme hijacked by cancer cells to acquire invasive and migratory properties. During EMT, epithelial cells lose their polarity, cell-cell junctions (downregulation of E-cadherin, claudins, occludin), and epithelial markers (cytokeratins), and gain mesenchymal markers (vimentin, N-cadherin, fibronectin), motility, and resistance to apoptosis. EMT is driven by transcription factors Snail, Slug, Twist, and ZEB1/2, which directly repress E-cadherin transcription. Importantly, EMT is often partial and reversible: the reverse process (mesenchymal-to-epithelial transition, MET) may be required for tumour cells to colonise and form macrometastases at distant sites.

Why does loss of E-cadherin promote metastasis? E-cadherin is a calcium-dependent transmembrane protein that mediates homophilic cell-cell adhesion in epithelia. Its cytoplasmic domain binds β-catenin, linking it to the actin cytoskeleton. Loss of E-cadherin disrupts cell-cell adhesion, liberating cells from the primary tumour mass. Additionally, the released β-catenin can translocate to the nucleus and act as a transcriptional co-activator (Wnt signalling), further promoting proliferation and invasion. Germline mutation of CDH1 (E-cadherin gene) causes hereditary diffuse gastric cancer and lobular breast carcinoma.

The Pathologist's Eye

When evaluating a tumour for invasion on biopsy, look for: (1) irregular tumour borders with tongue-like projections extending into surrounding stroma; (2) desmoplastic stromal reaction (dense fibrosis around invasive glands, indicating a host response to invasion); (3) lymphovascular invasion (tumour emboli within endothelium-lined spaces); (4) perineural invasion (tumour cells wrapping around nerve fibres, common in pancreatic and prostatic adenocarcinoma). These features distinguish invasive carcinoma from in situ disease and are critical for staging and management.

Quick Recall: Invasion and Metastasis

EMT: loss of E-cadherin (↓epithelial markers) + gain of vimentin (↑mesenchymal markers); driven by Snail/Slug/Twist/ZEB.

MMP-2/9: degrade type IV collagen in basement membrane; critical for invasion.

Seed and soil: Paget's hypothesis; organ tropism explained by chemokine/receptor (CXCR4/CXCL12) and pre-metastatic niche.

CDH1 (E-cadherin) germline mutation: hereditary diffuse gastric cancer + lobular breast cancer.

Colonisation: most rate-limiting step; dormancy, angiogenesis, immune evasion required.

Recent Advances

Direct KRAS inhibitors. For decades, KRAS was considered "undruggable" because its smooth protein surface lacked a binding pocket for small molecules. The development of covalent inhibitors targeting the KRAS G12C mutant (sotorasib, adagrasib) marked a breakthrough. These drugs lock KRAS in the GDP-bound (inactive) state by exploiting the unique cysteine at position 12. Sotorasib was approved for previously treated KRAS G12C-mutant NSCLC. Inhibitors targeting other KRAS mutations (G12D, G12V) are in clinical development.

Liquid biopsy and circulating tumour DNA (ctDNA). Cell-free DNA shed by tumours into the bloodstream can be analysed by next-generation sequencing to identify actionable mutations, monitor treatment response, detect minimal residual disease, and identify resistance mutations, all without an invasive tissue biopsy. ctDNA-based assays (e.g., Guardant360, FoundationOne Liquid CDx) are increasingly incorporated into clinical practice for NSCLC, breast, and colorectal cancer.

Tumour mutational burden (TMB) and microsatellite instability (MSI) as biomarkers. TMB (the number of somatic mutations per megabase of sequenced DNA) and MSI-high status (resulting from defective mismatch repair, dMMR) predict response to immune checkpoint inhibitors (anti-PD-1/PD-L1) across tumour types. Pembrolizumab is approved for all MSI-high/dMMR solid tumours regardless of site of origin, the first "tissue-agnostic" approval in oncology, reflecting the primacy of molecular biology over anatomical classification in modern cancer therapy.

The key diagnostic clue in distinguishing a well-differentiated carcinoma from a benign neoplasm on biopsy: invasion. No amount of cytological atypia definitively diagnoses malignancy without evidence of stromal, vascular, or perineural invasion. Conversely, bland-looking neoplasms that penetrate the basement membrane (e.g., follicular thyroid carcinoma with capsular invasion) are malignant regardless of how "normal" the cells appear. The pathologist's search for invasion must be systematic: examine the tumour–stroma interface, look for desmoplastic reaction, and evaluate lymphovascular spaces.

When evaluating a tumour of uncertain lineage on small biopsy, the first-line IHC panel should establish the broad category: cytokeratin (epithelial), vimentin (mesenchymal), LCA/CD45 (haematolymphoid), S100 (melanocytic/neural), and synaptophysin/chromogranin (neuroendocrine). This "lineage panel" approach prevents the common error of ordering 20 markers without a diagnostic framework. Once lineage is established, targeted sub-panels refine the diagnosis.

International Frameworks

Hallmarks of cancer — 2022 update. Hanahan's 2022 update extends the original six hallmarks (sustained proliferative signalling, evasion of growth suppressors, resistance to cell death, replicative immortality, induced angiogenesis, activation of invasion and metastasis), the two enabling characteristics (genomic instability, tumour-promoting inflammation), and the two emerging hallmarks (deregulated cellular energetics, evasion of immune destruction). The 2022 framework adds phenotypic plasticity and disrupted differentiation as a discrete hallmark capability, and identifies non-mutational epigenetic reprogramming and polymorphic microbiomes as additional enabling characteristics. Senescent cells of varying origins are recognised as functionally significant components of the tumour microenvironment. The conceptual update has direct relevance for stratifying tumour biology beyond mutation profile in clinical reporting. Citation: Hanahan D. Cancer Discov 2022;12(1):31–46. PMID 35022204.

WHO Classification of Tumours, 5th edition — hierarchical taxonomy and integrated diagnosis. The 5th edition of the WHO Classification of Tumours (the "Blue Books"), inaugurated in 2019 with the Digestive System volume and continuing in successive organ-system volumes, replaces the discrete chapter-based structure of the 4th edition with a hierarchical taxonomy organised at five levels — site, category, family (or superfamily), type, and subtype. Each tumour entity is anchored to an ICD-O morphology code (M-XXXX/Y) in which the four-digit prefix specifies histological type and the suffix codes biological behaviour (/0 benign, /1 uncertain or borderline, /2 in situ, /3 malignant). The defining methodological shift is integrated diagnosis: where the 4th edition prioritised morphology with molecular findings as adjuncts, the 5th edition recognises certain entities as essentially molecularly defined — NUT carcinoma, SMARCB1-deficient carcinomas, DICER1-mutated tumours, and the BCOR- and CIC-rearranged sarcomas — such that morphology and a specified molecular alteration are jointly required for diagnosis. Grading conventions remain entity-specific rather than universal: the FNCLCC system for soft tissue sarcomas; ISUP Grade Groups (2014) for prostatic adenocarcinoma; the WHO/ISUP nucleolar grade (2016) for clear-cell and papillary renal cell carcinoma; the Nottingham (Bloom-Richardson) system for breast carcinoma; the WHO/ENETS scheme for neuroendocrine neoplasms (G1, G2, G3 stratified by mitotic count and Ki-67 index); and the WHO four-tier scheme of well, moderately, poorly differentiated, and undifferentiated carcinoma for hepatocellular carcinoma (replacing historical Edmondson-Steiner). The framework formalises three concepts that the FRCPath and international postgraduate examiner will probe directly — that benign and malignant counterparts of the same tumour family share a morphological spectrum, that hereditary tumour syndromes are listed as named entities with their causative germline alterations, and that "essential" diagnostic criteria are distinguished from "desirable" criteria in each entity description. This provides a reproducible standard for surgical-pathology reporting that aligns with the College of American Pathologists synoptic protocols and the International Collaboration on Cancer Reporting (ICCR) datasets adopted by the Royal College of Pathologists, the Royal College of Pathologists of Australasia, and the College of American Pathologists. Citation: Nagtegaal ID, Odze RD, Klimstra D, et al; WHO Classification of Tumours Editorial Board. The 2019 WHO classification of tumours of the digestive system. Histopathology 2020; 76: 182–188. PMID 31433515.

Ultra High-Yield Chapter Summary

Topic	Must Remember
Hallmarks of cancer	8 hallmarks + 2 enabling characteristics (Hanahan & Weinberg 2011)
Oncogenes	Dominant; gain-of-function; single allele sufficient.
RAS	Most commonly mutated oncogene; GTPase locked in GTP-bound active state; codons 12/13/61; KRAS G12C inhibitors
MYC	Transcription factor; t(8;14) Burkitt; NMYC amplification = poor prognosis in neuroblastoma
BCR-ABL	t(9;22) Philadelphia; CML; constitutive TK; imatinib; also in Ph+ ALL
HER2	Amplification in 20% breast cancers; trastuzumab; also gastric cancer
Tumour suppressors	Recessive; loss-of-function; both alleles must be lost (two-hit)
p53	Guardian of genome; most commonly mutated gene (>50% cancers); Li-Fraumeni; HPV E6 degrades it
RB	G1/S checkpoint; Knudson two-hit; retinoblastoma; HPV E7 degrades it
APC	Wnt/β-catenin; FAP; initiating event in adenoma-carcinoma sequence of CRC
BRCA1/2	Homologous recombination repair; hereditary breast-ovarian; PARP

	inhibitor sensitivity
VHL	HIF-1α degradation; clear cell RCC, haemangioblastoma, phaeo
CDK4/6-Cyclin D	G1 checkpoint; palbociclib/ribociclib in HR+ breast cancer; cyclin D1: MCL t(11;14)
p16/INK4a	CDK4/6 inhibitor; frequently deleted/methylated; p16 IHC = HPV surrogate in oropharyngeal SCC
Chemical carcinogenesis	Initiation (irreversible DNA damage) → promotion (clonal expansion) → progression (malignant)
Aflatoxin B1	p53 codon 249 mutation; HCC; synergy with HBV; aflatoxin grain contamination
HPV E6/E7	E6 degrades p53; E7 degrades RB; cervical, oropharyngeal SCC
EBV	Burkitt, NPC, HL, PTLD, NK/T-cell lymphoma; LMP1, EBNA2
H. pylori	Gastric adenocarcinoma (CagA+) and MALT lymphoma
EMT	E-cadherin loss + vimentin gain; Snail/Slug/Twist/ZEB; invasion and metastasis
Metastatic cascade	Invasion → intravasation → circulation → extravasation → colonisation (rate-limiting)
Seed and soil	Paget; organ tropism; CXCR4/CXCL12; pre-metastatic niche
Warburg effect	Aerobic glycolysis; ↑GLUT1; basis of FDG-PET
Epigenetic silencing	Promoter CpG methylation (p16, MLH1, BRCA1, VHL); HDAC inhibitors
KRAS G12C inhibitors	Sotorasib, adagrasib; first direct KRAS inhibitors; approved for NSCLC
TMB/MSI-H	Predict checkpoint inhibitor response; pembrolizumab approved tissue-agnostic for MSI-H/dMMR

Diagnostic thinking: self-sufficiency in growth signals + evasion of apoptosis + sustained angiogenesis → hallmarks of cancer (Hanahan-Weinberg)

Diagnostic thinking: stepwise accumulation of mutations (APC → KRAS → TP53) → adenoma-carcinoma sequence (CIN pathway)

Diagnostic thinking: loss of E-cadherin + nuclear beta-catenin + EMT markers → invasive/metastatic phenotype (Figure 6.7)

Chapter 7: Neoplasia Part 2: Diagnosis and Clinical Aspects

THE BIG PICTURE

Cancer diagnosis integrates morphology, immunohistochemistry, molecular testing, and clinical correlation. The pathologist provides the tissue diagnosis that determines classification, grading, staging, and treatment planningal chain, transforming tissue morphology, immunophenotype, and molecular profile into a diagnosis that determines whether a patient receives surgery, chemotherapy, immunotherapy, or palliation. This chapter bridges the gap between cancer biology (Chapter 6) and organ-specific tumour pathology (Part B), covering the agents that cause cancer, the clinical effects tumours produce, and the expanding arsenal of diagnostic tools available to the modern pathologist.

High-yield topics in this chapter:

Chemical, radiation, and microbial carcinogenesis; Paraneoplastic syndromes; Tumour grading and staging (TNM); Laboratory diagnosis of cancer (biopsy, FNAC, frozen section, IHC, FISH, molecular diagnostics, flow cytometry, liquid biopsy); Serum tumour markers; Prognostic and predictive markers; Cancer epidemiology and screening; Precision oncology and companion diagnostics.

Tissue diagnosis is the foundation of cancer management. It provides tumour type, grade, stage, margin status, and molecular profile — information essential for treatment planning. The diagnostic pathologist today works not only with haematoxylin and eosin but with immunohistochemistry panels, fluorescence in situ hybridisation, next-generation sequencing, and liquid biopsy platforms. Understanding these tools, their indications, their limitations, and the clinical questions they answer is as essential to the modern pathology postgraduate as understanding the morphology itself.

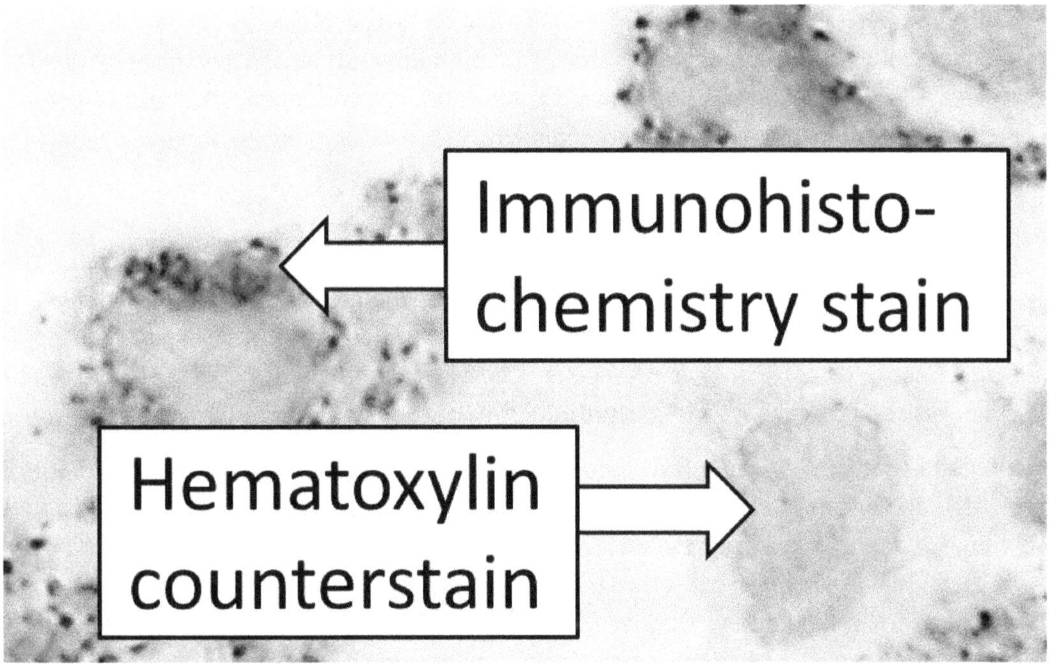

Figure 7.1: Immunohistochemistry — positive staining example showing brown DAB chromogen versus blue haematoxylin counterstain (Source: Mikael Häggström, Wikimedia Commons, CC0.)

Agents of Carcinogenesis

HIGH-YIELD TUMOR MARKERS

Marker	Tumor	Clinical Use
AFP	HCC, Yolk sac tumor, Teratoma	Diagnosis + monitoring
β-hCG	Choriocarcinoma, Testicular GCT	Diagnosis + follow-up
CEA	Colorectal Ca	Monitoring (not screening)
CA-125	Ovarian (serous)	Monitoring response
CA 19-9	Pancreatic Ca	Monitoring
PSA	Prostate Ca	Screening + monitoring
S-100	Melanoma, Schwannoma	IHC diagnosis
Chromogranin A	Neuroendocrine tumors	Serum + IHC
CD117 (c-KIT)	GIST	Diagnosis + imatinib eligibility
HER2/neu	Breast Ca	Prognosis + trastuzumab
BRCA1/2	Breast / Ovarian Ca	Risk + PARP inhibitor
ALK	NSCLC (adenocarcinoma)	Targeted Rx (crizotinib)
Calretinin	Mesothelioma	IHC (vs adenocarcinoma)
TTF-1	Lung adenoCa, Thyroid	IHC site of origin

Figure 7.2: High-Yield Tumor Markers. (Source: Author's original.)

The molecular hallmarks of cancer (see Chapter 6) are driven by specific aetiological agents. These agents, whether chemical, physical, or biological, share a common endpoint: they damage DNA, activate oncogenes, or disable tumour suppressor genes. Understanding carcinogenesis is fundamental both for cancer prevention and for interpreting the molecular profiles used in modern diagnosis.

Chemical Carcinogenesis

The concept of chemical carcinogenesis was established by Percivall Pott in 1775, who linked scrotal cancer in chimney sweeps to soot exposure. Since then, hundreds of chemical carcinogens have been identified and classified by the International Agency for Research on Cancer (IARC) into Group 1 (definite), Group 2A (probable), and Group 2B (possible) carcinogens. Chemical carcinogenesis proceeds through a well-characterised multistep process involving initiation, promotion, and progression.

The molecular mechanism of chemical carcinogenesis — the three-phase sequence of initiation (irreversible DNA damage by the ultimate carcinogen), promotion (reversible clonal expansion driven by non-mutagenic promoters), and progression (accumulation of mutations toward malignant phenotype) — is detailed in Chapter 6. The present section focuses on the clinical and agent-specific perspective: which chemicals cause which cancers, how they are classified for occupational and public health risk (IARC Group 1, 2A, 2B, 3), and the exam-testable carcinogen–tumour associations.

IARC (International Agency for Research on Cancer) classifies agents by strength of evidence for human carcinogenicity: Group 1 (definite carcinogen — sufficient evidence in humans; includes aflatoxin, benzene, tobacco, HPV, asbestos, ionising radiation, H. pylori), Group 2A (probable), Group 2B (possible), and Group 3 (not classifiable). Group 4 ("probably not carcinogenic") has historically contained a single agent and was phased out of routine use.

Table 7.2: Major Chemical Carcinogens and Associated Neoplasms

Carcinogen	Type	Associated Neoplasm
Aflatoxin B1 (Aspergillus flavus)	Indirect	Hepatocellular carcinoma
Benzo[a]pyrene (tobacco smoke, soot)	Indirect	Lung, laryngeal, oropharyngeal carcinomas
Beta-naphthylamine (aniline dyes)	Indirect	Urinary bladder carcinoma
Vinyl chloride	Indirect	Hepatic angiosarcoma
Nickel, chromium compounds	Indirect	Lung carcinoma
Arsenic	Indirect	Skin, lung carcinoma
Asbestos	Indirect	Mesothelioma, lung carcinoma (see Chapter 16)

Cyclophosphamide, busulphan	Direct	Leukaemias, bladder carcinoma
Nitrosamines (processed meats)	Indirect	Gastric, oesophageal carcinoma
Benzene	Indirect	Acute myeloid leukaemia (see Volume 1)

The key diagnostic clue in occupational cancer is the combination of an unusual tumour at an unusual site in a patient with a relevant exposure history: hepatic angiosarcoma in a vinyl chloride worker, mesothelioma in an asbestos-exposed individual, or bladder carcinoma in an aniline dye worker.

Radiation Carcinogenesis

The cellular mechanisms of radiation-induced DNA damage (direct strand breaks, indirect oxidative damage via ROS, pyrimidine-dimer formation by UV) are covered in Chapter 6. This section summarises the clinical spectrum of radiation-associated malignancies and the latency patterns that guide survivorship surveillance: UV-B causes basal cell carcinoma, squamous cell carcinoma, and melanoma of sun-exposed skin, with nucleotide excision repair (NER) defects (xeroderma pigmentosum) producing a several-thousand-fold risk increase. Ionising radiation produces leukaemia with a short latency of 5–7 years (atomic bomb survivors, therapeutic radiation) followed by solid tumours (thyroid, breast, lung, colon) with latencies of 10–20 years. Thyroid is especially radiosensitive in children (Chernobyl). There is no safe threshold — risk rises linearly with dose (linear no-threshold model).

Quick Recall: Radiation Carcinogenesis

UV-B: Pyrimidine dimers; C→T transitions; NER repairs; defective in xeroderma pigmentosum.

Ionising radiation: Double-strand breaks; leukaemia (short latency 5-7 yr) then solid tumours (long latency 10-20 yr).

Radiosensitive tissues: Thyroid, bone marrow, breast, lung, GI epithelium.

Microbial Carcinogenesis

Approximately 15 to 20% of all human cancers worldwide are attributable to infectious agents. In developing countries including India, the proportion is even higher owing to the burden of hepatitis B, hepatitis C, HPV, and *Helicobacter pylori* infections. The IARC classifies seven viruses, one bacterium, and three parasites as Group 1 carcinogens.

Oncogenic DNA Viruses

Human papillomavirus (HPV): High-risk HPV types (16, 18, 31, 33, 45) cause cervical, oropharyngeal, anal, vulvar, vaginal, and penile carcinomas. The oncogenic mechanism centres on two viral proteins: E6 (which binds and degrades p53 via the ubiquitin-proteasome pathway) and E7 (which binds and inactivates Rb, releasing E2F transcription factors). Integration of viral DNA into the host genome disrupts E2, the viral repressor of E6/E7 expression, leading to constitutive oncogene expression. HPV 16 predominates in squamous cell carcinomas, while HPV 18 is overrepresented in adenocarcinomas of the cervix (see Chapter 25, Chapter 32).

HPV E6 → Binds p53 → Ubiquitin-mediated degradation → Loss of p53 checkpoint

HPV E7 → Binds Rb → Release of E2F → Uncontrolled S-phase entry

Epstein-Barr virus (EBV): EBV is associated with Burkitt lymphoma (endemic form in Africa), nasopharyngeal carcinoma, Hodgkin lymphoma (mixed cellularity and lymphocyte-depleted subtypes), post-transplant lymphoproliferative disorder (PTLD), and a subset of gastric carcinomas. EBV infects B lymphocytes via the CD21 receptor and drives proliferation through latent membrane protein 1 (LMP-1), which mimics constitutive CD40 signalling and activates NF-κB, JAK/STAT, and PI3K/AKT pathways. In Burkitt lymphoma, EBV-driven B-cell proliferation increases the probability of the t(8;14) translocation that deregulates MYC (see Volume 1).

Hepatitis B virus (HBV) and Hepatitis C virus (HCV): Both viruses cause hepatocellular carcinoma (HCC), primarily through the pathway of chronic hepatitis, cirrhosis, and regenerative hyperplasia (see Chapter 20). HBV additionally has a direct oncogenic role through integration into the host genome and production of HBx protein, which activates multiple signalling pathways and inhibits p53. HCV, an RNA virus, does not integrate into the genome but promotes carcinogenesis through chronic inflammation, oxidative stress, and activation of growth factor pathways. India has intermediate HBV endemicity (3 to 4% carrier rate) and an estimated 12 to 18 million HCV-infected individuals.

Human herpesvirus 8 (HHV-8/KSHV): Causes Kaposi sarcoma and primary effusion lymphoma. Produces viral homologues of cyclin D and cytokines that drive angiogenesis and proliferation.

Human T-cell lymphotropic virus 1 (HTLV-1): An RNA retrovirus causing adult T-cell leukaemia/lymphoma, endemic in Japan and the Caribbean. The viral protein Tax activates NF-κB, drives proliferation, and impairs DNA repair. Disease latency is typically 20 to 30 years.

Oncogenic Bacteria and Parasites

Helicobacter pylori: Classified as a Group 1 carcinogen for gastric adenocarcinoma and gastric MALT lymphoma. Chronic gastritis induced by *H. pylori* progresses through the Correa cascade: chronic gastritis, intestinal metaplasia, dysplasia, and adenocarcinoma. The CagA protein, injected into gastric epithelial cells by the type IV secretion system, activates growth factor receptors and promotes epithelial proliferation (see Chapter 18).

Among the oncogenic parasites, *Schistosoma haematobium* causes squamous cell carcinoma of the urinary bladder (endemic in Egypt and sub-Saharan Africa), and the liver flukes *Clonorchis sinensis* and *Opisthorchis viverrini* cause cholangiocarcinoma (see Chapter 20).

Table 7.3: Infectious Agents and Associated Cancers

Agent	Mechanism	Associated Cancer
HPV 16, 18	E6 degrades p53; E7 inactivates Rb	Cervical, oropharyngeal, anal SCC
EBV	LMP-1 mimics CD40; NF-κB	Burkitt lymphoma, NPC, Hodgkin,

	activation	PTLD, gastric
HBV	HBx inactivates p53; genomic integration	Hepatocellular carcinoma
HCV	Chronic inflammation; oxidative stress	Hepatocellular carcinoma
HHV-8	Viral cyclin D; angiogenic cytokines	Kaposi sarcoma, primary effusion lymphoma
HTLV-1	Tax activates NF-κB	Adult T-cell leukaemia/lymphoma
H. pylori	CagA; chronic inflammation; Correa cascade	Gastric adenocarcinoma, MALT lymphoma
S. haematobium	Chronic cystitis; carcinogen concentration	SCC urinary bladder
Liver flukes	Chronic biliary inflammation	Cholangiocarcinoma

When faced with a question on biological carcinogenesis, the examiner expects the molecular mechanism for each agent: E6/E7 for HPV, LMP-1 for EBV, HBx for HBV, CagA for H. pylori, and Tax for HTLV-1.

Quick Recall: Agents of Carcinogenesis

Chemical: Initiation (irreversible DNA damage) → Promotion (reversible clonal expansion) → Progression (malignant conversion). Most carcinogens are indirect-acting (require P-450 activation).

Radiation: UV-B causes pyrimidine dimers; ionising radiation causes double-strand breaks. Leukaemia (short latency), solid tumours (long latency).

Microbial: HPV (E6/E7), EBV (LMP-1), HBV (HBx), HCV (chronic inflammation), HTLV-1 (Tax), H. pylori (CagA), parasites (chronic inflammation).

Integration: Microbial carcinogenesis connects to cervical pathology (Chapter 25), hepatobiliary pathology (Chapter 20), gastric pathology (Chapter 18), and the biology of viral oncoproteins discussed in Chapter 6.

Cancer Epidemiology

Cancer epidemiology provides the context within which diagnosis operates. Globally, the most common cancers by incidence are lung, breast, colorectal, prostate, and stomach. Regional cancer profiles differ significantly between high- and low/middle-income countries. South Asia accounts for a disproportionate share of the global burden of oral and cervical cancer. These epidemiological patterns reflect the combined influence of tobacco use (oral cancers), HPV infection (cervical), dietary habits (oesophageal, gastric), and increasing urbanisation and lifestyle changes (breast, colorectal).

Environmental and lifestyle factors account for the majority of cancers; only 5 to 10% of all cancers arise from inherited germline mutations. This is supported by migrant studies showing that cancer incidence in immigrant populations tends to converge with that of the host country within one to two generations, underscoring the dominance of environmental over genetic factors.

Predisposing conditions: Several non-hereditary conditions increase cancer risk: chronic inflammation (ulcerative colitis and colorectal carcinoma, chronic pancreatitis and pancreatic carcinoma), immunodeficiency (HIV-associated Kaposi sarcoma and lymphomas; post-transplant lymphoproliferative disorder), and precursor lesions (Barrett oesophagus, oral leukoplakia, cervical CIN). Immunodeficiency-associated carcinogenesis is particularly important given the global HIV burden and the increasing use of immunosuppressive therapies.

Clinical Effects of Neoplasia

The clinical effects of tumours extend far beyond the mass itself. Tumours produce symptoms through local effects, hormonal activity, and remote (paraneoplastic) phenomena.

Local and Systemic Effects

Local effects depend on the anatomical site and include obstruction (colonic carcinoma causing bowel obstruction, bronchogenic carcinoma causing atelectasis), compression (meningioma compressing brain parenchyma, pelvic tumours compressing ureters), ulceration and haemorrhage (gastric carcinoma, bladder carcinoma), pathological fracture (metastatic deposits or primary bone tumours), and perforation (gastric lymphoma during chemotherapy).

Cancer cachexia is a complex metabolic syndrome characterised by progressive weight loss, muscle wasting (sarcopenia), anorexia, and weakness that cannot be fully reversed by conventional nutritional support. Cachexia affects up to 80% of patients with advanced cancer and is a direct cause of death in approximately 20 to 30% of cancer patients. The pathogenesis involves tumour-derived factors (proteolysis-inducing factor, lipid-mobilising factor) and host-derived inflammatory cytokines, particularly TNF-α (previously called cachectin), IL-6, and IL-1. These mediators increase basal metabolic rate, promote skeletal muscle proteolysis via the ubiquitin-proteasome pathway, suppress appetite through hypothalamic effects, and induce adipose tissue lipolysis. Unlike simple starvation, where the body preferentially burns fat and preserves lean mass, cachexia consumes both fat and skeletal muscle.

A viva question that reliably distinguishes strong from average candidates: 'Why cannot cancer cachexia be reversed by nutritional supplementation alone?' The answer lies in the cytokine-driven catabolic state: TNF-α and IL-6 actively drive proteolysis and lipolysis regardless of caloric intake, making cachexia a metabolic reprogramming rather than mere malnutrition.

Paraneoplastic Syndromes

Paraneoplastic syndromes are symptom complexes that cannot be explained by local tumour spread or metastasis. They occur in approximately 10 to 15% of cancer patients and may be the **first clinical manifestation** of an occult malignancy. Recognising these syndromes is clinically important for three reasons: they may mimic metastatic disease and lead to unnecessary staging procedures; they may provide an early clue to an otherwise undetected cancer; and they may cause significant morbidity independent of the tumour itself. The major categories are endocrinopathies, neuromyopathies, dermatological, haematological, and renal syndromes.

Table 7.8: Major Paraneoplastic Syndromes

Syndrome	Mediator	Associated Tumour
Cushing syndrome	Ectopic ACTH or CRH	Small cell lung carcinoma, pancreatic carcinoma
SIADH (hyponatraemia)	Ectopic ADH	Small cell lung carcinoma, CNS tumours
Hypercalcaemia	PTHrP; 1,25$(OH)_2D_3$; osteolytic metastases	SCC lung, breast, renal, myeloma, lymphoma
Carcinoid syndrome	Serotonin (5-HT), histamine	Carcinoid tumours (especially with liver metastases)
Polycythaemia	Ectopic EPO	Renal cell carcinoma, HCC, cerebellar haemangioblastoma
Trousseau syndrome (migratory thrombophlebitis)	Mucin, tissue factor, procoagulants	Pancreatic carcinoma, lung, GI cancers
DIC	Procoagulants, tissue factor	APL, mucin-secreting adenocarcinomas
Non-bacterial thrombotic endocarditis (marantic)	Hypercoagulable state	Advanced mucin-secreting adenocarcinomas
Lambert-Eaton syndrome	Anti-presynaptic Ca^{2+} channel Ab	Small cell lung carcinoma
Myasthenia gravis	Anti-AChR antibodies	Thymoma

Dermatomyositis	Autoimmune (mechanism unclear)	Lung, breast, ovarian, GI carcinomas
Acanthosis nigricans	Growth factor secretion (?TGF-α)	Gastric and other GI carcinomas
Membranous nephropathy	Immune complex deposition	Lung, colon carcinomas
Hypertrophic osteoarthropathy	Mechanism unclear	Lung carcinoma (especially non-small cell)

The distinction from [differential] rests on three features: In paraneoplastic hypercalcaemia, PTHrP (parathyroid hormone-related protein) is the most common mediator, especially in squamous cell carcinomas. It activates the same receptor as PTH (PTH1R) but is immunologically distinct and not detected by standard PTH assays. This contrasts with hypercalcaemia due to primary hyperparathyroidism (elevated PTH) and that due to osteolytic bone metastases (where the mechanism is direct bone destruction with normal PTH and normal PTHrP).

Exam Pitfall

Paraneoplastic hypercalcaemia is humoral, not metastatic: PTHrP from SCC lung can cause severe hypercalcaemia without any bone metastasis. Do not confuse this with hypercalcaemia from osteolytic metastases (breast cancer, myeloma), which occurs through local bone destruction by tumour cells and is mediated by RANKL and other osteoclast-activating factors.

Quick Recall: Paraneoplastic Syndromes

Endocrine: Cushing (SCLC, ACTH), SIADH (SCLC, ADH), Hypercalcaemia (SCC, PTHrP), Polycythaemia (RCC, EPO).

Neurological: Lambert-Eaton (SCLC, anti-Ca^{2+} channel), Myasthenia (thymoma, anti-AChR), Cerebellar degeneration (anti-Yo, breast/ovary).

Haematological: Trousseau (pancreas, mucin), DIC (APL), NBTE (advanced adenocarcinomas).

Dermatological: Acanthosis nigricans (gastric), Dermatomyositis (lung, breast, ovary).

Integration: Paraneoplastic syndromes connect to endocrine pathology (Chapter 27), haemostatic disorders (Volume 1), neuromuscular pathology (Chapter 30), and dermatopathology (Chapter 28). DIC and Trousseau syndrome are discussed in detail in Volume 1.

Grading and Staging of Tumours

Accurate grading and staging of malignant tumours are essential for prognostication, treatment planning, and clinical trial stratification. **Grading** reflects the degree of differentiation of the tumour (how closely the tumour resembles the tissue of origin) and is assessed by the pathologist on histological examination. **Staging** describes the extent of tumour spread and is a composite clinical-pathological assessment incorporating imaging, surgical findings, and pathological examination.

Histological Grading

Most grading systems use a three-tier (well-differentiated, moderately differentiated, poorly differentiated) or four-tier classification (adding undifferentiated). Important organ-specific grading systems include:

Gleason grading system (prostate carcinoma, see Chapter 24): Based on architectural patterns scored 1 to 5. The Grade Group system (1 to 5) derived from Gleason scores is now standard. **Nottingham grading system** (breast carcinoma, see Chapter 26): Combines tubule formation, nuclear pleomorphism, and mitotic count. **Fuhrman/WHO-ISUP grading** (renal cell carcinoma, see Chapter 23): Based on nucleolar prominence. **FIGO grading** (endometrial carcinoma, see Chapter 25): Based on percentage of solid (non-squamous) growth. For sarcomas, the FNCLCC (Fédération Nationale des Centres de Lutte Contre le Cancer) system uses tumour differentiation, mitotic count, and necrosis (see Chapter 29).

Table 7.6: Master Grading Systems

System	Organ	Parameters	Grades	Key Rule
Gleason/ISUP Grade Group	Prostate	Architectural pattern (1-5)	GG1-5	Cribriform pattern always Gleason pattern 4 or higher
Nottingham (Elston-Ellis)	Breast	Tubule formation + nuclear pleomorphism + mitotic count	Grade 1-3 (3-5, 6-7, 8-9)	Each parameter scored 1-3; sum determines grade
WHO/ISUP (formerly Fuhrman)	RCC	Nucleolar prominence at 400x	Grade 1-4	G4: sarcomatoid/rhabdoid differentiation regardless of nucleoli
FNCLCC	Soft tissue sarcoma	Differentiation + mitotic count + necrosis	Grade 1-3	Each scored 1-3; total 2-3=G1, 4-5=G2, 6-8=G3
WHO NE grading	Neuroendocrine	Ki-67 index and mitotic rate	G1 (Ki-67 <=2%), G2 (3-20%), G3 (>20%); NEC separate	NET vs NEC: p53/Rb aberrant in NEC, intact in NET G3
Edmondson-Steiner	HCC	Nuclear size, N:C ratio, architecture	Grade 1-4	Higher grade correlates with vascular invasion risk

Tumour Staging: The TNM System

The TNM staging system, maintained by the American Joint Committee on Cancer (AJCC) and the Union for International Cancer Control (UICC), is the most widely used staging framework. It consists of three components:

T (Tumour): Size and/or extent of the primary tumour (T1-T4, with Tis for carcinoma in situ and T0 for no evidence of primary tumour). **N (Nodes):** Extent of regional lymph node involvement (N0-N3). **M (Metastasis):** Presence or absence of distant metastases (M0 or M1). The prefix 'p' denotes pathological staging (pT, pN, pM) based on surgical specimens; 'c' denotes clinical staging based on imaging and physical examination; 'y' denotes post-neoadjuvant therapy staging.

The TNM components are combined into an overall **Stage Group** (Stage I through Stage IV), with higher stages indicating more advanced disease and poorer prognosis. It is critical to remember that staging is the single most important prognostic factor for most solid malignancies, more powerful than grade, histological subtype, or molecular markers in determining overall survival.

Table 7.7: TNM Staging Principles (AJCC 8th Edition)

Component	Definition	Key Concepts
T (Tumour)	Size and/or depth of invasion of primary tumour (Tis, T1-T4)	Tis = carcinoma in situ. T criteria are organ-specific (size for breast/lung; depth for GI).
N (Nodes)	Regional lymph node involvement (N0-N3)	ITC: <0.2 mm or <200 cells (pN0). Micrometastasis: 0.2-2 mm (pN1mi). Macrometastasis: >2 mm. Sentinel LN biopsy determines pN.
M (Metastasis)	Distant metastasis (M0 vs M1)	M1 = Stage IV in most cancers regardless of T or N.
Prefixes	c = clinical, p = pathological, y = post-neoadjuvant, r = recurrence	ypTNM reflects treatment effect; ypT0N0 = pathological complete response (pCR).

> **Quick Recall: Grading and Staging**
>
> **Grading = differentiation** (pathologist assesses on histology): well, moderate, poor, undifferentiated.
>
> **Staging = extent of spread** (TNM system): T = tumour size/extent, N = nodes, M = metastasis.
>
> **Key principle:** Staging is the most important prognostic factor for most solid tumours. Grade and stage are complementary, not interchangeable (Figure 7.3).

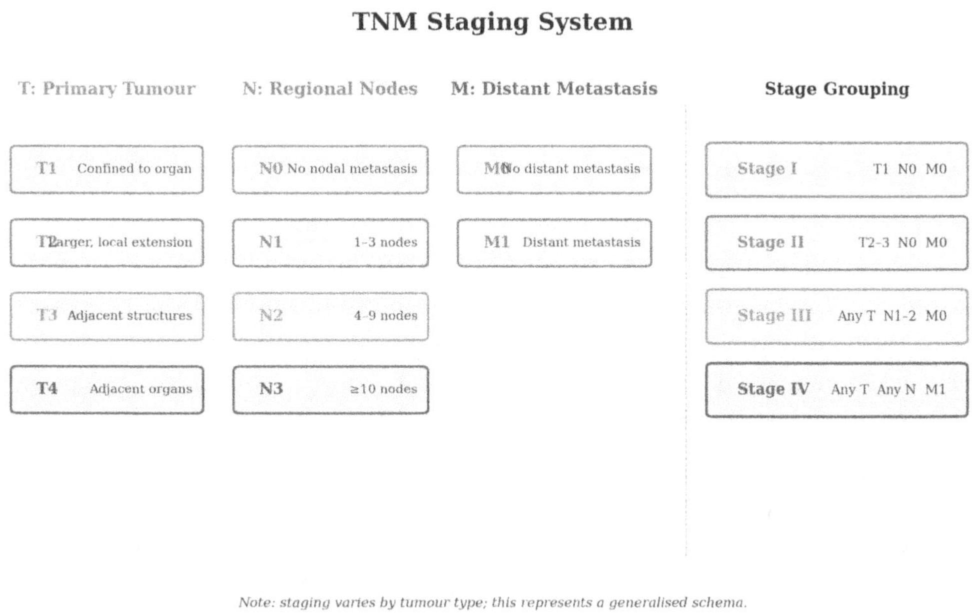

Figure 7.3: TNM staging concept. (Source: Author's original.)

WHO Histological Grading of Tumours (General Principles)

The WHO classification of tumours ("Blue Book" series, now in its 5th edition) provides site-specific histological diagnoses. Across most organ systems, histological grade is expressed as a 3- or 4-tier system assessing differentiation. Grade is distinct from stage: grade is "how the tumour looks" (pathologist, from morphology), stage is "how far it has spread" (clinician/radiologist/pathologist, from anatomy).

Table 7.3a: Generic WHO/AJCC 4-Tier Histological Grading

Grade	Differentiation	Glandular/structural resemblance	Prognostic implication
GX	Cannot be assessed	—	Not stratifiable
G1 — Well differentiated	Closely resembles tissue of origin	Glands/structures well-formed; nuclear atypia minimal	Best prognosis
G2 — Moderately differentiated	Intermediate resemblance	Glands/structures partially formed	Intermediate

G3 — Poorly differentiated	Barely recognisable lineage	Few glands/structures; high nuclear atypia; high mitotic rate	Worse
G4 — Undifferentiated / anaplastic	No recognisable lineage without ancillary tests	No glands/structures; bizarre pleomorphism	Worst; often behaves aggressively regardless of stage

Important site-specific grading modifications recognised by WHO include: Gleason score (prostate — 2+2 to 5+5, grouped into ISUP Grade Groups 1–5), Nottingham combined histological grade (breast — tubular formation + nuclear pleomorphism + mitotic count, each scored 1–3, total 3–9 mapped to Grade 1–3), FIGO grade (endometrioid endometrial carcinoma — Grade 1–3 by architecture + nuclear grade), Fuhrman/ISUP/WHO grade (renal cell carcinoma — Grade 1–4 by nucleolar prominence), and CNS WHO grade (1–4, where Grade 1 includes pilocytic astrocytoma, Grade 4 includes glioblastoma).

The WHO Classification of Tumours series is the authoritative global reference; the current (5th) edition transitioned in 2019–2024, standardising molecular-plus-morphology integrated diagnoses across all organ systems. Registrars should know the 5th-edition changes most relevant to their rotation chapters.

Laboratory Diagnosis of Cancer

The laboratory diagnosis of cancer encompasses a spectrum of techniques, from morphological assessment of tissue and cellular samples to sophisticated molecular profiling. The pathologist must select and interpret these tools in the clinical context, understanding that no single technique is sufficient in isolation.

Tissue Diagnosis: Biopsy and Fine Needle Aspiration Cytology

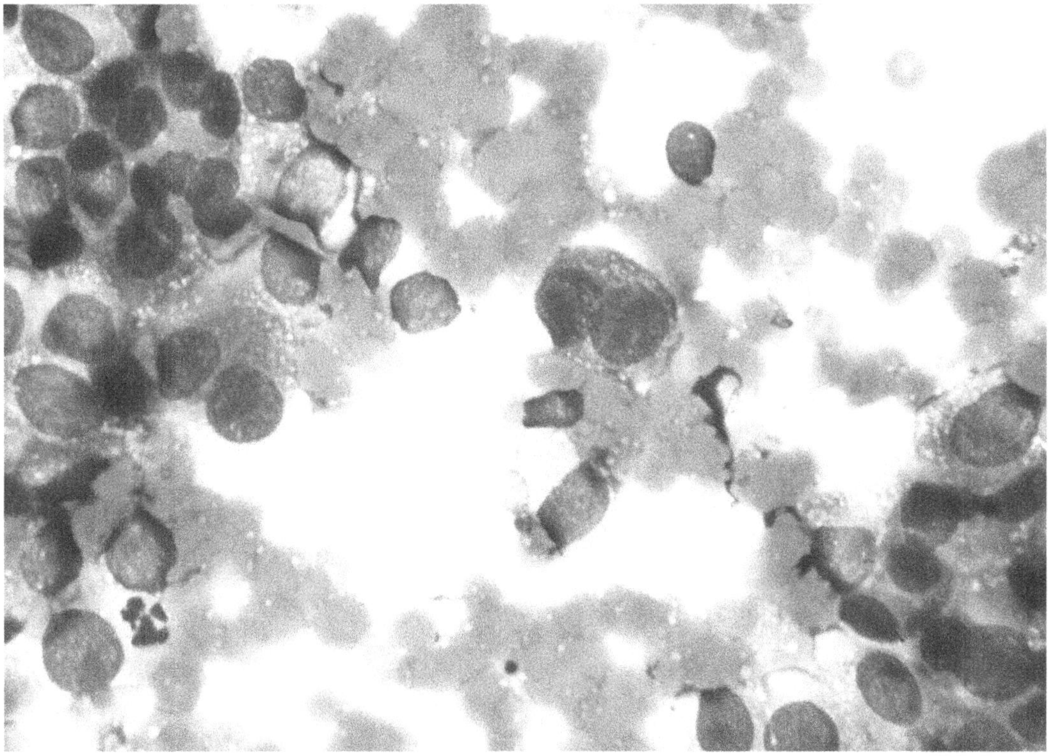

Figure 7.4: FNAC cytology — malignant melanoma cells. Field stain (similar to MGG). High nuclear-to-cytoplasmic ratio, irregular nuclear membranes, prominent nucleoli, melanin pigment (Source: Nephron, Wikimedia Commons, CC BY-SA 3.0.)

The definitive diagnosis of cancer requires morphological examination of tissue or cells. The main modalities are:

Excisional biopsy removes the entire lesion and provides the most complete material for histological assessment, grading, staging, and margin evaluation. It is the gold standard for lymph node assessment (lymphoma classification requires architectural assessment) and small superficial lesions. **Incisional biopsy** removes a representative portion and is used when complete excision is not feasible (large masses, deep-seated tumours). **Core needle biopsy (CNB)** provides a tissue core sufficient for histological subtyping and IHC; it is widely used for breast, liver, prostate, kidney, and lung lesions. Image-guided CNB (ultrasound, CT) has largely replaced open surgical biopsy for many deep lesions.

Fine needle aspiration cytology (FNAC) uses a 22-25 gauge needle to aspirate cells for cytological examination. It is rapid, inexpensive, minimally invasive, and does not require anaesthesia in most settings. FNAC is the initial investigation of choice for thyroid nodules (Bethesda system, see Chapter 33), superficial lymphadenopathy, breast lumps, and salivary gland swellings in routine clinical practice. However, FNAC has limitations: it does not provide architectural information (critical for lymphoma subclassification and grading of epithelial malignancies), and false-negative rates are significant in low-cellularity or fibrotic lesions.

The Pathologist's Eye

When choosing between FNAC and biopsy, the clinical question matters. For a suspected lymphoma, FNAC is insufficient for WHO classification; excisional biopsy is mandatory to assess nodal architecture. For a thyroid nodule, FNAC is the first-line investigation. For breast lumps, the triple test (clinical, radiological, pathological/FNAC or CNB) is the standard approach. The pathologist must guide the clinician to the appropriate sampling technique.

Frozen Section

Frozen section (cryostat section) is an intraoperative technique that provides a rapid histological diagnosis within 15 to 20 minutes. Fresh tissue is snap-frozen at -20 to -30°C, sectioned on a cryostat microtome, and stained (usually rapid H&E). The primary indications are: (1) determination of the nature of a lesion (malignant vs benign) to guide the extent of surgery; (2) assessment of surgical margins (especially in breast conservation surgery and head and neck surgery); (3) evaluation of sentinel lymph nodes; and (4) confirmation of adequate tissue sampling. Concordance rates between frozen section and final paraffin diagnosis exceed 95% in experienced hands, but limitations include freezing artefact (ice crystal formation that distorts cellular detail), sampling error, and difficulty with certain lesion types (lymphoid proliferations, some spindle cell lesions, follicular thyroid lesions where capsular invasion assessment is critical).

Clinical Pearl

Frozen-section reporting language is its own discipline. 'Consistent with' commits to the diagnosis; 'favour' acknowledges high probability with residual uncertainty; 'cannot exclude' flags a possibility that surgery should plan for; 'deferred to permanent' concedes the section is inadequate and intraoperative diagnosis is unsafe. Use the language deliberately. A surgeon who hears 'consistent with carcinoma, margins involved' will resect more tissue; a surgeon who hears 'deferred to permanent' will stop and wait. The careful pathologist never says 'benign' on frozen unless certain, because the permanent section sometimes reveals what the frozen could not.

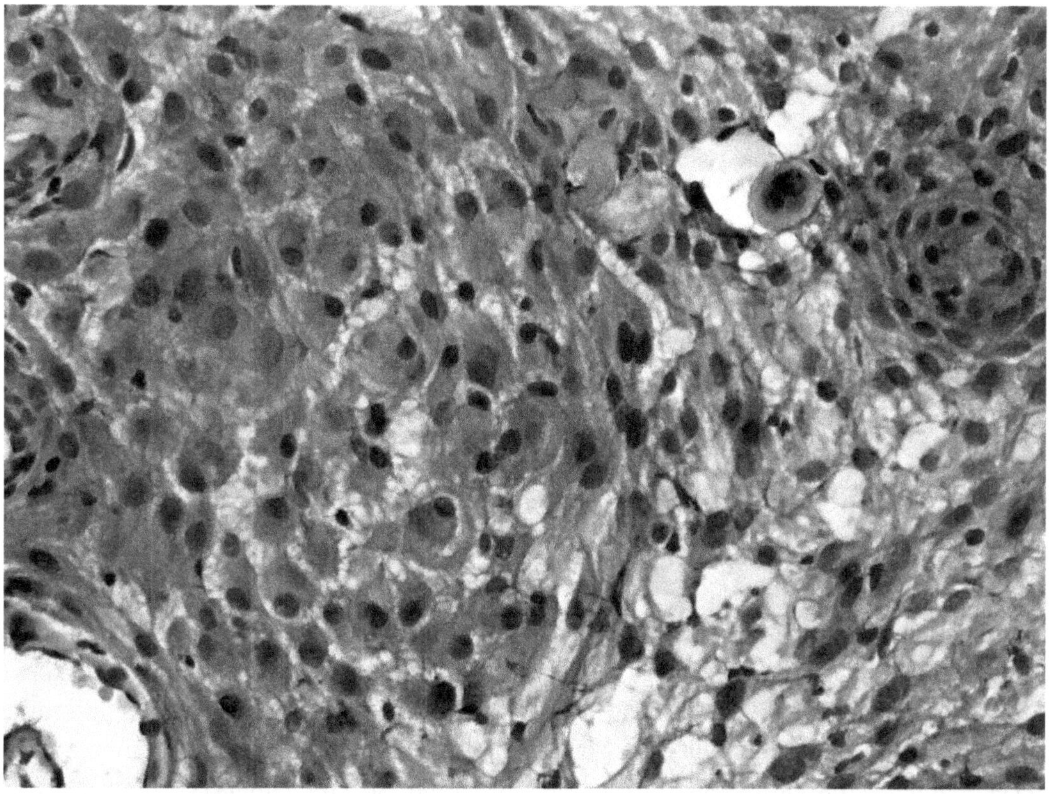

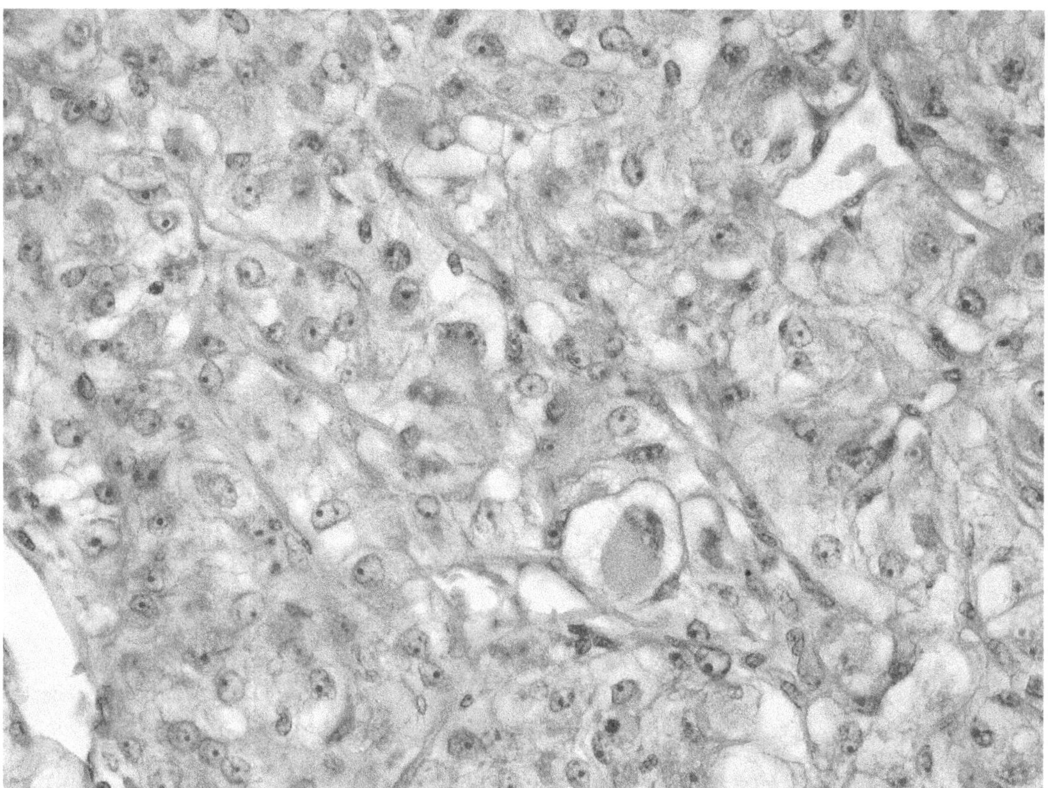

Figure 7.5: Frozen section versus permanent section — rhabdoid meningioma. Top: Cryostat (frozen) section showing ice crystal artefact and less crisp morphology. Bottom: Corresponding paraffin (permanent) section with clean, crisp histological detail. H&E (Sources: Top — Jensflorian, Wikimedia Commons, CC BY-SA 4.0; Bottom — Marvin 101, Wikimedia Commons, CC BY 3.0.)

Exam Pitfall

Frozen section is contraindicated in: (1) Follicular thyroid lesions (capsular/vascular invasion cannot be assessed on frozen section). (2) Lesions suspected of being lymphoma (architecture is disrupted by freezing). (3) Very small biopsies where tissue must be preserved for permanent sections and ancillary studies.

Immunohistochemistry

Immunohistochemistry (IHC) uses labelled antibodies to detect specific antigens in tissue sections. It is indispensable in modern diagnostic pathology and serves multiple roles: determination of lineage (epithelial, mesenchymal, melanocytic, lymphoid, neuroendocrine), identification of site of origin in metastatic carcinoma of unknown primary, assessment of prognostic and predictive markers (ER, PR, HER2, Ki-67 in breast cancer; PD-L1 in lung cancer), detection of specific molecular alterations (ALK rearrangement, microsatellite instability via MMR proteins), and classification of tumours according to WHO criteria. A detailed discussion of IHC principles and organ-specific panels is provided in Chapter 36.

Clinical Pearl

Ki-67: count the hot spot, not the whole field. Ki-67 proliferation index varies dramatically across a tumour, and a globally averaged value misses the prognostically important high-proliferation zone. Standard practice: scan the slide at low power, identify the area of densest nuclear positivity (the 'hot spot'), then count at least 500-1000 tumour cell nuclei in that zone, scoring positive vs negative. Whole-section averaging consistently underestimates the proliferation index in heterogeneous tumours; for breast, gastrointestinal neuroendocrine tumours, and CNS neoplasms, the hot-spot count is the method specified by current WHO and NICE guidance.

Table 7.9: Key IHC Markers by Diagnostic Category

Stain	Target	Positive Result	Key Use	Pitfall
PAS	Glycogen, fungal wall, BM	Magenta	Glycogen storage, fungal ID, BM thickening	Diastase removes glycogen; diastase-resistant = non-glycogen
Congo Red	Amyloid	Salmon pink; apple-green birefringence	Amyloid confirmation	Overstaining mimics positivity; polarised light essential

Ziehl-Neelsen	Acid-fast bacilli	Red against blue	TB, atypical mycobacteria	Fite for lepra bacilli; modified ZN for Nocardia
Reticulin	Type III collagen fibres	Black	Hepatic architecture, lymphoma vs carcinoma	Does not grade fibrosis; use Masson trichrome
Masson Trichrome	Collagen blue, muscle red	Blue collagen, red muscle	Fibrosis grading	Fixation-dependent colour intensity
Prussian Blue	Ferric iron (haemosiderin)	Blue-green granules	Iron overload, sideroblasts	Formalin pigment mimics iron
GMS	Fungal cell wall polysaccharides	Black against green	Fungal ID (PCP, Aspergillus)	Non-specific; also stains BM
Alcian Blue pH 2.5	Acid mucins	Blue	Mucinous tumours, Barrett	pH 2.5 = all acid mucins; pH 1.0 = sulphated only
Mucicarmine	Epithelial mucin	Magenta	Mucinous adenoCA, Cryptococcus	Does not stain connective tissue mucins
Fontana-Masson	Melanin, argentaffin granules	Black	Melanoma, carcinoid	Formalin pigment false positive
Oil Red O	Neutral lipid	Red droplets	Fatty change, fat embolism	Frozen sections only

Table 7.11: Special Stains Master Reference

Diagnostic Question	Key IHC Markers
Epithelial vs mesenchymal	Cytokeratins (AE1/AE3, CK7, CK20) vs Vimentin
Melanocytic lineage	S100, SOX10, HMB-45, Melan-A
Lymphoid lineage	CD45 (LCA), CD3 (T-cell), CD20 (B-cell)
Neuroendocrine differentiation	Synaptophysin, Chromogranin A, INSM1, CD56
Muscle differentiation	Desmin, SMA, Myogenin (rhabdomyosarcoma)

Vascular differentiation	CD31, CD34, ERG
Breast cancer prognostic panel	ER, PR, HER2, Ki-67
CUP: Lung primary	TTF-1, Napsin A
CUP: GI primary	CDX2, CK20+, CK7−
CUP: Thyroid primary	TTF-1, Thyroglobulin, PAX8
MMR/MSI screening	MLH1, MSH2, MSH6, PMS2
Soft tissue/small round cell panel	CD99 (Ewing), Myogenin (RMS), TLE1 (synovial sarcoma)

Cytogenetics and Fluorescence In Situ Hybridisation

Conventional cytogenetics (karyotyping) identifies chromosomal abnormalities including translocations, deletions, inversions, and amplifications. It requires viable, dividing cells and has been most widely applied in haematological malignancies (see Volume 1). In solid tumours, spectral karyotyping (SKY) and comparative genomic hybridisation (CGH) have extended cytogenetic analysis.

Fluorescence in situ hybridisation (FISH) uses fluorescently labelled DNA probes to detect specific chromosomal abnormalities in interphase cells, eliminating the need for cell culture. FISH can detect translocations (break-apart probes for ALK, ROS1 in lung adenocarcinoma; EWSR1 in Ewing sarcoma), amplifications (HER2 in breast cancer), and deletions (1p/19q co-deletion in oligodendroglioma). It can be performed on formalin-fixed, paraffin-embedded (FFPE) tissue, making it applicable to archival material. FISH is the gold standard for HER2 amplification assessment in equivocal (2+) IHC cases (see Chapter 26).

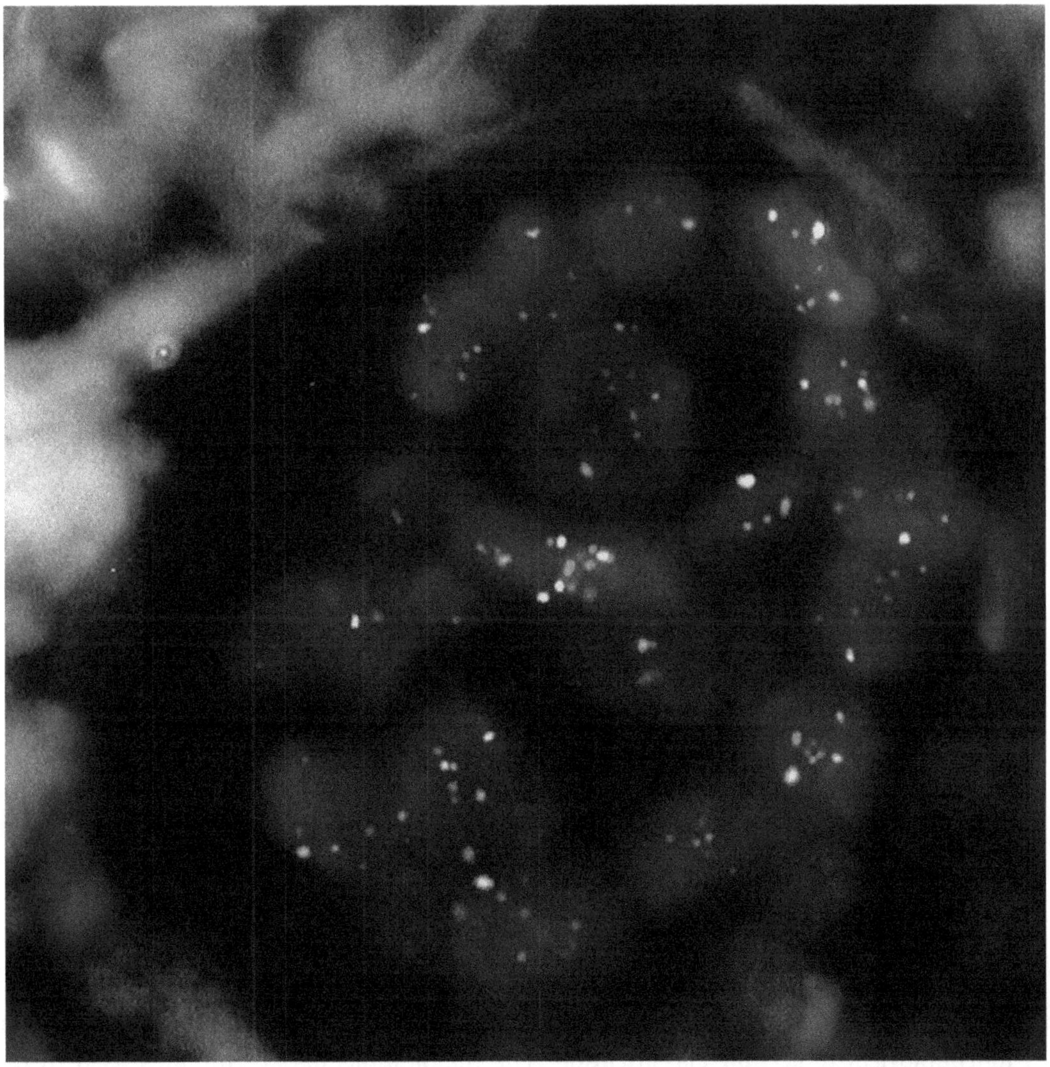

Figure 7.6: FISH — HER2 gene amplification. Multiple HER2 signals (red) relative to CEP17 reference signals (green) in tumour cell nuclei, indicating gene amplification (ratio ≥2.0) (Source: IrinaPav, Wikimedia Commons, CC BY-SA 4.0.)

Figure 7.7: Tuberculoid granuloma — well-formed epithelioid granuloma with central caseous necrosis. H&E. (Source: Humpath, Wikimedia Commons, CC BY-SA 3.0.)

Molecular Diagnostics

Molecular pathology has transformed cancer diagnosis from a purely morphological exercise to an integrated morphological-molecular classification. The major molecular techniques used in diagnostic pathology are:

Polymerase chain reaction (PCR): Amplifies specific DNA sequences for mutation detection, gene rearrangement analysis, and pathogen identification. Reverse transcription PCR (RT-PCR) detects fusion transcripts (BCR::ABL1 in CML, PML::RARA in APL; see Volume 1). Real-time quantitative PCR (qPCR) enables monitoring of minimal residual disease.

Next-generation sequencing (NGS): Massively parallel sequencing platforms that can interrogate hundreds of genes simultaneously. Targeted NGS panels (50 to 500 genes) are now standard of care for lung adenocarcinoma (EGFR, ALK, ROS1, BRAF, KRAS, MET, RET, NTRK), colorectal carcinoma (KRAS, NRAS, BRAF, MSI), melanoma (BRAF, NRAS, KIT), and many other tumour types. Whole-exome and whole-genome sequencing are increasingly used in research settings and for tumours of unknown primary. NGS also enables tumour mutational burden (TMB) assessment, a predictor of response to immune checkpoint inhibitors. NGS is widely available at major tertiary cancer centres internationally and through commercial laboratories.

Gene expression profiling: Microarray-based and RNA-sequencing platforms classify tumours into molecular subtypes with prognostic and therapeutic implications. The paradigm is breast cancer, where gene expression profiles define Luminal A, Luminal B, HER2-enriched, and Basal-like subtypes (see Chapter 26). The Oncotype DX and MammaPrint assays guide adjuvant chemotherapy decisions in early breast cancer.

Liquid biopsy: Analysis of tumour-derived material in peripheral blood, including circulating tumour DNA (ctDNA), circulating tumour cells (CTCs), and exosomes. Liquid biopsy enables non-invasive detection of actionable mutations (e.g., EGFR T790M resistance mutation in lung adenocarcinoma), monitoring of treatment response, detection of minimal residual disease, and early identification of resistance mechanisms. It does not replace tissue biopsy for primary diagnosis but serves as a complementary tool when tissue is unavailable or insufficient, and for longitudinal monitoring (Figure 7.8).

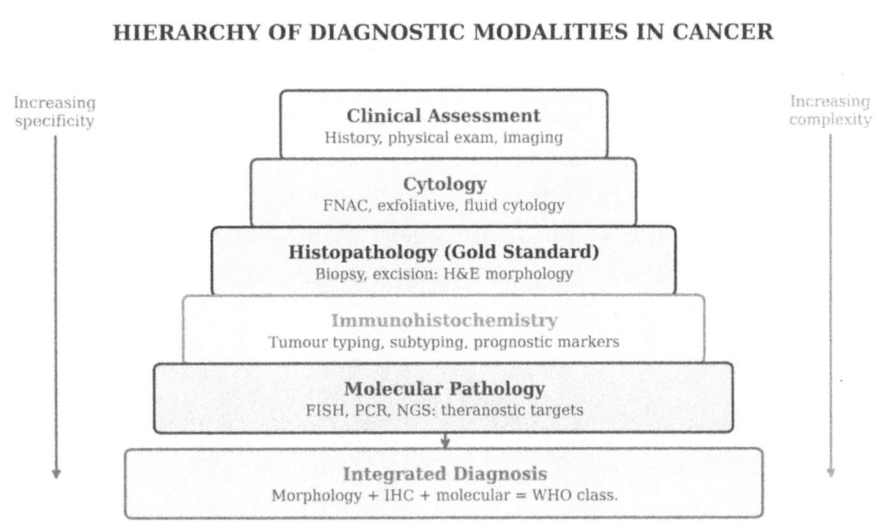

Figure 7.8: Hierarchy of diagnostic modalities in cancer. (Source: Author's original.)

Flow Cytometry

Flow cytometry (FCM) analyses the physical and immunophenotypic characteristics of individual cells in suspension. Cells labelled with fluorochrome-conjugated antibodies pass through a laser beam, and scattered light and fluorescence are measured. FCM is the standard technique for immunophenotyping haematological malignancies (see Volume 1): it rapidly distinguishes B-cell from T-cell lymphoproliferative disorders, identifies aberrant antigen expression patterns, and quantifies blast percentages. In solid tumour pathology, FCM has a more limited role, mainly in DNA ploidy analysis and cell cycle assessment. In body fluid cytology, FCM can identify lymphoma cells that are difficult to characterise on morphology alone (see Chapter 34).

> **Quick Recall: Laboratory Diagnosis of Cancer**
>
> **Tissue acquisition:** Excisional biopsy (gold standard for lymphoma), incisional biopsy, CNB (breast, liver, prostate), FNAC (thyroid, lymph node, breast).
>
> **Frozen section:** Intraoperative; 15-20 min; contraindicated in follicular thyroid lesions and lymphoma.
>
> **IHC:** Lineage, site of origin, prognostic/predictive markers, WHO classification. Panel-based approach.
>
> **FISH:** Translocations (ALK, EWSR1), amplifications (HER2), deletions (1p/19q). Works on FFPE tissue.
>
> **NGS:** Multi-gene panels for actionable mutations; TMB; standard of care in lung, CRC, melanoma.
>
> **Liquid biopsy:** ctDNA, CTCs; non-invasive monitoring; complementary to tissue biopsy.

Tumour Markers

Tumour markers are molecules (proteins, glycoproteins, enzymes, hormones, oncofetal antigens) produced by tumour cells or by the host in response to a tumour, detectable in blood, urine, or tissue. Despite their name, most tumour markers are neither sensitive nor specific enough for cancer screening in asymptomatic populations. Their primary clinical utility lies in four areas: monitoring treatment response, detecting recurrence, prognostication, and, in selected situations, aiding diagnosis.

Table 7.10: Clinically Important Serum Tumour Markers

Marker	Primary Tumour Association	Clinical Utility
CEA	Colorectal carcinoma	Monitoring recurrence; not screening (elevated in smoking, IBD, pancreatitis)
AFP	HCC; Yolk sac tumour (testicular/ovarian)	Diagnosis (HCC with AFP >400), monitoring, screening in cirrhotics
PSA	Prostate carcinoma	Screening (controversial), monitoring post-treatment
CA 125	Ovarian epithelial carcinoma (serous)	Monitoring treatment response; not screening (elevated in endometriosis, pregnancy, peritonitis)
CA 19-9	Pancreatic adenocarcinoma	Monitoring; not screening (elevated in obstructive jaundice, cholangitis)

CA 15-3 / CA 27.29	Breast carcinoma	Monitoring metastatic disease
hCG	Gestational trophoblastic disease; testicular germ cell tumours	Diagnosis, staging, monitoring, detecting recurrence
LDH	Lymphoma, germ cell tumours, melanoma	Prognostic marker; elevated in tumour lysis
Thyroglobulin	Differentiated thyroid carcinoma (post-thyroidectomy)	Monitoring for recurrence
Calcitonin	Medullary thyroid carcinoma	Diagnosis and monitoring; screening in MEN2 families
Chromogranin A	Neuroendocrine tumours	Diagnosis and monitoring
S100B	Melanoma	Prognostic; monitoring for metastatic disease

When faced with a question on tumour markers, the examiner expects the marker-tumour association and an understanding of limitations. CEA is elevated in smokers and inflammatory conditions; PSA screening remains controversial owing to overdiagnosis; CA 125 is elevated in multiple benign gynaecological conditions. No serum tumour marker is sufficiently sensitive and specific for population-based cancer screening, with the possible exceptions of AFP in high-risk cirrhotics and calcitonin in MEN2 kindreds.

Quick Recall: Tumour Markers

Oncofetal: CEA (colorectal), AFP (HCC, yolk sac tumour).
Glycoprotein: CA 125 (ovary), CA 19-9 (pancreas), CA 15-3 (breast).
Hormones: hCG (trophoblastic, germ cell), Calcitonin (medullary thyroid).
Enzymes: PSA (prostate), LDH (lymphoma, germ cell).
Key principle: Most markers are for monitoring, NOT screening. Tissue diagnosis remains mandatory.

Prognostic and Predictive Markers

A **prognostic marker** provides information about the likely outcome of the disease regardless of treatment (e.g., tumour stage, grade, lymphovascular invasion, Ki-67 proliferation index). A **predictive marker** provides information about the likely benefit from a specific therapy (e.g., ER positivity predicts response to tamoxifen; HER2 amplification predicts response to trastuzumab; EGFR mutations predict response to tyrosine kinase inhibitors; ALK rearrangement predicts response to crizotinib/alectinib; PD-L1 expression and MSI-H status predict response to immune checkpoint inhibitors). Some markers serve both prognostic and predictive functions.

The concept of **companion diagnostics** has emerged from the recognition that targeted therapies require matched diagnostic tests. A companion diagnostic is a test (IHC, FISH, PCR, or NGS) that identifies patients who are most likely to benefit from (or be harmed by) a specific drug. Examples include HER2 testing (IHC/FISH) as a companion diagnostic for trastuzumab, EGFR mutation testing for erlotinib/osimertinib, BRAF V600E testing for vemurafenib, and MMR/MSI testing for pembrolizumab. The pathologist is central to this paradigm, as the companion diagnostic test drives the treatment decision.

Table 7.5: Key Prognostic vs Predictive Markers

Marker	Prognostic	Predictive	Tumour
ER/PR	Yes (better prognosis if +)	Yes (endocrine therapy)	Breast
HER2	Yes (worse if amplified)	Yes (trastuzumab)	Breast, gastric
Ki-67	Yes (high = aggressive)	Uncertain	Multiple
EGFR mutation	Modest	Yes (TKIs)	Lung adenocarcinoma
ALK rearrangement	No	Yes (ALK inhibitors)	Lung adenocarcinoma
BRAF V600E	Yes (aggressive in CRC)	Yes (vemurafenib)	Melanoma, CRC, thyroid
MMR/MSI	Yes (better prognosis in CRC)	Yes (checkpoint inhibitors)	CRC, endometrial, multiple
PD-L1 (TPS/CPS)	Uncertain	Yes (pembrolizumab)	Lung, others
TMB	Uncertain	Yes (immunotherapy)	Pan-cancer

Cancer Screening

Cancer screening aims to detect malignancy at an early, curable stage in asymptomatic populations. An effective screening test must be sensitive, specific, affordable, and applicable to a disease with a significant preclinical detectable phase. Current evidence-based screening programmes include:

Cervical cancer: Pap smear (conventional or liquid-based cytology) and HPV DNA testing. VIA (visual inspection with acetic acid) is recommended as a cost-effective alternative in resource-limited settings. **Breast cancer:** Mammography (recommended from age 40-50 in various guidelines). Clinical breast examination is used in many national screening programmes. **Colorectal cancer:** Faecal occult blood test (FOBT/FIT), colonoscopy. **Lung cancer:** Low-dose CT (LDCT) for high-risk smokers (>30 pack-years). **Prostate cancer:** PSA testing remains controversial; shared decision-making is recommended. **Hepatocellular carcinoma:** AFP and ultrasound every 6 months in cirrhotics and HBV carriers.

Recent Advances

KEYNOTE-158 — tumour mutational burden as a tissue-agnostic predictive biomarker. The KEYNOTE-158 study established tumour mutational burden (TMB) as a tissue-agnostic predictive biomarker for response to programmed death-1 blockade with pembrolizumab (Marabelle et al. Lancet Oncology 2020; 21: 1353–1365; PMID 32919526). In a multi-cohort, open-label phase 2 trial across ten advanced solid-tumour cohorts (anal, biliary, cervical, endometrial, mesothelioma, neuroendocrine, salivary, small-cell lung, thyroid, and vulvar), TMB was measured on archival formalin-fixed paraffin-embedded tumour samples using the FoundationOne CDx assay. The prespecified threshold for high TMB was at least ten mutations per megabase. Among 790 patients evaluable for efficacy, 102 (13 per cent) had tTMB-high status. Objective response rates were 29 per cent (95 per cent CI 21–39) in the tTMB-high subgroup compared with 6 per cent (95 per cent CI 5–8) in the non-tTMB-high subgroup. The data supported the United States Food and Drug Administration's June 2020 tissue-agnostic accelerated approval of pembrolizumab for previously treated unresectable or metastatic solid tumours with TMB at least 10 mut/Mb.

DYNAMIC — ctDNA-guided adjuvant therapy in stage II colon cancer. The DYNAMIC trial demonstrated that circulating tumour DNA (ctDNA) status after curative-intent surgery for stage II colon cancer can guide adjuvant chemotherapy decisions without compromising recurrence-free survival (Tie et al. New England Journal of Medicine 2022; 386: 2261–2272; PMID 35657320). Four hundred and fifty-five patients across Australia and New Zealand were randomised 2:1 to either ctDNA-guided management — chemotherapy if ctDNA-positive at week 4 or 7 post-surgery and observation if ctDNA-negative — or standard clinicopathological management. ctDNA was assayed using a tumour-informed personalised assay anchored on multiplex PCR–targeted sequencing. At a median follow-up of 37 months only 15 per cent of patients in the ctDNA-guided arm received adjuvant chemotherapy versus 28 per cent in the standard arm (relative risk 1.82; 95 per cent CI 1.25–2.65), and two-year recurrence-free survival was non-inferior (93.5 versus 92.4 per cent). Three-year recurrence-free survival was 86.4 per cent in ctDNA-positive patients who received chemotherapy and 92.5 per cent in ctDNA-negative patients managed by observation alone, supporting post-operative molecular residual disease testing as a basis for adjuvant decision-making.

Precision oncology and pan-cancer approaches: The shift from tissue-of-origin to molecular classification is exemplified by tumour-agnostic approvals. The FDA approved pembrolizumab for any MSI-H/dMMR solid tumour regardless of site, and larotrectinib/entrectinib for any tumour harbouring an NTRK fusion. This represents a paradigm shift from 'where the cancer is' to 'what mutations the cancer has,' placing the molecular pathologist at the centre of treatment decisions.

Liquid biopsy and ctDNA: Circulating tumour DNA analysis is entering clinical practice for monitoring minimal residual disease (MRD) in colorectal and lung cancers. Multi-cancer early detection (MCED) tests, such as those based on cell-free DNA methylation patterns, aim to screen for multiple cancer types from a single blood draw. While promising, these require further validation before clinical adoption.

Artificial intelligence in pathology: Deep learning algorithms are being developed and validated for automated tumour detection (breast cancer metastases in sentinel lymph nodes), grading (Gleason grading in prostate cancer), quantification of biomarkers (Ki-67, PD-L1), and molecular subtype prediction from H&E morphology alone. AI is poised to augment, though not replace, the diagnostic pathologist (see Chapter 38) (Figures 7.8–7.10).

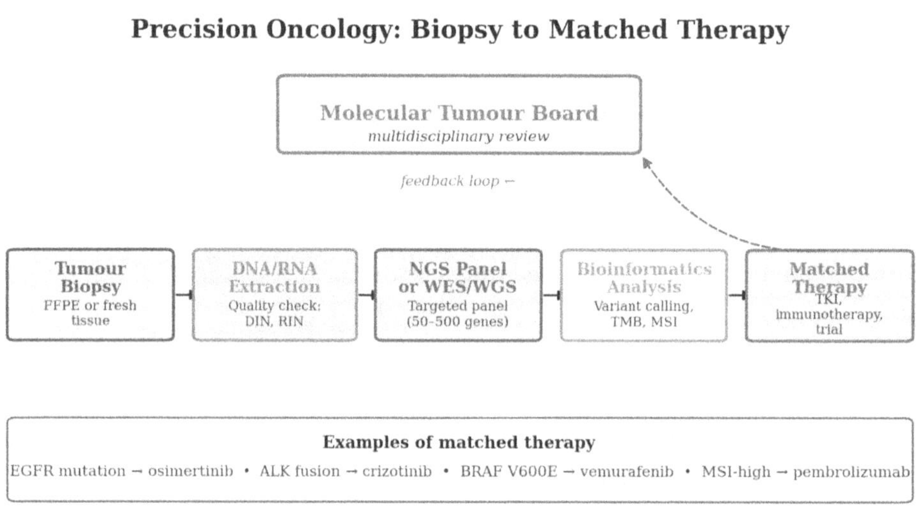

Figure 7.9: Concept diagram of precision oncology. (Source: Author's original.)

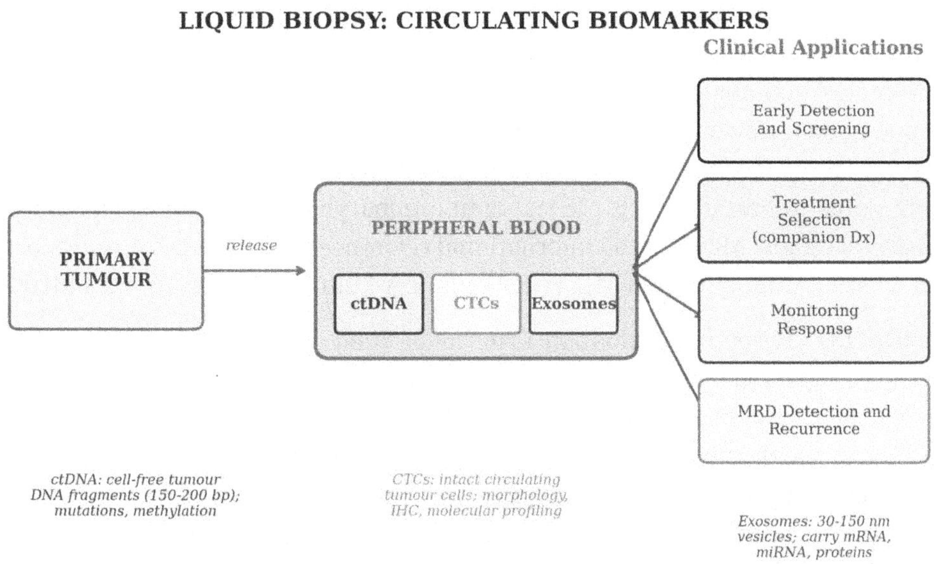

Figure 7.10: Liquid biopsy overview. (Source: Author's original.)

International Frameworks

AJCC 8th edition / UICC TNM 8 staging. The Eighth Edition of the AJCC Cancer Staging Manual (2017) and the parallel UICC TNM 8 framework moved cancer staging from a purely anatomic system toward a hybrid that incorporates non-anatomic prognostic factors where supported by evidence. Site-specific staging chapters now embed validated biomarkers and molecular factors alongside the classic T (primary tumour), N (regional lymph nodes), and M (distant metastasis) categories — for example, hormone receptor and HER2 status in breast cancer, p16 status in oropharyngeal carcinoma, and grade as a stage modifier in soft tissue sarcoma. AJCC 8 is the international reference for synoptic cancer reporting in CAP, ICCR, and RCPath datasets. Citation: Amin MB, et al. CA Cancer J Clin 2017;67(2):93–99. PMID 28094848.

RECIST 1.1 and iRECIST. Response Evaluation Criteria In Solid Tumours (RECIST 1.1, 2009) defines objective response in clinical trials of solid tumours. Up to five target lesions (maximum two per organ) are measured by their longest unidimensional diameter (short axis for nodes ≥15 mm), with the sum of diameters tracked across timepoints. Categories are complete response, partial response (≥30% decrease), stable disease, and progressive disease (≥20% increase plus an absolute ≥5 mm increase, or unequivocal new lesion). For trials of immune checkpoint inhibitors, the iRECIST modification (2017) requires confirmation of progression on a follow-up scan ≥4 weeks later, accommodating pseudo-progression and delayed responses; categories of unconfirmed progression (iUPD) and confirmed progression (iCPD) are introduced. Citation: Seymour L, et al. Lancet Oncol 2017;18(3):e143–e152. PMID 28271869.

Ultra High-Yield Chapter Summary

Table 7.4: Ultra High-Yield Summary; Neoplasia Part 2

Topic	Must Remember
Chemical carcinogenesis	Initiation (irreversible DNA damage) → Promotion (reversible clonal expansion) → Progression. Most carcinogens indirect-acting (P-450 activation).
Radiation carcinogenesis	UV-B: pyrimidine dimers, NER pathway. Ionising: double-strand breaks.
HPV carcinogenesis	E6 degrades p53; E7 inactivates Rb. Types 16, 18.
EBV carcinogenesis	LMP-1 mimics CD40; NF-κB activation.
HBV/HCV carcinogenesis	HBV: HBx protein, genomic integration. HCV: chronic inflammation pathway.
Cancer cachexia	TNF-α, IL-6 driven; proteolysis + lipolysis; NOT reversed by nutrition alone.
Paraneoplastic: Endocrine	SCLC: Cushing (ACTH), SIADH (ADH). SCC: Hypercalcaemia (PTHrP).

Paraneoplastic: Haematological	Trousseau (pancreas), DIC (APL), NBTE (adenocarcinomas).
Paraneoplastic: Neurological	Lambert-Eaton (SCLC, anti-Ca^{2+} channel), Myasthenia (thymoma).
Grading vs Staging	Grading = differentiation (pathologist). Staging = extent (TNM).
FNAC vs Biopsy	FNAC: rapid, cheap, first-line for thyroid/LN.
Frozen section	Intraoperative, 15-20 min.
IHC panel approach	Epithelial (CK), Melanocytic (S100/SOX10), Lymphoid (LCA), NE (Syn/CgA).
FISH	Translocations (ALK, EWSR1), amplifications (HER2), deletions (1p/19q).
NGS	Multi-gene panels; standard of care in lung, CRC, melanoma.
Liquid biopsy	ctDNA from blood; non-invasive; monitors MRD, detects resistance mutations.
CEA	Colorectal monitoring.
AFP	HCC (>400 diagnostic), yolk sac tumour.
CA 125	Ovarian serous carcinoma monitoring.
Prognostic vs Predictive	Prognostic: outcome regardless of Rx (stage, grade).
Companion diagnostics	Matched test + drug: HER2/trastuzumab, EGFR/osimertinib, BRAF/vemurafenib, MSI-H/pembrolizumab.
Precision oncology	Tumour-agnostic approvals: MSI-H → pembrolizumab; NTRK fusion → larotrectinib. 'What mutation' > 'which organ.'

Diagnostic thinking: elevated tumour marker + imaging mass + tissue biopsy → integrated diagnosis (never diagnose on marker alone)

Diagnostic thinking: CK7+/CK20– + TTF-1+ → lung primary; CK7–/CK20+ + CDX2+ → colorectal primary

Diagnostic thinking: high Ki-67 + p53 aberrant + loss of differentiation markers → high-grade malignancy (grade trumps subtype for prognosis)

Chapter 8: Genetic Disorders and Molecular Pathology

THE BIG PICTURE

Genetic diseases are far more common than traditionally appreciated. Beyond the classic single-gene and chromosomal disorders, virtually every human disease has a genetic component, whether through direct causation (sickle cell anaemia, cystic fibrosis), susceptibility (BRCA1 in breast cancer), or pharmacogenomic variation (drug metabolism polymorphisms). The pathologist encounters genetic disease across every organ system: from lysosomal storage diseases presenting as hepatosplenomegaly and developmental delay, to chromosomal abnormalities diagnosed on prenatal cytogenetics, to the molecular diagnostics that now define precision medicine. This chapter covers the principles of single-gene, chromosomal, and complex multigenic disorders, along with the molecular tools used to diagnose them.

High-yield topics in this chapter:
Mendelian disorders and enzyme defects; Lysosomal storage diseases (Gaucher, Niemann-Pick, Tay-Sachs, Fabry, MPS); Down syndrome and other chromosomal disorders; Turner and Klinefelter syndromes; Trinucleotide repeat disorders (Fragile X); Familial hypercholesterolaemia; Cystic fibrosis; Marfan syndrome; Genomic imprinting and Prader-Willi/Angelman; Non-coding DNA; Epigenetics; Molecular diagnostic techniques; Gene therapy.

Genetic disorders range from single-gene (Mendelian) defects to complex chromosomal abnormalities. A single nucleotide substitution causes sickle cell disease; an extra chromosome 21 produces Down syndrome; the expansion of a trinucleotide repeat silences a gene across generations. Genetic disease is not a niche subspeciality but a thread that runs through every branch of pathology, from the enzyme deficiencies that present in paediatric wards to the somatic mutations that drive cancer (see Chapter 6). The postgraduate pathologist must understand not only the diseases themselves but the molecular tools, from karyotyping to next-generation sequencing, that make their diagnosis possible.

Classification of Genetic Disorders

HIGH-YIELD NAMED SYNDROMES IN PATHOLOGY

Syndrome	Gene/Defect	Key Feature	System
Li-Fraumeni	TP53 (germline)	Multiple cancers < 45 yr	Onco
Lynch (HNPCC)	MLH1/MSH2/MSH6/PMS2	CRC + endometrial Ca	Onco
Beckwith-Wiedemann	IGF2 / 11p15.5	Macrosomia, omphalocele, Wilms	Peds
Von Hippel-Lindau	VHL (3p25)	RCC + hemangioblastoma + pheo	Onco
MEN 1 (Wermer)	MEN1 (menin)	Pituitary + Parathyroid + Pancreas	Endo
MEN 2A (Sipple)	RET proto-oncogene	MTC + Pheo + Parathyroid	Endo
MEN 2B	RET (M918T)	MTC + Pheo + Mucosal neuromas	Endo
Gardner	APC	FAP + osteomas + desmoids	GIT
Turcot	APC / MMR	FAP/Lynch + brain tumors	GIT
Peutz-Jeghers	STK11/LKB1	Hamartomatous polyps + pigmentation	GIT
DiGeorge	22q11.2 deletion	T-cell deficiency, hypoparathyroid	Immuno
Wiskott-Aldrich	WAS (Xp11)	Thrombocytopenia + eczema + immunodef.	Immuno
Chédiak-Higashi	LYST	Giant granules, recurrent infections	Immuno
Turner	45,X monosomy	Short stature, streak gonads	Genetics
Klinefelter	47,XXY	Tall, hypogonadism, gynecomastia	Genetics
Down	Trisomy 21	ALL risk, Alzheimer, endocardial cushion	Genetics
Marfan	FBN1 (fibrillin-1)	Aortic dissection, lens subluxation	CT
Ehlers-Danlos	COL5A1/COL3A1	Skin hyperextensibility, joint laxity	CT
Nephrotic (MCD)	Podocyte effacement	Selective proteinuria, children	Renal
Goodpasture	Anti-GBM (α3 Col IV)	Pulmonary hemorrhage + RPGN	Renal

Figure 8.1: High-Yield Named Syndromes in Pathology. (Source: Author's original.)

Genetic disorders can be broadly classified into four categories: (1) **single-gene (Mendelian) disorders,** caused by mutations in a single gene following autosomal dominant, autosomal recessive, or X-linked patterns of inheritance; (2) **chromosomal disorders,** involving changes in the number or structure of chromosomes; (3) **multifactorial (complex) disorders,** resulting from the interaction of multiple genes with environmental factors; and (4) **single-gene disorders with non-classical inheritance,** including trinucleotide repeat disorders, mitochondrial inheritance, and genomic imprinting.

Single-Gene (Mendelian) Disorders

Mendelian disorders result from mutations in a single gene and follow predictable patterns of inheritance. They are individually rare but collectively common, affecting approximately 1% of all live births. Single-gene disorders can be classified by the type of protein affected: structural proteins (Marfan syndrome, Ehlers-Danlos syndrome, osteogenesis imperfecta), receptor proteins (familial hypercholesterolaemia), channel proteins (cystic fibrosis), and enzyme proteins (lysosomal storage diseases, phenylketonuria).

Autosomal Dominant Disorders

Autosomal dominant (AD) disorders manifest when a single copy of the mutant allele is sufficient to produce disease. Key characteristics include: affected individuals usually have an affected parent; both males and females are affected equally; the disease does not skip generations (vertical transmission); and each offspring of an affected parent has a 50% risk of inheriting the mutation. Important concepts in AD inheritance include **variable expressivity** (the severity of disease varies among affected individuals), **incomplete penetrance** (not all individuals carrying the mutation express the disease), and **new mutations** (de novo mutations account for a proportion of cases, particularly in disorders affecting reproductive fitness such as achondroplasia).

Marfan Syndrome

Marfan syndrome is an AD disorder caused by mutations in the **FBN1** gene on chromosome 15, which encodes **fibrillin-1**, a glycoprotein component of extracellular microfibrils. Microfibrils serve as scaffolds for elastin deposition and also sequester TGF-β in the extracellular matrix. Loss of functional fibrillin-1 leads to two pathological consequences: structural weakness of connective tissues (particularly in the aorta, eye, and skeleton) and dysregulated TGF-β signalling, which contributes to aortic root dilation and skeletal overgrowth.

The classic triad involves the **skeletal system** (tall stature, long limbs, arachnodactyly, pectus deformities, scoliosis, joint hypermobility), the **eye** (bilateral superior subluxation of the lens [ectopia lentis], present in approximately 60% of patients), and the **cardiovascular system** (aortic root dilation, aortic dissection, mitral valve prolapse). Cystic medial degeneration (mucoid degeneration) of the aortic media is the histopathological hallmark, predisposing to dissecting aneurysm, the most common cause of death. Diagnosis is clinical (revised Ghent criteria); genetic testing for FBN1 mutations is confirmatory.

The distinction between Marfan syndrome and homocystinuria rests on three features: In homocystinuria, the lens subluxation is typically downward (inferior), there is a risk of thromboembolism (not aortic dissection), and intellectual disability is common. Marfan patients have upward lens subluxation, aortic root disease, and normal intelligence.

Diagnosis follows the revised Ghent criteria (2010), which give disproportionate weight to two cardinal features: aortic root dilation (Z-score ≥2 in adults) and ectopia lentis. In the absence of family history, both features together are sufficient for diagnosis; in the presence of a pathogenic FBN1 mutation, aortic root dilation alone suffices. The TGF-β signalling pathway is now a therapeutic target: losartan, an angiotensin II type 1 receptor blocker, reduces TGF-β activation and has been shown to slow aortic root dilation in clinical trials, though beta-blockers remain first-line prophylaxis against aortic complications.

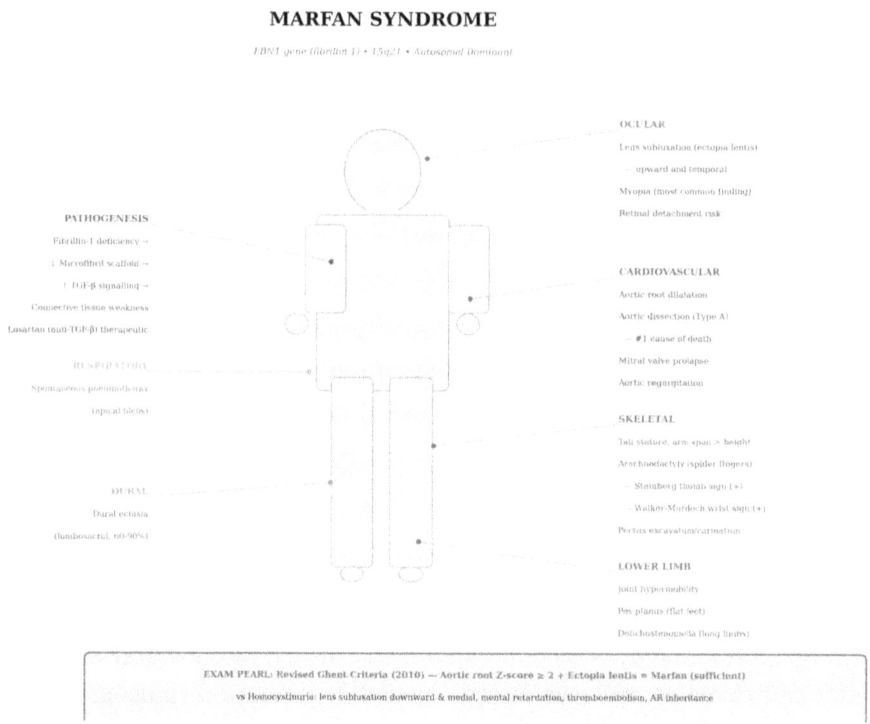

Figure 8.2: Marfan Syndrome: Clinical Features. (Source: Author's original.)

Ehlers-Danlos Syndromes

The Ehlers-Danlos syndromes (EDS) are a heterogeneous group of heritable connective tissue disorders characterised by joint hypermobility, skin hyperextensibility, and tissue fragility. The 2017 international classification recognises 13 subtypes. The two most important for examination purposes are classical EDS (cEDS, caused by mutations in COL5A1/COL5A2 encoding type V collagen, AD inheritance; features include markedly hyperextensible skin with atrophic 'cigarette-paper' scars, large joint hypermobility, and easy bruising) and vascular EDS (vEDS, caused by mutations in COL3A1 encoding type III collagen, AD; characterised by thin translucent skin, arterial/intestinal/uterine rupture, and a median life expectancy of 50 years). Vascular EDS is the most dangerous subtype because spontaneous rupture of medium-sized arteries, bowel, or gravid uterus can be rapidly fatal.

Hypermobile EDS (hEDS) is the most common subtype and the only one without an identified genetic basis. It is characterised by generalised joint hypermobility (assessed using the Beighton score), chronic pain, and frequent subluxations without the skin fragility of classical EDS. The pathologist should be aware that tissue biopsies in EDS patients may show abnormal collagen fibrils on electron microscopy (irregular fibre diameters, 'cauliflower' cross-sections in classical EDS), supporting diagnosis when genetic testing is inconclusive.

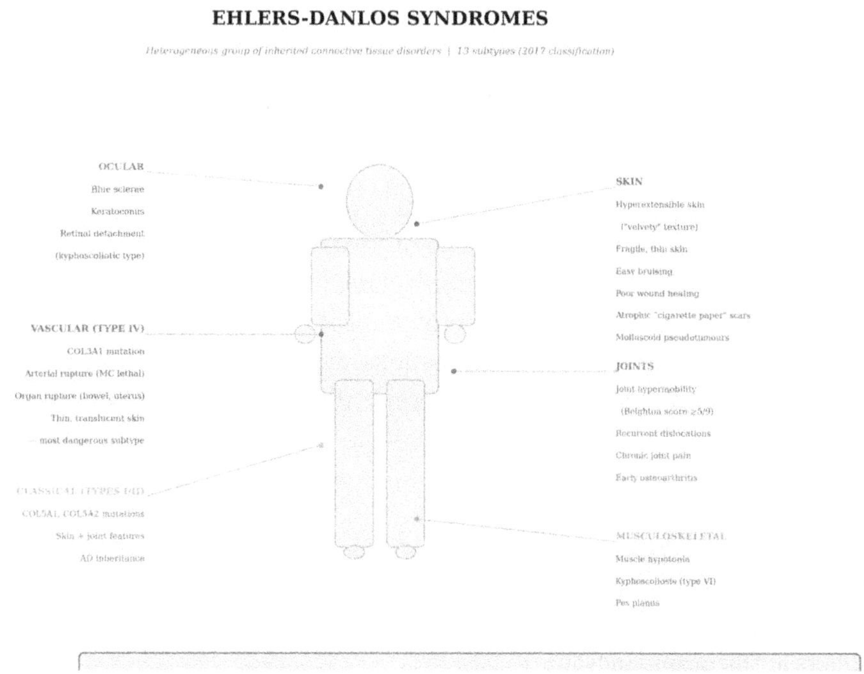

Figure 8.3: Ehlers-Danlos Syndromes: Clinical Features. (Source: Author's original.)

Osteogenesis Imperfecta

Osteogenesis imperfecta (OI, 'brittle bone disease') is a heterogeneous group of disorders caused predominantly by mutations in COL1A1 or COL1A2 genes encoding type I collagen, the principal structural protein of bone, skin, tendons, and sclera. Over 1,500 mutations have been identified. The clinical severity ranges from mild (OI type I: AD, most common; quantitative deficiency of type I collagen due to null allele; blue sclerae, easy fracturing after minimal trauma, normal stature, hearing loss in 50%) to lethal (OI type II: perinatal lethal; qualitative defect producing abnormal collagen; multiple intrauterine fractures, extreme skeletal fragility). Type III (progressively deforming) and type IV (moderate severity) complete the classical Sillence classification. Bisphosphonates (pamidronate, zoledronic acid) reduce fracture frequency in moderate-to-severe forms. Blue sclerae result from thinning of the collagen-deficient sclera, allowing the underlying choroidal pigment to show through.

Integration: *Connective tissue disorders connect to vascular pathology (aortic dissection, atherosclerosis in FH, Chapter 13), renal pathology (Alport syndrome, type IV collagen defect, Chapter 22), and skeletal pathology (osteogenesis imperfecta, EDS, Chapter 29).*

Familial Hypercholesterolaemia

Familial hypercholesterolaemia (FH) is an AD disorder caused by mutations in the **LDLR** gene (chromosome 19), encoding the LDL receptor. Less commonly, mutations in **APOB** (encoding apolipoprotein B-100, the LDL receptor ligand) or gain-of-function mutations in **PCSK9** (which promotes LDL receptor degradation) produce a similar phenotype. The LDL receptor is responsible for receptor-mediated endocytosis of LDL particles from the circulation. Heterozygous FH (1 in 250 to 500) causes moderate LDL elevation (300 to 500 mg/dL) and premature atherosclerosis, with myocardial infarction typically by the fourth or fifth decade. Homozygous FH (1 in a million) causes severe LDL elevation (>600 mg/dL), tendinous and cutaneous xanthomata in childhood, and myocardial infarction in the first two decades of life.

LDL receptor mutation → ↓LDL clearance → ↑Plasma LDL → Accelerated atherosclerosis → Premature MI

FH is the prototype for understanding receptor-mediated endocytosis. Over 2,000 different LDLR mutations have been identified, classified into five classes based on the step of receptor function affected: Class I (failure of synthesis), Class II (failure of transport from ER to Golgi), Class III (failure of LDL binding), Class IV (failure of receptor internalisation), and Class V (failure of receptor recycling). PCSK9 inhibitors (evolocumab, alirocumab) are a recent therapeutic advance that reduce LDL receptor degradation.

> **Quick Recall: Autosomal Dominant Disorders**
>
> **Marfan:** FBN1 (fibrillin-1); skeletal, eye (upward lens subluxation), cardiovascular (aortic dissection). Cystic medial degeneration.
>
> **FH:** LDLR gene; receptor-mediated endocytosis defect; 5 classes of mutations; premature atherosclerosis. PCSK9 inhibitors are therapeutic advances.
>
> **Other AD:** Huntington (HTT, CAG repeat), Neurofibromatosis (NF1/NF2), von Hippel-Lindau (VHL, see Chapter 23), ADPKD (PKD1/PKD2, see Chapter 23), Hereditary spherocytosis (see Volume 1).

Autosomal Recessive Disorders

Autosomal recessive (AR) disorders manifest only when both copies of the gene are mutated (homozygous or compound heterozygous). Carriers (heterozygotes) are phenotypically normal. AR disorders are characterised by horizontal transmission (siblings affected, parents unaffected carriers), equal male and female incidence, and higher incidence in consanguineous families. Most inborn errors of metabolism, including lysosomal storage diseases, are AR.

Phenylketonuria

Phenylketonuria (PKU) is the prototype inborn error of amino acid metabolism. It is an AR disorder caused by mutations in the PAH gene encoding phenylalanine hydroxylase, the hepatic enzyme that converts phenylalanine to tyrosine. Over 1,100 different PAH mutations have been identified. Deficiency of phenylalanine hydroxylase leads to accumulation of phenylalanine and its metabolites (phenylpyruvic acid, phenylacetic acid) in body fluids, with devastating effects on the developing brain. Untreated PKU causes severe intellectual disability (IQ typically below 50), seizures, fair skin and light hair (due to impaired melanin synthesis from the lack of tyrosine), musty body odour (from phenylacetic acid in sweat), and eczema.

PKU is the most successful example of newborn screening. The Guthrie test (bacterial inhibition assay) or tandem mass spectrometry (now the standard method in most developed countries) detects elevated phenylalanine in dried blood spots collected at 48-72 hours of life. Early dietary restriction of phenylalanine (started within the first two weeks of life) prevents intellectual disability and allows normal cognitive development. A less severe form, benign hyperphenylalaninaemia, requires monitoring but not dietary treatment. Maternal PKU (elevated phenylalanine during pregnancy in a PKU mother) can cause congenital heart defects, microcephaly, and intellectual disability in the fetus even if the fetus does not have PKU, emphasising the teratogenic effects of elevated phenylalanine. Sapropterin (BH4 supplementation) is effective in patients with BH4-responsive mutations.

The pathogenesis explains the morphology: because phenylalanine hydroxylase is deficient, phenylalanine cannot be converted to tyrosine. The resulting hyperphenylalaninaemia is directly toxic to the developing brain (inhibiting neurotransmitter synthesis, disrupting myelin formation, and generating oxidative stress). The lack of tyrosine explains the fair pigmentation (tyrosine is the precursor of melanin) and contributes to catecholamine deficiency.

Alpha-1 Antitrypsin Deficiency

Alpha-1 antitrypsin (A1AT) deficiency is an AR disorder caused by mutations in the SERPINA1 gene, encoding A1AT, the principal serum protease inhibitor (Pi). A1AT is synthesised in the liver and is the major inhibitor of neutrophil elastase in the lungs. The most clinically significant alleles are PiM (normal), PiS (mild deficiency), and PiZ (severe deficiency). The PiZZ genotype (homozygous Z allele) produces only 10-15% of normal A1AT levels and accounts for most clinically significant disease.

The disease manifests in two organs through distinct mechanisms. In the lungs, the lack of antiprotease protection allows unchecked neutrophil elastase activity, destroying alveolar walls and producing panacinar emphysema, characteristically affecting the lower lobes (in contrast to smoking-related centrilobular emphysema of the upper lobes; see Chapter 15). In the liver, the Z-mutant A1AT protein misfolds and polymerises within hepatocyte endoplasmic reticulum, where it accumulates as PAS-positive, diastase-resistant globular inclusions in periportal hepatocytes. This causes a toxic gain-of-function hepatopathy: neonatal hepatitis, childhood cirrhosis, and an increased risk of hepatocellular carcinoma in adults. The liver disease is a gain-of-function (protein accumulation), while the lung disease is a loss-of-function (protease-antiprotease imbalance).

A1AT deficiency is underdiagnosed. The Z allele frequency is lower in South Asian populations (approximately 1-2%) compared to Northern Europeans (4-5%), but the condition should be considered in unexplained early-onset emphysema or cryptogenic liver disease, particularly in non-smokers. Augmentation therapy (intravenous A1AT infusion) is available but expensive, with access varying between regions.

Lysosomal Storage Diseases

Lysosomal storage diseases (LSDs) are ~70 inherited metabolic disorders caused by deficiency of specific lysosomal enzymes, leading to substrate accumulation. Diagnosis relies on enzyme assay and genetic testing; enzyme replacement therapy (ERT) is available for Gaucher, Fabry, and Pompe diseases. Key enzyme–substrate pairs are in Table 8.1.**Table 8.1: Major Lysosomal Storage Diseases**

Disease	Enzyme Deficiency	Accumulated	Key Clinical Features

		Substrate	
Gaucher disease (Type 1, most common)	β-Glucocerebrosidase (GBA1)	Glucocerebroside	Hepatosplenomegaly, bone crises, Gaucher cells (crinkled paper cytoplasm), pancytopenia
Niemann-Pick A and B	Sphingomyelinase	Sphingomyelin	A: severe neurodegeneration, cherry-red spot. B: visceral, no CNS. Foam cells
Niemann-Pick C	NPC1/NPC2 (cholesterol transport)	Cholesterol, sphingolipids	Vertical supranuclear gaze palsy, ataxia, dementia
Tay-Sachs disease	Hexosaminidase A	GM2 ganglioside	Severe neurodegeneration, cherry-red spot (macula), no hepatosplenomegaly, Ashkenazi Jews
Fabry disease	α-Galactosidase A	Globotriaosylceramide (Gb3)	X-linked. Angiokeratomas, acroparaesthesia, renal failure, cardiac involvement
Gaucher Type 2 (acute)	β-Glucocerebrosidase	Glucocerebroside	Severe CNS involvement, death by age 2
Krabbe disease	Galactocerebrosidase	Galactocerebroside	Globoid cell leucodystrophy, severe white matter loss
Metachromatic leucodystrophy	Arylsulfatase A	Sulfatide	Progressive demyelination, detected by metachromatic staining (toluidine blue)

Gaucher disease deserves special attention as the most common LSD. Type 1 (non-neuronopathic, the vast majority of cases) presents with hepatosplenomegaly, bone disease (avascular necrosis, pathological fractures, Erlenmeyer flask deformity of the distal femur), and pancytopenia due to marrow infiltration. The hallmark histological finding is the **Gaucher cell:** a large macrophage (20 to 100 μm) with a distinctive 'wrinkled tissue paper' or 'crinkled paper' cytoplasmic appearance, resulting from the accumulation of glucocerebroside in distended lysosomes. Gaucher cells are strongly PAS-positive and are found in the spleen, liver, bone marrow, and lymph nodes. Enzyme replacement therapy (ERT) with imiglucerase and substrate reduction therapy (SRT) with eliglustat are available and effective treatments.

The key diagnostic clue in this setting is: A cherry-red spot at the macula is seen in Tay-Sachs disease and Niemann-Pick type A (and, less commonly, in Niemann-Pick C and some other LSDs). The cherry-red spot results from the contrast between the normal foveal area (which lacks ganglion cells and therefore does not accumulate substrate) and the surrounding retina, where swollen, lipid-laden ganglion cells appear pale. In Tay-Sachs, there is NO hepatosplenomegaly (the substrate accumulates in neurons, not visceral macrophages); in Niemann-Pick A, there IS hepatosplenomegaly.

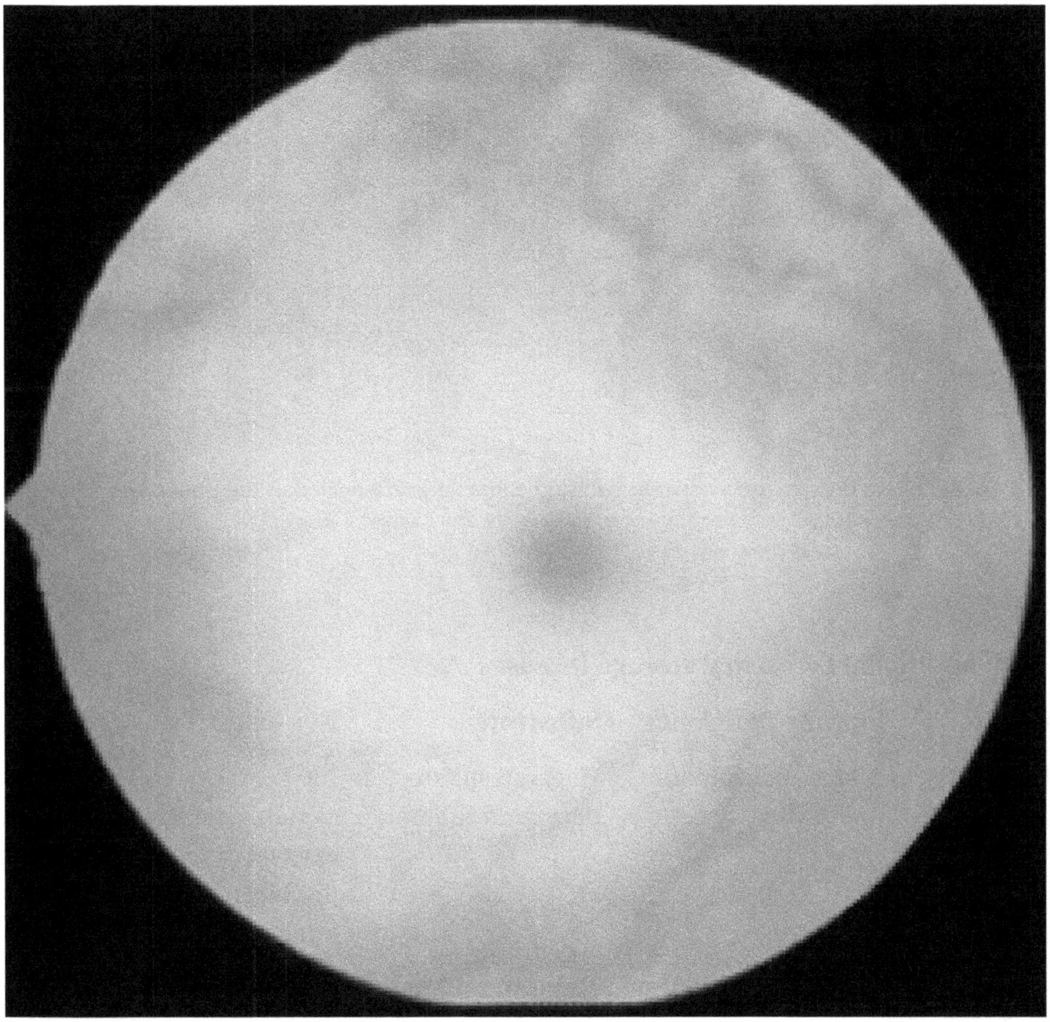

Figure 8.4: Tay-Sachs disease — cherry-red spot. Fundoscopy showing cherry-red fovea centralis surrounded by pale, swollen retinal ganglion cells laden with GM2 ganglioside. (Source: University of Michigan Kellogg Eye Center, Wikimedia Commons, Public Domain.)

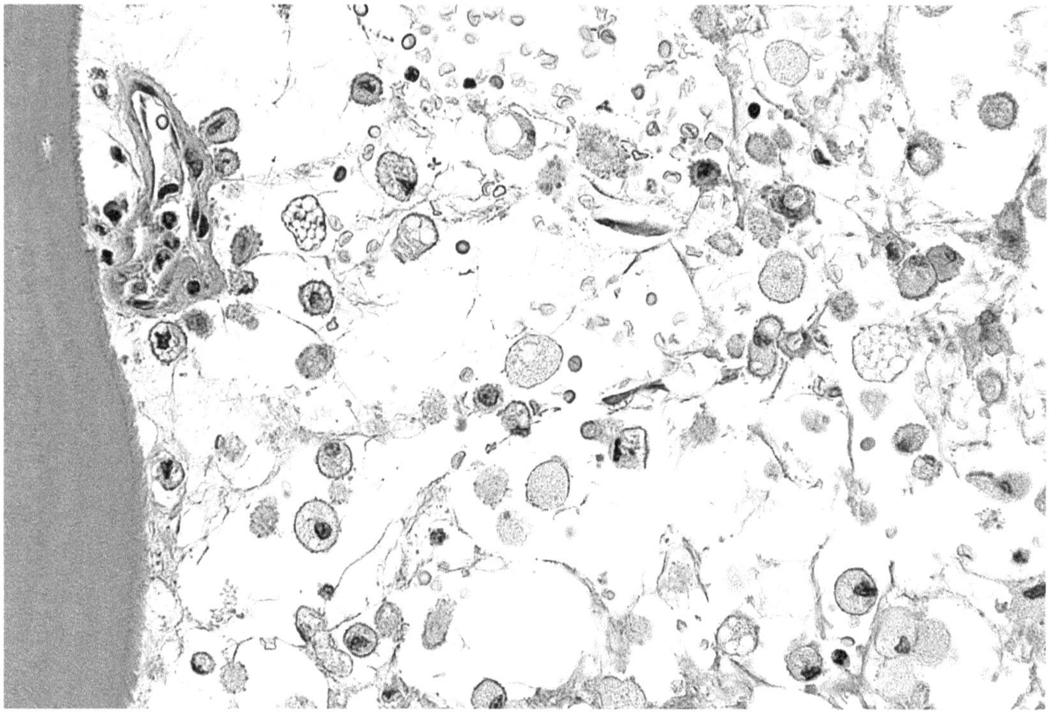

Figure 8.5: Gaucher cell in bone marrow aspirate showing characteristic wrinkled tissue paper cytoplasm. MGG (May–Grünwald Giemsa), ×1000. (Source: Nephron, Wikimedia Commons, CC BY-SA 3.0.)

The Pathologist's Eye

Table 8.1b: Additional Lysosomal Storage Diseases

Disease	Enzyme Deficiency	Substrate	Key Features
MPS I (Hurler/Scheie)	Alpha-L-iduronidase	Heparan sulfate, dermatan sulfate	AR. Coarse facies, corneal clouding, hepatosplenomegaly, skeletal dysostosis, intellectual disability (Hurler). Scheie: milder, normal intellect.
MPS II (Hunter)	Iduronate-2-sulfatase	Heparan sulfate, dermatan sulfate	X-linked recessive (only XL MPS). Similar to Hurler but NO corneal clouding. Pebbled skin lesion (ivory-coloured papules).
Krabbe disease	Galactocerebrosidase	Galactocerebroside	AR. Rapidly progressive CNS demyelination in infancy. Globoid cells (multinucleated macrophages) in white matter. No hepatosplenomegaly.

Metachromatic leukodystrophy	Arylsulfatase A	Sulfatide (cerebroside sulfate)	AR. Progressive demyelination. Metachromatic granules (brown with toluidine blue). Peripheral neuropathy + central demyelination.

In bone marrow aspirates, Gaucher cells must be distinguished from pseudo-Gaucher cells, which are macrophages with a similar crinkled appearance seen in CML, thalassaemia major, and other chronic haematological conditions with high cell turnover. True Gaucher cells are larger, have more uniform wrinkling, and stain strongly with PAS. The clinical context (hepatosplenomegaly in a child or young adult, Ashkenazi Jewish background) and confirmatory enzyme assay or GBA1 mutation analysis clinch the diagnosis.

Mucopolysaccharidoses

The mucopolysaccharidoses (MPS) result from deficiencies of enzymes degrading glycosaminoglycans (dermatan, heparan, keratan sulphate). Hurler (MPS I, α-L-iduronidase deficiency) is the prototype; Hunter (MPS II) is the only X-linked form. All show coarse facies, hepatosplenomegaly, and skeletal abnormalities. See table.

Niemann-Pick Type C: A Distinct Entity

Niemann-Pick type C results from NPC1/NPC2 mutations causing cholesterol trafficking defects, not sphingomyelinase deficiency. It presents with progressive neurodegeneration, vertical supranuclear gaze palsy, and hepatosplenomegaly. NPC has a variable age of onset, ranging from a severe neonatal form (with hydrops fetalis or neonatal cholestatic jaundice) to adult-onset neuropsychiatric disease. The classic presentation in late childhood includes progressive cerebellar ataxia, vertical supranuclear gaze palsy (VSGP, the most characteristic neurological sign, reflecting brainstem involvement), dystonia, dysarthria, dysphagia, and progressive dementia. Hepatosplenomegaly is common in early-onset cases but may be absent in adolescent or adult presentations. Gelastic cataplexy (sudden loss of muscle tone triggered by laughter) is a distinctive feature seen in approximately 20% of cases.

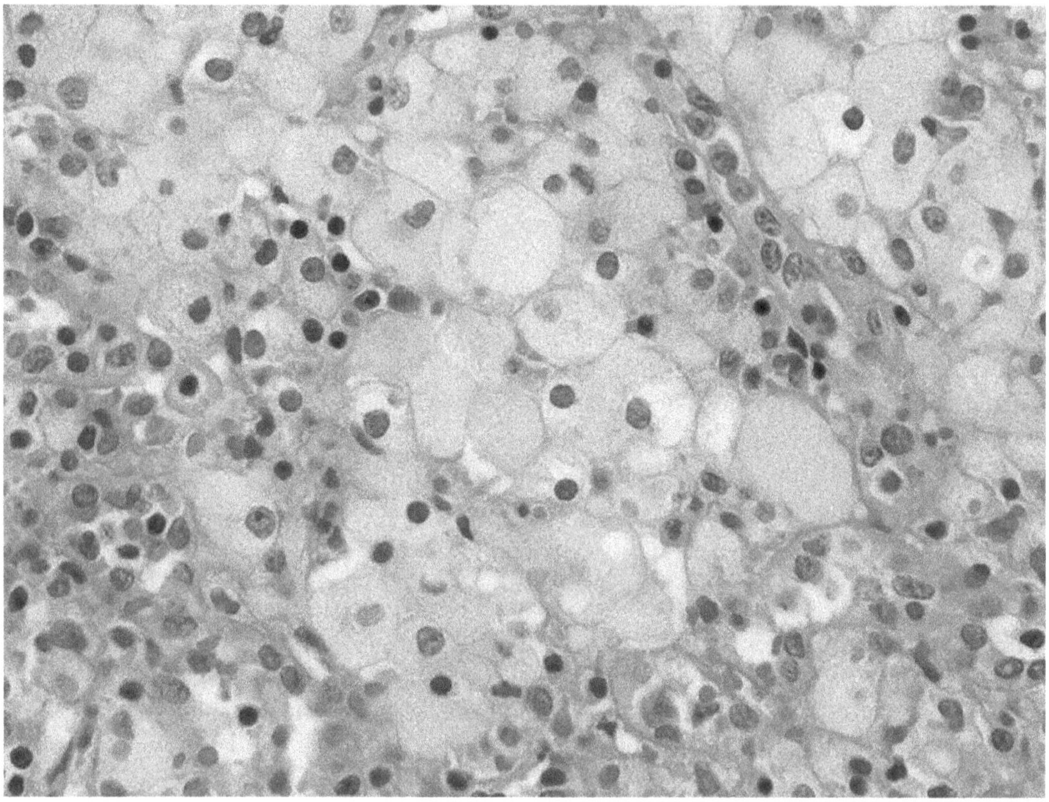

Figure 8.6: Niemann-Pick disease — Niemann-Pick cells (foam cells) in spleen. H&E, ×400. Large macrophages with abundant foamy, finely vacuolated cytoplasm (Source: W.CC, Wikimedia Commons, CC BY-SA 4.0.)

When faced with a child or adolescent with progressive ataxia, vertical gaze palsy, and hepatosplenomegaly, NPC should be high on the differential. The diagnosis is confirmed by filipin staining of cultured skin fibroblasts (showing perinuclear accumulation of unesterified cholesterol) or, increasingly, by biomarker assays (plasma oxysterols, particularly cholestane-3β,5α,6β-triol, or lysosphingomyelin-509) and NPC1/NPC2 gene sequencing. Miglustat, an inhibitor of glucosylceramide synthase, is the only approved disease-modifying therapy and has been shown to stabilise neurological progression in some patients.

A viva question that tests understanding of LSD pathophysiology: 'Why does enzyme replacement therapy work for Gaucher disease (Type 1) but not for Tay-Sachs?' The answer lies in the blood-brain barrier. In Gaucher Type 1, the pathology is visceral (macrophages in spleen, liver, bone marrow), and intravenously administered recombinant enzyme reaches these tissues effectively via mannose receptor-mediated uptake by macrophages. In Tay-Sachs, the pathology is neuronal: GM2 ganglioside accumulates in CNS neurons, which are inaccessible to intravenous enzyme because large proteins cannot cross the blood-brain barrier. This fundamental pharmacokinetic barrier explains why ERT has transformed outcomes in non-neuronopathic Gaucher disease but remains ineffective for the primary neurological LSDs.

Quick Recall: Lysosomal Storage Diseases

Gaucher: Most common LSD. β-Glucocerebrosidase deficiency. Wrinkled paper macrophages. Hepatosplenomegaly, bone disease, NO CNS in Type 1.

Tay-Sachs: Hex A deficiency. GM2 ganglioside. Cherry-red spot, NO hepatosplenomegaly.

Niemann-Pick A: Sphingomyelinase deficiency. Cherry-red spot WITH hepatosplenomegaly.

Fabry: X-linked. α-Gal A deficiency. Angiokeratomas, renal failure, cardiac disease.

MPS: GAG accumulation. Coarse facies, dysostosis multiplex.

Glycogen Storage Diseases

Glycogen storage diseases (GSDs) are inherited metabolic disorders caused by defects in enzymes of glycogen synthesis, degradation, or processing, leading to accumulation of glycogen (often abnormal in structure or location) in specific tissues. Liver and skeletal muscle are the two principal target organs, reflecting the two main physiological roles of glycogen — maintaining blood glucose between meals (liver) and fuelling anaerobic muscular work (muscle). Most GSDs are autosomal recessive; a notable exception is GSD IX (phosphorylase kinase deficiency), which is most often X-linked. Over 15 subtypes are described; the six numbered I–VI are the classical, exam-important forms.

Pathogenesis framework: Glycogenolysis defect → failure to release glucose → fasting hypoglycaemia (if liver enzyme) or exercise intolerance (if muscle enzyme). Glycogen synthesis or branching defect → structurally abnormal glycogen → cellular toxicity and organ failure.

Table 8.1c: Major Glycogen Storage Diseases

Type / Eponym	Enzyme Deficiency (Gene)	Primary Tissue	Key Clinical Features
GSD I (von Gierke)	Glucose-6-phosphatase (G6PC)	Liver, kidney	Severe fasting hypoglycaemia; massive hepatomegaly with "doll-like" rounded facies; lactic acidosis; hyperuricaemia (→ gout); hyperlipidaemia (→ eruptive xanthomas); risk of hepatic adenomas → HCC.
GSD II (Pompe)	Lysosomal acid α-glucosidase / acid maltase (GAA)	Heart, skeletal muscle (all tissues)	INFANTILE: cardiomegaly + hypotonia ("floppy infant") + macroglossia + short PR interval on ECG; death <2y without treatment. ADULT: limb-girdle-like myopathy with early diaphragmatic weakness. (Both GSD and LSD — see Integration.)
GSD III (Cori /	Debranching enzyme	Liver, muscle	Milder von Gierke-like picture + distal

Forbes)	(AGL)		myopathy in adulthood. Accumulated glycogen has abnormally short outer branches (limit dextrin).
GSD IV (Andersen)	Branching enzyme (GBE1)	Liver (also heart, muscle)	Failure to thrive, progressive hepatosplenomegaly, cirrhosis, death in infancy without liver transplant. Accumulated glycogen is amylopectin-like (long unbranched chains).
GSD V (McArdle)	Muscle glycogen phosphorylase (PYGM)	Skeletal muscle	Exercise intolerance with painful cramps and myoglobinuria; classic SECOND-WIND PHENOMENON (symptoms improve after brief rest). Forearm ischaemic exercise test: no rise in venous lactate. CK persistently elevated; normal life expectancy.
GSD VI (Hers)	Liver glycogen phosphorylase (PYGL)	Liver	Mild hepatomegaly, mild fasting hypoglycaemia, ketosis, growth retardation. Generally benign; symptoms often improve with age.

von Gierke disease (GSD I)

Genetics: Autosomal recessive. G6PC gene (chromosome 17q21) encoding glucose-6-phosphatase. Subtypes: Ia (~80%, pure G6PC deficiency) and Ib (~20%, SLC37A4 G6P transporter defect — adds neutropenia and inflammatory bowel disease).

Enzyme defect: Glucose-6-phosphatase is the final shared enzyme of both glycogenolysis and gluconeogenesis; its absence blocks both pathways simultaneously.

Biochemistry: Block at G6P → glucose causes (1) profound fasting hypoglycaemia within 3–4 hours of feeding, and (2) diversion of excess G6P into lactate (→ lactic acidosis), purine turnover (→ hyperuricaemia, precocious gout), and lipogenesis (→ hypertriglyceridaemia, eruptive xanthomas).

Clinical: Presents in infancy with hypoglycaemic seizures, lethargy, failure to thrive. Massive hepatomegaly; "doll-like" rounded facies due to cheek fat deposition. Bleeding diathesis from impaired platelet function.

Complications: Hepatic adenomas (5–75% of patients) with HCC transformation risk (~10%); renal Fanconi-like tubular dysfunction progressing to renal insufficiency; pulmonary hypertension.

Diagnosis: Molecular genetic testing (G6PC for Ia, SLC37A4 for Ib). Liver biopsy rarely required.

Management: Maintain euglycaemia: frequent daytime complex-carbohydrate feeds; uncooked cornstarch at bedtime (slow-release glucose, 4–6 hours). Avoid fructose and galactose. Liver transplant curative for hepatic manifestations.

Pompe disease (GSD II)

Classification: Unique dual classification — both a GSD (substrate is glycogen) and a lysosomal storage disease (enzyme is lysosomal).

Genetics: Autosomal recessive. GAA gene (chromosome 17q25.3).

Enzyme defect: Acid α-glucosidase (acid maltase), the lysosomal enzyme that hydrolyses glycogen to glucose within lysosomes.

Biochemistry: Glycogen accumulates within lysosomes, particularly in cardiac and skeletal muscle; lysosomal rupture releases degradative enzymes that damage surrounding cytoplasm.

Clinical — infantile: Presents within first months: "floppy baby" phenotype with profound hypotonia, macroglossia, feeding and respiratory difficulties, and massive hypertrophic cardiomyopathy (boot-shaped heart on CXR). ECG: short PR interval, high-voltage QRS. Death from cardiorespiratory failure by age 2 without enzyme replacement.

Clinical — adult: Limb-girdle-like progressive proximal myopathy; distinctive early diaphragmatic and paraspinal muscle involvement causing orthopnoea and sleep-disordered breathing.

Diagnosis: Reduced acid α-glucosidase activity on dried blood spot. Confirmation: GAA gene sequencing. Muscle biopsy: vacuolated fibres with PAS-positive glycogen and acid-phosphatase-positive lysosomal inclusions.

Management: Enzyme replacement therapy with alglucosidase alfa (approved 2006); earlier initiation improves survival. CRIM-negative patients (no endogenous enzyme) require immune tolerance induction. Newborn screening is now standard in many jurisdictions.

McArdle disease (GSD V)

Genetics: Autosomal recessive. PYGM gene (chromosome 11q13) encoding muscle glycogen phosphorylase.

Enzyme defect: Muscle glycogen phosphorylase — a tissue-specific isoenzyme distinct from the hepatic form.

Biochemistry: During anaerobic exercise, skeletal muscle cannot mobilise its glycogen stores. Symptoms develop within minutes of strenuous activity; resolve as bloodborne fuels (free fatty acids, hepatic glucose) take over — the "second-wind" phenomenon.

Clinical: Exercise intolerance with painful cramps, muscle stiffness, and in severe episodes acute rhabdomyolysis with myoglobinuria ("Coca-Cola" urine). Second-wind phenomenon is pathognomonic. Serum CK persistently elevated at rest.

Diagnosis: Forearm ischaemic exercise test (historical): failure of venous lactate to rise during ischaemic work, with normal rise in ammonia (confirming effort). Now largely replaced by PYGM gene sequencing. Muscle biopsy: subsarcolemmal PAS-positive vacuoles; absent histochemical staining for myophosphorylase.

Management: Graded aerobic exercise conditioning; oral sucrose before exercise may improve performance. No specific therapy. Normal life expectancy if severe rhabdomyolysis episodes are avoided.

Integration: Pompe disease straddles two classification systems. By substrate (glycogen) it is a GSD; by organelle (lysosome) it is an LSD. Both classifications appear in exam answers. The practical consequence: Pompe uniquely combines tissue-specific glycogen overload (like other GSDs) with lysosomal dysfunction and responsiveness to enzyme replacement (like other LSDs).

Diagnostic thinking: fasting hypoglycaemia + hepatomegaly + doll-like facies + lactic acidosis + hyperuricaemia + hyperlipidaemia → GSD I (von Gierke). Add neutropenia → GSD Ib subtype.

Diagnostic thinking: floppy infant + cardiomegaly + macroglossia + short PR on ECG → infantile Pompe (GSD II).

Diagnostic thinking: exercise intolerance + cramps + myoglobinuria + second-wind phenomenon + flat ischaemic-exercise lactate curve → McArdle (GSD V). No second-wind, fixed weakness → consider adult Pompe or mitochondrial myopathy.

Quick Recall: Glycogen Storage Diseases

von Gierke (GSD I): G6Pase deficiency. Liver + kidney. Fasting hypoglycaemia, massive hepatomegaly, doll-like facies, lactic acidosis, hyperuricaemia, hyperlipidaemia. Risk: hepatic adenomas → HCC.

Pompe (GSD II): Lysosomal acid α-glucosidase (GAA). Both GSD and LSD. INFANTILE: cardiomegaly + hypotonia + macroglossia + short PR. ADULT: LGMD-like + early diaphragmatic weakness. ERT = alglucosidase alfa.

Cori / Forbes (GSD III): Debranching enzyme. Milder von Gierke + adult myopathy. Limit dextrin accumulation.

Andersen (GSD IV): Branching enzyme. Infantile cirrhosis + liver failure. Amylopectin-like glycogen.

McArdle (GSD V): Muscle phosphorylase (PYGM). Exercise intolerance, cramps, myoglobinuria, SECOND-WIND phenomenon. Ischaemic exercise test: no lactate rise (normal ammonia).

Hers (GSD VI): Liver phosphorylase (PYGL). Mild hepatomegaly, mild hypoglycaemia, benign course.

Cystic Fibrosis

Cystic fibrosis (CF) is the most common lethal AR disorder in Caucasian populations (carrier frequency 1 in 25; disease frequency 1 in 2,500 live births). It is caused by mutations in the **CFTR** gene (chromosome 7), encoding the cystic fibrosis transmembrane conductance regulator, a chloride channel on epithelial cell surfaces. The most common mutation, **ΔF508** (deletion of phenylalanine at position 508), accounts for approximately 70% of CF alleles worldwide and causes a protein folding defect (Class II mutation) that prevents CFTR from reaching the cell surface.

Defective CFTR function leads to decreased chloride secretion and increased sodium (and water) absorption across epithelial surfaces, producing abnormally viscid secretions. The clinical consequences reflect this in multiple organ systems: **lungs** (thick mucus plugging, recurrent infections with *Pseudomonas aeruginosa* and *Staphylococcus aureus,* bronchiectasis, respiratory failure); **pancreas** (exocrine pancreatic insufficiency in 85-90%, leading to malabsorption and steatorrhoea); **liver** (focal biliary cirrhosis); **intestine** (meconium ileus in neonates); and **male reproductive tract** (obstructive azoospermia due to bilateral absence of the vas deferens, causing male infertility in >95%). The **sweat chloride test** (>60 mmol/L is diagnostic) remains the gold standard for diagnosis, supplemented by CFTR mutation analysis.

CFTR mutation → ↓Cl^- secretion / ↑Na^+ absorption → Dehydrated viscid secretions → Duct obstruction → Organ damage (lung, pancreas, liver)

A major therapeutic advance is the development of **CFTR modulators:** ivacaftor (potentiator, for gating mutations), lumacaftor/tezacaftor (correctors, help ΔF508 protein reach the surface), and the triple combination elexacaftor/tezacaftor/ivacaftor (Trikafta), which has dramatically improved outcomes for patients with at least one ΔF508 allele.

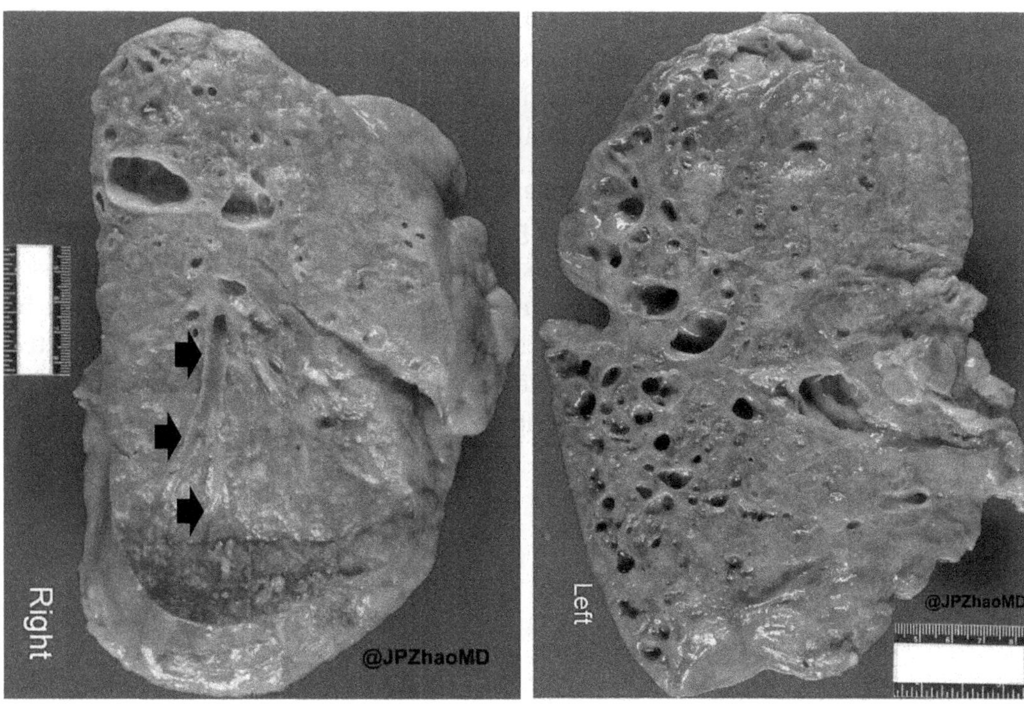

Figure 8.7: Cystic fibrosis — bilateral bronchiectasis, gross specimen. Dilated airways with inspissated mucus, extensive parenchymal destruction. (Source: JPZhaoMD, Wikimedia Commons/Flickr, CC BY 2.0.)

Integration: Cystic fibrosis connects to respiratory pathology (bronchiectasis, Chapter 15), pancreatic pathology (exocrine insufficiency, Chapter 21), and hepatobiliary pathology (focal biliary cirrhosis, Chapter 20).

Multifactorial (Complex) Disorders

Multifactorial disorders result from the combined effects of multiple genetic variants (each of individually small effect) interacting with environmental factors. They are the most common category of genetic disease and include conditions such as diabetes mellitus, hypertension, coronary artery disease, schizophrenia, neural tube defects, cleft lip/palate, and congenital heart disease. Unlike Mendelian disorders, multifactorial disorders do not follow simple inheritance patterns, but they do show familial clustering: first-degree relatives of an affected individual have a higher risk than the general population, and concordance rates in monozygotic twins exceed those in dizygotic twins, indicating a genetic contribution.

The genetic architecture of multifactorial diseases has been elucidated by genome-wide association studies (GWAS), which identify common single nucleotide polymorphisms (SNPs) associated with disease risk. Each individual SNP confers a modest increase in risk (typically odds ratios of 1.1-1.5), but the cumulative effect of many risk alleles can be substantial. Polygenic risk scores (PRS) aggregate the effects of thousands of SNPs to estimate an individual's genetic predisposition to a particular disease. PRS for coronary artery disease, breast cancer, and type 2 diabetes are entering clinical practice, though their utility in ethnically diverse populations underrepresented in GWAS databases remains under evaluation.

The concept of a liability threshold is central to understanding multifactorial inheritance. Each individual has a liability to a disease determined by the sum of genetic and environmental factors. When the liability exceeds a threshold, disease manifests. This model explains why: (1) the recurrence risk increases with the number of affected family members; (2) the recurrence risk is higher when the proband has severe disease; and (3) the recurrence risk is higher when the affected sex is the less commonly affected sex (e.g., pyloric stenosis is five times more common in males; an affected female must therefore have a higher genetic load, and her offspring carry higher risk) (Figure 8.8).

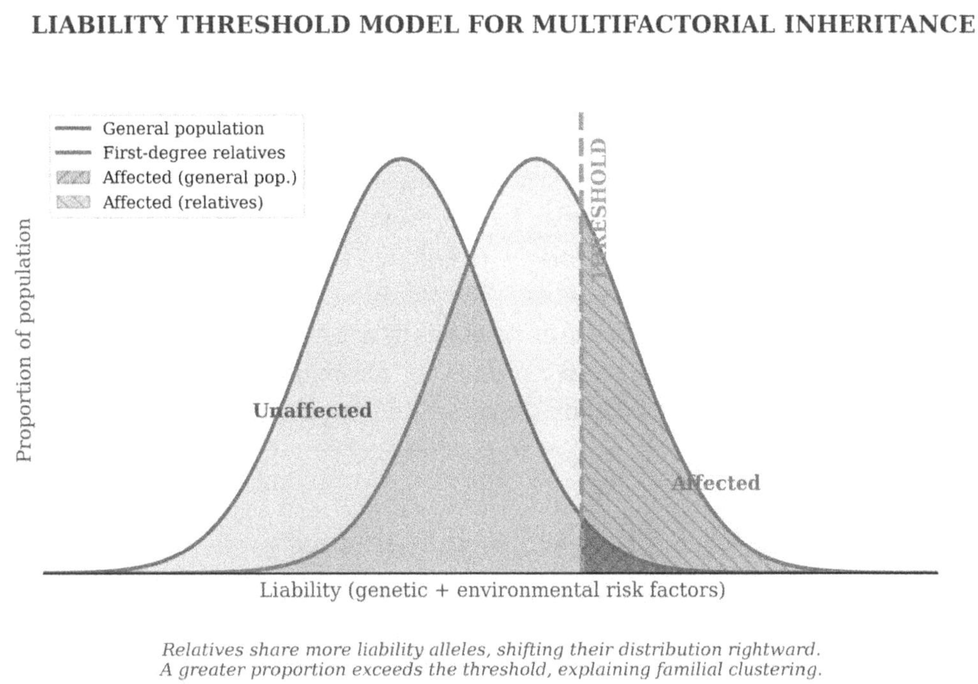

Figure 8.8: Liability threshold model for multifactorial inheritance. (Source: Author's original.)

Neural tube defects (NTDs; anencephaly, spina bifida) are the prototype multifactorial malformations. Both genetic factors (variants in folate metabolism genes including MTHFR C677T) and environmental factors (maternal folate deficiency, valproic acid exposure, maternal diabetes, maternal hyperthermia) contribute to risk. Periconceptional folic acid supplementation (400 µg/day for low-risk, 4 mg/day for high-risk women with a previously affected child) reduces the risk of NTDs by 50-70%, one of the most successful public health interventions in genetic disease prevention.

Chromosomal Disorders

Chromosomal disorders involve changes in the number (aneuploidy) or structure (translocations, deletions, inversions, ring chromosomes) of chromosomes and are a major cause of spontaneous abortions, congenital malformations, and intellectual disability. The normal human karyotype is 46,XX (female) or 46,XY (male), visualised by G-banding of metaphase chromosomes.

Down Syndrome (Trisomy 21)

Down syndrome is the most common chromosomal disorder and the most common genetic cause of intellectual disability, with an incidence of approximately 1 in 700 live births. Three cytogenetic patterns produce trisomy 21: **meiotic non-disjunction** (95% of cases; karyotype 47,XX,+21 or 47,XY,+21; maternal age is the strongest risk factor, rising sharply after age 35); **Robertsonian translocation** (4%; most commonly t(14;21), where the long arm of chromosome 21 is translocated to chromosome 14; this form may be inherited from a balanced carrier parent and has a recurrence risk of up to 15% if the mother is the carrier); and **mosaicism** (1%; 46,XX/47,XX,+21; milder phenotype).

Clinical features include a flat facial profile, upslanting palpebral fissures, epicanthal folds, Brushfield spots (speckled iris), single palmar crease (simian crease), sandal gap deformity of the toes, generalised hypotonia, and moderate to severe intellectual disability. **Congenital heart disease** is present in 40% of patients, with endocardial cushion defects (atrioventricular septal defect) being the most characteristic. There is a markedly increased risk of **acute leukaemia:** 10- to 20-fold increased risk of acute lymphoblastic leukaemia (ALL), and particularly a unique association with **transient abnormal myelopoiesis (TAM)** and **acute megakaryoblastic leukaemia (AMKL)** with GATA1 mutations in early childhood (see Volume 1). Early-onset **Alzheimer disease** (by age 40) is virtually universal, attributed to the presence of the APP gene (amyloid precursor protein) on chromosome 21. Increased susceptibility to infections, hypothyroidism, and atlantoaxial instability are additional clinical concerns (Figure 8.9).

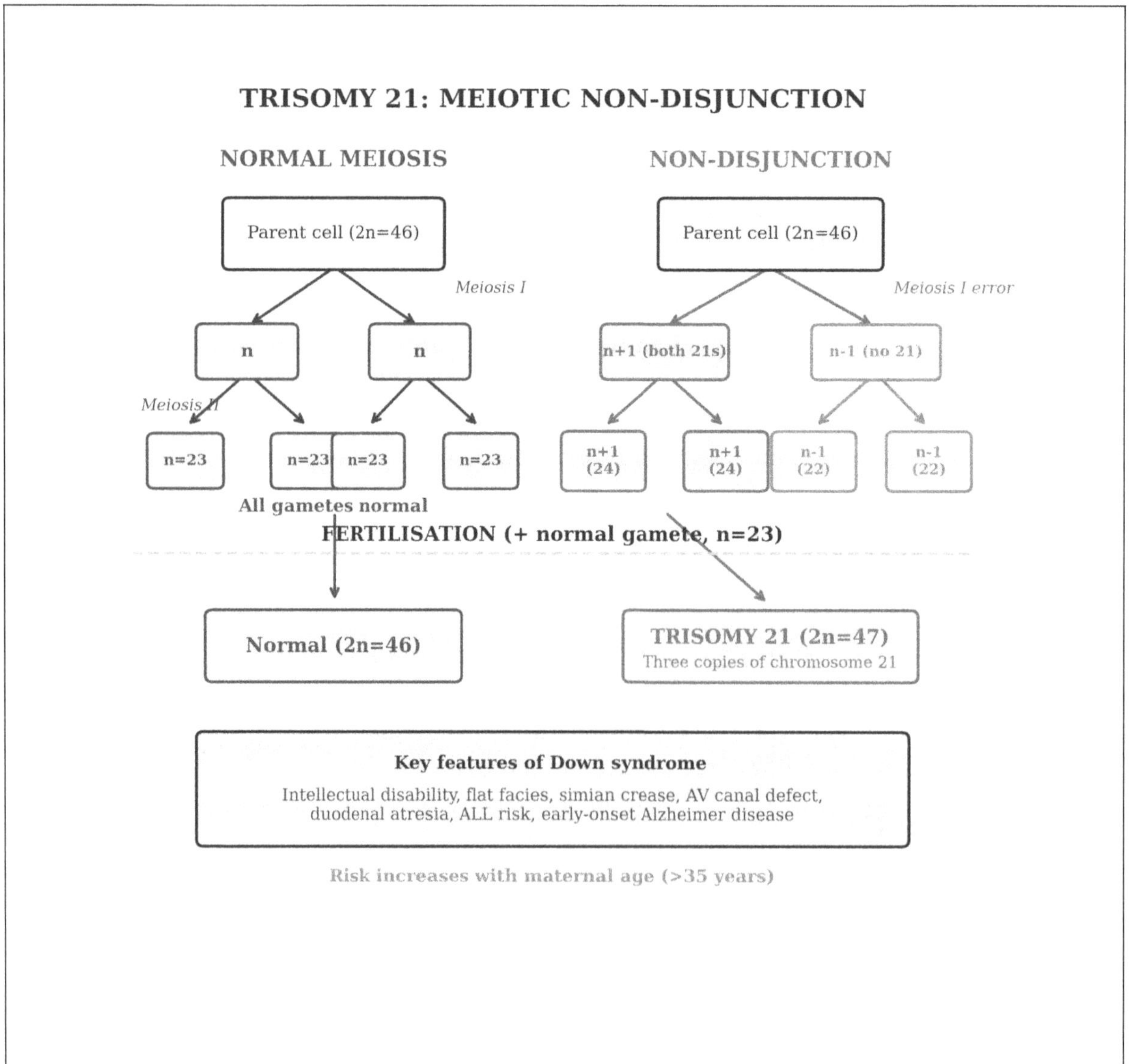

Figure 8.9: Karyotype showing trisomy 21 with mechanism of non-disjunction. (Source: Author's original.)

The molecular basis of the Down syndrome phenotype relates to gene dosage effects of chromosome 21. The Down syndrome critical region (DSCR) at 21q22.1-22.3 contains genes whose overexpression is responsible for specific features: DYRK1A (dual-specificity tyrosine phosphorylation-regulated kinase 1A) contributes to intellectual disability through effects on neuronal development, dendritic spine morphology, and tau phosphorylation (linking to the Alzheimer pathology seen in trisomy 21). DSCAM (Down syndrome cell adhesion molecule) affects cardiac development, contributing to the atrioventricular septal defect. Understanding these gene-dosage effects has opened therapeutic research into targeted kinase inhibitors for cognitive improvement.

Prenatal screening for Down syndrome has evolved through several generations. First-trimester combined screening (maternal age, nuchal translucency on ultrasound, and biochemical markers [β-hCG and PAPP-A]) offers detection rates of approximately 85-90% with a 5% false-positive rate. The quadruple test (AFP, β-hCG, unconjugated estriol, inhibin A) is used in the second trimester where first-trimester screening is unavailable. Non-invasive prenatal testing (NIPT) using cell-free fetal DNA in maternal blood has sensitivity and specificity exceeding 99% for trisomy 21, but remains a screening (not diagnostic) test; positive results require confirmatory amniocentesis or chorionic villus sampling (CVS) before clinical decision-making. Statutory limits on termination for fetal anomalies vary between jurisdictions, making timely prenatal diagnosis critical wherever termination is legally permitted.

Other Autosomal Trisomies

Edwards syndrome (Trisomy 18): Incidence 1 in 5,000. Severe intellectual disability, prominent occiput, micrognathia, low-set ears, overlapping fingers (clenched fist with index over third, fifth over fourth), rocker-bottom feet, congenital heart defects (VSD, PDA). Median survival 5 to 15 days; >90% die within the first year.

Patau syndrome (Trisomy 13): Incidence 1 in 15,000. Severe intellectual disability, microcephaly, microphthalmia, cleft lip/palate, polydactyly, congenital heart defects, holoprosencephaly. Median survival less than 10 days.

Sex Chromosome Disorders

Klinefelter syndrome (47,XXY): The most common sex chromosome aneuploidy in males, with an incidence of 1 in 660 males. Clinical features become apparent at puberty: tall stature, eunuchoid body habitus, small firm testes (testicular atrophy with hyalinised seminiferous tubules and Leydig cell hyperplasia), gynaecomastia, and infertility (azoospermia). There is increased risk of breast cancer (20-fold), metabolic syndrome, and osteoporosis. Most cases arise from maternal meiotic non-disjunction.

Turner syndrome (45,X): The most common sex chromosome abnormality in females, though 99% of 45,X conceptions end in spontaneous abortion. Incidence in live births is approximately 1 in 2,500 females. Karyotypic variants include 45,X (55%), 46,X,i(Xq) (isochromosome of the long arm, 15%), mosaics (45,X/46,XX), and others. Clinical features include short stature, webbed neck (cystic hygroma remnant), shield-shaped chest with widely spaced nipples, lymphoedema of hands and feet at birth, coarctation of the aorta (most characteristic cardiovascular defect), bicuspid aortic valve, streak gonads (bilateral ovarian failure), primary amenorrhoea, and infertility. Intelligence is usually normal.

Cytogenetic Nomenclature (ISCN)

Cytogenetic findings are reported using the International System for Human Cytogenomic Nomenclature (ISCN). The postgraduate pathologist should be familiar with standard ISCN notation. The format specifies the total chromosome number, the sex chromosome complement, and any abnormality. Examples: 47,XX,+21 (female with trisomy 21); 45,X (Turner syndrome); 47,XXY (Klinefelter syndrome); 46,XY,t(9;22)(q34;q11.2) (male with Philadelphia chromosome translocation); 46,XX,del(22)(q11.2) (female with 22q11.2 deletion/DiGeorge syndrome); 46,XY,inv(16)(p13.1q22) (male with pericentric inversion of chromosome 16, associated with acute myeloid leukaemia with eosinophilia, see Volume 1).

Structural chromosomal abnormalities include translocations (reciprocal and Robertsonian), deletions, duplications, inversions (pericentric and paracentric), isochromosomes, and ring chromosomes. Robertsonian translocations involve the fusion of two acrocentric chromosomes (13, 14, 15, 21, 22) at the centromere, with loss of the short arms. A carrier of a balanced Robertsonian translocation involving chromosome 21 (e.g., 45,XX,rob(14;21)(q10;q10)) is phenotypically normal but has a significant risk of producing offspring with trisomy 21 through meiotic segregation. The 22q11.2 deletion syndrome (DiGeorge/velocardiofacial syndrome) is the most common microdeletion syndrome (incidence 1 in 4,000) and is characterised by cardiac defects (especially conotruncal anomalies such as tetralogy of Fallot and interrupted aortic arch), thymic hypoplasia (T-cell immunodeficiency), parathyroid hypoplasia (neonatal hypocalcaemia), and facial dysmorphism. Detection requires FISH or CMA, as the deletion is below the resolution of conventional karyotyping.

Clinical Pearl

FISH probe design: break-apart versus fusion. Break-apart probes flank a single gene locus; the intact gene shows fused signals (yellow when red-green probes are used), the rearranged gene shows split signals. Use break-apart for genes with multiple known partner genes (ALK in lung, ROS1, RET, MYC, BCL2, BCL6). Fusion probes target two specific genes; co-localisation indicates the specific fusion. Use fusion probes when the partner is known (BCR-ABL1, EWS-FLI1, PML-RARA). The wrong probe design produces a false negative: a break-apart probe will not detect a balanced translocation if designed inside the breakpoint, and a fusion probe misses unusual partners.

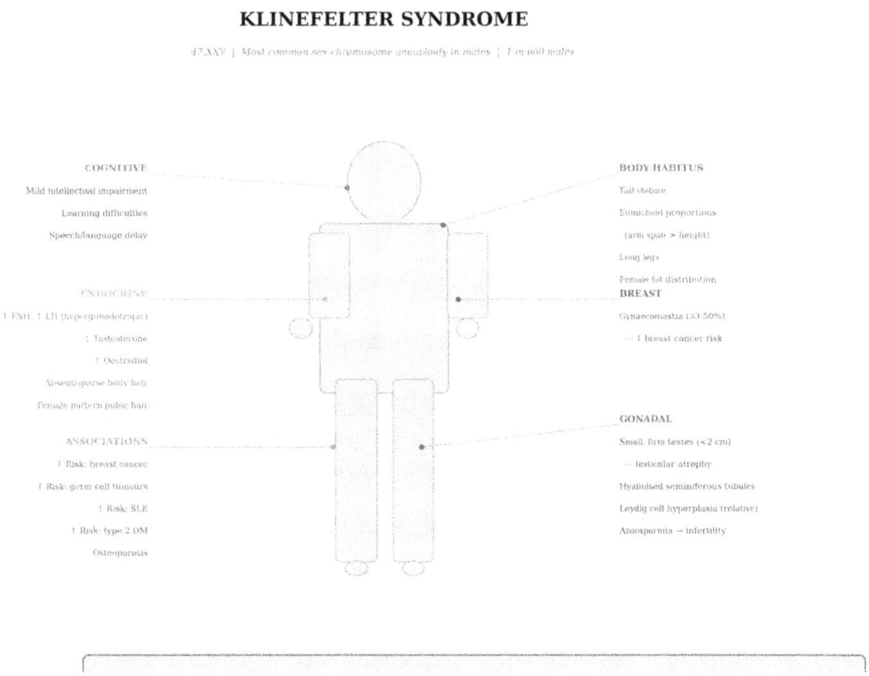

Figure 8.10: Klinefelter Syndrome (47,XXY): Clinical Features. (Source: Author's original.)

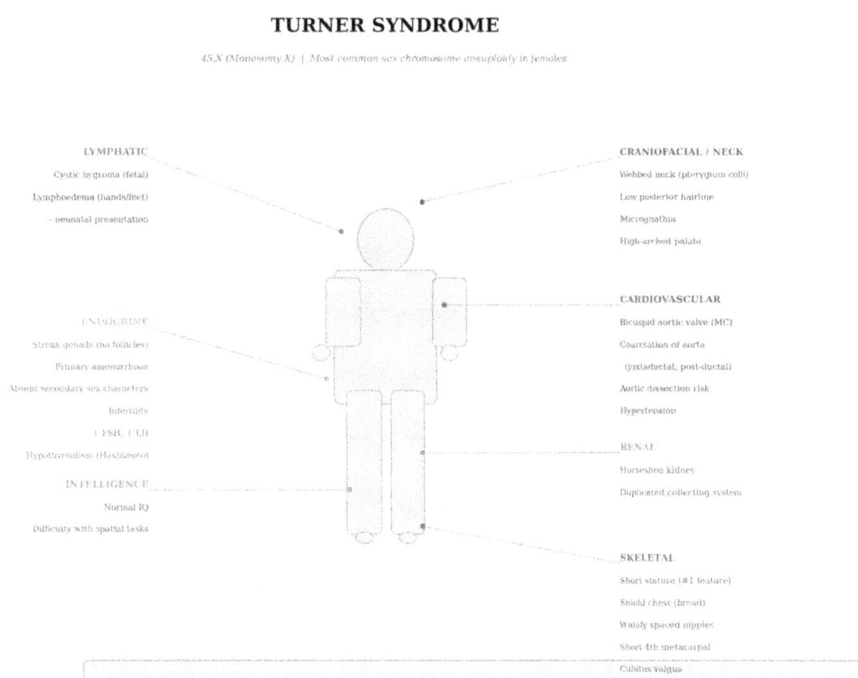

Figure 8.11: Turner Syndrome (45,X): Clinical Features. (Source: Author's original.)

Microdeletion Syndromes

Microdeletion syndromes are caused by chromosomal deletions too small to detect on conventional karyotyping (typically 1-3 Mb), requiring FISH or CMA for detection. In addition to the 22q11.2 deletion syndrome (discussed above), important microdeletion syndromes include Williams syndrome (7q11.23 deletion; ELN gene [elastin] loss; supravalvular aortic stenosis, 'elfin' facies, hypercalcaemia, gregarious personality, intellectual disability), Wolf-Hirschhorn syndrome (4p16.3 deletion; severe growth retardation, 'Greek warrior helmet' facies, seizures, severe ID), and Cri du Chat syndrome (5p15.2 deletion; high-pitched cat-like cry in infancy, microcephaly, severe ID). Contiguous gene syndromes reflect the deletion of multiple adjacent genes, producing a complex phenotype that may not be explained by a single gene defect.

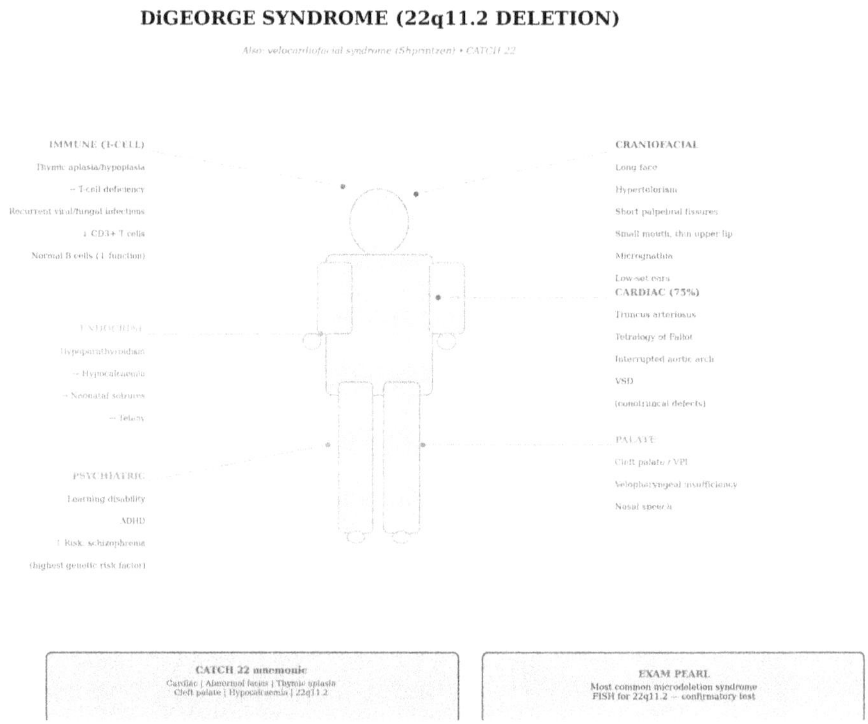

Figure 8.12: DiGeorge Syndrome (22q11.2 Deletion): Clinical Features. (Source: Author's original.)

Quick Recall: Chromosomal Disorders

Down (Trisomy 21): Non-disjunction (95%). AV canal defect. ALL/AMKL risk. Early Alzheimer.

Edwards (Trisomy 18): Clenched fist, rocker-bottom feet, VSD. >90% die within first year.

Patau (Trisomy 13): Cleft lip/palate, polydactyly, holoprosencephaly.

Klinefelter (47,XXY): Tall, small firm testes, gynaecomastia, infertility. ↑20× breast cancer risk.

Turner (45,X): Short stature, webbed neck, coarctation of aorta, streak gonads, primary amenorrhoea.

Single-Gene Disorders with Non-Classical Inheritance

Trinucleotide Repeat Disorders

Trinucleotide repeat (TNR) disorders are caused by the expansion of unstable microsatellite repeats beyond a threshold number. The expanded repeats are dynamic, tending to increase in size during meiosis, a phenomenon called **anticipation** (earlier onset and increasing severity in successive generations). TNR disorders can affect **coding regions** (CAG repeats encoding polyglutamine tracts, causing protein misfolding and aggregation, as in Huntington disease and spinocerebellar ataxias) or **non-coding regions** (CGG repeats in the 5' UTR causing gene silencing by methylation, as in Fragile X syndrome; GAA repeats in introns causing transcriptional silencing, as in Friedreich ataxia; CTG repeats in the 3' UTR causing toxic RNA gain-of-function, as in myotonic dystrophy).

Fragile X syndrome is the most common inherited cause of intellectual disability and the second most common genetic cause after Down syndrome. It results from expansion of a CGG trinucleotide repeat in the 5' UTR of the FMR1 gene on the X chromosome. Normal individuals have 6 to 45 repeats; premutation carriers have 55 to 200 repeats (at risk of fragile X-associated tremor/ataxia syndrome [FXTAS] and premature ovarian insufficiency); full mutation has >200 repeats, causing hypermethylation of the FMR1 promoter and silencing of FMRP (fragile X messenger ribonucleoprotein) expression. FMRP is an RNA-binding protein important for synaptic development and plasticity. Males with full mutations are more severely affected (moderate to severe intellectual disability, long face, large ears, macro-orchidism after puberty). The inheritance pattern shows the **Sherman paradox:** carrier males (premutation) transmit through phenotypically normal daughters, whose offspring are then at risk of full mutation through further expansion during maternal meiosis.

Importantly, the premutation state itself is not entirely benign. Two distinct clinical syndromes are associated with the FMR1 premutation: fragile X-associated tremor/ataxia syndrome (FXTAS) in older males (typically over 50 years), characterised by progressive cerebellar ataxia, intention tremor, parkinsonism, cognitive decline, and the pathognomonic finding of eosinophilic intranuclear inclusions in neurons and astrocytes; and fragile X-associated primary ovarian insufficiency (FXPOI), affecting approximately 20% of female premutation carriers, who develop ovarian failure before age 40. Both conditions are thought to result from a toxic gain-of-function of the expanded CGG mRNA rather than from loss of FMRP protein (which remains at normal or near-normal levels in premutation carriers). The risk of CGG expansion from premutation to full mutation during maternal transmission increases with the size of the maternal premutation allele: a premutation of 55-59 repeats carries approximately 4% risk of expanding to full mutation, whereas greater than 100 repeats carries virtually 100% risk.

Table 8.2: Important Trinucleotide Repeat Disorders

Disease	Gene	Repeat	Region	Key Feature
Fragile X syndrome	FMR1	CGG	5' UTR	Most common inherited intellectual disability; methylation silencing

Huntington disease	HTT	CAG	Coding	Caudate atrophy; polyglutamine aggregation; AD; anticipation via paternal transmission
Myotonic dystrophy	DMPK (DM1)	CTG	3' UTR	Toxic RNA; most common adult muscular dystrophy; cataracts, myotonia
Friedreich ataxia	FXN	GAA	Intron	AR (unique among TNR). Loss of frataxin; progressive ataxia; hypertrophic cardiomyopathy
Spinocerebellar ataxias	Various	CAG	Coding	AD; cerebellar degeneration; polyglutamine diseases

Exam Pitfall

Friedreich ataxia is the only common AR trinucleotide repeat disorder; all others (Huntington, Fragile X, myotonic dystrophy, SCA) are dominant. Friedreich ataxia also uniquely involves an intronic GAA repeat causing loss of frataxin (an iron-sulfur cluster assembly protein), leading to mitochondrial iron accumulation and oxidative damage.

Genomic Imprinting

Genomic imprinting is an epigenetic phenomenon in which certain genes are expressed in a parent-of-origin-specific manner. One allele (maternal or paternal) is silenced by DNA methylation, so the gene is effectively monoallelic. If the expressed (active) allele is mutated or deleted, disease results even though the other copy of the gene is structurally intact but silenced. The classic examples are:

Prader-Willi syndrome (PWS): Caused by loss of function of paternally expressed genes at chromosome 15q11-q13 (the maternal copy is normally imprinted/silenced). Mechanisms include paternal deletion (70%), maternal uniparental disomy (25%), and imprinting centre defects (5%). Features: hypotonia at birth, hyperphagia leading to obesity, short stature, hypogonadism, intellectual disability, behavioural issues.

Clinical Pearl

Imprinting versus uniparental disomy. Imprinting silences one parental copy of a gene by methylation; the surviving copy must function. Loss of the active copy by deletion produces disease. Uniparental disomy (UPD) is a different mechanism: both chromosomes derive from the same parent, the imprinted copies stay silent, and the gene is functionally absent. Prader-Willi can result from paternal 15q11 deletion (most common) OR from maternal UPD15 (silent paternal genes, no expression). Angelman is the mirror image: maternal 15q11 deletion or paternal UPD15. Methylation testing detects both mechanisms; FISH alone misses UPD. Order both.

Angelman syndrome: Caused by loss of function of the maternally expressed UBE3A gene at the same 15q11-q13 locus (the paternal copy is imprinted). Mechanisms: maternal deletion (70%), paternal UPD (2%), UBE3A point mutation (10%), imprinting defects. Features: severe intellectual disability, absent speech, seizures, ataxic gait ('puppet-like'), paroxysmal laughter, microcephaly.

A viva question that reliably separates strong candidates: 'A deletion at 15q11-q13 causes Prader-Willi or Angelman depending on the parent of origin. Explain.' The answer: the same chromosomal region contains both paternally expressed genes (relevant to PWS) and maternally expressed UBE3A (relevant to Angelman). A paternal deletion removes the active paternal genes while the maternal copies are imprinted, causing PWS. A maternal deletion removes active UBE3A while the paternal copy is imprinted, causing Angelman.

Mitochondrial Inheritance

Mitochondrial DNA (mtDNA) is a small (16.5 kb), circular, double-stranded DNA molecule encoding 13 proteins of the electron transport chain, 22 tRNAs, and 2 rRNAs. Mitochondrial inheritance follows a **maternal pattern** (all mitochondria are inherited from the ovum). Key features include **heteroplasmy** (a cell may contain a mixture of normal and mutant mitochondria, and the proportion determines disease severity), **threshold effect** (disease manifests when the proportion of mutant mtDNA exceeds a tissue-specific threshold), and **replicative segregation** (during cell division, mitochondria are distributed randomly, so daughter cells may have different proportions of mutant mtDNA). Mitochondrial diseases primarily affect organs with high energy demands: brain, skeletal muscle, heart, and kidney. Examples include MELAS (mitochondrial encephalomyopathy, lactic acidosis, stroke-like episodes), MERRF (myoclonus epilepsy with ragged red fibres), and Leber hereditary optic neuropathy (LHON).

Integration: Mitochondrial diseases connect to neuropathology (Chapter 30) and skeletal muscle pathology (Chapter 29). Ragged red fibres on modified Gomori trichrome stain are the histological hallmark of mitochondrial myopathies.

Molecular Tools in Genetic Diagnosis

The laboratory diagnosis of genetic disorders has been transformed by molecular techniques. The choice of technique depends on the clinical question: single-gene mutation testing, genome-wide screening, epigenetic analysis, or prenatal diagnosis.

Karyotyping (conventional cytogenetics): G-banded karyotype analysis detects numerical abnormalities (aneuploidy) and large structural abnormalities (>5-10 Mb). It remains the standard for suspected chromosomal disorders (Down syndrome, Turner, Klinefelter) and is performed on lymphocytes, amniocytes, or chorionic villi. Limitations: requires viable dividing cells, 7-14 day turnaround, low resolution.

FISH: Fluorescent probes detect specific chromosomal regions on interphase or metaphase nuclei. Used for rapid aneuploidy screening (13, 18, 21, X, Y), microdeletion syndromes (22q11.2 deletion/DiGeorge, Williams syndrome 7q11.23), and specific translocations. Results within 24-48 hours.

Chromosomal microarray (CMA): Array CGH or SNP arrays detect copy number variations (CNVs) across the entire genome at much higher resolution than karyotyping (>50-100 kb). CMA is now the recommended first-tier test for children with intellectual disability, developmental delay, autism spectrum disorder, and multiple congenital anomalies. It detects microdeletions and microduplications that are below the resolution of conventional karyotyping. Limitation: cannot detect balanced translocations or low-level mosaicism.

PCR-based techniques: PCR amplification followed by Sanger sequencing is the traditional approach for single-gene testing (CFTR, FBN1, GBA1). Methylation-specific PCR detects imprinting abnormalities (PWS/Angelman). Triplet repeat-primed PCR detects expanded repeats (Fragile X, Huntington, myotonic dystrophy).

Next-generation sequencing (NGS): Whole-exome sequencing (WES) and whole-genome sequencing (WGS) are increasingly used for undiagnosed genetic conditions, particularly when the phenotype is non-specific or when multiple genes could be responsible. Clinical exome panels targeting specific disease groups (e.g., epilepsy panels, skeletal dysplasia panels) offer a focused alternative. NGS has revolutionised the diagnosis of rare genetic diseases, with diagnostic yields of 25-40% in previously undiagnosed cases.

Non-invasive prenatal testing (NIPT): Analysis of cell-free fetal DNA (cffDNA) in maternal blood enables screening for common aneuploidies (trisomies 21, 18, 13) and sex chromosome abnormalities from 10 weeks of gestation. NIPT has sensitivity and specificity >99% for trisomy 21 but remains a screening test; positive results require confirmatory invasive testing (amniocentesis or chorionic villus sampling) before clinical decisions.

Genetic counselling is an integral component of genetic testing and diagnosis. Pre-test counselling ensures informed consent, discusses the implications of possible results (including variants of uncertain significance [VUS], incidental findings, and the psychological impact of predictive testing), and addresses reproductive options. Post-test counselling interprets results in the clinical context, discusses recurrence risks, and connects families with appropriate support services. The rise of direct-to-consumer genetic testing and expanded carrier screening panels has created new challenges for genetic counselling services, as patients may present with results they do not fully understand.

The choice of molecular test depends on the clinical scenario. For a dysmorphic neonate with suspected aneuploidy, karyotyping remains the first-line test. For a child with unexplained intellectual disability and normal karyotype, chromosomal microarray (CMA) is the recommended first-tier investigation. For a patient with a suspected Mendelian disorder where the gene is known, targeted gene sequencing or a focused panel is most efficient. For an undiagnosed patient with a complex phenotype, whole-exome sequencing offers the broadest yield. This algorithmic approach avoids unnecessary testing and maximises diagnostic efficiency.

Quick Recall: Molecular Diagnostic Tools in Genetics

Karyotype: Aneuploidy, large structural changes (>5 Mb). Slow (7-14 days).

FISH: Targeted; rapid (24-48 hr); aneuploidy screening, microdeletions, specific translocations.

CMA: Genome-wide CNV detection; first-tier for ID/DD/autism. Cannot detect balanced translocations.

NGS: WES/WGS for undiagnosed conditions; gene panels for specific phenotypes; 25-40% diagnostic yield.

NIPT: cffDNA from maternal blood; screening for trisomies from 10 weeks; confirmatory testing required.

Epigenetics and Non-Coding DNA

Less than 2% of the human genome encodes proteins. The remaining >98%, once dismissed as 'junk DNA,' is now recognised to contain functionally important elements including regulatory sequences, non-coding RNA genes, and structural DNA.

Non-coding DNA includes: promoters and enhancers that regulate gene transcription; genes encoding microRNAs (miRNAs, 18-25 nucleotides) that silence target mRNAs by degradation or translational inhibition; long non-coding RNAs (lncRNAs, >200 nucleotides) that regulate chromatin structure and gene expression; telomeric and centromeric DNA essential for chromosome stability and segregation; and introns that enable alternative splicing. Mutations in non-coding DNA increasingly are recognised as causes of disease, including cancer (enhancer hijacking, miRNA dysregulation) and genetic disorders.

Epigenetics refers to heritable changes in gene expression without DNA sequence alteration. The two principal mechanisms are DNA methylation (methyl groups at CpG dinucleotides, generally silencing transcription) and histone modification (acetylation, methylation, phosphorylation altering chromatin accessibility). Aberrant DNA methylation is a hallmark of cancer: global hypomethylation promotes genomic instability, while promoter hypermethylation silences tumour suppressors (e.g., MLH1 in MSI-H colorectal cancer, MGMT in glioblastoma). These modifications are therapeutically targetable with DNMT inhibitors (azacitidine, decitabine) and HDAC inhibitors (vorinostat).

The clinical significance of epigenetics extends beyond cancer. Epigenetic dysregulation underlies several genetic syndromes: Prader-Willi and Angelman syndromes (discussed above) are caused by imprinting defects; Rett syndrome results from mutations in MECP2, a protein that reads DNA methylation marks; ICF syndrome (immunodeficiency, centromeric instability, and facial anomalies) is caused by mutations in DNMT3B, a DNA methyltransferase. Epigenetic therapies are already in clinical use: azacitidine and decitabine (hypomethylating agents) are standard treatments for myelodysplastic syndromes (see Volume 1), and histone deacetylase (HDAC) inhibitors (vorinostat, romidepsin) are approved for T-cell lymphomas. The emerging field of environmental epigenetics studies how prenatal and early-life exposures (nutrition, toxins, stress) can alter epigenetic marks, with potential transgenerational effects on disease risk.

Gene Therapy

Gene therapy aims to treat disease by introducing, altering, or replacing genetic material within a patient's cells. Two broad strategies exist: **gene augmentation** (adding a functional copy of a deficient gene, the approach used in most current therapies) and **gene editing** (correcting or disrupting specific mutations using tools such as CRISPR-Cas9). Delivery vehicles (vectors) include adeno-associated viruses (AAV, the most widely used), lentiviruses, and non-viral methods (lipid nanoparticles).

Approved gene therapies include voretigene neparvovec (Luxturna) for RPE65-associated inherited retinal dystrophy, onasemnogene abeparvovec (Zolgensma) for spinal muscular atrophy, and ex vivo gene therapy for beta-thalassaemia (betibeglogene autotemcel/Zynteglo) and sickle cell disease (exagamglogene autotemcel/Casgevy, using CRISPR to reactivate fetal haemoglobin). CAR-T cell therapy (see Volume 1) represents a form of gene-modified cell therapy for haematological malignancies. Challenges include immunogenicity, insertional mutagenesis (with integrating vectors), limited cargo capacity (AAV carries only ~4.7 kb), high cost, and long-term durability of effect.

Key challenges in gene therapy include viral vector immunogenicity (pre-existing antibodies to AAV), insertional mutagenesis risk with integrating vectors (lentiviral), limited AAV packaging capacity (~4.7 kb), and delivery to target tissues. Genome-wide off-target analysis remains essential for CRISPR-based therapies.

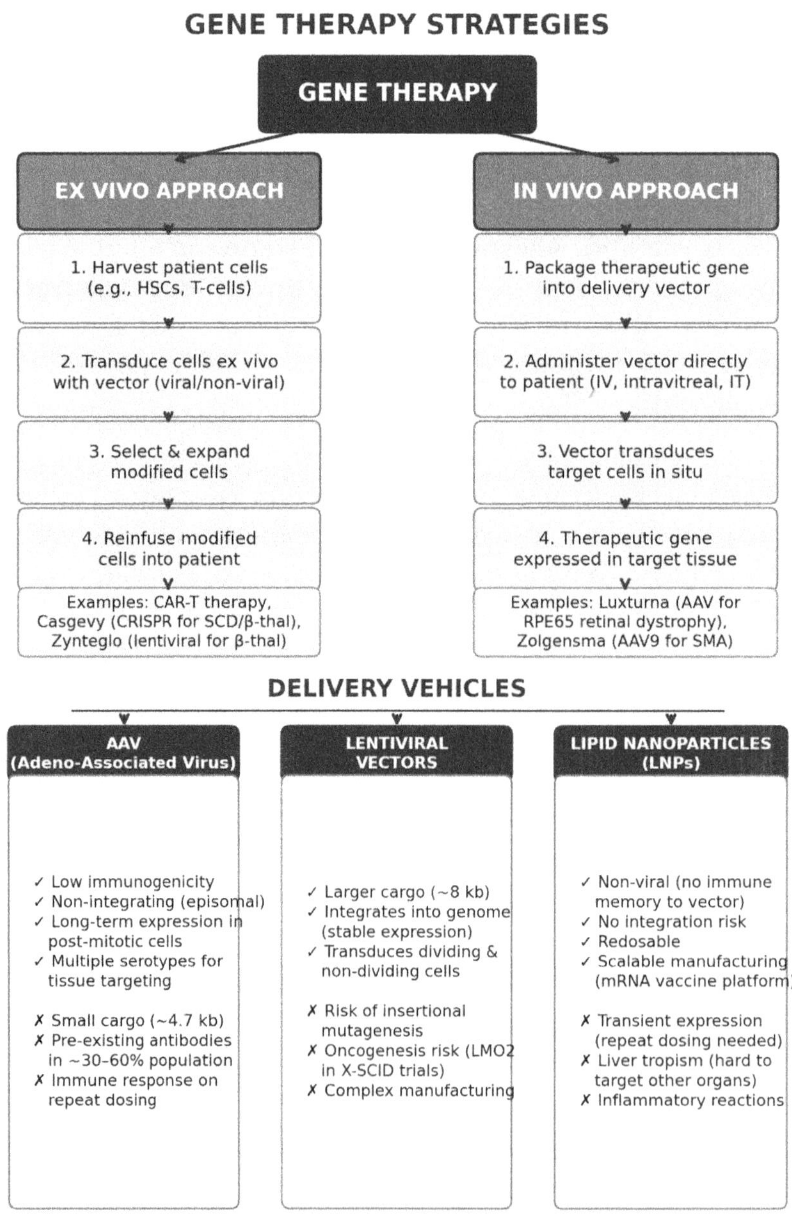

Figure 8.13: Overview of gene therapy strategies: ex vivo versus in vivo approaches, with comparison of AAV, lentiviral, and lipid nanoparticle delivery vehicles. (Source: Author's original.)

Recent Advances

CRISPR-based therapeutics: The approval of Casgevy (exagamglogene autotemcel) in 2023 for sickle cell disease and transfusion-dependent beta-thalassaemia marked the first regulatory approval of a CRISPR-Cas9-based gene therapy. This ex vivo approach edits the patient's haematopoietic stem cells to disrupt the BCL11A erythroid enhancer, reactivating fetal haemoglobin production. Base editing and prime editing, next-generation CRISPR tools that do not require double-strand breaks, are in clinical trials for multiple genetic conditions.

Genome-wide screening in newborns: Pilot programmes are evaluating the use of whole-genome or whole-exome sequencing in newborn screening, expanding beyond the traditional biochemical analyte panels. This raises both diagnostic opportunities (detecting hundreds of actionable conditions early) and ethical challenges (variants of uncertain significance, incidental findings, informed consent).

Pharmacogenomics: The integration of genetic testing into drug prescribing (e.g., CYP2D6 genotyping for codeine and tamoxifen, DPYD testing for fluorouracil, TPMT/NUDT15 for thiopurines) is becoming clinical reality, particularly in oncology and psychiatry, moving medicine closer to the promise of personalised prescribing.

The key diagnostic clue when molecular testing reveals a variant of uncertain significance (VUS): a VUS is not a positive result. Clinical decisions should not be based on a VUS alone. The pathologist's role is to integrate the molecular finding with morphology, IHC, clinical context, and family history. Reclassification of VUS to pathogenic or benign occurs as population databases grow (ClinVar, gnomAD); flagging a VUS for periodic reassessment is part of responsible molecular reporting.

When a child presents with intellectual disability, dysmorphic features, and a normal karyotype, the next diagnostic step is chromosomal microarray (CMA), not FISH. CMA detects submicroscopic deletions and duplications (copy number variants) across the entire genome in a single test and has replaced karyotyping as the first-tier cytogenetic investigation for intellectual disability. FISH is reserved for confirmation of specific suspected microdeletion syndromes (e.g., DiGeorge 22q11.2, Williams 7q11.23) or when a balanced rearrangement is suspected.

International Frameworks

ACMG/AMP 2015 germline variant classification. The 2015 American College of Medical Genetics and Genomics and Association for Molecular Pathology consensus is the international reference for interpreting germline sequence variants in Mendelian disorders. Variants are classified into five tiers — pathogenic, likely pathogenic, variant of uncertain significance, likely benign, and benign — using twenty-eight weighted criteria covering population frequency (PM2, BA1, BS1, BS2), computational predictions (PP3, BP4), functional studies (PS3, BS3), co-segregation (PP1, BS4), de novo data (PS2, PM6), allelic data (PM3, BP2), and clinical phenotype concordance (PP4). Subsequent Sequence Variant Interpretation (SVI) Working Group recommendations have refined individual criteria (notably PVS1 for null variants and PP3/BP4 for in-silico predictors). The framework should be distinguished from the AMP/CAP/ASCO tier I-IV system used for somatic variants in cancer. Citation: Richards S, et al. Genet Med 2015;17(5):405–424. PMID 25741868.

Hereditary tumour syndromes — gene-phenotype correlation and the pathologist's role. Approximately five to ten per cent of all cancers arise on a background of an identifiable hereditary cancer syndrome, with autosomal dominant inheritance predominating and a fifty per cent transmission risk to offspring. The syndromes most relevant to histopathology fall into a handful of well-characterised gene–phenotype pairings that the FRCPath candidate must recognise from morphology, immunohistochemistry, and family history. Lynch syndrome (germline pathogenic variants in MLH1, MSH2, MSH6, PMS2, or EPCAM) accounts for two to three per cent of colorectal carcinomas, produces a defective mismatch-repair phenotype recognisable as paired MLH1/PMS2 or MSH2/MSH6 loss on IHC and microsatellite instability on PCR or next-generation sequencing, and extends to endometrial, ovarian, gastric, urothelial, hepatobiliary, and small-bowel adenocarcinomas; universal IHC screening of all colorectal and endometrial carcinomas is now routine practice in many centres, complementing rather than displacing the legacy Amsterdam II and revised Bethesda criteria as case-finding tools. Hereditary breast and ovarian cancer syndrome (BRCA1, BRCA2; less commonly PALB2, ATM, CHEK2) accounts for roughly five per cent of breast carcinomas and fifteen per cent of high-grade serous ovarian carcinomas, and predicts response to platinum chemotherapy and PARP inhibitors. Li-Fraumeni syndrome (germline TP53) produces an early-onset spectrum of soft tissue sarcoma, osteosarcoma, breast carcinoma in young women, brain tumours, adrenocortical carcinoma, and leukaemia, with the Chompret criteria defining testing thresholds. Familial adenomatous polyposis (APC) and MUTYH-associated polyposis (MUTYH) produce hundreds to thousands of colorectal adenomas with progression to carcinoma by the third decade, with extracolonic manifestations including duodenal adenomas, desmoid tumours, and congenital hypertrophy of the retinal pigment epithelium. Peutz-Jeghers syndrome (STK11) produces hamartomatous gastrointestinal polyps with arborising smooth muscle cores and mucocutaneous melanotic pigmentation, with elevated risk of pancreatic, breast, ovarian, and gastrointestinal carcinoma. Cowden / PTEN hamartoma tumour syndrome (PTEN) predisposes to breast, follicular thyroid, endometrial, and renal carcinoma. Multiple endocrine neoplasia syndromes — MEN1 (MEN1: parathyroid, pancreatic islet, anterior pituitary), MEN2A and MEN2B (RET: medullary thyroid carcinoma with phaeochromocytoma and hyperparathyroidism in MEN2A; mucosal neuromas and Marfanoid habitus in MEN2B) — and von Hippel-Lindau disease (VHL: clear-cell renal cell carcinoma, phaeochromocytoma, retinal and central nervous system haemangioblastoma) round out the syndromes most often examined. The 5th edition WHO Classification of Tumours formally lists each syndrome's defining germline gene as part of the relevant tumour-entity description; synoptic reporting requires notation of universal MMR/MSI testing in colorectal and endometrial carcinoma. The pathologist's role is not to diagnose the syndrome — that is genetic counselling — but to flag the morphological, immunohistochemical, and family-history features that should prompt referral. Citation: Garutti M, Foffano L, Mazzeo R, et al. Hereditary cancer syndromes: a comprehensive review with a visual tool. Genes (Basel) 2023; 14: 1025. PMID 37239385.

Ultra High-Yield Chapter Summary

Table 8.3: Ultra High-Yield Summary; Genetic Disorders and Molecular Pathology

Topic	Must Remember
AD inheritance	50% risk per offspring; variable expressivity; incomplete penetrance; de novo mutations (achondroplasia).
Marfan syndrome	FBN1 (fibrillin-1); upward lens subluxation; cystic medial degeneration; aortic dissection.
Familial hypercholesterolaemia	LDLR gene; 5 classes of receptor mutations; premature atherosclerosis.
Cystic fibrosis	CFTR (Cl^- channel); ΔF508 (70%); viscid secretions; Pseudomonas lung infections; sweat Cl^- >60; CFTR modulators (Trikafta).
Gaucher disease	Most common LSD; β-glucocerebrosidase; wrinkled paper cells; HSM + bone disease; NO CNS in Type 1; ERT available.
Tay-Sachs	Hex A deficiency; GM2 ganglioside; cherry-red spot WITHOUT HSM; neurons

	only; Ashkenazi Jews.
Niemann-Pick A	Sphingomyelinase; cherry-red spot WITH HSM; foam cells; neurons + macrophages.
MPS	GAG accumulation; coarse facies; dysostosis multiplex.
Down syndrome	Trisomy 21; non-disjunction 95%; AV canal defect; ALL/AMKL (GATA1); early Alzheimer (APP on chr 21).
Turner syndrome	45,X; short stature; coarctation; streak gonads; cystic hygroma.
Klinefelter syndrome	47,XXY; small firm testes; azoospermia; gynaecomastia; ↑20× breast cancer.
Fragile X	FMR1 CGG repeat (>200); methylation silencing; most common inherited ID; macro-orchidism; Sherman paradox.
Huntington disease	HTT CAG repeat; coding region; polyglutamine aggregation; caudate atrophy; AD; paternal anticipation.
Friedreich ataxia	FXN GAA repeat; intronic; AR (unique among TNR); frataxin loss; hypertrophic cardiomyopathy.
Genomic imprinting	Prader-Willi (paternal deletion 15q) vs Angelman (maternal deletion 15q/UBE3A).
Mitochondrial inheritance	Maternal; heteroplasmy; threshold effect. MELAS, MERRF, LHON.
CMA	First-tier test for ID/DD/autism; detects CNVs genome-wide; cannot detect balanced translocations.
NIPT	cffDNA in maternal blood; screens trisomies 21/18/13 from 10 weeks; confirmatory invasive testing needed.
Gene therapy	AAV vector most common; CRISPR-Cas9 approved (Casgevy for SCD/thalassaemia).

CRISPR-Cas9 Gene Editing

Clustered Regularly Interspaced Short Palindromic Repeats (CRISPR) with the Cas9 nuclease is a revolutionary gene-editing tool with both research and therapeutic applications. A synthetic guide RNA (gRNA) directs the Cas9 endonuclease to a specific genomic locus complementary to the gRNA sequence. Cas9 creates a double-strand break (DSB) at the target site. Two repair pathways follow. Non-homologous end joining (NHEJ) introduces insertions or deletions (indels) that disrupt gene function (gene knockout). Homology-directed repair (HDR) uses a supplied DNA template to introduce precise corrections (gene correction). The first approved CRISPR therapy targets sickle cell disease and beta-thalassaemia: exagamglogene autotemcel (exa-cel, approved 2023) disrupts BCL11A in autologous haematopoietic stem cells to reactivate foetal haemoglobin. Other applications under investigation include transthyretin amyloidosis (in vivo liver-directed CRISPR) and CAR-T cell engineering (Figures 8.13–8.14).

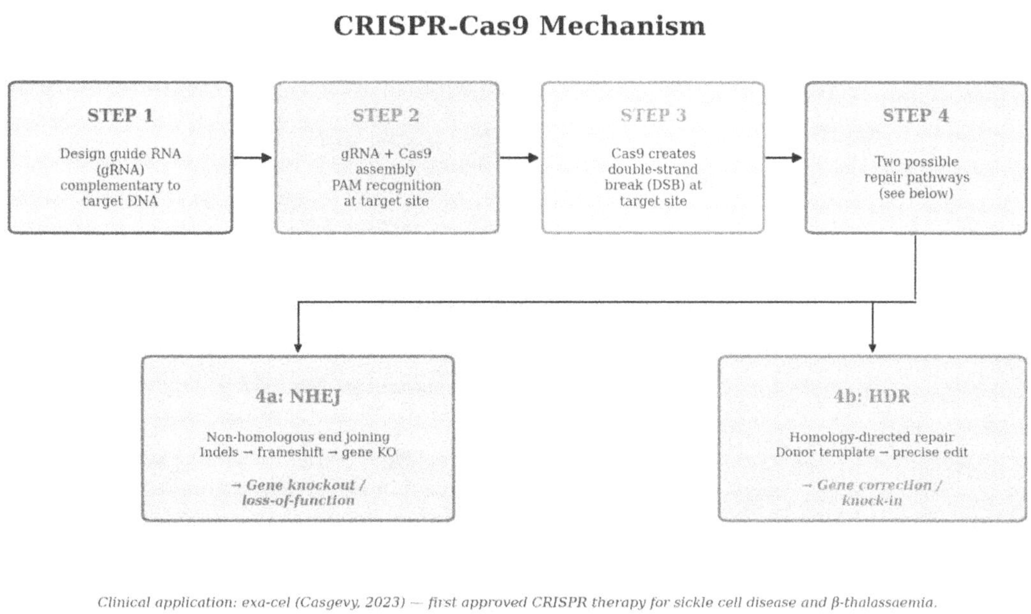

Figure 8.14: CRISPR-Cas9 Mechanism. (Source: Author's original.)

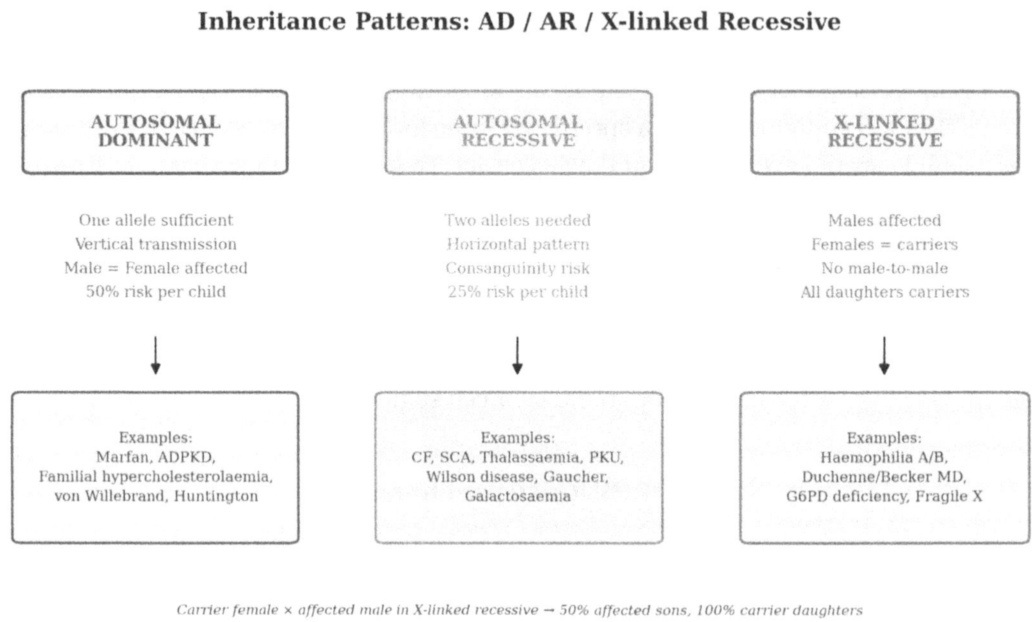

Figure 8.15: Inheritance Patterns: Autosomal Dominant, Autosomal Recessive, and X-linked Recessive. (Source: Author's original.)

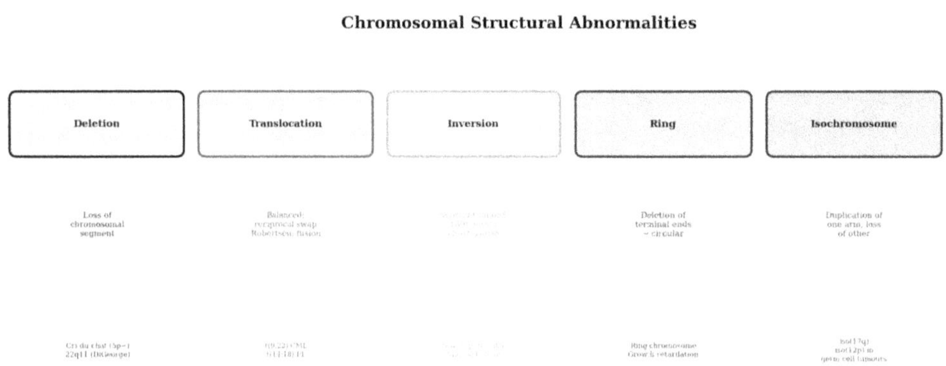

Figure 8.16: Chromosomal Structural Abnormalities. (Source: Author's original.)

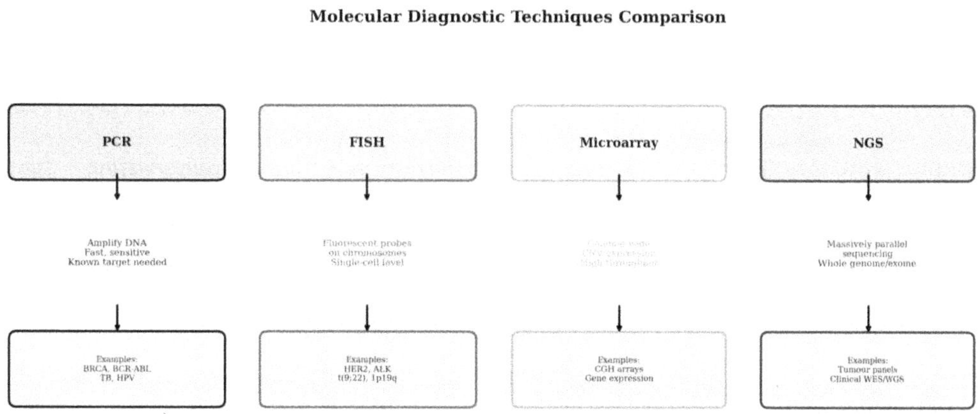

Figure 8.17: Molecular Diagnostic Techniques Comparison. (Source: Author's original.)

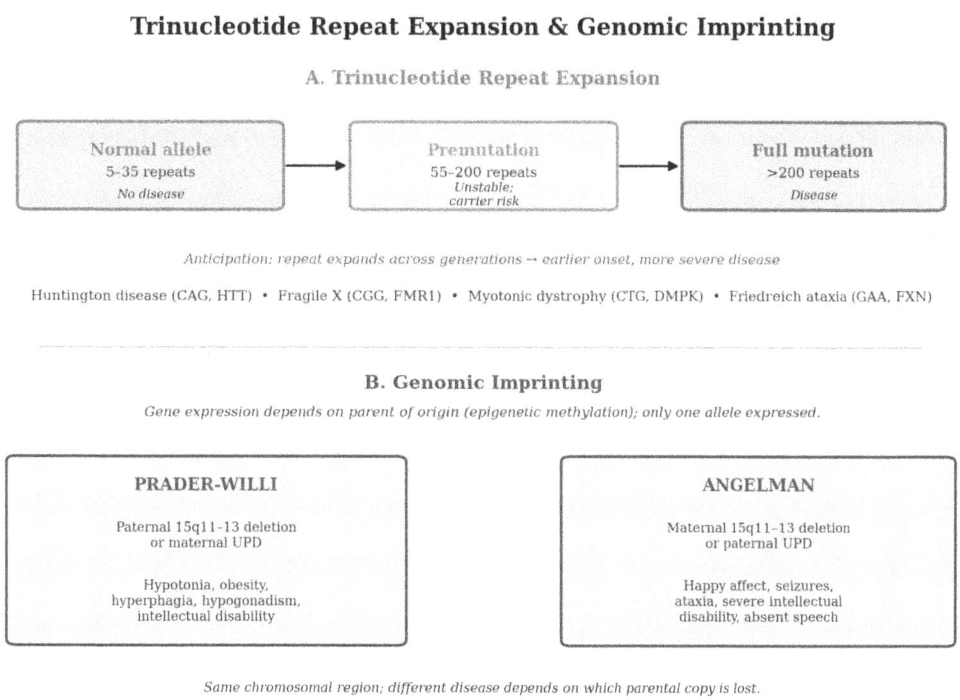

Figure 8.18: Trinucleotide Repeat Expansion and Genomic Imprinting. *(Source: Author's original.)*

Diagnostic thinking: consanguinity + autosomal recessive pattern + enzyme deficiency → inborn error of metabolism (common in consanguineous populations)

Diagnostic thinking: intellectual disability + dysmorphic facies + single palmar crease → trisomy 21 (confirm with karyotype/FISH)

Diagnostic thinking: trinucleotide repeat expansion + anticipation + neurodegeneration → trinucleotide repeat disorder (Huntington, fragile X, myotonic dystrophy) (Figure 8.18)

Chapter 9: Infectious Disease Pathology

THE BIG PICTURE

Infectious diseases remain among the leading causes of morbidity and mortality in low- and middle-income countries. The pathologist plays a central role in infectious disease diagnosis — from recognising the tissue reaction patterns that suggest particular classes of organisms, to identifying pathognomonic morphological features (caseating granulomas in tuberculosis, foamy Virchow cells in lepromatous leprosy, owl-eye inclusions in CMV, ingested erythrocytes in Entamoeba trophozoites, tachyzoites in toxoplasmosis), to directing the appropriate ancillary investigations (special stains, immunohistochemistry, CBNAAT, serology). This chapter approaches infectious disease from the pathologist's perspective, organised around the tissue reaction patterns that form the diagnostic starting point for any suspected infection.

High-yield topics in this chapter: Tissue reaction patterns in infection (suppurative, granulomatous, cytopathic/cytoproliferative, necrotising, chronic with fibrosis); tuberculosis (primary vs secondary, Ghon focus and complex, miliary TB, granuloma morphology, CBNAAT, regional epidemiology); leprosy spectrum (tuberculoid to lepromatous, Ridley–Jopling classification, lepra reactions); HIV/AIDS pathology and opportunistic infections; syphilis (primary, secondary, tertiary, congenital) and serological diagnosis; fungal infections (Aspergillus vs Mucor, Histoplasma, Cryptococcus, Candida); tropical parasitic infections (malaria with artemisinin resistance, visceral leishmaniasis, amoebiasis, cysticercosis, hydatid disease, filariasis); sexually transmitted infections.

The unifying principle of infectious disease pathology is that the morphological pattern reflects both the organism and the host response. The same organism can produce different patterns in different hosts — Mycobacterium tuberculosis causes well-formed caseating granulomas in the immunocompetent host but poorly formed granulomas with disseminated miliary disease in the immunocompromised host; Mycobacterium leprae produces tuberculoid granulomas in patients with preserved cell-mediated immunity and foamy macrophage infiltrates in those with anergic responses. Recognising the pattern, narrowing to the likely organism, and confirming with appropriate special stains or molecular tests is the diagnostic workflow this chapter teaches.

General Principles: Host Tissue Reaction Patterns

The host response to infection can be classified into five broad histopathological patterns, each associated with specific categories of organisms. Recognising these patterns on biopsy narrows the differential diagnosis and guides further investigation.

Table 9.1: Tissue Reaction Patterns in Infection

Pattern	Histology	Typical Organisms
Suppurative (pyogenic)	Neutrophilic infiltrate, abscess formation, tissue destruction	Staphylococcus, Streptococcus, Gram-negative bacilli, Nocardia
Granulomatous	Epithelioid macrophages, Langhans giant cells, +/- caseation	Mycobacterium tuberculosis, Leprosy, Fungi (Histoplasma, Coccidioides), Syphilis, Sarcoidosis (non-infectious)

Cytopathic/cytoproliferative	Viral inclusions, multinucleated cells, cell lysis or proliferation	CMV, HSV, HPV, Adenovirus, Measles, Polyomavirus
Necrotising	Tissue necrosis, vascular thrombosis, minimal inflammation	Clostridium (gas gangrene), Mucor/Rhizopus (angioinvasive fungi), Naegleria
Chronic inflammation/fibrosis	Lymphoplasmacytic infiltrate, fibrosis, scarring	HBV, HCV (chronic hepatitis), Schistosomiasis (pipe-stem fibrosis)

The key diagnostic clue in this setting is: When a granuloma is identified on biopsy, the first question is whether caseation (caseous necrosis) is present. Caseating granulomas strongly suggest tuberculosis (or, less commonly, fungal infection). Non-caseating granulomas have a broader differential including sarcoidosis, Crohn disease, foreign body reaction, and drug reaction. Notably, TB can occasionally produce non-caseating granulomas, particularly in immunocompromised patients (Figure 9.1).

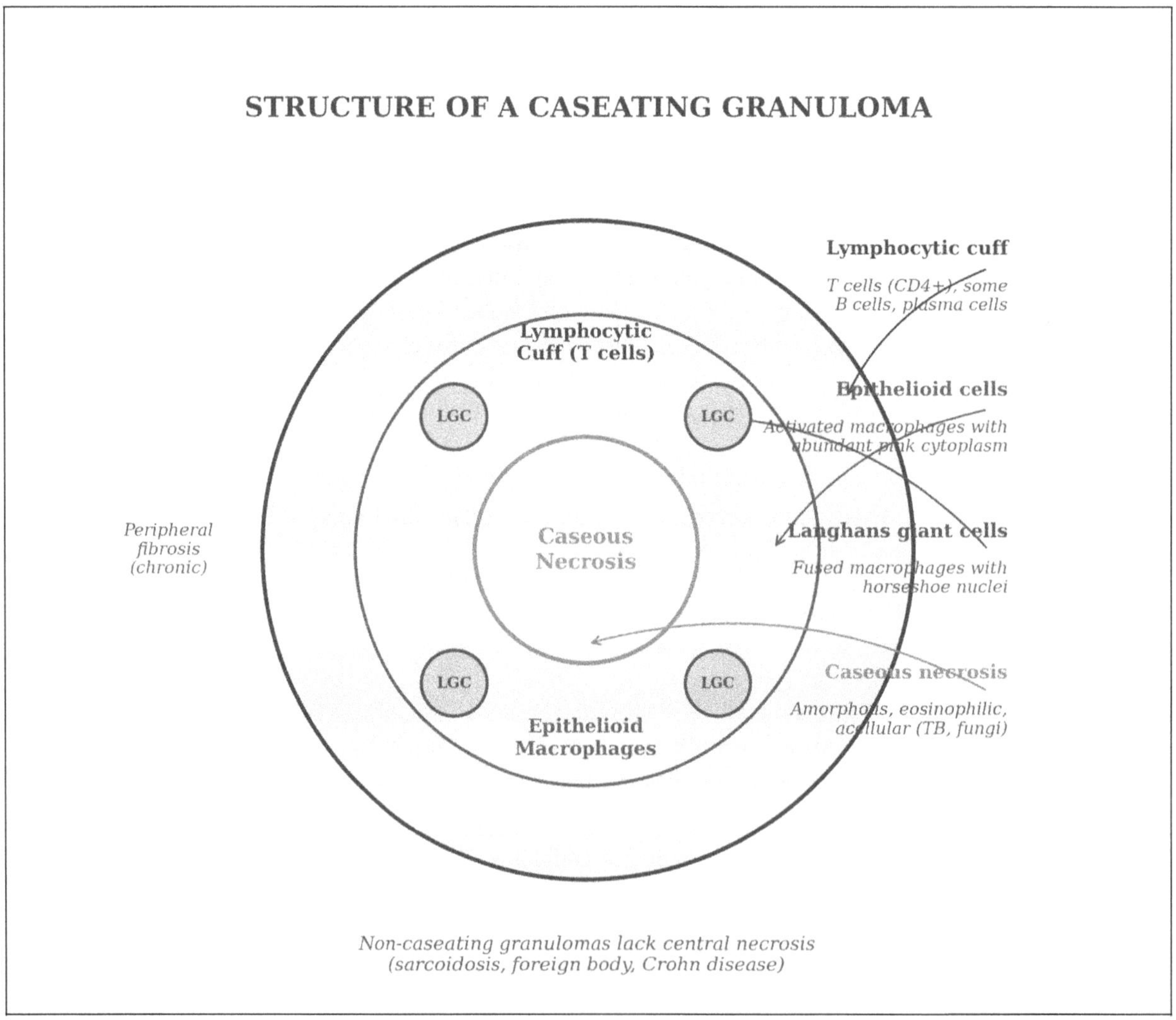

Figure 9.1: Schematic of a granuloma. (Source: Author's original.)

Tuberculosis

South Asia carries a disproportionate share of the global tuberculosis (TB) burden (approximately 30% of cases per the Global TB Report 2023). TB remains one of the most important infectious diseases in pathology practice across endemic regions, and understanding its pathogenesis, morphology, and diagnostic modalities is non-negotiable.

Pathogenesis

Mycobacterium tuberculosis is an aerobic, acid-fast bacillus with a lipid-rich cell wall containing mycolic acids, which confer acid-fastness and resistance to killing. The pathogenesis of TB involves a complex interplay between the bacillus and the host immune response, particularly cell-mediated immunity (Th1-type). **Primary TB** occurs in previously unexposed individuals: inhaled bacilli are phagocytosed by alveolar macrophages, which fail to kill the bacillus owing to its cell wall lipids (cord factor, lipoarabinomannan). Infected macrophages produce IL-12, activating CD4+ T cells to produce IFN-γ, which activates macrophages and leads to granuloma formation. The combination of the primary parenchymal lesion (Ghon focus, typically subpleural in the mid-zone or lower lobe) and the draining hilar lymph node constitutes the **Ghon complex.** In most immunocompetent individuals, the infection is contained, and the Ghon complex heals by fibrosis and calcification (Ranke complex).

> **Diagnostic Thinking**
>
> Ghon focus (subpleural parenchymal lesion) + hilar lymph node involvement = Ghon complex → primary TB. Healed Ghon complex with calcification = Ranke complex.

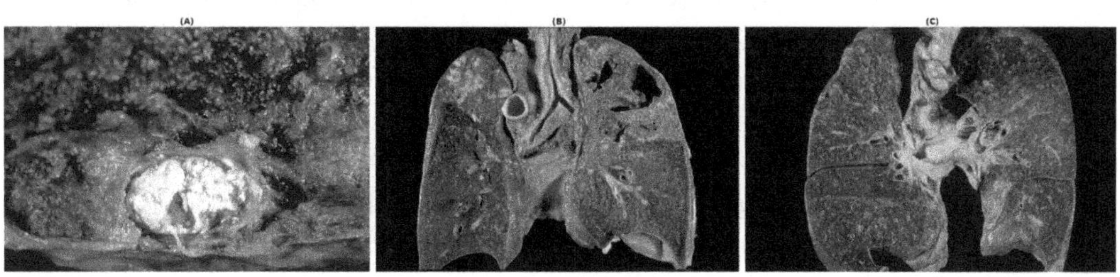

Figure 9.2: Gross pathology of tuberculosis. (A) Primary TB — subpleural Ghon focus with central caseous necrosis. (B) Secondary (reactivation) TB — apical cavitary disease with extensive caseation and cavitation. (C) Miliary TB — innumerable 1–2 mm millet seed-like granulomas throughout both lung fields following haematogenous dissemination. (Source: Yale Rosen, Wikimedia Commons, CC BY-SA 2.0.)

Inhalation → Alveolar macrophage phagocytosis → IL-12 → Th1 response (IFN-γ) → Macrophage activation → Granuloma formation → Containment or progression

Secondary (reactivation) TB occurs when latent bacilli reactivate, typically in the apices of the lungs (where high oxygen tension favours mycobacterial growth). Reactivation produces cavitary disease with caseating granulomas, cavitation (due to liquefaction of caseous material and its discharge into airways), and fibrosis. Complications include haemoptysis, bronchopleural fistula, and miliary dissemination.

> **Diagnostic Thinking**
>
> Apical cavitary lesion + caseating granulomas + AFB-positive → secondary/reactivation TB. Apical localisation reflects high oxygen tension favouring mycobacterial growth (Figure 9.2B).

Extrapulmonary Tuberculosis

Extrapulmonary TB accounts for 15 to 20% of all TB cases and is more common in immunocompromised patients (HIV-TB coinfection). Important sites include: **lymph node TB** (scrofula; the most common extrapulmonary site; cervical lymph nodes most frequently involved); **intestinal TB** (ileocaecal region; must be distinguished from Crohn disease, see Chapter 19); **skeletal TB** (Pott spine; vertebral involvement with cold abscess and spinal deformity); **genitourinary TB** (sterile pyuria is a classic clue); **CNS TB** (TB meningitis, tuberculoma); and **miliary TB** (haematogenous dissemination with innumerable small granulomas in multiple organs, seen as 1-2 mm millet seed-like nodules grossly).

> **Exam Pitfall**
>
> **Intestinal TB vs Crohn disease:** Both produce granulomatous inflammation in the ileocaecal region. TB granulomas are confluent, large, and caseating; Crohn granulomas are discrete, small, and non-caseating. TB ulcers are circumferential (transverse); Crohn ulcers are longitudinal.

Laboratory Diagnosis of Tuberculosis

The diagnostic armamentarium for TB includes microscopy (Ziehl-Neelsen acid-fast staining, auramine-rhodamine fluorescent staining), culture (Lowenstein-Jensen medium, BACTEC MGIT liquid culture), molecular methods (GeneXpert MTB/RIF [CBNAAT], which simultaneously detects *M. tuberculosis* and rifampicin resistance within 2 hours; TrueNat; line probe assays [LPA] for first- and second-line drug resistance), tuberculin skin test (Mantoux), interferon-gamma release assays (IGRA: QuantiFERON-TB Gold, T-SPOT.TB), and histopathology (caseating granulomas with Langhans giant cells, ZN stain for AFB). **MDR-TB** (resistance to at least isoniazid and rifampicin) and **XDR-TB** (MDR-TB plus resistance to a fluoroquinolone and at least one injectable agent; or, by the 2021 WHO definition, MDR-TB plus resistance to a fluoroquinolone) are growing challenges. The WHO-endorsed rapid molecular tests (GeneXpert, LPA) have transformed MDR-TB diagnosis by providing same-day results.

Molecular Diagnostics for TB: CBNAAT and Truenat

Cartridge-based nucleic acid amplification testing (CBNAAT, marketed as GeneXpert MTB/RIF) has revolutionised TB diagnosis globally. The GeneXpert system is a real-time PCR platform that simultaneously detects Mycobacterium tuberculosis DNA and rifampicin resistance (by identifying mutations in the rpoB gene) directly from sputum or other clinical specimens within 2 hours, without the need for prior culture or specialist laboratory infrastructure. Sensitivity is approximately 98% for smear-positive TB and 67-72% for smear-negative, culture-positive TB, with near-100% specificity. In TB-endemic settings, GeneXpert has been deployed under national TB programmes, replacing smear microscopy as the initial diagnostic test for presumptive TB patients.

Truenat MTB (developed by Molbio Diagnostics, Goa) is a chip-based, battery-operable point-of-care molecular test endorsed by WHO in 2020. It uses real-time micro-PCR technology and requires only 0.5 mL of sputum processed with a simple lysis step (TruePrep). Truenat MTB detects M. tuberculosis in approximately 1 hour; a reflex Truenat MTB-RIF Dx test on positive samples detects rifampicin resistance. Its portability and minimal infrastructure requirements make it suitable for peripheral health centres where GeneXpert deployment may not be feasible. Both CBNAAT and Truenat have been incorporated into the NTEP diagnostic algorithm as initial tests for all TB suspects.

The TB diagnostic hierarchy in current practice in TB-endemic regions: Truenat/CBNAAT (initial molecular test for all presumptive TB patients) → if positive and rifampicin-resistant, second-line drug susceptibility testing by line probe assay (LPA, detecting isoniazid and fluoroquinolone resistance) or phenotypic DST on MGIT → if CBNAAT/Truenat negative but clinical suspicion persists, liquid culture (MGIT/BACTEC, result in 1-6 weeks, gold standard for sensitivity). ZN smear microscopy retains a role for monitoring treatment response (sputum conversion at 2 and 5 months).

Sputum from presumptive TB → CBNAAT/Truenat (2 hr) → MTB detected + Rif resistance? → If Rif-resistant: LPA/phenotypic DST → Tailored MDR-TB regimen

Quick Recall: Tuberculosis

Primary TB: Ghon focus (subpleural) + hilar LN = Ghon complex. Heals as Ranke complex (fibrosis + calcification).

Secondary TB: Apical cavitary disease. Caseating granulomas.

Extrapulmonary: LN (most common), intestinal (ileocaecal), Pott spine, GU (sterile pyuria), CNS, miliary.

Diagnosis: ZN stain, Culture (LJ/MGIT), GeneXpert (2hr, detects Rif resistance), IGRA. MDR = INH+Rif resistant.

WHO Drug-Resistance Classification (2021 revised)

The WHO drug-resistance classification, revised in January 2021, stratifies M. tuberculosis resistance for treatment selection under the Programmatic Management of Drug-Resistant TB (PMDT).

Table 9.1a: WHO Drug-Resistance TB Classification (2021)

Category	Definition	Treatment implication (broad)
Drug-susceptible TB (DS-TB)	M. tuberculosis susceptible to all first-line drugs (H, R, Z, E)	Standard 6-month HRZE regimen
Isoniazid-resistant TB (Hr-TB)	Resistance to isoniazid; rifampicin-susceptible	6-month regimen of RZE + levofloxacin
Rifampicin-resistant TB	Resistance to rifampicin (with or without H	All-oral shorter MDR regimen

(RR-TB)	resistance); detected by Xpert MTB/RIF, Truenat MTB-RIF	
Multidrug-resistant TB (MDR-TB)	Resistance to at least both H and R	All-oral shorter MDR regimen (BPaLM or modified) per drug-susceptibility testing
Pre-extensively drug-resistant TB (pre-XDR-TB)	MDR-TB with additional resistance to any fluoroquinolone (levofloxacin or moxifloxacin)	Longer individualised regimen with bedaquiline, linezolid, pretomanid
Extensively drug-resistant TB (XDR-TB)	Pre-XDR-TB with additional resistance to at least one of: linezolid OR bedaquiline	Individualised regimen using remaining active drugs (delamanid, meropenem/clavulanate, clofazimine, cycloserine)

The 2021 update redefined XDR-TB (previously required resistance to a second-line injectable). Pre-XDR-TB is a new formal category. Both bedaquiline and linezolid are now "essential" drugs — resistance to either escalates the case. These cases are notified and treated under national tuberculosis programmes (e.g., India's NTEP/PMDT, WHO End TB Strategy).

Leprosy (Hansen Disease)

Leprosy, caused by *Mycobacterium leprae,* remains endemic in South Asia, which accounts for the majority of new leprosy cases globally. The disease presents as a clinicopathological spectrum determined by the host immune response, described by the **Ridley-Jopling classification:** at one pole, **tuberculoid leprosy (TT)** reflects a strong Th1 response with well-formed granulomas, few bacilli, and limited skin and nerve involvement; at the opposite pole, **lepromatous leprosy (LL)** reflects anergy (absent Th1 response) with diffuse macrophage infiltration (foamy macrophages/Virchow cells/lepra cells), massive bacillary load, and widespread skin, nerve, and visceral involvement. Between these poles lie borderline forms (BT, BB, BL) with intermediate features.

Table 9.2: Ridley-Jopling Spectrum of Leprosy

Feature	Tuberculoid (TT/BT)	Lepromatous (LL/BL)
Immune response	Strong Th1 (cell-mediated)	Anergic; Th2 dominant
Skin lesions	Few (<5), well-defined, anaesthetic	Numerous, diffuse, leonine facies
Nerve involvement	Early, asymmetric, thickened nerves	Late, symmetric, glove-and-stocking anaesthesia

Histology	Well-formed granulomas (epithelioid, Langhans)	Diffuse macrophage infiltrate (foamy/Virchow cells)
AFB on slit-skin smear	Few or absent (paucibacillary)	Abundant, globi (multibacillary)
Lepromin test	Positive	Negative
Reactions	Type 1 (reversal reaction, CMI)	Type 2 (ENL, immune complex-mediated)

Nerve involvement is the hallmark of leprosy. *M. leprae* has a unique tropism for Schwann cells of peripheral nerves, entering via the PGL-1 (phenolic glycolipid-1) interaction with laminin-α2 on the Schwann cell surface. Thickened, palpable peripheral nerves (ulnar, lateral popliteal, great auricular) are a cardinal clinical sign. Nerve damage leads to anaesthesia, motor weakness, and trophic changes (claw hand, wrist drop, foot drop) that cause the deformities traditionally associated with leprosy.

Lepra reactions are immunologically mediated acute episodes that cause significant morbidity. **Type 1 (reversal reaction)** is a delayed-type hypersensitivity reaction seen in borderline forms, causing inflammation in existing skin lesions and acute neuritis. **Type 2 (erythema nodosum leprosum, ENL)** is an immune complex-mediated vasculitis seen in LL/BL, causing painful subcutaneous nodules, fever, iridocyclitis, orchitis, and glomerulonephritis.

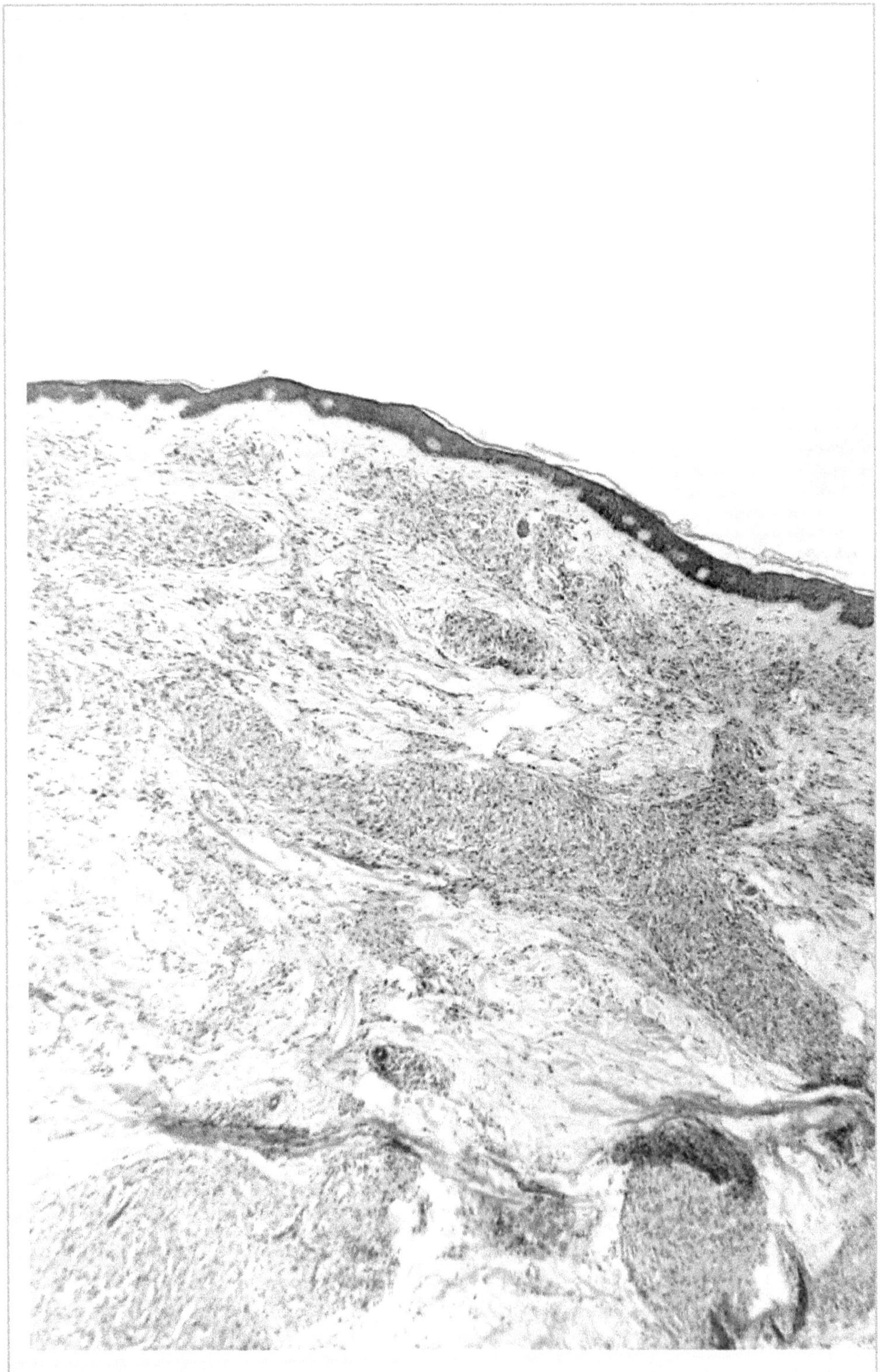

Figure 9.3: Lepromatous leprosy: dermal infiltrate of foamy macrophages (Virchow cells) with Grenz zone. Inset: Fite-Faraco stain showing acid-fast bacilli within macrophages. H&E + Fite-Faraco (inset), ×400 + ×1000 (inset). (Source: Calicut Medical College, Wikimedia Commons, CC BY-SA 4.0.)

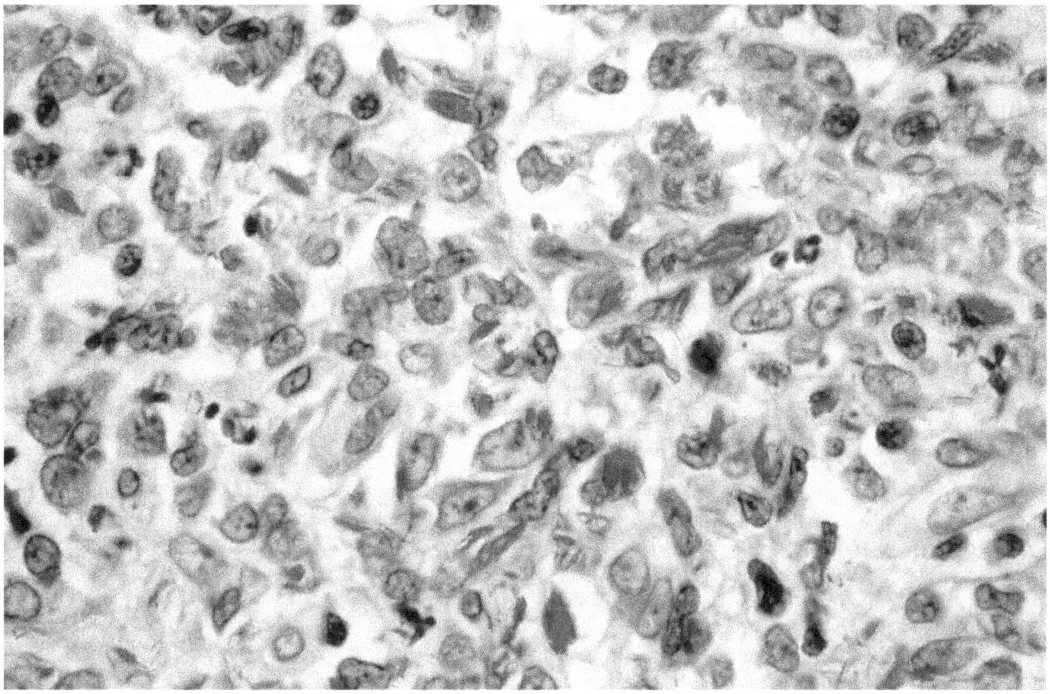

Figure 9.3 (inset): Lepromatous leprosy: Fite-Faraco stain showing abundant acid-fast bacilli (red) within foamy macrophages (Virchow cells). ×1000. (Source: SB Lucas, Wellcome Collection, CC0 1.0.)

WHO Operational Classification (for MDT decisions)

For field decisions on multidrug therapy (MDT), the WHO introduced a simplified operational classification based on skin-lesion count (or, if smears available, bacillary load). It complements the Ridley-Jopling spectrum (Table 9.2), which remains the histopathological standard.

Table 9.2a: WHO Operational Classification of Leprosy

Category	Criteria (field)	Ridley-Jopling equivalent	WHO MDT regimen (adult)
Paucibacillary (PB)	≤5 skin lesions; AFB negative on slit-skin smear (if available)	TT, BT (and indeterminate)	Rifampicin 600 mg monthly + Dapsone 100 mg daily × 6 months
Multibacillary (MB)	>5 skin lesions OR any AFB-positive smear OR nerve trunk involvement	BB, BL, LL	Rifampicin 600 mg monthly + Clofazimine (300 mg monthly + 50 mg daily) + Dapsone 100 mg daily × 12 months
Single-lesion PB	Exactly 1 skin lesion, smear-negative, no nerve involvement	TT/indeterminate	Single-dose ROM: Rifampicin 600 mg + Ofloxacin 400 mg + Minocycline 100 mg (if MDT

			unavailable)

Exam point: the WHO classification is operational (treatment-oriented); Ridley-Jopling is immunopathological. Both are asked in theory and viva. The shift from Ridley-Jopling to PB/MB was designed for field workers who lack histopathology access.

Integration: The leprosy spectrum illustrates the critical role of the host immune response in determining disease pattern, a principle that recurs in the pathogenesis of TB, sarcoidosis (Chapter 15), and fungal infections. Nerve pathology is detailed in Chapter 30.

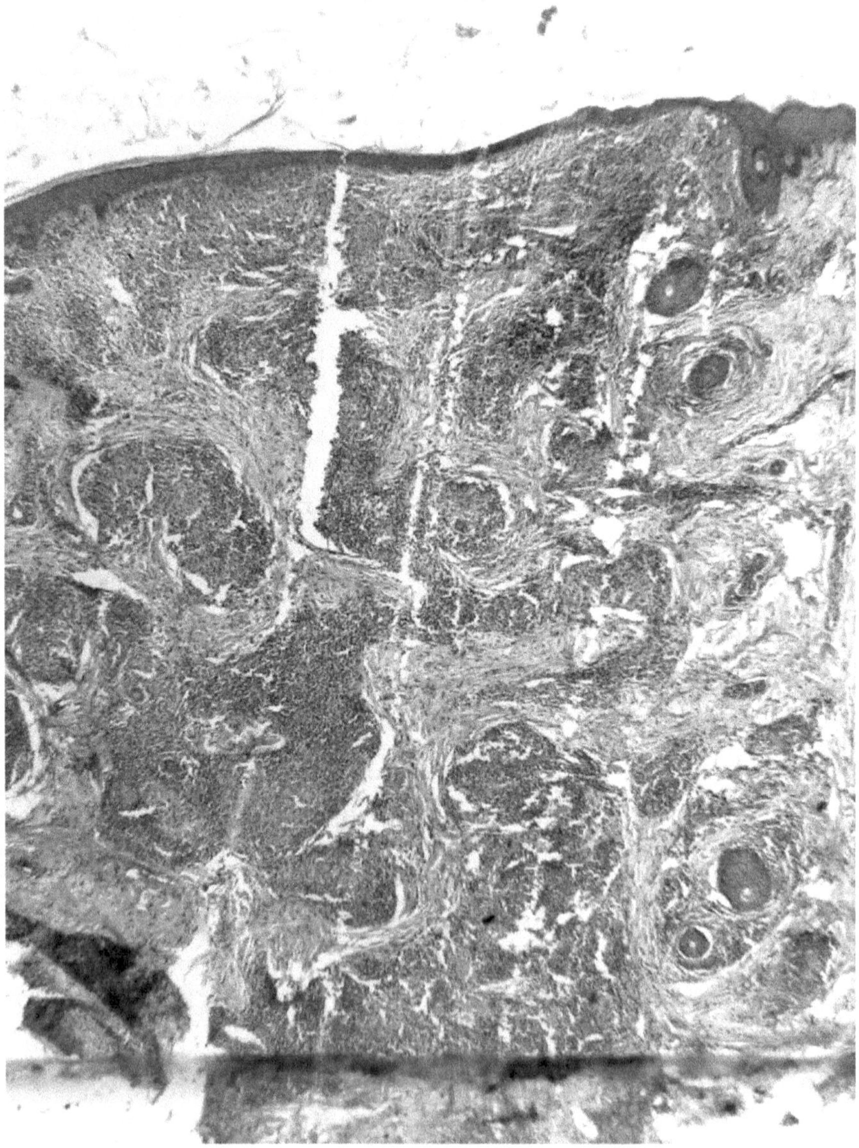

Figure 9.4: Tuberculoid leprosy: skin biopsy showing well-formed epithelioid granulomas with Langhans giant cells surrounding dermal nerves. No caseation. H&E. (Source: Calicut Medical College, Wikimedia Commons, CC BY-SA 4.0.)

HIV/AIDS Pathology

Human immunodeficiency virus (HIV) selectively infects and destroys CD4+ T-helper lymphocytes, leading to progressive immunodeficiency. The virus (an RNA lentivirus) binds the CD4 molecule and a co-receptor (CCR5 in early infection, CXCR4 in late-stage disease) to enter target cells. After reverse transcription, proviral DNA integrates into the host genome. The natural history proceeds through three phases: **acute retroviral syndrome** (high viraemia, flu-like illness, transient CD4 drop), **clinical latency** (years of asymptomatic viral replication with progressive CD4 decline), and **AIDS** (CD4 <200 cells/µL, with opportunistic infections and malignancies).

HIV gp120 binds CD4 + co-receptor (CCR5/CXCR4) → Fusion → Reverse transcriptase → Proviral DNA integration → Latency + replication → CD4 depletion → AIDS

AIDS-defining conditions include opportunistic infections (*Pneumocystis jirovecii* pneumonia, cerebral toxoplasmosis, cryptococcal meningitis, CMV retinitis, disseminated *Mycobacterium avium-intracellulare* [MAI], oesophageal candidiasis, progressive multifocal leukoencephalopathy [PML]) and malignancies (Kaposi sarcoma [HHV-8], primary CNS lymphoma, non-Hodgkin lymphoma, cervical carcinoma). The lymph node shows a characteristic sequence of changes: follicular hyperplasia (early), follicle lysis and involution (progressive), and lymphocyte depletion (advanced/burnt-out). Bone marrow may show dysplasia, granulomas, haemophagocytosis, and infection-associated changes (see Volume 1).

Stool Examination in AIDS

The investigation of chronic diarrhoea in HIV/AIDS patients requires a systematic approach to stool examination, as the differential diagnosis encompasses multiple opportunistic pathogens. In patients with CD4 counts below 200 cells/µL, the major aetiological agents include Cryptosporidium parvum (the most common cause of persistent watery diarrhoea in AIDS; oocysts are detected by modified ZN stain [acid-fast, 4-6 µm] or immunofluorescence), Isospora belli (large oocysts, 25-30 µm, modified ZN-positive, responds to co-trimoxazole), Microsporidium species (tiny spores, 1-2 µm, detected by modified trichrome/Weber stain or calcofluor white), Cyclospora cayetanensis (oocysts 8-10 µm, variably acid-fast, autofluorescent under UV), cytomegalovirus (causes colonic ulceration with characteristic owl-eye intranuclear inclusions on biopsy), and Mycobacterium avium complex (MAI/MAC, detected by ZN stain of stool concentrate or by blood culture in disseminated disease).

Clinical Pearl

Modified ZN is the often-missed stain. Standard Ziehl-Neelsen uses 20% sulphuric acid as the decolouriser and detects Mycobacterium tuberculosis. Modified (Kinyoun, weak ZN) uses 1% sulphuric acid and detects partially acid-fast organisms: Nocardia, Cryptosporidium, Cyclospora, Isospora, and Rhodococcus. A clinical scenario of chronic diarrhoea in an HIV-positive patient with negative routine stool examination should always prompt a modified ZN stain on stool. Likewise, suppurative pulmonary or cerebral lesions in immunocompromised patients should be stained with modified ZN before concluding 'no acid-fast organisms identified.'

The stool examination protocol in a suspected AIDS patient with diarrhoea should include: (1) routine microscopy for ova and parasites (wet mount and iodine preparation); (2) modified ZN stain for Cryptosporidium, Isospora, and Cyclospora; (3) modified trichrome stain for Microsporidium; (4) bacterial culture for Salmonella, Shigella, and Campylobacter; (5) Clostridium difficile toxin assay if there is antibiotic exposure; and (6) GeneXpert/Truenat if intestinal TB is suspected. If stool examination is negative but symptoms persist, colonoscopy with biopsy is indicated to detect CMV colitis, MAI, Kaposi sarcoma, or lymphoma.

Why does tuberculosis in HIV-positive patients often show atypical histological features? As CD4 counts decline, the host loses the capacity to mount the characteristic Th1-mediated granulomatous response. In advanced AIDS (CD4 below 50-100 cells/µL), tissue biopsies from TB-infected sites may show poorly formed or absent granulomas, minimal caseation, and instead reveal sheets of foamy macrophages packed with acid-fast bacilli ('lepromatous' pattern of TB). This paradoxical abundance of organisms with minimal inflammatory response reflects immune failure. The pathologist must maintain a high index of suspicion: any chronic inflammatory infiltrate in an HIV-positive patient, even without classical granulomas, should prompt ZN staining and culture.

Syphilis

Syphilis, caused by the spirochaete *Treponema pallidum,* is a sexually transmitted infection with a protean clinicopathological presentation across three stages. **Primary syphilis** manifests as a chancre (painless ulcer with raised, indurated borders and a clean base) at the site of inoculation, accompanied by painless inguinal lymphadenopathy. Histologically, the chancre shows a dense perivascular plasma cell infiltrate with obliterative endarteritis (intimal proliferation and luminal narrowing of small vessels). **Secondary syphilis** (6-8 weeks later) is a systemic phase characterised by condylomata lata (moist, flat, wart-like lesions in the anogenital region), mucocutaneous rash (maculopapular, including palms and soles), lymphadenopathy, and spirochaetaemia. **Tertiary syphilis** (years to decades later) produces gummas (granulomatous lesions with central coagulative necrosis, surrounded by epithelioid cells, giant cells, and plasma cells), cardiovascular syphilis (aortitis with tree-bark appearance of the aortic intima, aneurysm of the ascending aorta, aortic regurgitation), and neurosyphilis (tabes dorsalis, general paresis). Obliterative endarteritis and the plasma cell-rich infiltrate are the histological hallmarks across all stages.

> **Quick Recall: Syphilis**
>
> **Histological hallmark:** Obliterative endarteritis + perivascular plasma cell infiltrate (all stages).
>
> **Primary:** Painless chancre. Secondary: Condylomata lata, palmar rash.
>
> **Diagnosis:** Screening: VDRL/RPR (non-treponemal). Confirmatory: FTA-ABS/TPHA (treponemal).

Serological Diagnosis of Syphilis: The Algorithm

Serological testing is the mainstay of syphilis diagnosis, as Treponema pallidum cannot be cultured in vitro. Two categories of tests are used: non-treponemal tests (VDRL, RPR) and treponemal tests (FTA-ABS, TPHA/TPPA, EIA/CLIA). Non-treponemal tests detect antibodies (reagin) against cardiolipin-lecithin-cholesterol antigen released from damaged host cells and treponemes. They are inexpensive, rapid, and quantitative (titre correlates with disease activity), making them ideal for screening and monitoring treatment response. However, they have limitations: false negatives in very early primary syphilis (before seroconversion, 1-3 weeks) and in the prozone phenomenon (false negative due to antibody excess in secondary syphilis, overcome by serum dilution); and false positives in conditions including SLE, antiphospholipid syndrome, pregnancy, acute febrile illness, HIV, and intravenous drug use (biological false positives).

Treponemal tests detect antibodies specifically directed against T. pallidum antigens. FTA-ABS (fluorescent treponemal antibody absorption test) is the traditional confirmatory test; TPHA/TPPA (T. pallidum haemagglutination/particle agglutination) is widely used internationally. Automated treponemal EIA/CLIA assays are now used for high-throughput screening in many laboratories, prompting a shift from the traditional algorithm (screen with RPR, confirm with treponemal test) to the reverse algorithm (screen with treponemal EIA, confirm with RPR, resolve discordant results with TPPA).

Traditional algorithm: Screen (VDRL/RPR) → Positive → Confirm (FTA-ABS/TPHA) → Positive = syphilis confirmed

Reverse algorithm: Screen (treponemal EIA/CLIA) → Positive → Quantitative RPR → If RPR positive: active/recent syphilis → If RPR negative: TPPA to resolve (positive TPPA = past treated syphilis or late latent; negative TPPA = likely EIA false positive). The reverse algorithm is increasingly adopted in laboratories with automated platforms but is not yet universal. Dark-field microscopy of chancre fluid (visualising live spirochaetes) is the definitive test in primary syphilis but is rarely available outside specialised STI clinics. In tissue sections, Warthin-Starry silver stain identifies spirochaetes, though sensitivity is low (30-70%); immunohistochemistry for T. pallidum has superior sensitivity and is available in reference laboratories.

Malaria

Malaria, caused by *Plasmodium* species (*P. falciparum, P. vivax, P. malariae, P. ovale, P. knowlesi*), remains one of the most important parasitic diseases globally. *P. falciparum* causes the most severe disease (falciparum malaria, malignant tertian) and accounts for the majority of malaria-related deaths. The life cycle involves the female *Anopheles* mosquito (definitive host) and humans (intermediate host), with hepatic (pre-erythrocytic) and erythrocytic stages.

The pathogenesis of severe *P. falciparum* malaria centres on two mechanisms: **cytoadherence** (parasitised red blood cells [pRBCs] express PfEMP-1 [*P. falciparum* erythrocyte membrane protein 1] on knob-like protrusions, which bind to endothelial receptors including ICAM-1, CD36, and chondroitin sulfate A [in the placenta], causing sequestration of pRBCs in the microvasculature of the brain [cerebral malaria], kidneys, lungs, and placenta) and **rosetting** (parasitised RBCs bind to uninfected RBCs, forming rosettes that further impair microvascular flow). The result is microvascular obstruction, tissue hypoxia, and organ dysfunction.

Pathological findings include splenomegaly (hyperplasia of splenic macrophages with haemozoin [malaria pigment] deposition), hepatomegaly, Kupffer cell hyperplasia with haemozoin, anaemia (haemolysis + dyserythropoiesis), cerebral oedema (in cerebral malaria; ring haemorrhages around occluded vessels), acute kidney injury, blackwater fever (massive intravascular haemolysis with haemoglobinuria), and placental malaria. Diagnosis relies on thick and thin peripheral blood smear examination (gold standard), rapid diagnostic tests (RDTs, detecting HRP-2 or pLDH), and PCR for species identification and low-level parasitaemia.

Why is P. falciparum more pathogenic than other species? Three features: (1) it can infect red cells of all ages (not limited to reticulocytes as *P. vivax*), leading to higher parasitaemia; (2) cytoadherence/sequestration causes microvascular obstruction (unique to *P. falciparum*); and (3) rosetting further impairs blood flow. *P. vivax* and *P. ovale* form hypnozoites in the liver (dormant hepatic stage), causing relapses; *P. malariae* causes recrudescences from persistent low-level erythrocytic infection.

> Quick Recall: Malaria
>
> **P. falciparum virulence:** PfEMP-1/knobs → cytoadherence to ICAM-1/CD36 → sequestration → cerebral malaria, organ failure. Infects all RBC ages.
>
> **Pathology:** Splenomegaly (haemozoin), ring haemorrhages (brain), blackwater fever, placental malaria.
>
> **Diagnosis:** Thick smear (detection), thin smear (speciation), RDT (HRP-2), PCR. Banana-shaped gametocytes = P. falciparum.

Recent Advances in Malaria Diagnosis and Resistance

Rapid diagnostic tests (RDTs) have transformed malaria diagnosis in resource-limited settings. RDTs are immunochromatographic lateral flow assays that detect parasite-specific antigens in a finger-prick blood sample within 15-20 minutes. Two target antigens are widely used: HRP-2 (histidine-rich protein 2, specific to P. falciparum; persists in blood for 2-4 weeks after treatment, so cannot distinguish active from recently treated infection) and pLDH (parasite lactate dehydrogenase, produced by all Plasmodium species; clears rapidly after treatment, so can monitor therapeutic response). The emergence of HRP-2/HRP-3 gene deletions in P. falciparum parasites (particularly in the Horn of Africa and South America) threatens the reliability of HRP-2-based RDTs, as these parasites produce no HRP-2 and therefore yield false-negative results. WHO has recommended surveillance for HRP-2 deletions and the use of dual-antigen RDTs (HRP-2 plus pLDH) in areas where deletions exceed 5%.

Artemisinin-based combination therapies (ACTs) remain the cornerstone of falciparum malaria treatment globally. However, partial artemisinin resistance (characterised by delayed parasite clearance with a parasite clearance half-life greater than 5 hours, associated with mutations in the PfKelch13 gene, particularly C580Y) has emerged in Southeast Asia and has now been confirmed in East Africa (Rwanda, Uganda) and, alarmingly, in sporadic reports from India (northeastern states). Kelch13 mutations do not cause complete treatment failure when partner drugs (lumefantrine, piperaquine) remain effective, but the concern is the eventual loss of ACT efficacy. Molecular surveillance of Kelch13 mutations is now a WHO priority.

Fungal Infections

Fungal infections (mycoses) are increasingly important in immunocompromised patients. They are classified by depth of invasion: **superficial** (dermatophytes), **subcutaneous** (sporotrichosis, mycetoma, chromoblastomycosis), **deep/systemic** (histoplasmosis, coccidioidomycosis, blastomycosis, paracoccidioidomycosis, cryptococcosis, candidiasis), and **opportunistic** (Aspergillus, Mucor/Rhizopus, Pneumocystis).

Aspergillosis causes a spectrum of disease: allergic bronchopulmonary aspergillosis (ABPA, in asthmatics), aspergilloma (fungal ball in pre-existing cavities), and invasive aspergillosis (in immunocompromised patients, characterised by angioinvasive septate hyphae with acute-angle [45-degree] branching causing vascular thrombosis and infarction). **Mucormycosis (zygomycosis),** caused by Mucor, Rhizopus, and related genera, gained renewed clinical importance after the global surge of COVID-19-associated mucormycosis (CAM) in 2021. Mucor hyphae are characteristically broad, ribbon-like, pauci-septate (or aseptate), with irregular, right-angle branching, and are angioinvasive, causing tissue infarction. Risk factors include uncontrolled diabetes mellitus (diabetic ketoacidosis), corticosteroid use, and immunosuppression. The rhino-orbito-cerebral form is the most common clinical presentation.

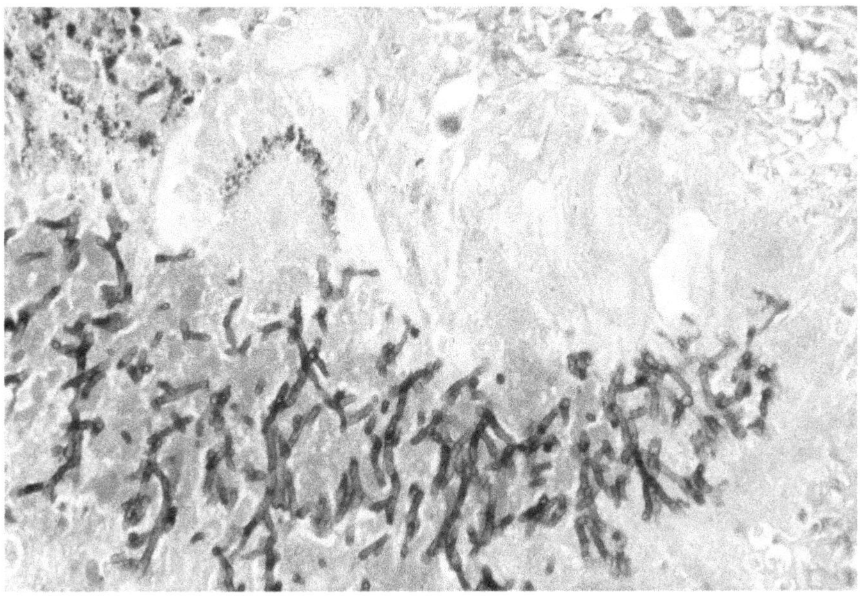

Figure 9.5: Aspergillosis: septate hyphae with acute-angle (45°) dichotomous branching, highlighted on Grocott methenamine silver (GMS) stain. Granulomatous tissue reaction. (Source: Wikimedia Commons, CC BY-SA 3.0.)

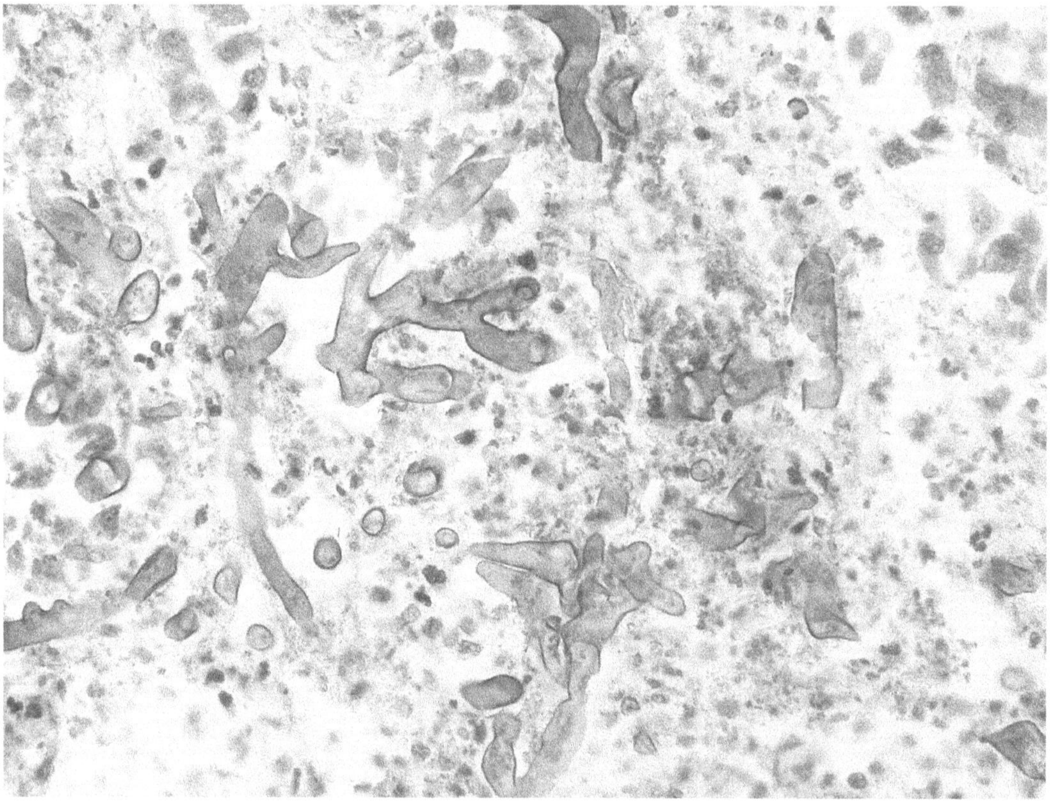

Figure 9.6: Mucormycosis (zygomycosis): broad, ribbon-like, pauci-septate hyphae with right-angle (90°) branching amid necrotic tissue. H&E. (Source: Wikimedia Commons, CC BY-SA 3.0.)

The Pathologist's Approach to Special Stains in Infectious Disease

When a tissue biopsy shows an inflammatory pattern suggestive of infection, the pathologist must select the appropriate panel of special stains. The choice is guided by the histological pattern: a granulomatous pattern mandates ZN stain (for mycobacteria), GMS stain (for fungi), and consideration of Warthin-Starry (for spirochaetes and Bartonella). A pattern of necrotising inflammation with vascular thrombosis should prompt GMS and PAS for angioinvasive fungi (Aspergillus, Mucor). A dense plasma cell infiltrate in any tissue should raise suspicion for syphilis and prompt Warthin-Starry staining and clinical correlation. The brown-pigmented organisms seen on H&E (Cryptococcus capsule appears as a clear halo; malaria pigment is refractile brown-black) may not require special stains for recognition, but mucicarmine (highlighting Cryptococcus capsule in red) and Fontana-Masson (melanin-like pigment) can confirm the identification.

Clinical Pearl

Histoplasma versus Pneumocystis on GMS. Both stain black with Grocott methenamine silver; both are found in immunocompromised patients; both produce alveolar-pattern lung disease. Distinguish them morphologically. Histoplasma capsulatum: 2-4 micrometre yeast forms, intracellular, located within macrophage cytoplasm, narrow-based budding, and uniform size. Pneumocystis jirovecii: 5-8 micrometre cysts, extracellular, free-lying in foamy alveolar exudate, with a characteristic intracystic dot or comma (the 'parenthesis' or 'crushed ping-pong ball' appearance). Size, location, and the central dot decide it. PAS distinguishes further: Histoplasma is PAS-positive, Pneumocystis is PAS-negative.

In TB-endemic settings, the minimum stain panel for a granulomatous lesion is: ZN stain (for acid-fast bacilli), GMS or PAS stain (for fungal organisms), and polarised light examination (for foreign body material). If ZN and GMS are negative but clinical suspicion for TB remains high, additional steps include Fite-Faraco stain (modified acid-fast stain with higher sensitivity for paucibacillary TB and essential for leprosy bacilli, which are poorly detected by standard ZN), CBNAAT/Truenat on fresh tissue (if available), and mycobacterial culture. The diagnostic yield of tissue culture for TB (60-80%) exceeds that of histological staining alone (approximately 30-50% in paucibacillary disease).

The Pathologist's Eye: A common pitfall is the failure to request special stains on a granulomatous lesion because the clinical team has already 'diagnosed' sarcoidosis. In TB-endemic regions, sarcoidosis remains a diagnosis of exclusion. Every granulomatous lesion must have AFB and GMS stains performed regardless of the clinical impression. The converse pitfall is equally dangerous: assuming every caseating granuloma is TB without considering fungal infection (histoplasmosis, coccidioidomycosis), which can produce identical histology and requires different treatment.

Integration: *Special stains for infections connect to histopathology laboratory techniques (Chapter 35). The GMS stain and PAS stain are also used for non-infectious purposes: GMS highlights basement membranes in renal biopsies (Chapter 22), and PAS highlights glycogen, neutral mucins, and basement membranes across multiple organ systems. Understanding the chemistry of these stains (GMS is a silver-based stain that oxidises polysaccharides in fungal cell walls; PAS uses periodic acid to oxidise vicinal diols to aldehydes, which then react with Schiff reagent) helps the pathologist interpret staining patterns and troubleshoot false-positive results.*

Viral Inclusions and Cytopathic Effects

Several viruses produce characteristic intracellular inclusions detectable on routine H&E-stained sections or cytological preparations. Recognising these inclusions is a core competency for the diagnostic pathologist.

Table 9.3: Viral Inclusions and Cytopathic Effects

Special Stains for Infectious Organisms

Table 9.4: Special Stains in Infectious Disease Pathology

Stain	Target Organism	Key Features
Ziehl-Neelsen (ZN)	Mycobacteria	Red bacilli on blue background; acid-fast
Fite-Faraco (modified ZN)	M. leprae	Gentler decolourisation preserves M. leprae (which is less strongly acid-fast)
GMS (Grocott methenamine silver)	Fungi, Pneumocystis	Black organisms on green background; best for detecting fungal elements

PAS (Periodic acid-Schiff)	Fungi, Whipple (T. whipplei)	Magenta staining of carbohydrate-rich cell walls
Warthin-Starry / Steiner	Spirochaetes (Treponema), H. pylori, Bartonella	Black organisms on yellow background (silver stain)
Giemsa	Protozoa (Leishmania, malaria), Helicobacter	Visualises intracellular organisms and morphological detail
Mucicarmine	Cryptococcus	Stains the thick mucopolysaccharide capsule magenta
India ink	Cryptococcus (CSF)	Negative staining; clear halo around yeast in dark background
Brown and Brenn / Gram (tissue)	Bacteria	Blue (Gram-positive) or red (Gram-negative) organisms in tissue sections

Parasitic Infections of Pathological Importance

Leishmaniasis

Leishmaniasis, caused by *Leishmania* species transmitted by the sandfly (*Phlebotomus*), presents as a clinical spectrum determined by the species and host immune response. **Visceral leishmaniasis (kala-azar),** caused by *L. donovani* in South Asia and East Africa, is characterised by hepatosplenomegaly (massive), pancytopenia, fever, and hypergammaglobulinaemia. The bone marrow, spleen, and liver show parasitised macrophages containing **Leishman-Donovan (LD) bodies:** amastigotes (2-4 µm) with a nucleus and a rod-shaped kinetoplast, visible on Giemsa-stained smears. **Cutaneous leishmaniasis** (*L. tropica, L. major*) produces localised skin ulcers with granulomatous inflammation. **Mucocutaneous leishmaniasis** (*L. braziliensis*) causes destructive naso-oropharyngeal lesions.

Bihar and eastern Uttar Pradesh are endemic zones for visceral leishmaniasis in India. Diagnosis relies on demonstration of LD bodies in bone marrow or splenic aspirates, serological tests (rK39 rapid test), and PCR. Amphotericin B (liposomal) and miltefosine are the primary treatments.

Cysticercosis

Cysticercosis is caused by the larval stage (cysticercus) of the pork tapeworm *Taenia solium.* Humans become the intermediate host by ingesting eggs from contaminated food or water (faecal-oral transmission). The larvae encyst in tissues, most importantly the **brain** (neurocysticercosis, the most common cause of acquired epilepsy in endemic regions, including India), **eye,** and **skeletal muscle.** On histology, the cysticercus is identified as a fluid-filled cyst containing an invaginated scolex with hooklets, surrounded by a fibrous capsule and a host inflammatory response (granulomatous inflammation, eosinophils) that becomes prominent as the larva degenerates. Calcified cysticerci are frequently incidental findings on radiological imaging. Neurocysticercosis is staged as vesicular (viable cyst, minimal inflammation), colloidal (degenerating, intense inflammation), granular-nodular, and calcified.

Filariasis

Lymphatic filariasis, caused by *Wuchereria bancrofti* (most common in tropical regions) and *Brugia malayi,* is transmitted by *Culex* mosquitoes. Adult worms reside in lymphatic vessels, causing lymphatic obstruction, lymphoedema, and eventually elephantiasis (chronic massive lymphoedema, particularly of the lower extremities and genitalia). Histologically, the lymphatics show adult worms within dilated channels, with surrounding granulomatous inflammation, fibrosis, and endothelial proliferation. Microfilariae are detected in peripheral blood (nocturnal periodicity for *W. bancrofti*) by thick smear (Giemsa stain) or concentration techniques. Rapid antigen-based card tests (ICT) are used for field diagnosis.

Other Important Parasites

Amoebiasis: *Entamoeba histolytica* causes amoebic colitis (flask-shaped ulcers in the caecum and ascending colon) and amoebic liver abscess (anchovy sauce pus). Trophozoites with ingested RBCs are the diagnostic hallmark on PAS staining. **Hydatid disease:** *Echinococcus granulosus* produces hydatid cysts (liver most common, lung second), characterised by a laminated acellular wall and daughter cysts containing brood capsules with protoscolices (hydatid sand). Casoni test and specific serology (ELISA for echinococcal antibodies) aid diagnosis. **Toxoplasmosis:** *Toxoplasma gondii* causes congenital infection (TORCH), encephalitis in AIDS (ring-enhancing lesions), and lymphadenitis (Piringer-Kuchinka pattern: follicular hyperplasia + epithelioid cell clusters + monocytoid B-cell hyperplasia).

Amoebiasis: Intestinal and Hepatic

Entamoeba histolytica infection remains a significant cause of morbidity in tropical regions. Intestinal amoebiasis presents as amoebic dysentery with characteristic flask-shaped ulcers: the organism penetrates the colonic mucosa through collagenase and cysteine protease secretion, spreading laterally in the submucosa to produce ulcers with a narrow mucosal opening and broad undermined base. The cecum and ascending colon are most commonly affected. Histologically, the ulcer base shows necrotic debris with trophozoites (15-30 µm, with ingested erythrocytes, a pathognomonic feature distinguishing E. histolytica from non-pathogenic E. dispar). Amoebic liver abscess, the most common extraintestinal manifestation, produces a cavity filled with 'anchovy paste' or 'chocolate sauce' material (liquefied necrotic liver tissue) with trophozoites found at the periphery of the abscess wall, not in the necrotic centre. Diagnosis combines serology (anti-amoebic antibodies, sensitivity >90% for liver abscess), stool microscopy (trophozoites with ingested RBCs), and stool antigen detection (E. histolytica-specific lectin antigen ELISA). Ultrasound-guided aspiration of liver abscess is both diagnostic and therapeutic (Figure 9.7).

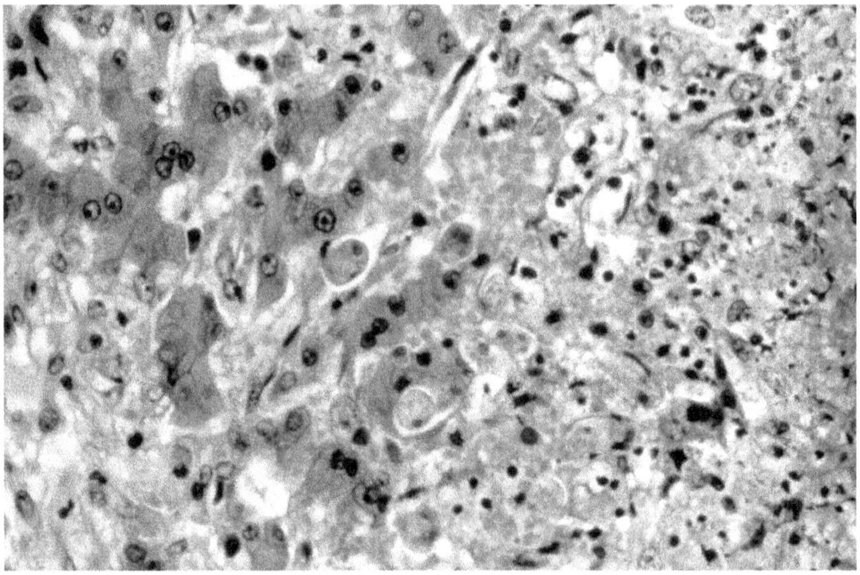

Figure 9.7: Amoebic liver abscess. Trophozoites of Entamoeba histolytica with ingested erythrocytes (pathognomonic feature) amid necrotic hepatocytes and inflammatory debris. H&E. (Source: Wellcome Collection, CC BY 4.0.)

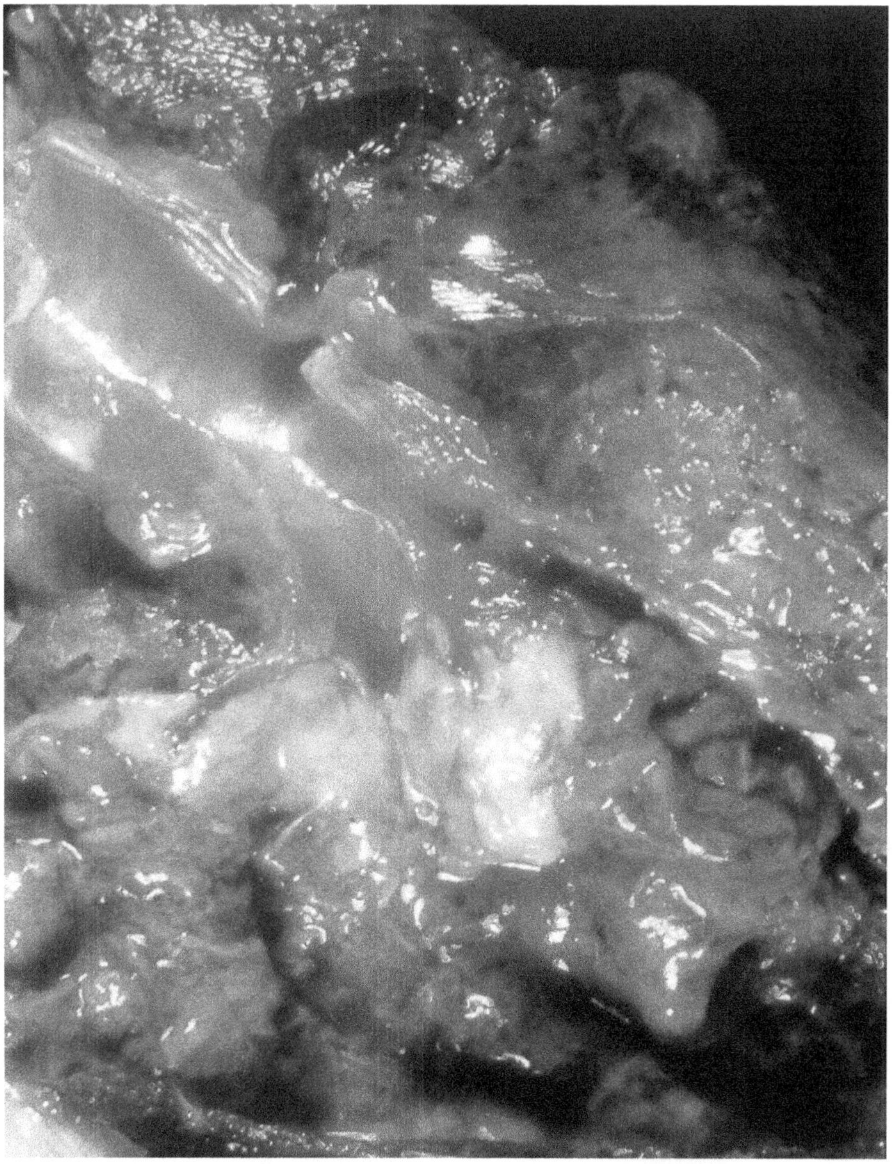

Figure 9.8: Amoebic liver abscess, gross: cut surface of liver showing abscess cavity with characteristic "anchovy paste" necrotic material. (Source: Yale Rosen, Flickr/Wikimedia Commons, CC BY-SA 2.0.)

Hydatid Disease

Hydatid disease, caused by the larval stage of Echinococcus granulosus (cystic echinococcosis) or E. multilocularis (alveolar echinococcosis), is endemic in pastoral regions where the dog-sheep life cycle is maintained. The liver (60-70%) and lungs (20-30%) are the most commonly affected organs. The hydatid cyst has a characteristic three-layered structure: an outer pericyst (host fibrous response), a middle laminated membrane (acellular, eosinophilic, PAS-positive), and an inner germinal layer (from which brood capsules containing protoscoleces develop). Protoscoleces and hooklets ('hydatid sand') are visible on aspiration cytology and are diagnostic. Daughter cysts may form within the mother cyst. Rupture of a hydatid cyst can cause anaphylaxis (due to release of cyst fluid containing parasite antigens into the systemic circulation) and dissemination of protoscoleces (secondary echinococcosis). Imaging (ultrasound classification by WHO/CE stages), serology (IgG ELISA, arc-5 test), and histology of the laminated membrane are diagnostic. Surgery (pericystectomy) or PAIR (percutaneous aspiration, injection of hypertonic saline/albendazole, re-aspiration) are treatment options.

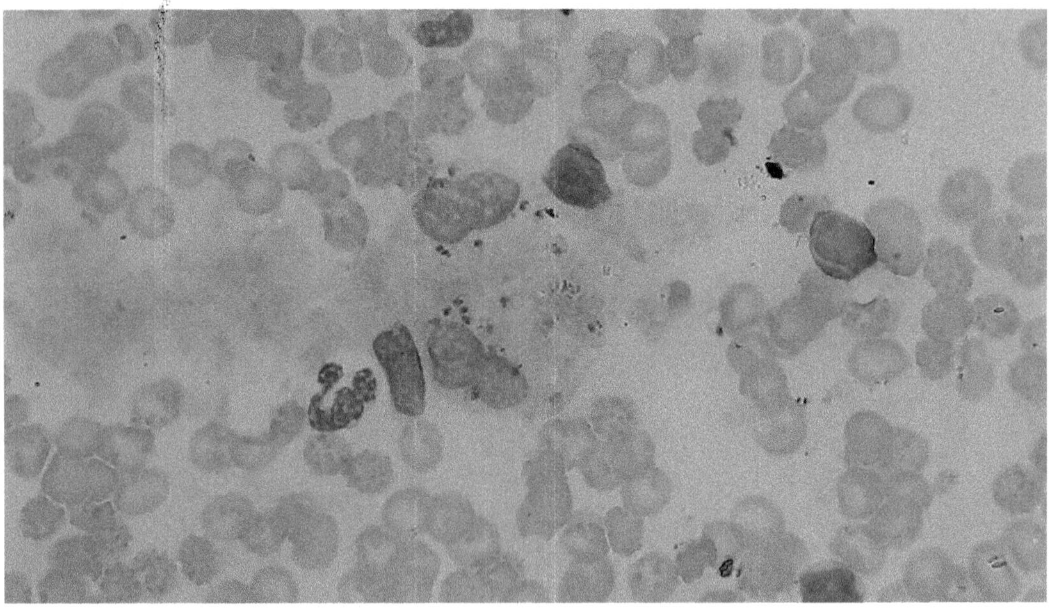

Figure 9.9: Visceral leishmaniasis: macrophage filled with Leishmania donovani amastigotes (LD bodies) showing characteristic nucleus and kinetoplast, with extracellular amastigotes. Giemsa. (Source: Ajay Kumar Chaurasiya, Wikimedia Commons, CC BY-SA 4.0.)

Integration: Parasitic infections connect to hepatobiliary pathology (amoebic abscess, hydatid, liver flukes; Chapter 20), neuropathology (neurocysticercosis, cerebral malaria, toxoplasmosis; Chapter 30), and renal pathology (malarial nephropathy, filarial nephropathy; Chapter 22).

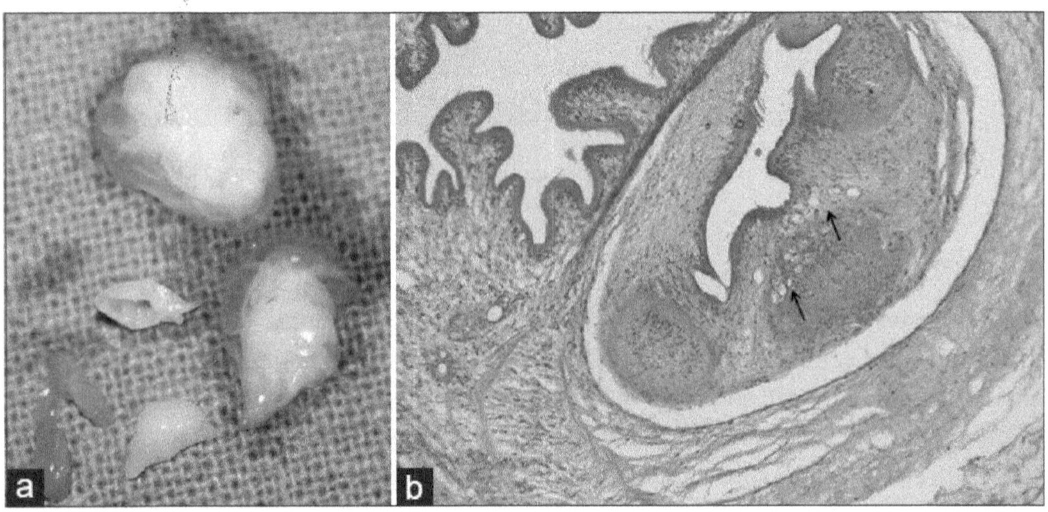

Figure 9.10: Cysticercosis: (a) Gross cysticerci excised from tissue. (b) H&E section showing cysticercus larva with scolex (arrows) surrounded by host tissue reaction. (Source: Bansal S, Suri A, Sharma MC, Kakkar A., Wikimedia Commons, CC BY-SA 3.0.)

Sexually Transmitted Infections: A Diagnostic Overview

Beyond syphilis (discussed above), the pathologist encounters several STIs in tissue and cytological specimens. **Gonorrhoea** (*Neisseria gonorrhoeae*) produces acute suppurative inflammation of the urethra, cervix, rectum, and pharynx; Gram stain of urethral discharge shows intracellular Gram-negative diplococci. **Chlamydial infections** (*Chlamydia trachomatis*) cause urethritis, cervicitis, pelvic inflammatory disease, lymphogranuloma venereum (LGV), and trachoma. LGV produces stellate microabscesses within lymph nodes, a pattern also seen in cat-scratch disease (*Bartonella henselae*) and tularaemia. **Granuloma inguinale** (donovanosis, caused by *Klebsiella granulomatis*) produces painless genital ulcers with characteristic **Donovan bodies** (organisms within macrophages, visible as safety-pin-shaped bipolar staining bodies on Giemsa stain). **Chancroid** (*Haemophilus ducreyi*) produces painful genital ulcers with ragged undermined edges and painful inguinal lymphadenopathy (buboes).

Table 9.5b: Differential Diagnosis of Genital Ulcers

STI	Ulcer Character	Lymphadenopathy	Diagnostic Clue
Syphilis (T. pallidum)	Painless, indurated, clean base	Painless, bilateral	Obliterative endarteritis, plasma cells; dark-field microscopy
Chancroid (H. ducreyi)	Painful, soft, ragged, purulent	Painful, unilateral (bubo)	School of fish arrangement on culture
LGV (C. trachomatis)	Small, painless (may go unnoticed)	Painful, matted, draining sinuses	Stellate microabscesses in LN
Granuloma inguinale (K. granulomatis)	Painless, beefy-red, bleeds easily	Pseudo-buboes (subcutaneous granulomas)	Donovan bodies in macrophages (Giemsa)
Herpes (HSV-2)	Painful, grouped vesicles/shallow ulcers	Tender, bilateral	Multinucleated cells, Cowdry A inclusions; Tzanck smear

The Pathologist's Eye

When evaluating granulomatous inflammation in a biopsy, a systematic approach avoids diagnostic pitfalls. First, determine the pattern: caseating (TB, fungi) vs non-caseating (sarcoidosis, Crohn, foreign body) vs suppurative (cat-scratch, LGV, fungi). Second, order special stains: ZN for AFB, GMS/PAS for fungi, Warthin-Starry for spirochaetes and Bartonella. Third, consider the clinical context: a cervical lymph node with caseating granulomas in a patient from a TB-endemic region is TB until proven otherwise; a hilar lymph node with non-caseating granulomas in a young adult may be sarcoidosis. Fourth, always examine polarised light for foreign material.

Congenital Infections: The TORCH Complex

The TORCH complex (Toxoplasma, Others, Rubella, CMV, HSV) causes transplacental/perinatal infection. Key features: CMV = most common congenital infection (periventricular calcifications, hearing loss); Rubella = PDA, cataracts, deafness; Toxoplasma = diffuse intracranial calcifications; HSV = encephalitis, vesicles. See accompanying table. Congenital rubella syndrome (CRS), though now rare in countries with high vaccination coverage, remains relevant in regions where rubella immunisation was added to national programmes only recently. The classic triad comprises sensorineural deafness (most common manifestation, 60-75%), congenital heart disease (PDA and pulmonary artery stenosis are characteristic), and cataracts. Additional features include thrombocytopenic purpura ('blueberry muffin' rash from dermal erythropoiesis), hepatosplenomegaly, microcephaly, and intellectual disability. CRS results from viral-induced inhibition of cell division and vasculitis in the developing fetus.

Congenital CMV is the most common congenital viral infection worldwide (0.5-1% of live births). Most congenital CMV infections are asymptomatic at birth, but approximately 10-15% of infected neonates are symptomatic, with features including petechial rash, hepatosplenomegaly, jaundice, microcephaly, periventricular calcifications (distinguishing from Toxoplasma, which produces diffuse/scattered calcifications), chorioretinitis, and sensorineural hearing loss (the most common long-term sequela, occurring in 10-15% of even asymptomatic congenital CMV). Diagnosis is by detection of CMV DNA by PCR in urine or saliva within the first 3 weeks of life (after 3 weeks, a positive result may reflect postnatal acquisition).

Congenital toxoplasmosis results from primary maternal Toxoplasma gondii infection during pregnancy. The classic triad (present in only a minority of symptomatic neonates) comprises chorioretinitis, hydrocephalus, and diffuse intracranial calcifications. The risk of fetal transmission increases with gestational age at maternal infection (10% in the first trimester, 60-80% in the third), but severity decreases: first-trimester transmission causes severe disease while late transmission is usually subclinical at birth. Congenital syphilis, if untreated, causes early manifestations (rhinitis/snuffles, hepatosplenomegaly, osteochondritis, periostitis, desquamating rash) and late manifestations (Hutchinson teeth, interstitial keratitis, eighth nerve deafness, saddle nose, sabre shins, Clutton joints).

Integration: *TORCH infections connect to diseases of infancy and childhood (Chapter 11), neuropathology (congenital CMV, toxoplasma, Chapter 30), and female genital tract pathology (placental pathology, villitis of unknown aetiology, Chapter 25). The pathologist examining a placenta should look for chronic villitis, plasma cell deciduitis, and funisitis as markers of intrauterine infection.*

Laboratory Errors and Quality in Infectious Disease Diagnosis

Pre-analytical, analytical, and post-analytical errors in infectious disease testing can have critical consequences, including missed diagnoses and inappropriate treatment. Key pre-analytical errors include improper specimen collection (e.g., collecting blood cultures after antibiotic administration, reducing sensitivity by 30-40%), inadequate specimen transport (delay in inoculating culture media, allowing fastidious organisms to die), and mislabelling. Analytical errors include failure to use appropriate special stains (e.g., not performing ZN stain on a granulomatous lesion), misidentification of organisms on Gram stain, and contamination of culture media. Post-analytical errors include failure to communicate critical results promptly (e.g., positive blood cultures) and misinterpretation of serology (e.g., not recognising the prozone phenomenon in syphilis testing).

Quality assurance in the microbiology laboratory requires internal quality control (daily media checks, ATCC reference strains, stain controls) and external quality assessment (EQAS participation, proficiency testing panels). The pathologist should ensure that turnaround times meet clinical needs: Gram stain and preliminary blood culture results should be available within the same working day. The introduction of MALDI-TOF mass spectrometry has reduced organism identification time from 24-48 hours to minutes and is increasingly available in tertiary centres globally. Antimicrobial stewardship, guided by accurate susceptibility testing and appropriate consultation between pathologist and clinician, is essential to combat antimicrobial resistance.

Mpox (Monkeypox)

Mpox, caused by the monkeypox virus (an orthopoxvirus), was declared a global public health emergency in 2022-2023. The virus causes a vesiculopustular rash progressing through macules, papules, vesicles, pustules, and crusts (resembling smallpox but less severe). Histologically, the skin lesions show ballooning degeneration of keratinocytes, intracytoplasmic eosinophilic Guarnieri bodies (aggregates of viral particles), and multinucleated giant cells in the epidermis. The dermis shows mixed inflammation with vasculitis. Diagnosis is by PCR from lesion fluid or crust. The pathologist may encounter mpox in skin biopsies from patients presenting with atypical rashes, particularly in the context of HIV co-infection where the clinical presentation may be more severe and atypical (larger, more numerous lesions, secondary bacterial superinfection). Awareness of orthopoxvirus cytopathic effects on histology is important for differential diagnosis from herpes simplex and varicella-zoster infections.

Zika Virus

Zika virus (ZIKV, a flavivirus transmitted primarily by Aedes aegypti mosquitoes) gained global prominence during the 2015-2016 epidemic in Brazil due to its association with congenital Zika syndrome (CZS). ZIKV has a tropism for neural progenitor cells, and maternal infection during the first trimester can cause severe fetal microcephaly, intracranial calcifications (particularly periventricular and subcortical), ventriculomegaly, cortical thinning, ocular anomalies (macular scarring, optic nerve hypoplasia), and arthrogryposis. The virus crosses the placenta and directly infects and destroys neural progenitor cells in the fetal brain, leading to impaired neurogenesis and neuronal migration. In adults, ZIKV infection is usually mild (fever, rash, conjunctivitis, arthralgia), but Guillain-Barré syndrome is a recognised complication. Diagnosis relies on RT-PCR of blood or urine within the first 2 weeks of illness, followed by serological testing (IgM), which cross-reacts with other flaviviruses (dengue) and requires confirmatory plaque reduction neutralisation testing (PRNT). There is no approved vaccine or specific antiviral therapy.

Influenza A (H1N1) Pathology

The 2009 H1N1 pandemic ('swine flu') provided important pathological insights into influenza pneumonia. Unlike seasonal influenza, which primarily causes disease in the elderly and immunocompromised, the 2009 H1N1 pandemic disproportionately affected young adults and pregnant women. The pathology centres on viral tropism for the lower respiratory tract epithelium, particularly type II pneumocytes and bronchiolar epithelial cells, causing necrotising tracheobronchitis and diffuse alveolar damage (DAD). Autopsy findings include extensive DAD with hyaline membranes, pulmonary oedema, haemorrhage, and secondary bacterial pneumonia (Staphylococcus aureus, including MRSA, and Streptococcus pneumoniae). Viral antigen is detectable in alveolar epithelium by immunohistochemistry. Diagnosis in living patients uses nasopharyngeal swab RT-PCR. Seasonal H1N1 outbreaks recur annually in many regions, and the pathologist should be aware of the DAD pattern when evaluating autopsy lungs from fatal pneumonia cases during influenza season.

Recent Advances

Global burden of bacterial antimicrobial resistance — GRAM 2019. The Global Research on Antimicrobial Resistance (GRAM) collaborators produced the first comprehensive estimate of the worldwide burden of bacterial antimicrobial resistance (Murray et al. The Lancet 2022; 399: 629–655; PMID 35065702). The systematic analysis covered 204 countries and territories, 23 pathogens, and 88 pathogen–drug combinations, drawing on 471 million individual records and isolates. In 2019, an estimated 1.27 million deaths globally were directly attributable to bacterial antimicrobial resistance and 4.95 million deaths were associated with it — a burden exceeding both HIV/AIDS and malaria. Six pathogens — Escherichia coli, Staphylococcus aureus, Klebsiella pneumoniae, Streptococcus pneumoniae, Acinetobacter baumannii, and Pseudomonas aeruginosa — accounted for 73 per cent of attributable deaths. Resistance to fluoroquinolones and beta-lactam antibiotics dominated the burden. The all-age age-standardised mortality rate was highest in western sub-Saharan Africa and lowest in Australasia. The estimate is now the principal reference for international antimicrobial-stewardship policy and for prioritising investment in novel antimicrobials, vaccines, and diagnostic capacity.

Clinical metagenomic sequencing of cerebrospinal fluid. Wilson and colleagues prospectively evaluated metagenomic next-generation sequencing of cerebrospinal fluid for the diagnosis of meningitis and encephalitis (Wilson et al. New England Journal of Medicine 2019; 380: 2327–2340; PMID 31189036). The one-year, eight-centre study enrolled 204 hospitalised paediatric and adult patients; 48.5 per cent had been admitted to intensive care and 30-day mortality was 11.3 per cent. Among 58 nervous-system infections diagnosed in 57 patients, metagenomic sequencing identified 13 (22 per cent) that were not detected by clinical testing at the source hospital, and made concurrent diagnoses in 19 of the remaining 45. Eight of the 13 sequencing-only diagnoses had a likely clinical effect, with seven guiding treatment changes. Pathogens uniquely identified included St Louis encephalitis virus, Cryptococcus neoformans, Streptococcus agalactiae, Nocardia farcinica, and hepatitis E virus. The study established metagenomic sequencing as a diagnostically useful adjunct to conventional microbiology in the workup of suspected neurologic infection, and informed subsequent CDC and ESCMID positioning on actionable applications of clinical metagenomics.

Syndromic multiplex PCR panels: Platforms like BioFire FilmArray can simultaneously detect dozens of bacterial, viral, and fungal pathogens from a single specimen (blood, CSF, respiratory, GI) within one hour, transforming the speed of infectious disease diagnosis in critical care settings.

Metagenomic next-generation sequencing (mNGS): Unbiased sequencing of all nucleic acids in a clinical sample can identify unexpected, rare, or novel pathogens that conventional tests miss. mNGS of CSF has proven particularly useful in diagnosing encephalitis of unknown aetiology, identifying organisms such as Balamuthia, novel arenaviruses, and atypical Mycobacterium species.

COVID-19 pathology: SARS-CoV-2 infection revealed a distinctive pattern of diffuse alveolar damage (DAD) with prominent microthrombi, reflecting endothelial activation and a prothrombotic state. Post-mortem studies demonstrated multi-organ tropism (lung, heart, kidney, brain, vasculature). The pandemic also drove the mucormycosis epidemic in South Asia and underscored the importance of autopsy pathology in understanding emerging infections (see Chapter 39).

Ultra High-Yield Chapter Summary

Table 9.5: Ultra High-Yield Summary; Infectious Disease Pathology

Topic	Must Remember
Tissue reaction patterns	Suppurative (pyogenic bacteria), Granulomatous (TB, fungi, syphilis), Cytopathic (viruses), Necrotising (Mucor, Clostridium).
TB pathogenesis	Th1 response; IFN-γ activates macrophages. Ghon complex = parenchymal focus + hilar LN.
Secondary TB	Apical cavitary disease; caseating granulomas; Langhans giant cells.
Extrapulmonary TB	LN (most common), intestinal (ileocaecal, vs Crohn), Pott spine, GU (sterile pyuria), CNS, miliary.
TB diagnosis	ZN stain, LJ/MGIT culture, GeneXpert (2 hr, detects Rif resistance).
Leprosy spectrum	TT: Th1, few bacilli, granulomas, lepromin +.
Lepra reactions	Type 1 (reversal): DTH, borderline.
HIV pathogenesis	CD4 + CCR5/CXCR4; reverse transcriptase; progressive CD4 depletion.
AIDS-defining	PCP, cerebral toxoplasma, cryptococcal meningitis, CMV retinitis, Kaposi (HHV-8), PCNS lymphoma.
Syphilis histology	Obliterative endarteritis + plasma cells (all stages).
Malaria (P. falciparum)	PfEMP-1 → cytoadherence → sequestration → cerebral malaria. Infects all RBC ages.
Aspergillus vs Mucor	Aspergillus: septate, 45° branching. Mucor: pauci-septate, 90°, ribbon-like.
CMV inclusion	Owl-eye intranuclear + cytoplasmic basophilic granules.
HSV inclusion	Cowdry A (eosinophilic); multinucleation; nuclear moulding.
Koilocyte	HPV cytopathic effect: perinuclear halo, wrinkled nucleus.
Key stains	ZN (TB), Fite (leprosy), GMS (fungi), PAS (fungi, Whipple), Warthin-Starry

	(spirochaetes), Mucicarmine (Crypto).
Kala-azar (VL)	L. donovani; massive HSM; LD bodies (amastigotes with kinetoplast) in marrow/spleen; rK39 rapid test.
Neurocysticercosis	T. solium larvae; most common cause of acquired epilepsy in endemic regions; scolex with hooklets; staged vesicular→calcified.
Filariasis	W. bancrofti; lymphatic obstruction → elephantiasis; nocturnal microfilaraemia; ICT card test.
Genital ulcer DDx	Painless = syphilis or granuloma inguinale. Painful = chancroid or herpes.
Granuloma approach	Caseating (TB, fungi) vs non-caseating (sarcoidosis, Crohn) vs suppurative (cat-scratch, LGV).

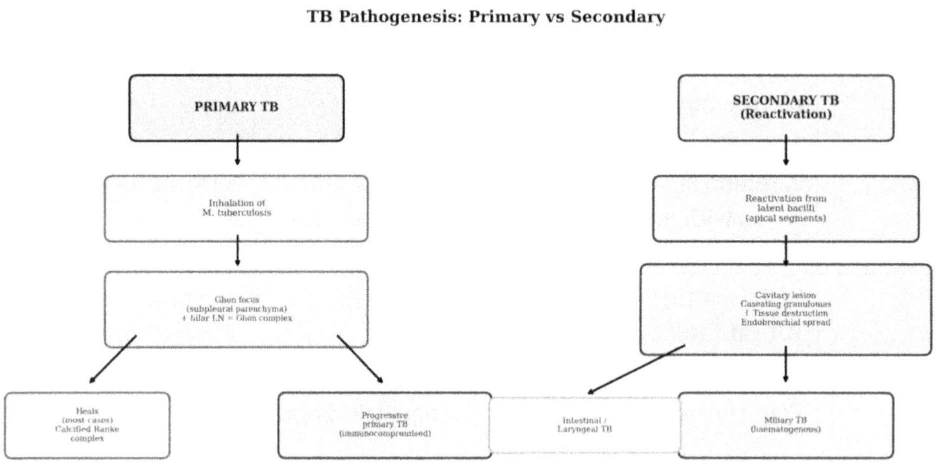

Figure 9.11: TB Pathogenesis: Primary vs Secondary. (Source: Author's original.)

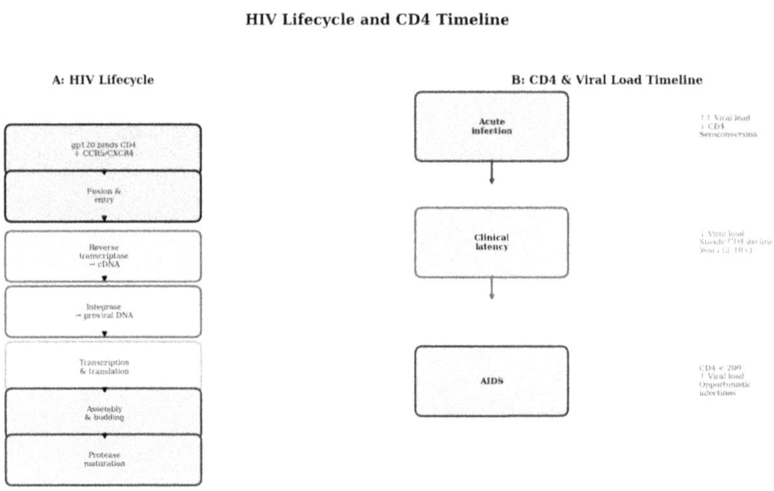

Figure 9.12: HIV Lifecycle and CD4 Timeline. (Source: Author's original.)

Diagnostic thinking: caseating granuloma + AFB positivity + Mantoux positive → tuberculosis (most common granulomatous disease in endemic regions)

Diagnostic thinking: owl-eye nuclear inclusions + immunocompromised host → CMV infection

Diagnostic thinking: non-caseating granuloma + asteroid/Schaumann bodies + exclusion of TB → sarcoidosis (see Chapter 15 for sarcoidosis)

Chapter 10: Environmental and Nutritional Pathology

THE BIG PICTURE

Human disease does not arise solely from intrinsic genetic programmes or microbial invasion. A vast and largely preventable burden of morbidity and mortality stems from what we breathe, eat, drink, and are exposed to, whether through occupation, lifestyle, or the broader environment. Environmental pathology encompasses the cellular and tissue responses to physical agents (radiation, thermal injury), chemical toxins (lead, arsenic, alcohol, tobacco), and occupational exposures (silica, asbestos). Nutritional pathology addresses the consequences of both deficiency and excess, from protein-energy malnutrition in developing nations to the obesity epidemic driving metabolic syndrome and cancer globally. Understanding these mechanisms is fundamental to preventive medicine and public health pathology.

High-yield topics in this chapter: Obesity and its pathogenesis (leptin, adipokines, cancer link); pathology of alcohol abuse (hepatic and systemic); fat-soluble vitamin deficiency and excess; protein-energy malnutrition (kwashiorkor vs marasmus); lead poisoning; radiation injury (deterministic vs stochastic effects, acute radiation syndrome); occupational lung diseases (pneumoconioses); diet and cancer; environmental and chemical carcinogenesis; adverse drug reactions.

The environment is not merely a backdrop to disease; it is an active participant. From the silica particle lodging in an alveolar macrophage to the excess calorie tipping an adipocyte into inflammatory dysfunction, environmental and nutritional insults operate through defined molecular pathways that produce predictable, examinable patterns of tissue injury. Where occupational health regulations are still evolving and the dual burden of malnutrition and obesity coexists, this chapter carries both clinical and public health weight. What follows examines these pathways with diagnostic relevance and exam calibration at the forefront.

Environmental Diseases

Tobacco and Smoking

Tobacco remains the single most preventable cause of death worldwide. Cigarette smoke contains over 7,000 chemical compounds, of which at least 70 are established carcinogens. The pathological effects of tobacco are mediated through three principal mechanisms: direct chemical carcinogenesis, promotion of atherosclerosis and thrombosis, and chronic airway inflammation.

Carcinogenesis: Polycyclic aromatic hydrocarbons (PAHs) and nitrosamines in tobacco smoke are metabolically activated by cytochrome P450 enzymes (particularly CYP1A1 and CYP1B1) to form DNA adducts. Benzo[a]pyrene, a major PAH, directly induces G:C to T:A transversions in the *TP53* gene, a mutation signature characteristic of smoking-related cancers. Nitrosamines, notably NNK (4-(methylnitrosamino)-1-(3-pyridyl)-1-butanone), are particularly implicated in lung adenocarcinoma.

Beyond the lung, tobacco is causally linked to cancers of the oral cavity, larynx, oesophagus, pancreas, bladder, kidney, and cervix (see Chapters 16, 17, 18, 23, 24, 25).

Cardiovascular effects: Nicotine promotes sympathetic activation, raises blood pressure, and increases platelet adhesiveness. Carbon monoxide displaces oxygen from haemoglobin, promoting endothelial hypoxia and dysfunction. These synergistic effects accelerate atherosclerosis (see Chapter 13). Smoking is the single strongest modifiable risk factor for peripheral vascular disease.

Respiratory effects: Chronic irritation leads to goblet cell hyperplasia, squamous metaplasia of bronchial epithelium, impaired mucociliary clearance, and recurrent infections. Progressive destruction of alveolar walls produces centrilobular emphysema through protease-antiprotease imbalance: smoke-activated neutrophils and macrophages release elastase, while oxidants in smoke inactivate alpha-1 antitrypsin (see Chapter 15).

Maternal and fetal effects: Smoking during pregnancy causes intrauterine growth restriction, placental abruption, preterm delivery, and increased risk of sudden infant death syndrome (see Chapter 11).

E-cigarettes and vaping: Electronic nicotine delivery systems (ENDS) produce aerosols containing nicotine, flavouring agents, and thermal decomposition products including formaldehyde and acrolein. E-cigarette or vaping product use-associated lung injury (EVALI) emerged as a distinct clinicopathological entity in 2019, characterised by acute fibrinous organising pneumonia or diffuse alveolar damage; vitamin E acetate used as a diluent in tetrahydrocannabinol-containing cartridges was identified as the primary causative agent (Figure 10.1).

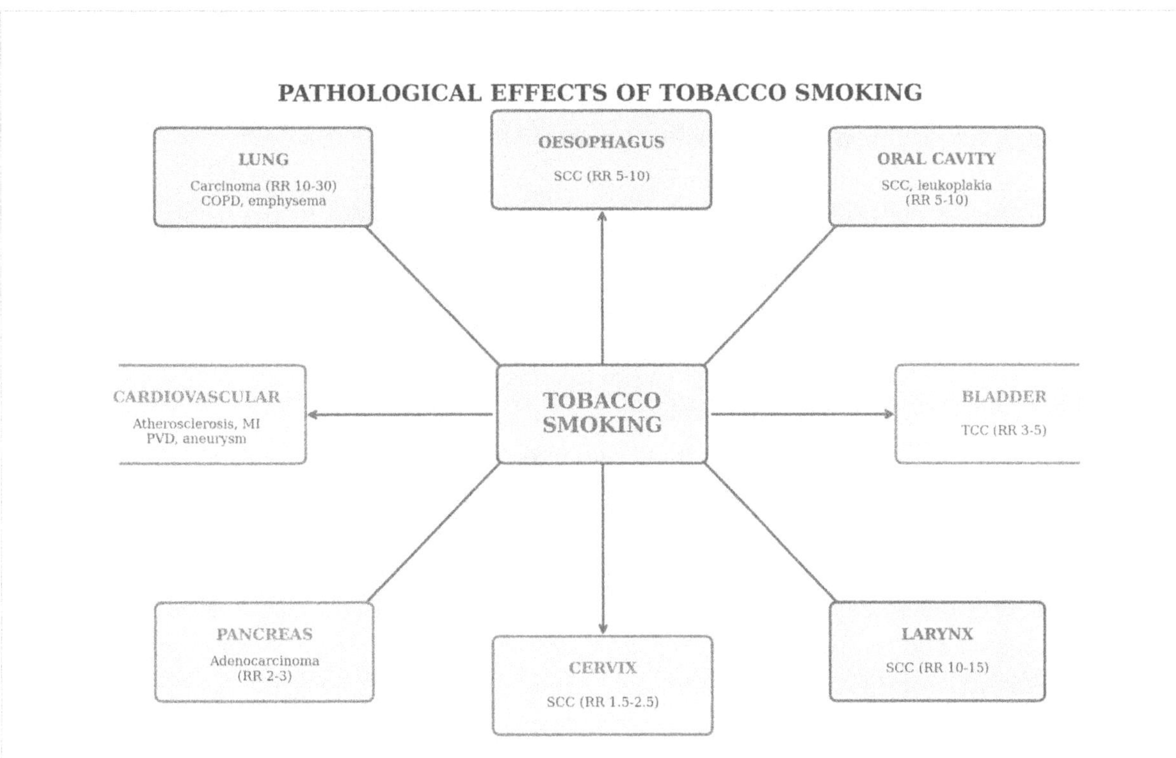

Figure 10.1: Pathological effects of tobacco smoking. (Source: Author's original.)

Pathology of Alcohol Abuse

Alcohol (ethanol) is metabolised primarily in the liver by three enzymatic systems: alcohol dehydrogenase (ADH) in the cytosol, the microsomal ethanol-oxidising system (MEOS/CYP2E1) in the smooth endoplasmic reticulum, and catalase in peroxisomes. All three pathways generate acetaldehyde, a highly reactive and toxic metabolite that forms protein adducts, promotes lipid peroxidation, and damages DNA.

Ethanol → Acetaldehyde (via ADH/CYP2E1) → Acetate (via ALDH2) → CO_2 + H_2O

The key diagnostic clue in alcoholic liver disease is the progression from steatosis (fatty change) to steatohepatitis to cirrhosis, driven by acetaldehyde toxicity, oxidative stress, and CYP2E1-mediated free radical generation.

Hepatic pathology: Alcoholic steatosis (fatty liver) is the earliest and most common change, characterised by macrovesicular fat accumulation in hepatocytes. The mechanisms include increased NADH/NAD+ ratio (from ADH and ALDH reactions) favouring fatty acid synthesis over oxidation, impaired lipoprotein assembly and secretion, and increased peripheral lipolysis. With continued exposure, alcoholic hepatitis develops, featuring hepatocyte ballooning, Mallory-Denk bodies (damaged cytokeratin intermediate filaments, particularly CK8 and CK18), neutrophilic infiltration (a distinctive feature distinguishing it from most other forms of hepatitis), and perivenular/perisinusoidal fibrosis. Progression to cirrhosis occurs in 10 to 15 percent of chronic heavy drinkers. The fibrosis pattern is characteristically perivenular and pericellular ("chicken-wire" pattern) initially, evolving into micronodular cirrhosis (see Chapter 20 for detailed hepatic pathology).

Clinical Pearl

Mallory-Denk bodies are not specific to alcohol. These eosinophilic cytoplasmic inclusions, composed of damaged keratin 8/18 intermediate filaments and ubiquitinated p62, are seen in alcoholic steatohepatitis but also in metabolic dysfunction-associated steatohepatitis (MASH), Wilson disease, primary biliary cholangitis, hepatocellular carcinoma, chronic cholestatic liver disease, and amiodarone toxicity. The morphology is identical across causes. Diagnosis of alcoholic versus metabolic steatohepatitis requires clinical history, BMI, lipid profile, and sometimes HFE genetic testing, not microscopy alone.

Systemic effects of chronic alcohol abuse extend well beyond the liver. Dilated cardiomyopathy ("alcoholic cardiomyopathy") results from direct toxic effects of acetaldehyde on myocardial cells and thiamine deficiency. Acute and chronic pancreatitis result from premature activation of pancreatic enzymes and acinar cell injury (see Chapter 21). Peripheral neuropathy and Wernicke encephalopathy are thiamine-deficiency mediated. Wernicke encephalopathy presents with the classic triad of ophthalmoplegia, ataxia, and confusion; untreated, it progresses to Korsakoff psychosis (confabulatory amnesia). Cerebellar degeneration affects the anterior vermis. Fetal alcohol spectrum disorder (FASD) includes microcephaly, cardiac defects, and characteristic facies (smooth philtrum, thin upper lip, short palpebral fissures). Chronic alcohol use increases risk of cancers of the oral cavity, oesophagus, liver, and breast, partly through acetaldehyde-DNA adducts and partly through CYP2E1-mediated activation of procarcinogens.

Integration: Alcoholic liver disease connects to hepatic pathology (Chapter 20), pancreatitis (Chapter 21), dilated cardiomyopathy (Chapter 14), and thiamine deficiency (discussed below in this chapter).

Why does chronic alcohol use cause both fatty liver and peripheral neuropathy through different mechanisms? Fatty liver (steatosis) results from the direct metabolic effects of ethanol oxidation: the increased NADH/NAD+ ratio generated by ADH and ALDH shifts hepatic lipid metabolism towards fatty acid synthesis and away from beta-oxidation, while also impairing VLDL secretion. Peripheral neuropathy, by contrast, is an indirect consequence: chronic alcohol use depletes thiamine (vitamin B1) through poor dietary intake, impaired intestinal absorption, and reduced hepatic storage. Thiamine pyrophosphate is essential for peripheral nerve energy metabolism (as a cofactor for pyruvate dehydrogenase and transketolase), and its deficiency leads to axonal degeneration. Thus, the liver injury is a direct toxic effect of ethanol metabolites, while the neuropathy is a nutritional deficiency consequence of the alcoholic lifestyle (see thiamine deficiency, below in this chapter, and Chapter 3 for wound healing implications of nutritional deficiencies).

Quick Recall: Alcohol Pathology

Diagnostic thinking: perivascular lymphocytic infiltrate + ceroid-laden macrophages → alcoholic hepatitis pathway

Metabolism: ADH (cytosol), CYP2E1/MEOS (SER), catalase (peroxisomes); all produce acetaldehyde.
Hepatic progression: Steatosis → Steatohepatitis (Mallory-Denk bodies, neutrophils, perivenular fibrosis) → Micronodular cirrhosis.
CYP2E1 induction: Generates free radicals, activates procarcinogens, potentiates drug toxicity (paracetamol).
NADH/NAD+ ratio: Increased ratio shunts metabolism toward fatty acid synthesis; explains steatosis.
Systemic: Cardiomyopathy, pancreatitis, Wernicke-Korsakoff, FASD, cancers (oral, oesophageal, liver, breast).

Lead Poisoning

Lead is one of the most important environmental toxicants. In low- and middle-income settings, exposure sources include lead-acid battery recycling, traditional cosmetics (surma, kajal), adulterated spices (lead chromate used as a colourant in turmeric), lead-glazed pottery, and contaminated water from old plumbing. Children are especially vulnerable because of higher gastrointestinal absorption rates (up to 50% in children versus 15% in adults) and a developing nervous system that is exquisitely sensitive to lead toxicity.

Mechanisms of toxicity: Lead exerts its effects through multiple pathways. It binds to sulfhydryl groups on proteins, inactivating enzymes involved in haem synthesis: delta-aminolevulinic acid dehydratase (ALA dehydratase, also called ALAD) and ferrochelatase. Inhibition of ALA dehydratase causes accumulation of ALA in serum and urine. Inhibition of ferrochelatase prevents incorporation of iron into protoporphyrin IX, causing accumulation of zinc protoporphyrin (ZPP) and free erythrocyte protoporphyrin (FEP). The result is microcytic hypochromic anaemia with characteristic basophilic stippling of red blood cells (aggregates of degraded ribosomal RNA due to inhibition of pyrimidine 5' nucleotidase). Lead also interferes with calcium-dependent processes, disrupting neurotransmitter release and synaptic function. In the kidney, it damages proximal tubular epithelial cells, producing intranuclear lead inclusions (acid-fast on staining) and eventually chronic interstitial nephritis and "saturnine gout" from impaired urate excretion.

Lead → Inhibits ALA dehydratase + ferrochelatase → ↑ALA, ↑ZPP/FEP → Microcytic anaemia with basophilic stippling

System	Pathological Effects	Diagnostic Clue
Haematopoietic	Microcytic anaemia, basophilic stippling, ringed sideroblasts, inhibited haem synthesis	↑FEP/ZPP, ↑ALA in urine, basophilic stippling on PBS
Nervous system	Children: encephalopathy, cognitive impairment, behavioural disorders. Adults: peripheral neuropathy (wrist/foot drop), headache	Blood lead level; cognitive testing in children
Renal	Proximal tubular damage, intranuclear inclusions (acid-fast), chronic interstitial nephritis, "saturnine gout"	Fanconi-like syndrome, hyperuricaemia
GI tract	Colicky abdominal pain ("lead colic"), "lead line" on gingival margin (Burton line)	Burton line on examination
Reproductive	Infertility, spontaneous abortion, reduced sperm quality	Occupational history
Skeletal	"Lead lines" on metaphyses of long bones (radiographic finding in children)	X-ray long bones

Table 10.1: Systemic Effects of Lead Poisoning

Quick Recall: Lead Poisoning

Key enzymes inhibited: ALA dehydratase and ferrochelatase (haem synthesis pathway).

Blood film: Microcytic hypochromic anaemia with basophilic stippling (pyrimidine 5' nucleotidase inhibition).

Kidney: Intranuclear inclusions (acid-fast), proximal tubular damage, saturnine gout.

CNS: Children: encephalopathy and cognitive impairment at lower levels than adults.
South Asian sources: Surma, adulterated turmeric, battery recycling. CDC threshold: 3.5 μg/dL (2021).

Other Environmental Toxicants

Arsenic: Chronic arsenic exposure through contaminated groundwater is a major public health crisis in West Bengal, Bangladesh, Bihar, and Uttar Pradesh. Arsenic inhibits pyruvate dehydrogenase and other mitochondrial enzymes by binding to sulfhydryl groups. Chronic arsenicosis manifests as a characteristic sequence of skin changes: diffuse hyperpigmentation ("raindrop" pattern of melanosis), keratoses on palms and soles, and progression to squamous cell carcinoma and basal cell carcinoma of the skin. Arsenic is also a recognised carcinogen for lung and bladder cancers and is associated with peripheral neuropathy and "blackfoot disease" (peripheral vascular disease). *The key diagnostic clue in chronic arsenicosis is the combination of skin hyperpigmentation, palmar/plantar keratoses, and a history of contaminated groundwater exposure in endemic regions.*

Mercury: Mercury exists in three forms: elemental (vapour), inorganic salts, and organic (methylmercury). Methylmercury bioaccumulates in the food chain and is the form responsible for Minamata disease, characterised by cerebellar ataxia, visual field constriction, sensory neuropathy, and teratogenicity. Inorganic mercury targets the kidney, causing membranous nephropathy and acute tubular necrosis.

Carbon monoxide: CO binds haemoglobin with 200-fold greater affinity than oxygen, forming carboxyhaemoglobin (COHb). At 20 to 30 percent COHb, headache and confusion develop; above 60 percent, coma and death ensue. A distinctive feature is cherry-red discolouration of skin and viscera at autopsy. The brain and heart, being most sensitive to hypoxia, bear the brunt of injury. Bilateral globus pallidus necrosis is the classic neuropathological finding in survivors.

Adverse Drug Reactions

Adverse drug reactions (ADRs) are a significant cause of iatrogenic disease and are broadly classified into two types. **Type A (augmented)** reactions are dose-dependent, predictable, and represent exaggerations of the drug's pharmacological action (e.g., bleeding with anticoagulants, hypoglycaemia with insulin). They account for approximately 80% of all ADRs. **Type B (bizarre)** reactions are dose-independent, unpredictable, and often immune-mediated (e.g., drug hypersensitivity, idiosyncratic hepatotoxicity, Stevens-Johnson syndrome). Major drug-induced organ injuries include hepatotoxicity (paracetamol is the leading cause of acute liver failure in Western countries; isoniazid and anti-tubercular drugs are major causes in TB-endemic regions), nephrotoxicity (aminoglycosides, NSAIDs, cisplatin), pulmonary toxicity (bleomycin, amiodarone, methotrexate causing interstitial lung disease), and bone marrow suppression (chemotherapeutic agents, chloramphenicol). A detailed discussion of drug-induced liver injury (DILI) appears in Chapter 20.

Exam Pitfall: Adverse Drug Reactions

Do not confuse Type A and Type B reactions. Type A = Augmented, dose-dependent, predictable, common. Type B = Bizarre, dose-independent, unpredictable, often immune-mediated.

Remember that paracetamol hepatotoxicity is dose-dependent (Type A) and involves CYP2E1-mediated formation of NAPQI (N-acetyl-p-benzoquinone imine), which is detoxified by glutathione. N-acetylcysteine works by replenishing glutathione stores.

Physical Injuries: Thermal and Electrical

Thermal injury: Burns are classified by depth. Superficial (first-degree) burns affect only the epidermis (erythema, pain). Partial-thickness (second-degree) burns extend into the dermis (blistering, severe pain). Full-thickness (third-degree) burns destroy the entire dermis and appendages (white or charred, painless due to nerve destruction). Systemic effects of extensive burns (>20% total body surface area) include hypovolaemic shock (massive fluid loss from increased vascular permeability mediated by histamine, prostaglandins, and complement activation), sepsis (loss of the skin barrier; Pseudomonas aeruginosa and Staphylococcus aureus are the most common organisms), hypermetabolic state, and curling ulcers (acute gastric stress ulcers from splanchnic vasoconstriction). Inhalation injury in fires causes thermal damage to the upper airway, chemical injury to the lower airway from toxic fumes, and carbon monoxide poisoning.

Heat stroke occurs when core body temperature exceeds 40°C, overwhelming thermoregulatory mechanisms. The pathology includes widespread endothelial damage, rhabdomyolysis (release of myoglobin causing acute tubular necrosis), disseminated intravascular coagulation (DIC), and multi-organ failure. Neuropathological findings include cerebellar Purkinje cell loss, which may be the basis of persistent ataxia in survivors. **Hypothermia** below 32°C causes loss of consciousness; cardiac arrhythmias (particularly ventricular fibrillation) are the most dangerous consequence. Frostbite produces vasoconstriction, extracellular ice crystal formation (drawing water out of cells), and vascular endothelial damage leading to thrombosis and gangrene.

Electrical injury: Electrical current causes injury through direct disruption of cardiac conduction (ventricular fibrillation is the most common cause of death), resistive heating along the current path (deep burns along blood vessels and nerves), and tetanic muscle contraction. The entry and exit wound pattern is characteristic. Lightning strike can produce a distinctive arborising skin pattern (Lichtenberg figures).

Radiation Injury

Ionising radiation includes electromagnetic radiation (X-rays, gamma rays) and particulate radiation (alpha particles, beta particles, neutrons). The biological effects depend on the type of radiation, dose, dose rate, and tissue sensitivity. Radiation injury results primarily from two mechanisms: **direct damage** to DNA (strand breaks, base modifications) and **indirect damage** through radiolysis of water producing hydroxyl free radicals (·OH), which are the most important mediators of radiation-induced cellular injury.

Ionising radiation → Radiolysis of H_2O → ·OH free radicals → DNA double-strand breaks → Cell death or mutagenesis

Deterministic vs stochastic effects: This distinction is fundamental. **Deterministic effects** have a threshold dose below which they do not occur; above the threshold, severity increases with dose. Examples include skin erythema (threshold approximately 2 Gy), cataracts (approximately 2 Gy), and the acute radiation syndromes. **Stochastic effects** have no threshold (any dose carries some risk); the probability, not severity, increases with dose. The two principal stochastic effects are carcinogenesis and heritable genetic mutations.

The distinction from thermal or chemical injury rests on the latent period: radiation damage may manifest days to decades after exposure, depending on whether the effect is deterministic or stochastic.

Tissue radiosensitivity follows the law of Bergonié and Tribondeau: cells that are rapidly dividing, have a long mitotic future, and are undifferentiated are the most radiosensitive. In order of decreasing sensitivity: lymphocytes and haematopoietic precursors (most sensitive), germ cells, GI epithelium, vascular endothelium, and mature neurons and muscle cells (most resistant). The notable exception is the lymphocyte, which undergoes apoptosis at very low doses despite being a non-dividing cell, through p53-mediated mechanisms.

Acute Radiation Syndrome

Acute radiation syndrome (ARS) occurs following whole-body exposure to high doses of penetrating radiation delivered over a short period. It progresses through four phases: prodromal (nausea, vomiting within hours), latent (apparent improvement), manifest illness, and recovery or death. Three clinical sub-syndromes are recognised, depending on dose:

Sub-syndrome	Dose (Gy)	Latent Period	Key Features	Prognosis
Haematopoietic	2–10	2–3 weeks	Pancytopenia, infections, haemorrhage; bone marrow aplasia	Potentially survivable with supportive care and stem cell transplant
Gastrointestinal	>6	3–5 days	Mucosal denudation, bloody diarrhoea, sepsis from gut bacterial translocation	High mortality; superimposed haematopoietic failure
Cerebrovascular (CNS)	>20	Hours	Cerebral oedema, vasculitis, obtundation, seizures, death within	Invariably fatal

			1–2 days	

Table 10.2: Acute Radiation Syndromes

Radiation carcinogenesis: Radiation is a well-established carcinogen (stochastic effect). The most important radiation-induced malignancies include leukaemias (particularly AML and CML, with peak incidence 5 to 7 years post-exposure, as documented in Japanese atomic bomb survivors), thyroid cancer (especially in children exposed to radioactive iodine, as seen after Chernobyl), breast cancer, lung cancer, and sarcomas in previously irradiated fields. The latency period for solid tumours is typically 10 to 30 years. DNA double-strand breaks leading to chromosomal translocations and point mutations are the principal mechanisms (see Chapter 6 for carcinogenesis).

Late effects of radiation on tissues: Chronic radiation injury to blood vessels produces obliterative endarteritis with intimal fibrosis and luminal narrowing, leading to ischaemic atrophy and fibrosis of the affected tissue. Radiation fibrosis of the lung, radiation nephritis, and radiation enteritis are important clinical entities. In the skin, chronic radiation dermatitis features epidermal atrophy, dermal fibrosis, telangiectasia, and a risk of squamous cell carcinoma in the irradiated field.

Quick Recall: Radiation Injury

Deterministic: Threshold exists; severity increases with dose. Examples: ARS, cataracts, skin burns.

Stochastic: No threshold; probability increases with dose. Examples: cancer, heritable mutations.

ARS progression: Haematopoietic (2–10 Gy) → GI (>6 Gy) → CNS (>20 Gy). Fatal at higher doses.

Most radiosensitive: Lymphocytes and haematopoietic precursors (Bergonié-Tribondeau law).

Leukaemia latency: 5–7 years. Solid tumour latency: 10–30 years.

Chronic vascular: Obliterative endarteritis → ischaemic atrophy and fibrosis (Figure 10.2).

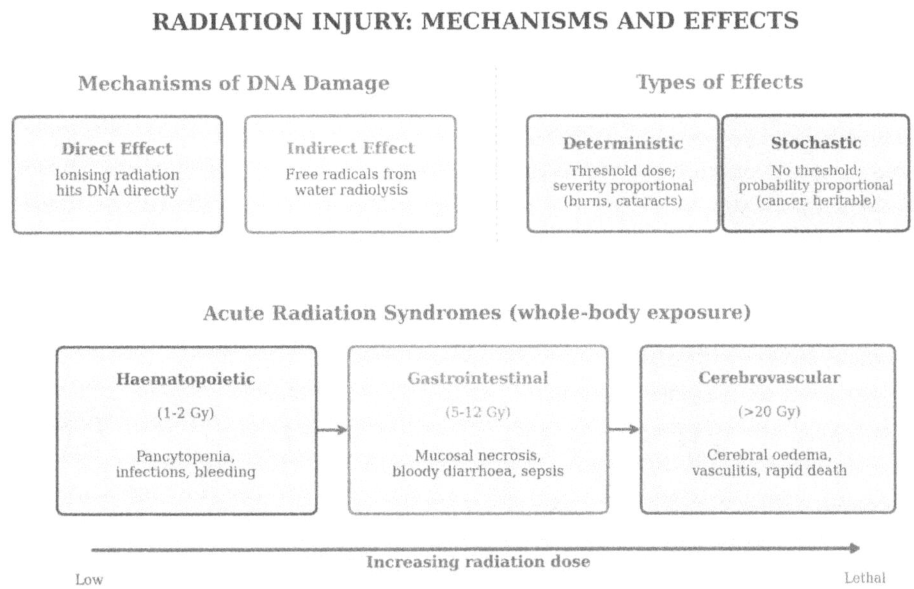

Figure 10.2: Radiation injury mechanisms and effects. (Source: Author's original.)

Occupational Lung Diseases (Pneumoconioses)

Pneumoconioses are non-neoplastic lung diseases caused by inhalation of mineral dusts in the occupational setting. The reaction depends on the type of dust (fibrogenic vs non-fibrogenic), the size of particles (1 to 5 μm is the most dangerous range, as these particles reach the terminal airways and alveoli), and the duration and intensity of exposure. The lung's response to inhaled particles is mediated primarily by alveolar macrophages, which phagocytose the dust and release fibrogenic cytokines, reactive oxygen species, and inflammatory mediators.

Silicosis

Silicosis, the most prevalent chronic occupational disease worldwide, results from inhalation of crystalline silicon dioxide (quartz). Occupations at risk include sandblasting, stone cutting, mining, tunnelling, and ceramic work. *Silicosis is particularly prevalent among stone quarry, agate, slate, and ceramic workers in low- and middle-income settings without effective respiratory protection.*

Pathogenesis: Silica particles are phagocytosed by alveolar macrophages but cannot be degraded, leading to macrophage activation and death with release of lysosomal enzymes. The cycle of phagocytosis, activation, and macrophage death perpetuates inflammation. Silica activates the NLRP3 inflammasome, leading to IL-1β and IL-18 release, which drives fibrosis. Silica also has direct cytotoxic effects on macrophages by disrupting phagolysosomal membranes.

Morphology: The hallmark is the silicotic nodule: a whorled pattern of concentrically arranged hyalinised collagen fibres surrounded by dust-laden macrophages. Under polarised light, birefringent silica particles are visible. Early disease affects the upper lobes and hilar lymph nodes. Progressive massive fibrosis (PMF) represents coalescence of nodules into large fibrotic masses exceeding 2 cm, typically in the upper zones. Eggshell calcification of hilar lymph nodes is a characteristic radiographic finding.

Complications: Silicosis markedly increases susceptibility to tuberculosis (silicotuberculosis), a combination of particular importance in TB-endemic regions. The impaired macrophage function in silicotic lungs creates a permissive environment for *Mycobacterium tuberculosis*. Other associations include Caplan syndrome (rheumatoid pneumoconiosis), increased risk of lung cancer (IARC Group 1 carcinogen for crystalline silica), and progressive massive fibrosis.

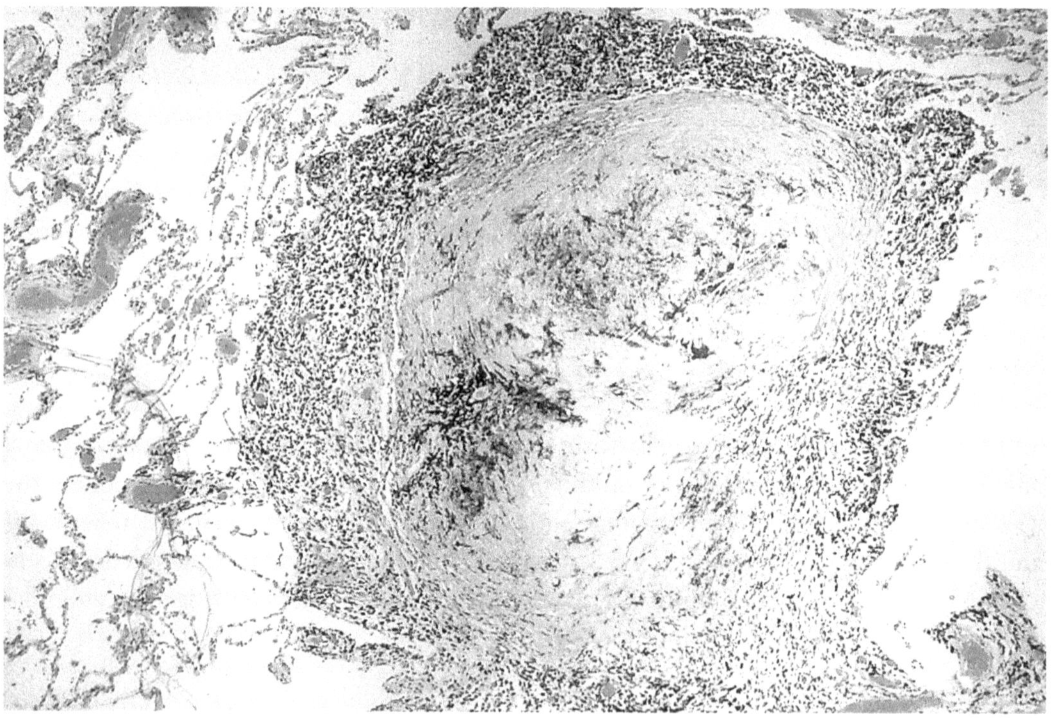

Figure 10.3: Silicotic nodule: whorled, concentrically layered hyalinised collagen with peripheral dust-laden macrophages and surrounding lung parenchyma. H&E. (Source: Yale Rosen, Wikimedia Commons, CC BY-SA 2.0.)

Asbestosis and Asbestos-Related Diseases

Asbestos is a family of fibrous silicates classified into two groups: serpentine (chrysotile, the most commonly used) and amphibole (crocidolite, amosite, tremolite). Amphibole fibres are more pathogenic because their straight, stiff configuration allows deeper penetration into the lung and greater resistance to clearance. The key asbestos-related diseases are:

Disease	Pathology	Latency	Key Features

Asbestosis	Diffuse interstitial fibrosis, lower lobe predominance	10–20 years	Ferruginous (asbestos) bodies; honeycombing in advanced disease
Pleural plaques	Well-circumscribed plaques of dense collagen on parietal pleura	10+ years	Most common asbestos-related finding; bilateral; often calcified
Pleural effusion	Serous or serosanguinous effusion	5–10 years	Earliest asbestos-related manifestation
Malignant mesothelioma	Malignant tumour of mesothelial cells (pleura > peritoneum)	25–45 years	Strongly associated with amphibole (crocidolite); BAP1 loss; see Chapter 16
Bronchogenic carcinoma	All histological types; synergistic risk with smoking	10–30 years	Asbestos + smoking = multiplicative risk (50–90×); see Chapter 16

Table 10.3: Spectrum of Asbestos-Related Diseases

Ferruginous bodies (asbestos bodies when the core fibre is asbestos) are golden-brown, fusiform structures with a beaded or dumbbell appearance, formed by iron and protein coating of asbestos fibres by macrophages. They are best visualised with Prussian blue stain. *When faced with a histological section showing interstitial fibrosis with ferruginous bodies, the diagnosis of asbestosis is straightforward; the challenge is distinguishing early asbestosis from other causes of lower lobe fibrosis such as UIP.*

Coal Workers' Pneumoconiosis

Coal workers' pneumoconiosis (CWP) results from inhalation of coal dust. Simple CWP is characterised by coal macules (1 to 2 mm aggregates of carbon-laden macrophages around respiratory bronchioles) and coal nodules (larger, with surrounding fibrosis). The coal macule produces focal emphysema by weakening the bronchiolar wall. Complicated CWP (progressive massive fibrosis) develops when nodules coalesce into large black fibrotic masses in the upper lobes. Caplan syndrome (rheumatoid pneumoconiosis) occurs in coal miners (and silica-exposed workers) with rheumatoid arthritis, producing necrobiotic nodules with a peripheral zone of coal dust.

Integration: Pneumoconioses connect to respiratory pathology (Chapter 15 for interstitial lung disease classification, Chapter 16 for mesothelioma and lung carcinoma), immunopathology (Chapter 5 for Caplan syndrome/RA), and inflammation (Chapter 2 for NLRP3 inflammasome).

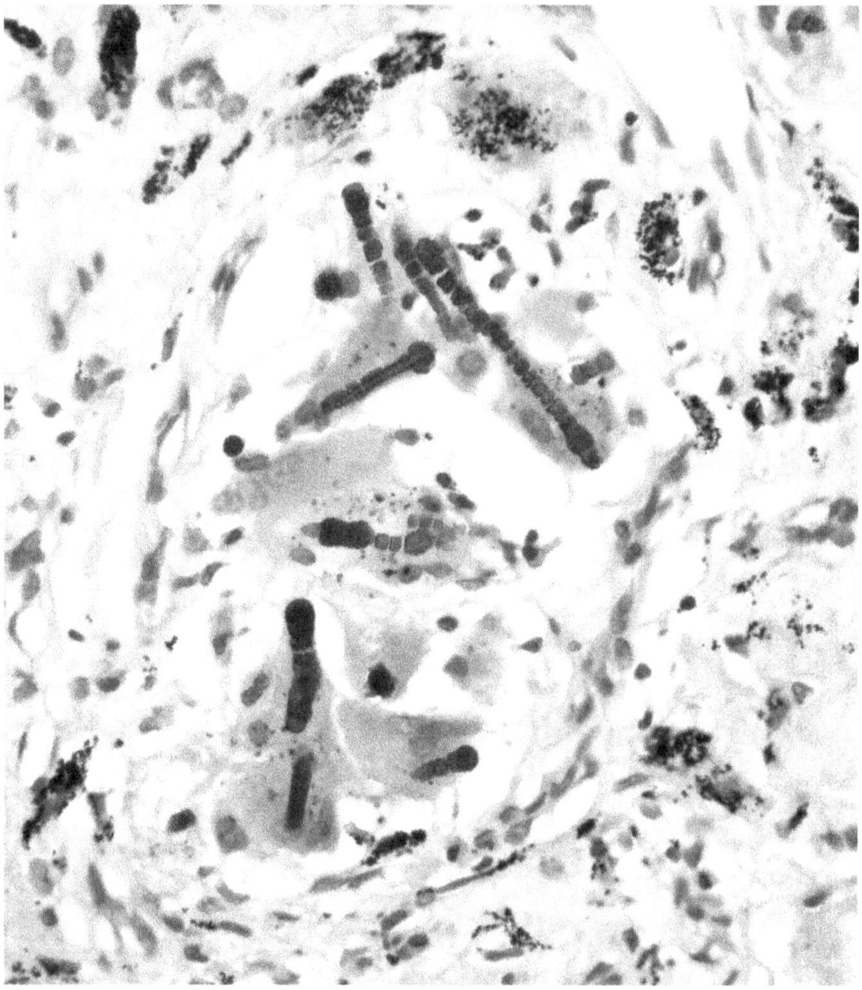

Figure 10.4: Ferruginous (asbestos) bodies: golden-brown, beaded, dumbbell-shaped structures representing iron-coated asbestos fibres within lung parenchyma. The segmented iron encrustation (Prussian blue positive) around a transparent asbestos core is pathognomonic. H&E. (Source: Nephron, Wikimedia Commons, CC BY-SA 3.0.)

Nutritional Diseases

Protein-Energy Malnutrition

Protein-energy malnutrition (PEM) remains a major public health problem across the developing world. PEM manifests as a spectrum ranging from marasmus (predominantly caloric deficiency) to kwashiorkor (predominantly protein deficiency), with marasmic kwashiorkor as an intermediate form. Recent national surveys in South Asia have documented stunting prevalence of approximately 30% and wasting of approximately 18% in children under five, underscoring the persistent severity of the problem.

Feature	Marasmus	Kwashiorkor
Primary deficiency	Total caloric deficit	Protein deficit (calories may be adequate)
Age of onset	< 1 year (typically)	1–3 years (typically, post-weaning)
Oedema	Absent	Present (pitting oedema, often pedal → generalised)
Body habitus	Severe wasting, loss of subcutaneous fat, "skin and bones"	Relative preservation of subcutaneous fat; pot belly (ascites/hepatomegaly)
Liver	Small, atrophic	Enlarged, fatty (fatty change due to impaired apolipoprotein synthesis)
Skin and hair	Thin, wrinkled skin; lanugo hair	Flaky paint dermatosis, flag sign (alternating bands of pigmented/depigmented hair)
Serum albumin	Decreased but less severely	Markedly decreased (→ oedema)
Thymus	Atrophied (most consistent finding in both)	Atrophied (most consistent finding in both)
Immune function	Cell-mediated immunity depressed; ↑ infections	Cell-mediated immunity depressed; ↑ infections
Appetite	Preserved (hungry child)	Anorexia (miserable, apathetic child)

Table 10.4: Marasmus vs Kwashiorkor

Pathology of PEM: The most consistent pathological finding in severe PEM is thymic atrophy with depletion of T lymphocytes, referred to as "nutritional thymectomy." This results in profound depression of cell-mediated immunity, explaining the high susceptibility to infections (measles, tuberculosis, diarrhoeal diseases). In kwashiorkor, the liver shows marked fatty change (macrovesicular steatosis) due to impaired synthesis of apolipoproteins needed for VLDL export; this is a critical distinction from marasmus where the liver is small and atrophic. Bone marrow may show hypoplasia or gelatinous transformation. Small bowel mucosa demonstrates villous atrophy and loss of brush border enzymes, compounding malabsorption.

The pathogenesis explains the morphology: because protein synthesis is selectively impaired in kwashiorkor, the hepatocyte cannot assemble VLDL to export triglycerides, and the liver becomes fatty; because albumin synthesis falls, oncotic pressure drops and oedema develops.

The Pathologist's Eye: Liver Biopsy in PEM

In a liver biopsy from a malnourished child, the pattern of steatosis provides the clue. Kwashiorkor produces diffuse macrovesicular steatosis, often severe, with preserved lobular architecture. This must be distinguished from MASLD (older age group, metabolic risk factors) and alcoholic steatosis (adult, relevant history). In settings with high prevalence of nutritional deficiency, always correlate with nutritional history, serum albumin, and anthropometry.

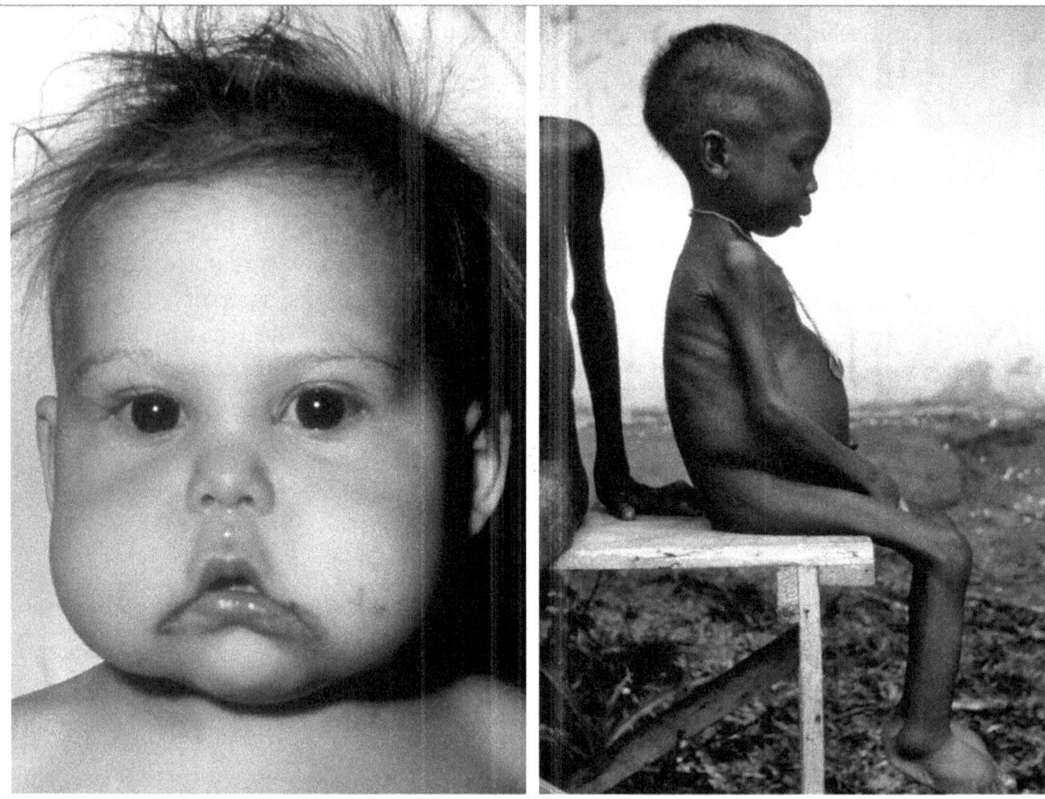

Figure 10.5: Protein-energy malnutrition: (a) Kwashiorkor — characteristic moon facies with oedema and sparse depigmented hair. (b) Marasmus — severe wasting with loss of subcutaneous fat and muscle, distended abdomen. (Source: CDC/Wikimedia Commons, Public Domain.)

Quick Recall: Protein-Energy Malnutrition

Most consistent finding: Thymic atrophy with T-cell depletion (→ depressed cell-mediated immunity → infections).

Kwashiorkor liver: Fatty (impaired VLDL/apolipoprotein synthesis). Marasmus liver: atrophic.

Kwashiorkor oedema: Due to hypoalbuminaemia (↓ oncotic pressure).

Flag sign: Alternating bands of pigmented and depigmented hair (kwashiorkor).
South Asia survey data: ~30% stunted, ~18% wasted in children <5 years.

WHO Classification of Child Malnutrition (2006 Standards)

The WHO 2006 Child Growth Standards define malnutrition using z-scores against a reference population (multi-country study of exclusively breastfed infants). Severe acute malnutrition (SAM) and moderate acute malnutrition (MAM) determine treatment pathway.

Table 10.4a: WHO Classification of Acute Malnutrition in Children 6–59 Months

Category	Weight-for-height Z-score (WHZ)	MUAC (mid-upper arm circumference)	Oedema	Management
Severe acute malnutrition (SAM)	< −3 SD	<115 mm	Any bilateral pitting oedema = SAM regardless of anthropometry	Inpatient or outpatient therapeutic feeding (RUTF); F-75 → F-100 if complicated
Moderate acute malnutrition (MAM)	−3 to < −2 SD	115 — <125 mm	Absent	Supplementary feeding programme (SFP); fortified blended food
No acute malnutrition	≥ −2 SD	≥125 mm	Absent	Routine nutrition counselling

Complementary WHO classifications include: stunting (height-for-age Z-score < −2 SD — chronic malnutrition), wasting (weight-for-height Z-score < −2 SD — acute), and underweight (weight-for-age Z-score < −2 SD — composite). In recent national surveys from South Asia, stunting prevalence in children under 5 has been reported at 30-36%, wasting 18-20%, and underweight 30-33% — among the highest globally.

Fat-Soluble Vitamins

The fat-soluble vitamins (A, D, E, K) share the property of absorption with dietary lipids, requiring bile salts and pancreatic lipase for absorption. Deficiency therefore accompanies any condition causing fat malabsorption (coeliac disease, chronic pancreatitis, cholestasis, cystic fibrosis). Unlike water-soluble vitamins, fat-soluble vitamins are stored in the liver and adipose tissue, so deficiency develops slowly but toxicity from excess is also possible.

Vitamin A exists as preformed retinol (animal sources) and provitamin A carotenoids (beta-carotene). It functions in vision (retinal in rhodopsin), epithelial differentiation, and immune regulation. Deficiency progression: night blindness → Bitot spots → corneal xerosis → keratomalacia. See table. Vitamin D undergoes hepatic 25-hydroxylation and renal 1α-hydroxylation to active $1,25(OH)_2D_3$ (calcitriol), which promotes intestinal calcium/phosphate absorption and bone mineralisation. Deficiency causes rickets (children) and osteomalacia (adults). See flow notation and table.**7-dehydrocholesterol (skin + UV-B) → Cholecalciferol (D3) → 25(OH)D3 (liver) → $1,25(OH)_2$D3/Calcitriol (kidney)**

Deficiency in children causes **rickets** (failure of mineralisation of growth plate cartilage and osteoid, producing craniotabes, rachitic rosary, Harrison sulcus, bowing of legs) and in adults causes **osteomalacia** (defective mineralisation of newly formed osteoid on existing bone, producing bone pain, proximal myopathy, and pathological fractures). Laboratory findings include decreased serum calcium, decreased phosphorus, elevated alkaline phosphatase, and elevated PTH (secondary hyperparathyroidism).

Non-skeletal roles of vitamin D: Calcitriol has immunomodulatory properties, promoting innate immunity (cathelicidin production in macrophages) and modulating adaptive immunity. Epidemiological associations link vitamin D deficiency to increased susceptibility to tuberculosis, autoimmune diseases (type 1 diabetes, multiple sclerosis), cardiovascular disease, and certain cancers, though causality remains debated for most non-skeletal outcomes. *This is a frequently tested topic ("Role of vitamin D in health and disease") and the examiner expects both skeletal and non-skeletal functions.*

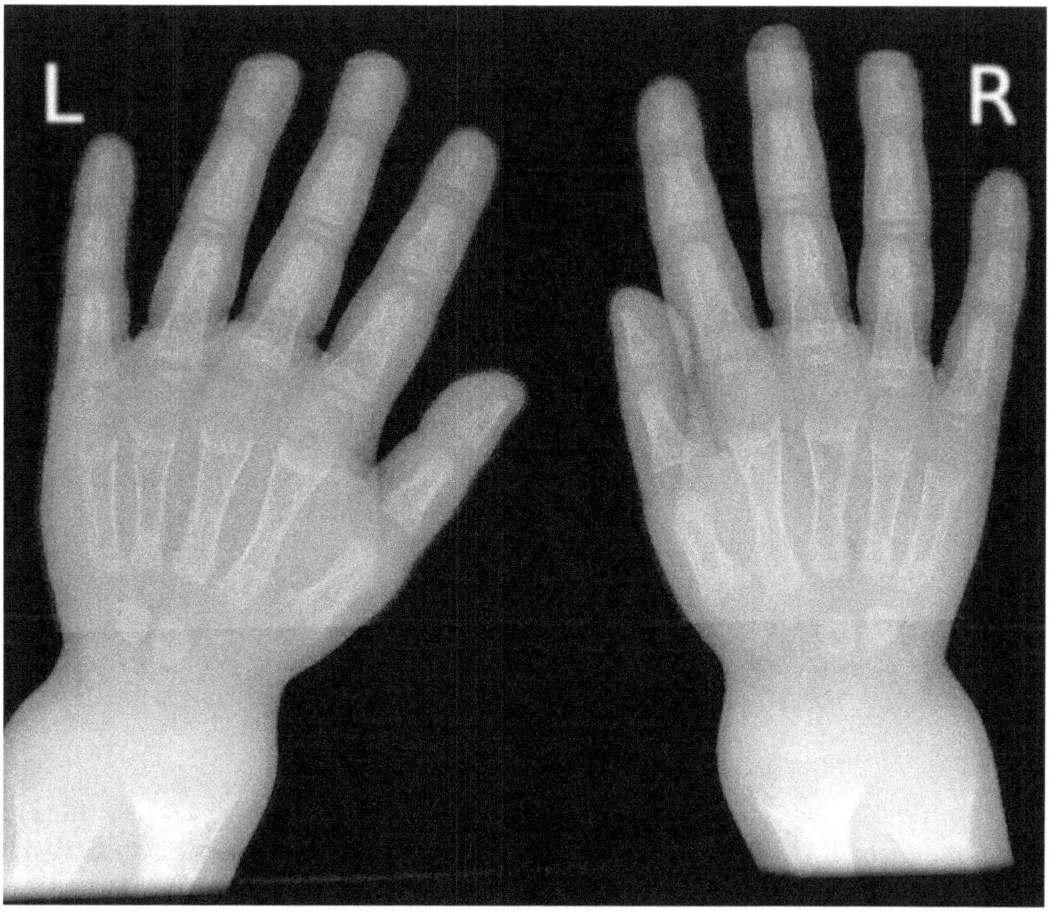

Figure 10.6: Rickets: radiograph of hands showing widened, irregular, cupped metaphyses with fraying and reduced bone density due to defective mineralisation of growth plates. (Source: Frank Gaillard, Wikimedia Commons, CC BY-SA 3.0.)

Vitamin E (Alpha-tocopherol): Vitamin E is the most important lipid-soluble antioxidant, protecting cell membrane polyunsaturated fatty acids from peroxidation by scavenging free radicals. Deficiency is rare in adults but occurs in fat malabsorption states, abetalipoproteinaemia, and premature neonates. Manifestations include spinocerebellar degeneration (posterior column and spinocerebellar tract demyelination), peripheral neuropathy, skeletal myopathy, and haemolytic anaemia in neonates (increased RBC membrane fragility from lipid peroxidation).

Vitamin K is essential for γ-carboxylation of clotting factors II, VII, IX, X and proteins C/S. Deficiency causes bleeding diathesis; haemorrhagic disease of the newborn results from poor placental transfer and sterile neonatal gut. Warfarin inhibits vitamin K epoxide reductase. See table.

Vitamin	Active Form	Key Functions	Deficiency	Excess/Toxicity
A (Retinol)	Retinoic acid, retinal	Vision, epithelial differentiation, immunity	Night blindness, Bitot spots, keratomalacia, squamous metaplasia	Pseudotumour cerebri, hepatotoxicity,

				teratogenicity
D (Calciferol)	1,25(OH)2D3 (calcitriol)	Ca/PO4 homeostasis, bone mineralisation, immunity	Rickets (children), osteomalacia (adults)	Hypercalcaemia, metastatic calcification
E (Tocopherol)	Alpha-tocopherol	Lipid-soluble antioxidant, membrane protection	Spinocerebellar degeneration, peripheral neuropathy, haemolytic anaemia (neonates)	Generally non-toxic; may potentiate anticoagulants
K (Phylloquinone)	Reduced vitamin K (KH2)	γ-carboxylation of II, VII, IX, X, protein C/S	VKDB (neonates), bleeding diathesis, ↑PT	Neonatal jaundice with synthetic K (historical)

Table 10.5: Fat-Soluble Vitamins: Functions, Deficiency, and Toxicity

Water-Soluble Vitamins

Thiamine (Vitamin B1): Thiamine pyrophosphate (TPP) is a cofactor for pyruvate dehydrogenase, alpha-ketoglutarate dehydrogenase, and transketolase (pentose phosphate pathway). Deficiency (beriberi) occurs in polished rice-dependent diets and chronic alcoholism. **Wet beriberi** features high-output cardiac failure with peripheral oedema and dilated cardiomyopathy. **Dry beriberi** manifests as peripheral neuropathy (symmetrical, ascending, sensorimotor). **Wernicke encephalopathy** (ophthalmoplegia, ataxia, confusion) is a medical emergency, particularly in alcoholics, requiring urgent parenteral thiamine before glucose administration (glucose without thiamine worsens the encephalopathy by consuming remaining thiamine stores).

Niacin (Vitamin B3): Niacin is a precursor of NAD and NADP. Deficiency causes pellagra, classically presenting with the 4 Ds: Dermatitis (photosensitive, symmetrical, Casal necklace around the neck), Diarrhoea, Dementia, and Death. Pellagra occurs in maize-dependent diets (maize niacin is bound in an unavailable form; alkali treatment as in Mexican nixtamalisation releases it), carcinoid syndrome (tryptophan diverted to serotonin synthesis), isoniazid therapy (interferes with tryptophan-niacin conversion), and Hartnup disease (defective tryptophan absorption).

Vitamin B12 (Cobalamin) and Folate: These are discussed in detail in Volume 1 (haematopathology). Briefly, deficiency of either causes megaloblastic anaemia (impaired DNA synthesis affecting rapidly dividing cells). Vitamin B12 deficiency additionally causes subacute combined degeneration of the spinal cord (demyelination of posterior columns and lateral corticospinal tracts). The most important cause of B12 deficiency is pernicious anaemia (autoimmune destruction of gastric parietal cells → loss of intrinsic factor → impaired ileal B12 absorption); see Volume 1.

Clinical Pearl

In low- and middle-income settings, multiple micronutrient deficiencies frequently coexist. A patient presenting with B12 deficiency commonly has accompanying folate, iron, and vitamin D deficiency, and frequently subclinical pyridoxine (B6) deficiency as well. Vegetarian dietary patterns predispose to B12, iron, and to a lesser extent zinc deficiency; the B12 deficiency masks the underlying iron deficiency (macrocytosis offsets microcytosis, producing a normocytic blood picture). Always check ferritin, B12, folate, and vitamin D together. Treating B12 alone in this setting unmasks florid iron-deficiency anaemia within weeks of starting cobalamin replacement.

Vitamin C (Ascorbic acid): Vitamin C is essential for the hydroxylation of proline and lysine residues in collagen synthesis by prolyl hydroxylase and lysyl hydroxylase. Deficiency causes scurvy: defective collagen leads to haemorrhagic manifestations (perifollicular haemorrhages, ecchymoses, gingival swelling and bleeding, subperiosteal haemorrhages in children), impaired wound healing, and bone disease ("scorbutic rosary"). Vitamin C also enhances non-haem iron absorption and serves as an antioxidant.

Vitamin	Active Form/Cofactor	Deficiency Syndrome	Classic Finding
B1 (Thiamine)	Thiamine pyrophosphate (TPP)	Beriberi (wet/dry), Wernicke encephalopathy	High-output cardiac failure (wet); peripheral neuropathy (dry); ophthalmoplegia + ataxia + confusion (Wernicke)
B2 (Riboflavin)	FAD, FMN	Ariboflavinosis	Angular cheilitis, glossitis, corneal vascularisation
B3 (Niacin)	NAD, NADP	Pellagra	4 Ds: Dermatitis, Diarrhoea, Dementia, Death; Casal necklace
B6 (Pyridoxine)	Pyridoxal phosphate (PLP)	Peripheral neuropathy, sideroblastic anaemia	Isoniazid-induced neuropathy (INH inhibits PLP); convulsions in infants
B9 (Folate)	Tetrahydrofolate (THF)	Megaloblastic anaemia; neural tube defects (NTDs)	Macrocytic anaemia; no neurological signs (unlike B12)
B12 (Cobalamin)	Methylcobalamin, adenosylcobalamin	Megaloblastic anaemia + SACD	Subacute combined degeneration (posterior + lateral columns); pernicious anaemia
C (Ascorbic acid)	Ascorbic acid	Scurvy	Perifollicular haemorrhage, gingival bleeding, impaired wound healing

Table 10.6: Water-Soluble Vitamins: Key Deficiency Syndromes

Exam Pitfall: Vitamin Deficiencies

Folate deficiency causes megaloblastic anaemia WITHOUT neurological signs. B12 deficiency causes megaloblastic anaemia WITH subacute combined degeneration of the spinal cord. This distinction is a perennial exam favourite.

Wernicke encephalopathy in alcoholics: always give thiamine BEFORE glucose. Glucose infusion without thiamine worsens the encephalopathy by consuming remaining B1 stores.

Vitamin D deficiency in children = rickets (growth plate pathology). In adults = osteomalacia (osteoid mineralisation defect on existing bone). Osteoporosis is NOT vitamin D deficiency; it is reduced bone mass with normal mineralisation.

Quick Recall: Vitamins (Selected High-Yield)

Vitamin A progression: Night blindness → Bitot spots → Corneal xerosis → Keratomalacia; squamous metaplasia.

Vitamin D activation: Skin (UV) → Liver (25-OH) → Kidney (1,25-$(OH)_2D_3$/calcitriol). Non-skeletal: immunity, TB susceptibility.

Vitamin K: γ-carboxylation of factors II, VII, IX, X, protein C/S. VKDB in neonates.

Thiamine: Cofactor for PDH, α-KGDH, transketolase. Wet beriberi (cardiac), dry beriberi (neuropathy), Wernicke encephalopathy.

Pellagra: 4 Ds (Dermatitis, Diarrhoea, Dementia, Death); Casal necklace; maize-dependent diets, carcinoid syndrome, isoniazid.

Scurvy: Defective collagen (proline/lysine hydroxylation); perifollicular haemorrhage, gingival bleeding, impaired wound healing.

Obesity

Obesity is defined as a body mass index (BMI) of 30 kg/m^2 or above, with overweight defined as BMI 25 to 29.9. **For Asian populations, lower cut-offs are used: overweight at BMI 23 and obesity at BMI 25, reflecting the higher metabolic risk at lower BMI in South Asians.** Many low- and middle-income countries now face a paradoxical dual burden: persistent undernutrition in rural populations coexisting with rapidly rising obesity in urban areas, with hundreds of millions of people obese by Asian criteria.

Pathogenesis of Obesity

The pathogenesis of obesity is multifactorial, involving an imbalance between energy intake and expenditure, modulated by genetic, hormonal, neural, and environmental factors.

Leptin and the neurohumoral regulation of energy balance: Leptin, a 16 kDa protein hormone secreted by adipocytes in proportion to fat mass, is the central mediator of the body's energy homeostasis. Leptin acts on the hypothalamic arcuate nucleus through two opposing neuronal populations. It stimulates POMC/CART neurons (anorexigenic: suppress appetite, increase energy expenditure through alpha-MSH acting on MC4R) and inhibits NPY/AgRP neurons (orexigenic: stimulate appetite, decrease energy expenditure). Ghrelin, secreted by the stomach during fasting, opposes leptin by stimulating NPY/AgRP neurons. Insulin, like leptin, has a long-term anorexigenic effect on the hypothalamus.

In most obese individuals, leptin levels are paradoxically elevated, indicating **leptin resistance** rather than deficiency. Leptin resistance may result from: (1) impaired transport across the blood-brain barrier; (2) defective receptor signalling through SOCS3-mediated inhibition (suppressor of cytokine signalling 3, upregulated by chronic hyperleptininaemia); or (3) post-receptor signalling defects. True leptin deficiency (ob/ob) is extremely rare and causes severe early-onset obesity that is dramatically responsive to exogenous leptin administration.

Adipocyte → ↑Leptin → Hypothalamus: ↑POMC/CART (satiety) + ↓NPY/AgRP (appetite) → ↓Food intake + ↑Energy expenditure

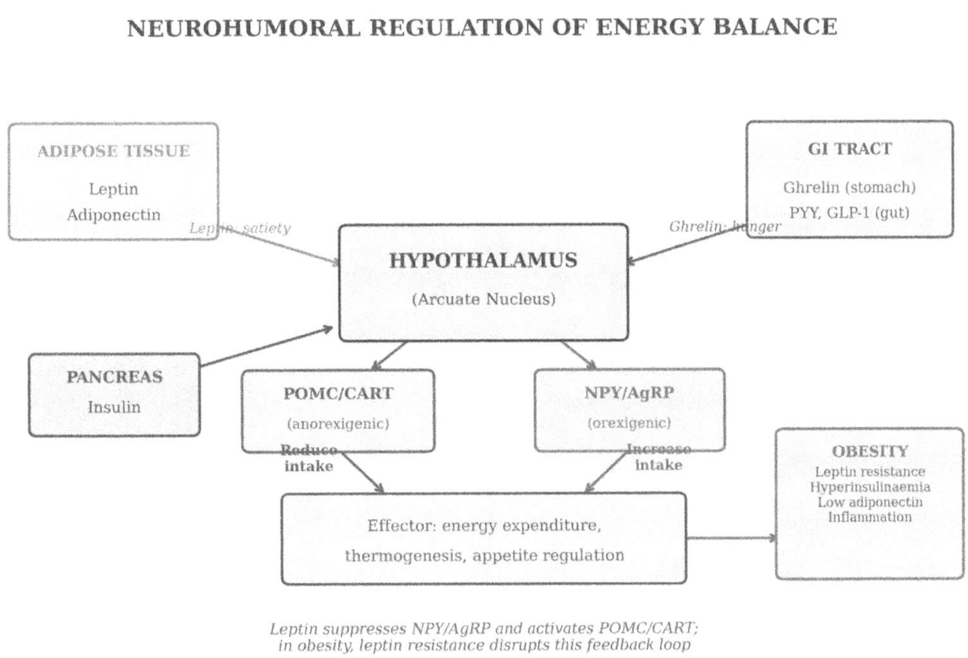

Figure 10.7: Neurohumoral regulation of energy balance. (Source: Author's original.)

Adipose tissue as an endocrine organ: Beyond leptin, adipocytes secrete a range of bioactive molecules collectively termed adipokines. Adiponectin (anti-inflammatory, insulin-sensitising, anti-atherogenic) is **decreased** in obesity, while pro-inflammatory adipokines (TNF-α, IL-6, resistin, MCP-1) are **increased**. This chronic low-grade inflammatory state, termed "metaflammation" (metabolically triggered inflammation), is the pathophysiological bridge linking obesity to insulin resistance, type 2 diabetes, atherosclerosis, MASLD, and cancer. TNF-α directly promotes insulin resistance by phosphorylating serine residues on the insulin receptor substrate (IRS-1), inhibiting downstream signalling. Macrophage infiltration of adipose tissue ("crown-like structures" around necrotic adipocytes) amplifies the inflammatory milieu.

Genetic factors: Genome-wide association studies (GWAS) have identified over 300 loci associated with BMI and fat distribution. The FTO gene (fat mass and obesity-associated) is the strongest common genetic determinant, influencing appetite regulation through effects on hypothalamic function. Rare monogenic obesity syndromes include leptin deficiency, leptin receptor mutations, MC4R mutations (the most common monogenic cause of obesity, accounting for 2 to 5 percent of severe childhood obesity), POMC deficiency, and PCSK1 mutations.

Consequences of Obesity

System/Disease	Mechanism/Association
Metabolic syndrome	Central obesity + insulin resistance + dyslipidaemia + hypertension + hyperglycaemia. Defined by IDF/NCEP-ATP III criteria; ≥3 of 5 criteria required
Type 2 diabetes mellitus	Insulin resistance mediated by adipokine dysregulation (↓adiponectin, ↑TNF-α, serine phosphorylation of IRS-1); eventual β-cell exhaustion
Atherosclerosis and CVD	Dyslipidaemia, chronic inflammation, endothelial dysfunction, prothrombotic state (elevated PAI-1)
MASLD (formerly NAFLD)	Hepatic steatosis → MASH → cirrhosis; insulin resistance drives hepatic lipogenesis (see Chapter 20)
Cholelithiasis	Increased cholesterol secretion in bile
Hypoventilation syndrome	Pickwickian syndrome: reduced chest compliance, hypercapnia, somnolence, obstructive sleep apnoea
Osteoarthritis	Mechanical stress on weight-bearing joints + adipokine-mediated synovial inflammation
Cancer	See below

Table 10.7: Systemic Consequences of Obesity

Obesity and Cancer

Obesity is now recognised as a significant and modifiable risk factor for at least 13 cancer types (IARC 2016). The cancers most strongly associated with obesity include endometrial (strongest association; risk increases 2- to 4-fold), oesophageal adenocarcinoma, hepatocellular carcinoma, renal cell carcinoma, postmenopausal breast cancer, colorectal, pancreatic, gallbladder, ovarian, thyroid, gastric cardia, meningioma, and multiple myeloma.

The mechanisms linking obesity to cancer include: (1) **Hyperinsulinaemia and IGF-1 signalling:** Chronic hyperinsulinaemia activates IGF-1 receptor and downstream PI3K/AKT/mTOR pathways, promoting cell proliferation and inhibiting apoptosis. (2) **Chronic inflammation:** Adipokine-mediated NF-κB activation and pro-inflammatory cytokine production (TNF-α, IL-6) create a tumour-promoting microenvironment. (3) **Increased oestrogen production:** Peripheral aromatisation of androgens in adipose tissue by aromatase (CYP19A1) produces excess oestrogen, explaining the strong endometrial and postmenopausal breast cancer link. (4) **Altered gut microbiome:** Dysbiosis produces pro-carcinogenic metabolites including secondary bile acids and trimethylamine N-oxide (TMAO). (5) **Adipokine imbalance:** Reduced adiponectin removes its anti-proliferative and pro-apoptotic effects mediated through AMPK signalling.

Obesity → ↑Insulin/IGF-1 + ↑Oestrogen (aromatase) + ↑Inflammation (TNF-α, IL-6) + ↓Adiponectin → ↑Cell proliferation + ↓Apoptosis → Cancer

The Pathologist's Eye: Adipose Tissue in Surgical Specimens

While obesity itself is rarely diagnosed histologically, its consequences are frequently encountered. In liver biopsies, steatosis exceeding 5% of hepatocytes warrants comment and correlation with metabolic risk factors for MASLD. In endometrial biopsies from obese patients, the threshold for concern regarding hyperplasia should be lower (excess oestrogen from adipose aromatase). In breast specimens, note that adipose tissue abundance can affect surgical margins and that crown-like structures (macrophage infiltration of breast adipose) have been associated with poor prognosis. The pathologist should also be aware that specimen fixation and processing may be suboptimal in markedly obese patients due to the large volume of adipose tissue, which resists formalin penetration.

Quick Recall: Obesity

Definition: BMI ≥30 (WHO); Asian cut-off: BMI ≥25. South Asian dual burden: rural malnutrition + urban obesity.

Leptin: Adipocyte hormone → hypothalamus (POMC/CART stimulation, NPY/AgRP inhibition). Obese = leptin resistance (↑leptin, impaired signalling via SOCS3).

Adipokines: ↓Adiponectin + ↑TNF-α/IL-6/resistin = "metaflammation" → insulin resistance, atherosclerosis.

Cancer link: 13 cancers (IARC 2016); strongest = endometrial. 5 mechanisms: insulin/IGF-1, oestrogen (aromatase), inflammation, microbiome, ↓adiponectin.

Metabolic syndrome: Central obesity + insulin resistance + dyslipidaemia + HTN + hyperglycaemia (≥3/5 criteria).

MC4R mutations: Most common monogenic cause of obesity (2–5% of severe childhood obesity).

WHO BMI Classification and Asian/Indian Cut-offs

The WHO global BMI categories were derived from studies in Western populations. For South Asian populations, cardiovascular and diabetes risk rises at lower BMI owing to higher body-fat percentage and visceral adiposity at equivalent BMI — the "Asian Indian phenotype." The WHO Expert Consultation (2004) and Indian consensus (2009) recommend lower cut-offs for Indians.

Table 10.5a: BMI Classification — WHO Global vs Asian/Indian

Category	WHO global (kg/m^2)	Asian/Indian (kg/m^2)	Cardiometabolic risk
Underweight	<18.5	<18.5	Increased (infection, osteoporosis, PEM)
Normal	18.5 — 24.9	18.0 — 22.9	Average
Overweight / At risk	25.0 — 29.9	23.0 — 24.9	Increased
Obese I	30.0 — 34.9	25.0 — 29.9	Moderate
Obese II	35.0 — 39.9	≥30.0	Severe
Obese III (morbid)	≥40.0	—	Very severe

Waist circumference (WC) cut-offs for central obesity also differ: WHO global ≥102 cm (men), ≥88 cm (women); South Asian consensus (e.g., 2009 South Asian Consensus) ≥90 cm (men), ≥80 cm (women); waist-to-height ratio >0.5 is used as a simpler alternative for metabolic-syndrome screening in many South Asian guidelines. Note: the BMI and waist cut-offs applied in South Asian clinical practice are lower than WHO global values.

Diet and Systemic Disease

Dietary Factors and Cancer

The relationship between diet and cancer operates through several mechanisms. **Exogenous carcinogens in food:** Aflatoxin B1, produced by *Aspergillus flavus* contaminating grains and peanuts (particularly in tropical regions including India), is a potent hepatocarcinogen. It causes a characteristic G:T transversion at codon 249 of *TP53* (p53 R249S mutation), a "molecular fingerprint" of aflatoxin exposure (see Chapter 20). Nitrosamines in processed and smoked meats are implicated in gastric and colorectal carcinogenesis. Heterocyclic amines formed during high-temperature cooking of meat (grilling, charring) are potent mutagens.

Endogenous factors: A high-fat diet increases bile acid secretion; colonic bacteria convert primary bile acids to secondary bile acids (deoxycholic acid, lithocholic acid), which act as tumour promoters in colorectal carcinogenesis. Caloric excess drives the insulin/IGF-1 axis (see obesity and cancer above). Deficiency of protective micronutrients (folate deficiency impairs DNA methylation and repair; selenium and antioxidant vitamins reduce oxidative DNA damage) contributes to cancer susceptibility.

Protective dietary factors: High fibre intake accelerates colonic transit time, dilutes carcinogens, and promotes butyrate production by colonic bacteria (butyrate is a histone deacetylase inhibitor with anti-proliferative effects). Fresh fruits and vegetables provide antioxidants and phytochemicals. The "Mediterranean diet" pattern, rich in olive oil, fish, fruits, and vegetables, is associated with reduced cardiovascular and cancer risk.

Habits and Customs in Cancer Predisposition

Culturally determined habits are particularly relevant across South Asia. **Betel nut (areca nut) chewing**, often combined with tobacco and slaked lime in "paan" or "gutka," is the leading cause of oral submucous fibrosis (OSF) and oral squamous cell carcinoma across the South Asian belt (see Chapter 17). The alkaloids in areca nut (arecoline, arecaidine) promote fibroblast proliferation and collagen deposition, producing the characteristic progressive trismus and mucosal blanching of OSF. Gutka (combined tobacco + areca nut) contains both nitrosamines and areca alkaloids, providing a synergistic carcinogenic stimulus. Similarly, the practice of reverse smoking (lit end inside the mouth, prevalent in parts of Andhra Pradesh) is associated with palatal carcinoma. Consumption of very hot beverages (chai at scalding temperatures) has been classified by IARC as "probably carcinogenic" (Group 2A) for oesophageal cancer due to chronic thermal injury to the oesophageal mucosa (see Chapter 18).

Climate Change and Health

Climate change is an emerging determinant of disease burden with implications for pathology. Rising temperatures expand the geographical range of vector-borne diseases (dengue, malaria, chikungunya) into previously temperate zones. Heat-related mortality, including heat stroke (characterised by rhabdomyolysis, DIC, and multi-organ failure), is increasing. Air pollution, exacerbated by climate change, is a major risk factor for chronic respiratory disease and lung cancer; the WHO estimates that ambient air pollution causes 4.2 million premature deaths annually. Particulate matter (PM2.5) penetrates to the alveoli and induces chronic airway inflammation, oxidative stress, and systemic inflammatory responses. In South Asia, the health burden of air pollution is particularly heavy: a Lancet Commission estimate attributed approximately 1.67 million deaths in India alone to air pollution in 2019.

Integration: Diet and cancer connects to chemical carcinogenesis (Chapter 6), oral pathology (Chapter 17), hepatobiliary pathology/aflatoxin (Chapter 20), and colorectal pathology (Chapter 19). Climate change connects to infectious diseases (Chapter 9) and respiratory pathology (Chapters 15, 16).

Recent Advances

Microplastics and nanoplastics in atheromas — first cardiovascular outcome study. Marfella and colleagues reported the first prospective cohort study to associate microplastic and nanoplastic contamination of human atherosclerotic plaque with cardiovascular outcomes (Marfella et al. New England Journal of Medicine 2024; 390: 900–910; PMID 38446676). Carotid plaque specimens were obtained from 304 asymptomatic patients undergoing carotid endarterectomy at a single Italian centre and analysed by pyrolysis–gas chromatography–mass spectrometry, stable-isotope analysis, and electron microscopy. Polyethylene was detected in plaque from 150 of 257 patients (58.4 per cent) followed up to a mean of 33.7 months, and polyvinyl chloride in 31 patients (12.1 per cent). Plaque-specimen electron microscopy demonstrated jagged-edged particles within macrophages and embedded in the extracellular matrix. Compared with patients without detectable polyethylene, those with polyethylene-positive plaque had a 4.53-fold higher risk of a composite cardiovascular endpoint (myocardial infarction, stroke, or death from any cause; 95 per cent CI 2.00–10.27). The study established a measurable, mechanistically plausible biological signal linking environmental plastic exposure to atherosclerotic disease.

Microplastics and nanoplastics have emerged as environmental contaminants of increasing concern. Recent studies have detected microplastic particles in human blood, placenta, lung tissue, and atherosclerotic plaques. A landmark 2024 study in the New England Journal of Medicine found that patients with carotid artery plaques containing polyethylene microplastics had a significantly higher risk of cardiovascular events compared to those without detectable microplastics. The pathological mechanisms under investigation include chronic inflammation (microplastic-induced macrophage activation), oxidative stress, endocrine disruption (leaching of bisphenol A and phthalates), and potential direct cellular toxicity. This is a rapidly evolving field with implications for environmental, cardiovascular, and reproductive pathology.

GLP-1 receptor agonists and the obesity paradigm shift: Semaglutide and tirzepatide (a dual GIP/GLP-1 receptor agonist) have demonstrated sustained weight loss of 15 to 25 percent of body weight in clinical trials (STEP and SURMOUNT programmes), fundamentally changing the therapeutic landscape of obesity. From a pathological perspective, this has implications for the future incidence of obesity-related cancers, MASLD progression, and metabolic syndrome complications. Whether weight loss induced by GLP-1 receptor agonists reduces cancer risk to the same degree as surgically induced weight loss (bariatric surgery has demonstrated reduced cancer incidence in long-term follow-up) remains an active area of investigation.

Exposome and environmental epigenetics: The concept of the "exposome," encompassing the totality of environmental exposures from conception to death, is gaining traction as a framework for understanding gene-environment interactions. Epigenetic modifications (DNA methylation, histone modification, non-coding RNA regulation) induced by environmental exposures such as air pollution (PM2.5 alters global DNA methylation patterns), heavy metals (arsenic disrupts DNA methylation through SAM depletion), and endocrine-disrupting chemicals (bisphenol A, phthalates) may mediate disease risk across generations through transgenerational epigenetic inheritance. This represents an important frontier connecting environmental pathology to molecular and genetic pathology (see Chapters 8 and 41).

Ultra High-Yield Chapter Summary

Topic	Must Remember
Tobacco carcinogenesis	PAHs/nitrosamines → CYP450 activation → DNA adducts; benzo[a]pyrene → TP53 G:C to T:A transversion
Alcohol metabolism	ADH (cytosol), CYP2E1 (SER), catalase (peroxisomes); all produce acetaldehyde; ↑NADH/NAD+ ratio
Alcoholic liver disease	Steatosis → Steatohepatitis (Mallory-Denk bodies, neutrophils, perivenular fibrosis) → Micronodular cirrhosis
Lead: haem synthesis	Inhibits ALA dehydratase + ferrochelatase → ↑ALA, ↑FEP/ZPP → microcytic anaemia, basophilic stippling
Lead: CNS	Children: encephalopathy, cognitive impairment at low levels. Adults: peripheral neuropathy (wrist drop).
Arsenic	Groundwater contamination (India); raindrop melanosis, palmar keratoses, cancers (skin, lung, bladder)
Radiation: deterministic vs stochastic	Deterministic: threshold, severity ↑ with dose.
Radiation: ARS	Haematopoietic (2–10 Gy) → GI (>6 Gy) → CNS (>20 Gy); latent period between phases
Silicosis	Upper lobe whorled collagen nodules, birefringent silica, NLRP3 inflammasome, eggshell calcification, ↑TB risk
Asbestosis	Lower lobe fibrosis, ferruginous bodies (Prussian blue +); pleural plaques (most common finding); mesothelioma (amphibole)
Asbestos + smoking	Multiplicative risk for lung cancer (50–90×); NOT for mesothelioma
Kwashiorkor vs Marasmus	Kwashiorkor: protein deficit, oedema, fatty liver, flag sign.

PEM: most consistent finding	Thymic atrophy with T-cell depletion (→ ↓cell-mediated immunity → infections)
Vitamin A	Night blindness → Bitot spots → keratomalacia; squamous metaplasia.
Vitamin D	Calcitriol (1,25-$(OH)_2$D3) via liver then kidney hydroxylation; rickets/osteomalacia.
Vitamin K	γ-carboxylation of II, VII, IX, X, protein C/S; VKDB in neonates; warfarin = K antagonist
Scurvy	Defective collagen (proline/lysine hydroxylation); perifollicular haemorrhage, gingival bleeding
Pellagra	4 Ds: Dermatitis, Diarrhoea, Dementia, Death; Casal necklace; niacin (B3) deficiency; carcinoid, isoniazid
Obesity: leptin	Adipocyte → hypothalamus: POMC/CART (↑satiety) + NPY/AgRP (↓appetite); resistance via SOCS3 in obesity
Obesity and cancer	13 cancers (IARC); strongest = endometrial.
Metabolic syndrome	Central obesity + insulin resistance + dyslipidaemia + HTN + hyperglycaemia (≥3/5 criteria)
Aflatoxin B1	Aspergillus flavus; TP53 codon 249 G:T transversion (R249S); hepatocellular carcinoma
Oral cancer (India)	Betel/areca nut + tobacco (gutka) → OSF → SCC; most common cancer in South Asian males

Table 10.8: Ultra High-Yield Chapter Summary

Diagnostic thinking: occupational dust exposure + upper lobe fibrosis + eggshell calcification → silicosis

Diagnostic thinking: ferruginous bodies + asbestos exposure + pleural plaques → asbestosis (watch for mesothelioma)

Chapter 11: Diseases of Infancy and Childhood

THE BIG PICTURE

Diseases of infancy and childhood differ fundamentally from adult pathology. Congenital anomalies, prematurity-related complications, perinatal infections, and a distinctive spectrum of neoplasms dominate this age group. Genetic and developmental factors carry far greater weight than the degenerative and environmental influences that drive adult disease. The perinatal period (from 28 weeks of gestation to 7 days after birth) carries the highest mortality risk of any period in life. An understanding of congenital malformations, TORCH infections, neonatal respiratory distress syndrome, hydrops fetalis, and childhood tumours is essential for the pathologist and for the postgraduate examination.

High-yield topics in this chapter: Congenital anomalies and teratogenesis (TORCH infections); neonatal respiratory distress syndrome (hyaline membrane disease); hydrops fetalis (immune and non-immune); sudden infant death syndrome (SIDS); tumours of infancy and childhood (neuroblastoma, Wilms tumour, retinoblastoma); small round cell tumour differential diagnosis; Potter sequence; necrotising enterocolitis.

The child is not a miniature adult. This foundational principle of paediatric pathology shapes every diagnostic consideration in this chapter. From the surfactant-deficient lung of the premature neonate to the embryonal tumours that recapitulate organogenesis gone wrong, the pathology of infancy and childhood reflects a developing organism in which the interplay of genetic programming, epigenetic regulation, and environmental insult produces disease patterns without parallel in adult medicine.

Congenital Anomalies

Congenital anomalies (birth defects) are structural defects present at birth, though they may not be clinically apparent until later. They are a leading cause of infant mortality globally. Terminology is important: a **malformation** is an intrinsic error of morphogenesis (e.g., congenital heart defect, neural tube defect); a **disruption** is destruction of a previously normal structure (e.g., amniotic band syndrome); a **deformation** is an abnormality caused by mechanical forces on a normally developing structure (e.g., clubfoot from oligohydramnios); and a **sequence** is a cascade of anomalies stemming from a single initiating event (e.g., Potter sequence from oligohydramnios).

Causes of congenital anomalies: Approximately 25% are due to genetic causes (chromosomal abnormalities, single-gene mutations), 15% are attributable to environmental causes (teratogens), and the remaining 60 to 65% are of unknown or multifactorial aetiology.

The classification of congenital anomalies into malformations, disruptions, deformations, and sequences is fundamental to understanding their pathogenesis and has direct clinical implications for recurrence risk counselling. A malformation is an intrinsic error of morphogenesis, meaning the developmental programme itself is faulty. Examples include ventricular septal defects, neural tube defects, and polydactyly. Because malformations arise from genetic or early embryonic events, they carry a measurable recurrence risk in subsequent pregnancies, and multifactorial inheritance models apply to many common malformations.

A disruption, by contrast, is the destruction of a previously normal structure by an extrinsic process. The classic example is amniotic band syndrome, in which strands of ruptured amnion encircle and constrict developing limbs or digits, causing amputation or ring constrictions. Because disruptions are extrinsic accidents, the recurrence risk is negligible. A deformation results from abnormal mechanical forces acting on an otherwise normally formed structure. Oligohydramnios, for instance, restricts fetal movement and leads to limb positional defects and facial compression (Potter facies). Deformations are generally correctable after birth if the underlying cause is addressed.

A sequence refers to a cascade of anomalies stemming from a single initiating event. Potter sequence exemplifies this concept: bilateral renal agenesis leads to oligohydramnios, which in turn causes pulmonary hypoplasia, limb compression defects, and characteristic facies. Recognising a sequence is diagnostically important because it directs the clinician to identify the primary event rather than treating each anomaly independently. Dysplasia, in the context of congenital anomalies, refers to abnormal cellular organisation within a tissue (distinct from the epithelial dysplasia of Chapter 6). Skeletal dysplasias such as achondroplasia (FGFR3 gain-of-function mutation) and thanatophoric dysplasia are prototypical examples.

The key diagnostic clue in congenital anomalies is the pattern of involvement: isolated single-organ defects suggest a malformation with specific genetic aetiology, whereas multiple anomalies in seemingly unrelated organ systems raise suspicion for a chromosomal abnormality or an early-acting teratogen. The syndromic approach, correlating the combination of anomalies with known genetic syndromes, remains the cornerstone of dysmorphology assessment.

Teratogens

A teratogen is any agent that produces a permanent structural or functional abnormality in the developing embryo or fetus. The susceptibility to teratogenic effects depends critically on the timing of exposure relative to gestational age. The **embryonic period (weeks 3 to 8)** is the period of maximal susceptibility, as this is the window of organogenesis. Exposure during the first two weeks typically results in either death or no effect ("all-or-none" phenomenon). Exposure during the fetal period (after week 8) primarily causes growth retardation and functional disturbances rather than major structural anomalies.

Teratogen	Major Anomalies
Alcohol (ethanol)	Fetal alcohol spectrum disorder (FASD): microcephaly, smooth philtrum, thin upper lip, short palpebral fissures, cardiac defects (VSD, ASD), cognitive impairment
Thalidomide	Phocomelia (limb reduction defects), cardiac, GI anomalies

Isotretinoin (Vit A)	Craniofacial (microtia, cleft palate), cardiac (conotruncal), CNS (hydrocephalus) defects
Warfarin	Nasal hypoplasia, stippled epiphyses (chondrodysplasia punctata), CNS defects
Phenytoin	Fetal hydantoin syndrome: craniofacial dysmorphism, nail/digit hypoplasia, cardiac defects
Valproic acid	Neural tube defects (spina bifida), craniofacial anomalies
Maternal diabetes	Caudal regression syndrome, cardiac defects (TGA), macrosomia, neural tube defects
Rubella (TORCH)	"Blueberry muffin" rash, PDA, cataracts, sensorineural deafness, microcephaly
CMV (TORCH)	Most common congenital infection; periventricular calcifications, microcephaly, hepatosplenomegaly, sensorineural hearing loss
Toxoplasma (TORCH)	Intracranial calcifications (diffuse/scattered), chorioretinitis, hydrocephalus
Ionising radiation	Microcephaly, growth retardation, cognitive impairment (dose-dependent)

Table 11.1: Major Teratogens and Their Effects

Quick Recall: Congenital Anomalies

Malformation: intrinsic morphogenesis error (VSD, NTD); recurrence risk present. Disruption: extrinsic destruction (amniotic bands); low recurrence. Deformation: mechanical forces (oligohydramnios); correctable.

Teratogen susceptibility: weeks 3 to 8 (organogenesis) = maximal risk. Before week 2 = all-or-none.

Most common teratogen: alcohol (FASD). Most common congenital infection: CMV. Most common genetic cause of intellectual disability: Down syndrome.

TORCH Infections

TORCH is an acronym for Toxoplasmosis, Other (syphilis, varicella, parvovirus B19), Rubella, Cytomegalovirus, and Herpes simplex. These infections are united by their ability to cross the placenta and cause congenital disease. **CMV is the most common congenital infection worldwide**, affecting approximately 0.5 to 1% of all live births. Most infected neonates are asymptomatic at birth, but 10 to 15% develop symptomatic disease with hepatosplenomegaly, jaundice, petechiae ("blueberry muffin" baby, also seen in rubella), microcephaly, and periventricular calcifications. Sensorineural hearing loss is the most common long-term sequela. Histologically, CMV produces characteristic large intranuclear inclusions ("owl-eye" inclusions) surrounded by a clear halo, with smaller granular cytoplasmic inclusions in epithelial cells of multiple organs (kidney, liver, lung, salivary glands).

Congenital syphilis: *Treponema pallidum* crosses the placenta, typically after the 16th week of gestation (the Langhans layer of the cytotrophoblast is protective earlier). **Early congenital syphilis** (manifesting before 2 years) presents with rhinitis ("snuffles"), mucocutaneous lesions, hepatosplenomegaly, and osteochondritis. **Late congenital syphilis** (manifesting after 2 years) produces the classic **Hutchinson triad**: interstitial keratitis, Hutchinson teeth (peg-shaped, notched upper central incisors), and eighth nerve deafness.

The key diagnostic clue in TORCH infections is the triad of hepatosplenomegaly, microcephaly, and petechiae/jaundice in a neonate. The pattern of intracranial calcifications helps distinguish the agent: periventricular (CMV) vs diffuse/scattered (toxoplasmosis).

Clinical Pearl

Intracranial calcification pattern decides between CMV and Toxoplasma. Periventricular calcifications, microcephaly, and sensorineural hearing loss point to congenital CMV; diffuse or scattered intracranial calcifications, hydrocephalus, and chorioretinitis point to congenital toxoplasmosis. The serological corollary is equally examined: Toxoplasma maternal infection is screened by the Sabin-Feldman dye test or IgG/IgM ELISA, with a fourfold rise or seroconversion confirming acute infection; congenital infection is confirmed by neonatal IgM (does not cross the placenta, so a positive neonatal IgM is the baby's, not the mother's). For CMV, neonatal urine viral culture or PCR within the first three weeks of life confirms congenital infection.

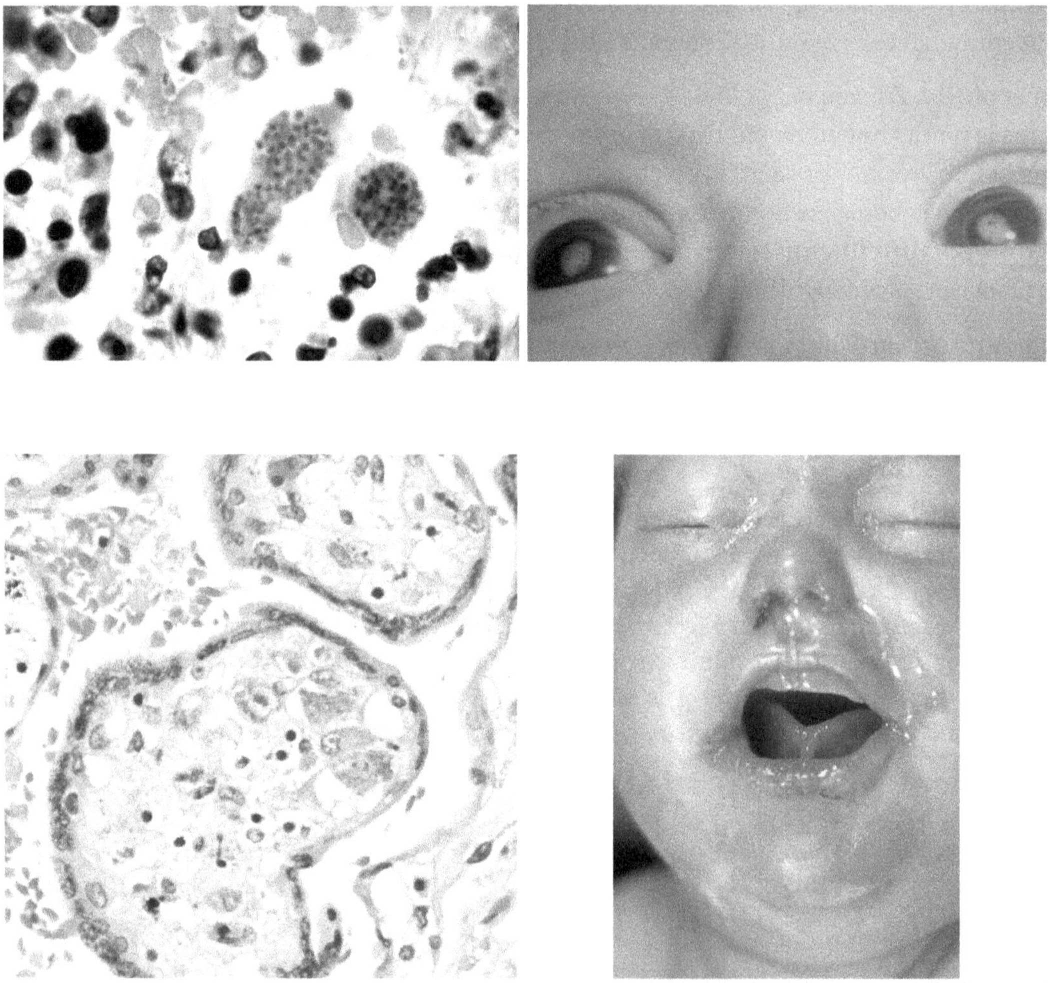

Figure 11.1: TORCH infections. (A) Toxoplasmosis: tachyzoites within a pseudocyst in brain tissue, H&E. (Source: Yale Rosen, CC BY-SA 2.0.) (B) Congenital rubella syndrome: bilateral cataracts. (Source: CDC, Public Domain.) (C) CMV placentitis: enlarged cells with owl-eye intranuclear inclusions in placental villi, H&E. (Source: Nephron, CC BY-SA 3.0.) (D) Congenital syphilis: neonatal snuffles (mucopurulent rhinitis). (Source: CDC/Dr. Norman Cole, Public Domain.)

Integration: TORCH infections connect to infectious disease pathology (Chapter 9 for individual organisms), hepatobiliary pathology (Chapter 20 for neonatal hepatitis), and neuropathology (Chapter 30 for CNS infections). Congenital cardiac defects connect to Chapter 14.

Prematurity and Diseases of the Neonatal Period

Neonatal Respiratory Distress Syndrome

Neonatal respiratory distress syndrome (RDS), also known as hyaline membrane disease (HMD), is the most common cause of respiratory failure in premature neonates. It results from **deficiency of pulmonary surfactant** due to immaturity of type II pneumocytes. Surfactant, a complex of phospholipids (predominantly dipalmitoyl phosphatidylcholine/lecithin) and surfactant proteins (SP-A, SP-B, SP-C, SP-D), reduces alveolar surface tension, preventing alveolar collapse at end-expiration.

Risk factors: Prematurity is the single most important risk factor (incidence inversely proportional to gestational age; approximately 60% at <28 weeks). Male sex, maternal diabetes (fetal hyperinsulinaemia inhibits surfactant synthesis), and caesarean section without labour (labour promotes cortisol release, which stimulates surfactant production) increase risk. Maternal corticosteroid administration (betamethasone) accelerates fetal lung maturation by stimulating type II pneumocyte surfactant production, and is the most important preventive intervention.

Surfactant deficiency → ↑Alveolar surface tension → Atelectasis → Hypoxia + CO_2 retention → Pulmonary vasoconstriction → Endothelial/epithelial damage → Plasma protein exudation → Hyaline membranes

Morphology: Grossly, the lungs are solid, airless, and dark red. Microscopically, the hallmark is **hyaline membranes**: eosinophilic, glassy membranes lining the alveolar ducts and respiratory bronchioles. These membranes are composed of fibrin, necrotic epithelial cell debris, and plasma proteins. The alveoli are diffusely atelectatic. In survivors, organisation of the membranes can lead to bronchopulmonary dysplasia (BPD), characterised by alveolar simplification, interstitial fibrosis, and dysmorphic vasculature.

Complications: Retinopathy of prematurity (ROP) results from oxygen therapy causing retinal vascular injury and abnormal neovascularisation. Intraventricular haemorrhage (IVH) arises from the fragile germinal matrix vasculature (subependymal germinal matrix haemorrhage), particularly in neonates <32 weeks. Necrotising enterocolitis (NEC) is the most common serious GI emergency in premature neonates, resulting from mucosal ischaemia, bacterial colonisation, and formula feeding; it presents with pneumatosis intestinalis (air in the bowel wall) and may progress to perforation and peritonitis.

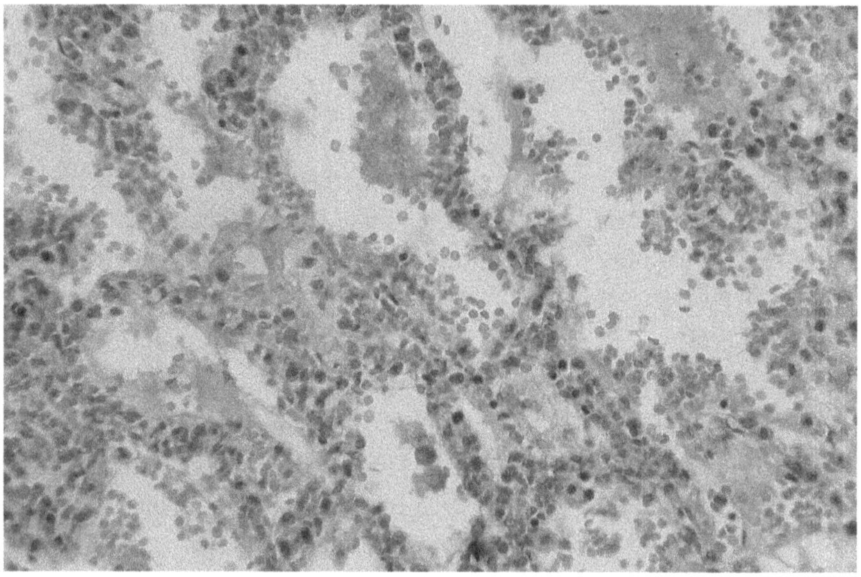

Figure 11.2: Neonatal RDS (hyaline membrane disease) with hyaline membranes lining atelectatic alveoli (H&E, ×100). (Source: Wikimedia Commons, CC BY-SA 3.0.)

Quick Recall: Neonatal RDS

Cause: Surfactant deficiency (type II pneumocyte immaturity). Key phospholipid: dipalmitoyl phosphatidylcholine (lecithin).

Risk factors: Prematurity (most important), male sex, maternal diabetes, C-section without labour.

Prevention: Maternal corticosteroids (betamethasone). Treatment: exogenous surfactant replacement.

Morphology: Eosinophilic hyaline membranes lining alveolar ducts/respiratory bronchioles; diffuse atelectasis.

L/S ratio: ≥2 indicates lung maturity (lecithin/sphingomyelin ratio in amniotic fluid). Phosphatidylglycerol confirms maturity.

Necrotising Enterocolitis

Necrotising enterocolitis (NEC) is the most common gastrointestinal emergency in premature neonates, with incidence rising sharply with decreasing gestational age. The pathogenesis involves a triad of intestinal immaturity (underdeveloped mucosal barrier, reduced secretory IgA, immature motility), microbial colonisation (abnormal gut flora, particularly with formula feeding), and ischaemic injury (mucosal hypoperfusion from perinatal asphyxia or haemodynamic instability).

The pathological hallmark is coagulative necrosis of the intestinal mucosa, which may extend transmurally. Bacterial gas production within the necrotic wall produces pneumatosis intestinalis, the pathognomonic radiological sign. Portal venous gas indicates extensive disease. Grossly, affected bowel is distended, haemorrhagic, and friable. Perforation with pneumoperitoneum occurs in severe cases.

Breast milk feeding is the single most important protective factor, providing secretory IgA, lactoferrin, lysozyme, and prebiotic oligosaccharides that promote commensal colonisation. Probiotics have shown benefit in meta-analyses.

Hydrops Fetalis

Hydrops fetalis is defined as the accumulation of oedema fluid in two or more fetal body compartments (skin/subcutaneous tissue, pleural cavity, pericardium, peritoneum). It is classified as immune or non-immune.

Immune hydrops (erythroblastosis fetalis): Results from maternal alloantibodies (most commonly anti-D/Rh) crossing the placenta and causing haemolysis of fetal red blood cells. The Rh-negative mother is sensitised during a previous pregnancy with an Rh-positive fetus (fetomaternal haemorrhage at delivery). In subsequent Rh-positive pregnancies, maternal IgG anti-D antibodies cross the placenta and opsonise fetal RBCs for splenic destruction. The consequences include severe fetal anaemia, extramedullary haematopoiesis (hepatosplenomegaly, circulating erythroblasts), high-output cardiac failure, generalised oedema (hydrops), and hyperbilirubinaemia causing **kernicterus** (bilirubin encephalopathy with selective damage to basal ganglia, hippocampus, and brainstem nuclei). Administration of anti-D immunoglobulin (RhoGAM) to Rh-negative mothers at 28 weeks and within 72 hours of delivery has dramatically reduced the incidence of immune hydrops.

Non-immune hydrops: Now accounts for over 90% of hydrops cases. Causes include cardiovascular anomalies (the most common cause), chromosomal abnormalities (Turner syndrome/45,X with cystic hygroma; trisomy 21), fetal anaemia (alpha-thalassaemia, parvovirus B19 infection of erythroid precursors causing transient aplastic crisis), twin-to-twin transfusion syndrome, and congenital infections (TORCH, particularly syphilis and CMV).

When faced with a case of hydrops fetalis, the first question to ask is: is it immune or non-immune? Non-immune causes now predominate (>90%) due to anti-D prophylaxis, and a systematic evaluation of cardiac, chromosomal, haematological, and infectious causes is required.

Exam Pitfall: Hydrops Fetalis

Non-immune hydrops is now more common than immune hydrops due to anti-D prophylaxis. Do not default to "Rh incompatibility" as the answer for hydrops without considering the full differential.

Kernicterus (bilirubin encephalopathy) affects basal ganglia selectively, not the cerebral cortex. The unconjugated bilirubin crosses the blood-brain barrier in neonates because of immature BBB and low albumin binding capacity.

Parvovirus B19 causes hydrops by infecting erythroid precursors in the bone marrow (affinity for P antigen/globoside), not by haemolysis.

Hydrops workup: Maternal blood group + antibody screen → Positive = immune → Negative = non-immune → Karyotype/microarray + TORCH serology + Hb electrophoresis (α-thal) + Fetal echo + Kleihauer-Betke

The morphological assessment of hydrops fetalis at autopsy requires systematic evaluation. Fluid collections should be documented in all compartments. The placenta in immune hydrops is characteristically large, pale, and oedematous, with immature villi showing stromal oedema and erythroblastosis in fetal capillaries. In non-immune hydrops due to alpha-thalassaemia major (homozygous deletion of all four alpha-globin genes, Hb Barts hydrops fetalis), fetal blood contains predominantly Hb Barts (gamma-4 tetramers) with extremely high oxygen affinity, resulting in tissue hypoxia and high-output cardiac failure.

Parvovirus B19-associated hydrops is potentially reversible with intrauterine transfusion. The virus infects erythroid precursors via the P antigen (globoside) receptor, causing transient aplastic crisis. In the fetus, where red cell turnover is physiologically high, this rapidly produces severe anaemia. The characteristic finding is giant proerythroblasts with nuclear clearing and peripheral chromatin margination (lantern cells). IHC or in situ hybridisation for parvovirus B19 confirms the diagnosis.

Potter Sequence

Potter sequence (oligohydramnios sequence) results from severe, prolonged oligohydramnios (decreased amniotic fluid), regardless of the underlying cause. Amniotic fluid is essential for fetal lung development (fetal breathing movements), cushioning, and allowing fetal movement. The most common causes of oligohydramnios are bilateral renal agenesis (classic Potter sequence), urinary tract obstruction (posterior urethral valves), and chronic amniotic fluid leakage. The resulting phenotype includes: **pulmonary hypoplasia** (the most important and usually lethal consequence), flattened facies (Potter facies: receding chin, flattened nose, low-set ears), limb deformities from compression, and growth restriction. Death typically results from pulmonary insufficiency.

Sudden Infant Death Syndrome (SIDS)

SIDS is defined as the sudden unexpected death of an apparently healthy infant under 1 year of age that remains unexplained after a thorough investigation including a complete autopsy, death scene investigation, and review of clinical history. Peak incidence is 2 to 4 months of age. The "triple risk model" proposes that SIDS occurs at the intersection of three factors: (1) a vulnerable infant (brainstem abnormality in serotonergic neurons affecting cardiorespiratory control and arousal), (2) a critical developmental period, and (3) an exogenous stressor (prone sleeping position, overheating, co-sleeping, soft bedding). **The "Back to Sleep" campaign (supine sleeping position) has reduced SIDS incidence by over 50%.** Risk factors include prematurity, male sex, maternal smoking during pregnancy, and low socioeconomic status. Autopsy findings are characteristically subtle: petechiae on thymic, pleural, and pericardial surfaces are common but non-specific.

Integration: Neonatal RDS connects to respiratory pathology (Chapter 15 for adult RDS/ARDS comparison) and surfactant biology. Hydrops fetalis connects to haematopathology (Volume 1

for Rh isoimmunisation, thalassaemia) and genetic disorders (Chapter 8 for chromosomal abnormalities).

Diagnostic thinking: hyaline membranes + collapsed alveoli in premature neonate → NRDS (surfactant deficiency)

Tumours of Infancy and Childhood

Childhood tumours differ from adult cancers in several fundamental ways. Embryonal (blastoma) and mesenchymal tumours predominate, in contrast to the epithelial carcinomas that dominate adult oncology. Many childhood tumours are linked to developmental abnormalities or inherited predisposition syndromes. Leukaemias (particularly ALL) are the most common childhood malignancies overall (see Volume 1), followed by CNS tumours and lymphomas. Among solid organ tumours, the characteristic childhood neoplasms include neuroblastoma, Wilms tumour (nephroblastoma), retinoblastoma, hepatoblastoma, rhabdomyosarcoma, and Ewing sarcoma.

Small Round Blue Cell Tumours

The "small round blue cell tumour" (SRBCT) differential is one of the most important diagnostic challenges in paediatric pathology. These tumours share a morphological pattern of sheets of small, round cells with high nuclear-to-cytoplasmic ratio, hyperchromatic nuclei, and scant cytoplasm. Distinction requires IHC, cytogenetics, and molecular studies.

Tumour	Age/Site	Key IHC	Molecular/ Cytogenetic	Distinguishing Features
Neuroblastoma	Adrenal/ sympathetic chain; <5 yrs	NSE, chromogranin, synaptophysin; CD99 negative	MYCN amplification; 1p del; 17q gain	Homer-Wright rosettes, neuropil, ↑VMA/HVA
Wilms tumour	Kidney; 2–5 yrs	WT1+, PAX8+	WT1 mutation (11p13); WTX; CTNNB1	Triphasic: blastemal + epithelial + stromal
Ewing sarcoma	Bone (diaphysis), soft tissue; 10–20 yrs	CD99 (MIC2)+, NKX2.2+, FLI-1+	EWSR1-FLI1 t(11;22) (85%); EWSR1-ERG	Membranous CD99; PAS+ glycogen
Rhabdomyosarcoma	Head/neck, GU tract; <10 yrs	Desmin+, myogenin+, MyoD1+	PAX3-FOXO1 t(2;13) (alveolar RMS)	Cross-striations (rare); botryoid variant (grape-

				like)
Lymphoblastic lymphoma/ALL	Mediastinum, BM; children	TdT+, CD99+, CD10+	Various translocations (see Vol 1)	TdT is the key marker; see Volume 1
Medulloblastoma	Posterior fossa; <10 yrs	Synaptophysin+, NeuN+	WNT, SHH, Group 3, Group 4 molecular subgroups	Homer-Wright rosettes; see Chapter 30
Retinoblastoma	Eye; <3 yrs	Synaptophysin+, NSE+	RB1 biallelic inactivation (13q14)	Flexner-Wintersteiner rosettes (true rosettes)

Table 11.2: Small Round Blue Cell Tumours of Childhood: Differential Diagnosis

> **The Pathologist's Eye: Approaching the Small Round Blue Cell Tumour**
>
> When faced with a biopsy of a small round blue cell tumour in a child, the systematic approach begins with clinical context (age, site, imaging) and proceeds to a tiered IHC panel. Step 1: CD99 and TdT. If TdT+, think lymphoblastic lymphoma/ALL. If CD99 membranous positive and TdT negative, Ewing sarcoma is likely (confirm with EWSR1 FISH). Step 2: If CD99 negative, apply neuroendocrine markers (synaptophysin, chromogranin) for neuroblastoma, skeletal muscle markers (desmin, myogenin) for rhabdomyosarcoma, and WT1 for Wilms tumour. Step 3: Molecular confirmation is increasingly required for definitive diagnosis (EWSR1 rearrangement, MYCN amplification, PAX-FOXO1 fusion).

Neuroblastoma

Neuroblastoma is the most common extracranial solid tumour of childhood, arising from neural crest-derived cells of the sympathetic nervous system. The adrenal medulla is the most common primary site (40%), followed by extra-adrenal sympathetic ganglia (retroperitoneum, posterior mediastinum, neck, pelvis). The median age at diagnosis is 18 months. Neuroblastoma is remarkable for its clinical heterogeneity: it can undergo spontaneous regression (particularly in stage 4S disease in infants), mature into benign ganglioneuroma, or behave as an aggressively metastatic tumour.

Why can neuroblastoma spontaneously regress while most other childhood cancers cannot? Spontaneous regression in neuroblastoma (particularly stage 4S in infants under 18 months) involves delayed activation of apoptotic pathways normally active during sympathetic nervous system development. Neuroblasts with favourable biology (hyperdiploidy, whole-chromosome gains, no MYCN amplification) retain capacity for terminal differentiation or apoptosis. This underlies the paradox of stage 4S: despite widespread metastases to liver, skin, and bone marrow, the tumour may regress completely, representing one of the most striking examples of tumour biology dictating outcome.

Morphology: Classic neuroblastoma consists of small round blue cells forming Homer-Wright pseudorosettes (tumour cells surrounding a central core of neuropil, which is a tangle of neuritic processes; these are "pseudo" rosettes because there is no central lumen, unlike the true Flexner-Wintersteiner rosettes of retinoblastoma). The tumour cells may show variable differentiation toward ganglion cells. The Shimada classification (International Neuroblastoma Pathology Classification, INPC) categorises tumours by the amount of Schwannian stroma, degree of differentiation, mitosis-karyorrhexis index (MKI), and patient age into favourable and unfavourable histology groups.

Prognostic factors: The most important prognostic factors are: (1) **MYCN amplification** (present in 25 to 30% of cases; strongly adverse prognosis regardless of stage); (2) **Age at diagnosis** (<18 months favourable; >18 months unfavourable); (3) **Stage** (INRGSS staging system); (4) **Tumour ploidy** (hyperdiploidy/near-triploidy favourable in infants; diploidy/near-tetraploidy unfavourable); (5) **1p deletion and 17q gain** (adverse); (6) **Histology** (Shimada: favourable vs unfavourable). Elevated urinary catecholamine metabolites (VMA and HVA) are present in over 90% of cases and serve as useful tumour markers.

Wilms Tumour (Nephroblastoma)

Wilms tumour is the most common renal tumour of childhood, with peak incidence at 2 to 5 years. It arises from nephrogenic rests (persistent metanephric blastema), which are found in the adjacent kidney in 40% of unilateral and nearly 100% of bilateral cases. **The hallmark morphology is triphasic: blastemal (sheets of small blue cells), epithelial (tubular/glomeruloid structures), and stromal (fibroblastic, myxoid, skeletal muscle) components.** The proportion of each component varies, and blastemal predominance (particularly after chemotherapy) carries a worse prognosis.

Genetics: WT1 (11p13) is a tumour suppressor gene mutated in approximately 15 to 20% of sporadic Wilms tumours. WT1 mutations are associated with **WAGR syndrome** (Wilms tumour, Aniridia, Genitourinary anomalies, mental Retardation; 11p13 deletion) and **Denys-Drash syndrome** (Wilms tumour, diffuse mesangial sclerosis, male pseudohermaphroditism; WT1 point mutation). **Beckwith-Wiedemann syndrome** (11p15.5; IGF-2 overexpression due to loss of imprinting) carries a 5% risk of Wilms tumour and also predisposes to hepatoblastoma. CTNNB1 (beta-catenin) and WTX are other commonly mutated genes.

Retinoblastoma

Retinoblastoma is the most common intraocular malignancy of childhood, with peak incidence before 3 years. It arises from biallelic inactivation of RB1 on 13q14, making it the paradigmatic example of the Knudson two-hit hypothesis. Approximately 40% are hereditary (germline RB1 mutation), presenting with bilateral, multifocal tumours at younger age. Sporadic cases (60%) involve two somatic mutations and are unilateral.

Clinical Pearl

Bilateral or multifocal retinoblastoma means germline RB1 mutation until proven otherwise. The germline form (40% of cases) presents earlier, is bilateral or multifocal, and carries a 50% lifetime risk of second non-ocular primary malignancy: osteosarcoma is the most frequent (especially in the femur and tibia), followed by soft-tissue sarcomas, melanoma, and brain tumours. Sporadic somatic-only retinoblastoma (60%) is unilateral, presents later, and does not carry the same second-primary risk. The clinical implication is concrete: every bilateral retinoblastoma family needs RB1 germline testing, genetic counselling, and lifelong surveillance for sarcoma. The 'trilateral retinoblastoma' (bilateral retinoblastoma plus pinealoblastoma) is a rare but examined complication of germline RB1 loss.

Morphology: small round blue cells forming Flexner-Wintersteiner rosettes (true rosettes with a central lumen lined by photoreceptor-like cells) and Homer-Wright pseudorosettes (neuropil core without a lumen). Flexner-Wintersteiner rosettes are relatively specific for retinoblastoma. Fleurettes represent higher photoreceptor differentiation and indicate better prognosis. Calcification is common on CT.

Rosette distinctions: Flexner-Wintersteiner = true rosettes with central lumen (specific for retinoblastoma); Homer-Wright = neuropil core without lumen (shared with neuroblastoma, medulloblastoma); fleurettes = bouquet-like photoreceptor clusters (unique to retinoblastoma, better prognosis).

Hepatoblastoma

Hepatoblastoma is the most common primary hepatic malignancy of childhood, typically presenting before age 3 as an abdominal mass with markedly elevated AFP. It is associated with Beckwith-Wiedemann syndrome (11p15.5 imprinting abnormalities) and familial adenomatous polyposis (APC mutations). The epithelial component recapitulates hepatocyte development: fetal pattern (small uniform hepatocytes in thin trabeculae, most common and most favourable), embryonal pattern (less differentiated), and small cell undifferentiated pattern (worst prognosis).

Pure fetal histology with fewer than 2 mitoses per 10 HPF has excellent prognosis with surgery alone. The PRETEXT staging system guides planning. Cisplatin-based neoadjuvant chemotherapy has improved resectability.

Quick Recall: Childhood Tumours

Neuroblastoma: Adrenal/sympathetic chain; <5 yrs; Homer-Wright rosettes; MYCN amplification (worst prognosis); ↑VMA/HVA; can spontaneously regress (stage 4S).

Wilms tumour: Kidney; 2–5 yrs; triphasic (blastemal + epithelial + stromal); WT1 (WAGR, Denys-Drash); Beckwith-Wiedemann (IGF2).

Retinoblastoma: Eye; <3 yrs; Flexner-Wintersteiner rosettes (true); RB1 biallelic loss (13q14); bilateral = germline.

Ewing sarcoma: Bone (diaphysis); 10–20 yrs; EWSR1-FLI1 t(11;22); CD99 membranous+; NKX2.2+; PAS+ glycogen.

Rhabdomyosarcoma: Head/neck, GU; <10 yrs; desmin+, myogenin+; alveolar RMS = PAX3-FOXO1 t(2;13), worse prognosis.

Hepatoblastoma: Liver; <3 yrs; ↑AFP; associated with Beckwith-Wiedemann and FAP.

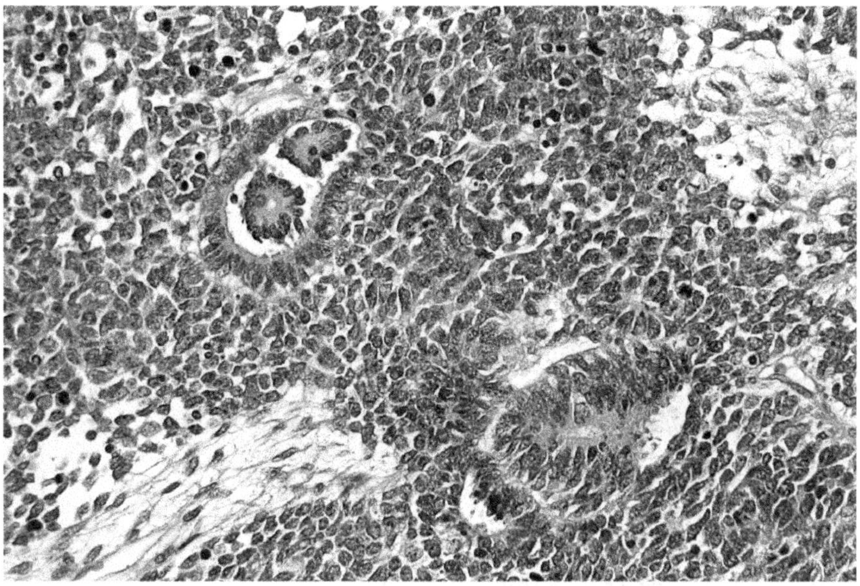

Figure 11.3: Wilms tumour showing triphasic pattern with blastemal, epithelial, and stromal components (H&E, ×200). (Source: Wikimedia Commons, CC BY-SA 3.0.)

International Neuroblastoma Pathology Classification (INPC / Shimada System)

The INPC, derived from the Shimada classification, stratifies neuroblastic tumours by age, histological differentiation, mitosis-karyorrhexis index (MKI), and Schwannian stromal development. It assigns tumours to "favourable" or "unfavourable" histology categories that drive risk stratification together with stage, MYCN status, and ploidy.

Table 11.2a: INPC Classification of Peripheral Neuroblastic Tumours

Category	Histology	Typical age / Prognosis
Neuroblastoma (Schwannian stroma-	Undifferentiated / poorly differentiated / differentiating. MKI graded low	Commonest form. Favourable/unfavourable

poor)	(<100/5000), intermediate (100–200/5000), high (>200/5000).	depends on age + differentiation + MKI (e.g., <1.5 yr + differentiating + low MKI = favourable).
Ganglioneuroblastoma, intermixed (Schwannian stroma-rich)	Well-developed Schwannian stroma (>50%) with microscopic foci of neuroblasts intermixed.	Always favourable histology.
Ganglioneuroblastoma, nodular (composite, stroma-rich/stroma-dominant and stroma-poor)	Macroscopic nodules of stroma-poor neuroblastoma within ganglioneuroma/ganglioneuroblastoma-intermixed background.	Favourable or unfavourable based on INPC rules applied to the nodule.
Ganglioneuroma (Schwannian stroma-dominant)	Maturing (scattered mature ganglion cells in stroma) or mature (only mature ganglion cells, no neuroblasts).	Always favourable histology; typically cured by resection.

Favourable vs unfavourable assignment, combined with stage (INRGSS: L1, L2, M, MS) and molecular markers (MYCN amplification — unfavourable; 11q aberration; DNA ploidy in infants), determines treatment intensity. MYCN amplification almost always = unfavourable outcome regardless of histology. Exam point: the four INPC categories and the MYCN/age axis together are the most frequently asked neuroblastoma prognostic concepts.

Wilms Tumour — SIOP vs COG Approach and WHO Histological Classification

Wilms tumour (nephroblastoma) has two parallel treatment protocols internationally. Both achieve excellent outcomes (>90% overall survival for favourable-histology tumours) but approach the tumour differently.

Table 11.3a: SIOP vs COG Approach to Wilms Tumour

Aspect	SIOP (Europe / most of world including India)	COG (North America)
Initial diagnosis	Radiological diagnosis; pre-operative chemotherapy without biopsy	Pre-treatment biopsy or upfront nephrectomy
Sequence	Pre-op chemo (4–6 weeks) → nephrectomy → post-op chemo ± RT	Upfront nephrectomy → staging → post-op chemo ± RT (biopsy first if unresectable)
Staging moment	Post-chemotherapy (at nephrectomy	Pre-treatment (at nephrectomy

	specimen)	specimen)
Histological risk stratification	Low risk / intermediate risk / high risk (assessed on post-chemo specimen — accounts for chemo-induced changes including blastemal regression)	Favourable histology / unfavourable histology (anaplasia focal or diffuse)
Key prognostic factor	Blastemal predominance after chemotherapy = high-risk (chemoresistant blastema)	Diffuse anaplasia = unfavourable histology

Under the WHO Classification of Tumours (Urinary and Male Genital Organs, 5th edition, 2022), childhood renal tumours include: Wilms tumour (nephroblastoma — most common, triphasic blastemal/epithelial/stromal), clear cell sarcoma of kidney (CCSK — "bone metastasising tumour of childhood"), malignant rhabdoid tumour of kidney (SMARCB1/INI1 loss — worst prognosis), congenital mesoblastic nephroma (most common renal tumour under 3 months — classical and cellular variants; cellular = ETV6-NTRK3 fusion, same as infantile fibrosarcoma), and metanephric tumours (adenoma/adenofibroma/stromal tumour).

In low- and middle-income settings: Wilms remains the most common renal malignancy of childhood; SIOP protocol predominates. Bilateral disease (~5%) mandates nephron-sparing surgery. WAGR syndrome (WT1 deletion 11p13), Denys-Drash (WT1 missense), and Beckwith-Wiedemann (11p15 IGF2) are the classic predisposing syndromes — all exam-testable.

Integration: Paediatric tumour genetics connects to Knudson two-hit hypothesis and tumour suppressor biology (Chapter 6), MYCN and oncogene biology (Chapter 6), Beckwith-Wiedemann and genomic imprinting (Chapter 8), and familial cancer syndromes (Chapter 7). Retinoblastoma is the prototype for inherited cancer predisposition. TORCH infections link to Chapter 9 (organism-specific pathogenesis) and Chapter 30 (CNS manifestations). Hydrops connects to haemolytic disease (Volume 1) and cardiovascular pathology (Chapter 14).

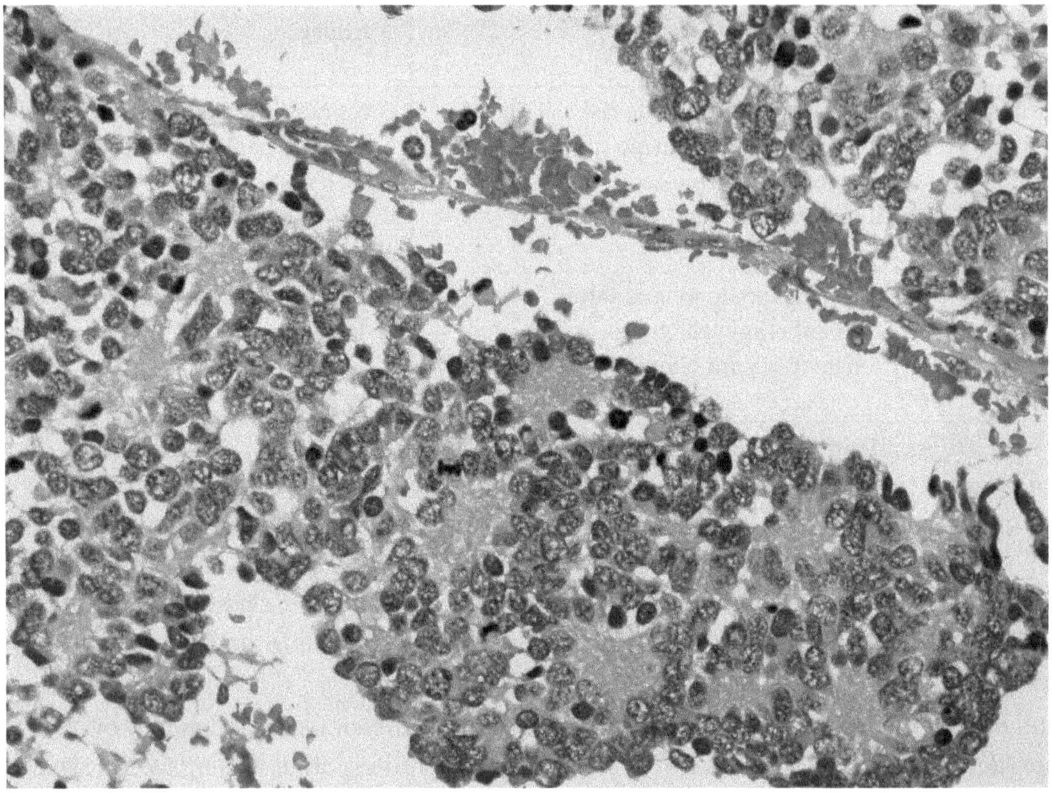

Figure 11.4: Neuroblastoma: Homer-Wright pseudorosettes with central neuropil core surrounded by small round blue cells. H&E. (Source: Wikimedia Commons, CC BY-SA 3.0.)

Recent Advances

International incidence of childhood cancer (IICC-3, 2001–10). The third International Incidence of Childhood Cancer study reported population-based incidence rates for cancer in children and adolescents from 153 cancer registries across 62 countries, covering 2001–10 (Steliarova-Foucher et al. The Lancet Oncology 2017; 18: 719–731; PMID 28410997). Among children aged 0–14 years, the worldwide age-standardised incidence rate was 140.6 per million person-years; among adolescents aged 15–19 years, 185.3 per million person-years. The leading childhood cancers globally were leukaemias (46.4 per million), central nervous system tumours (28.2 per million), and lymphomas (15.2 per million); among adolescents, lymphomas (37.9 per million) and epithelial tumours and melanoma (33.6 per million) led the distribution. Substantial geographic variation was documented, including higher rates in high-income regions and incomplete ascertainment in low-income registries, with implications for case-finding and survival reporting. The IICC-3 dataset is the principal international reference for paediatric oncology epidemiology and underpins WHO and IARC priority-setting in childhood cancer.

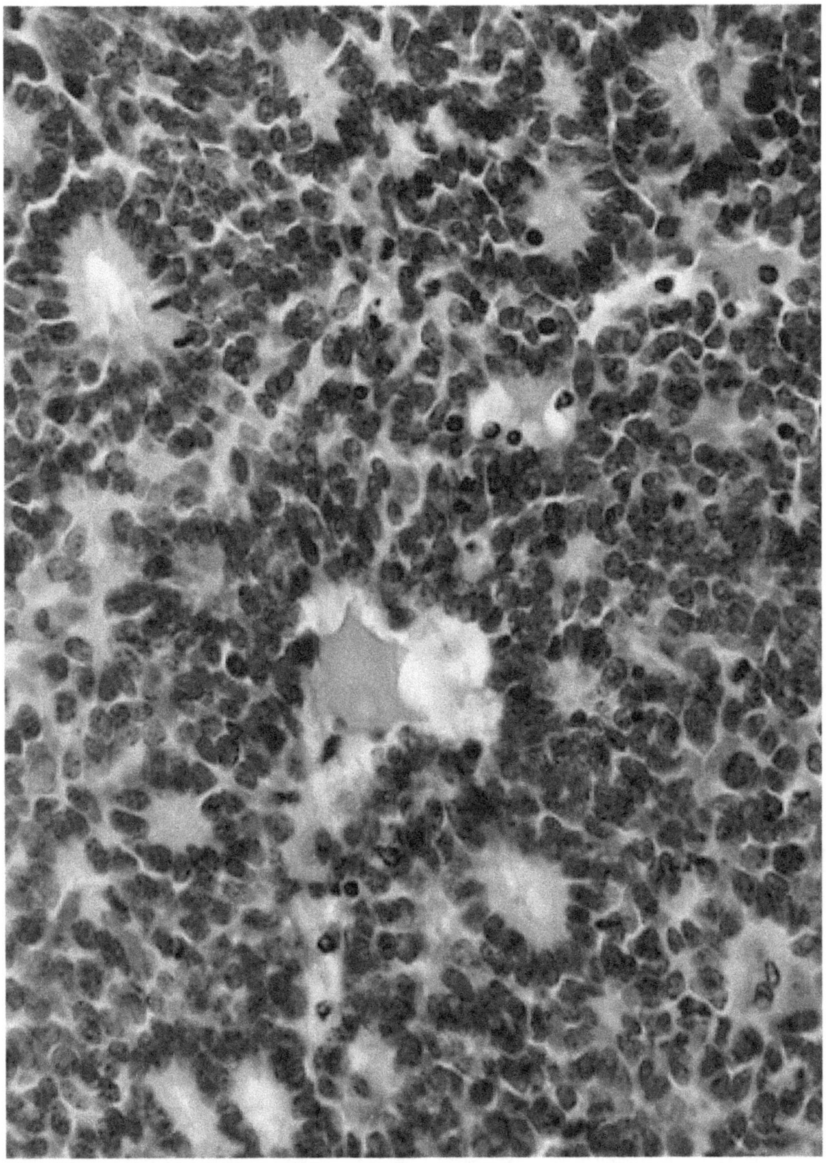

Figure 11.5: Retinoblastoma: Flexner-Wintersteiner rosettes (true rosettes) with central lumen lined by tumour cells. H&E. (Source: Wikimedia Commons, CC BY-SA 3.0.)

Molecular classification of paediatric cancers: The WHO 5th Edition Classification of Tumours has increasingly integrated molecular markers into the classification of childhood tumours. Medulloblastoma is now classified into four molecular subgroups (WNT, SHH, Group 3, Group 4) with distinct prognoses and therapeutic implications. Ewing sarcoma-like tumours with non-EWSR1 fusions (e.g., CIC-DUX4, BCOR-CCNB3) are recognised as distinct entities. Infant-type hemispheric gliomas harbouring ALK, ROS1, NTRK, or MET fusions are now distinguished from adult diffuse gliomas and are amenable to targeted therapy.

Liquid biopsy in paediatric oncology: Cell-free DNA (cfDNA) and circulating tumour DNA (ctDNA) are being evaluated for non-invasive monitoring of minimal residual disease and treatment response in neuroblastoma, Ewing sarcoma, and paediatric brain tumours. Detection of MYCN amplification in cfDNA has shown promise as a prognostic biomarker in neuroblastoma.

Newborn screening expansion: Programmes such as India's Rashtriya Bal Swasthya Karyakram (RBSK) are expanding newborn screening for inborn errors of metabolism in low- and middle-income settings. Tandem mass spectrometry-based screening can detect over 40 metabolic disorders from a dried blood spot, enabling early intervention before irreversible organ damage occurs. Several states have begun implementing universal newborn screening programmes.

Newborn screening (NBS) in low- and middle-income countries: pilot programmes using tandem mass spectrometry (covering 30 to 50 inborn errors of metabolism) are operational in selected tertiary centres. Universal implementation remains challenging due to infrastructure, cost, and follow-up logistics. Most national paediatric societies recommend at least congenital hypothyroidism, hearing loss, and critical congenital heart disease as priority screens.

Precision medicine in paediatric oncology: ALK inhibitors (crizotinib, lorlatinib) for ALK-amplified neuroblastoma and larotrectinib/entrectinib for NTRK fusion-positive infantile fibrosarcoma represent paradigmatic examples of precision oncology in children. The Pediatric MATCH trial has demonstrated that molecularly matched therapies produce responses in heavily pre-treated patients. In low- and middle-income settings, comprehensive genomic panels for paediatric solid tumours are progressively becoming available at major cancer centres.

Liquid biopsy in paediatric oncology: cfDNA and ctDNA are being evaluated for non-invasive monitoring of minimal residual disease, treatment response, and relapse detection. These approaches are attractive because they reduce the need for repeated tissue biopsies in young children. Methylation-based classification of paediatric CNS tumours (Heidelberg classifier) is transforming diagnostic accuracy and enabling identification of novel molecular subgroups with distinct biology and outcomes (see Chapter 30).

Ultra High-Yield Chapter Summary

Topic	Must Remember
Malformation vs disruption vs deformation	Malformation: intrinsic error. Disruption: destruction of normal structure. Deformation: mechanical forces.
Embryonic period	Weeks 3–8: maximal teratogenic susceptibility (organogenesis). <2 weeks: all-or-none
CMV (congenital)	Most common congenital infection; owl-eye inclusions; periventricular calcifications; hearing loss = most common sequela
Toxoplasma	Diffuse intracranial calcifications (vs periventricular in CMV);

	chorioretinitis; hydrocephalus
Congenital syphilis	Hutchinson triad (late): interstitial keratitis + Hutchinson teeth + 8th nerve deafness
Neonatal RDS	Surfactant deficiency (type II pneumocyte immaturity); hyaline membranes; prevention: maternal corticosteroids
L/S ratio	≥2 = lung maturity. Phosphatidylglycerol confirms.
NEC	Most common GI emergency in prematures; pneumatosis intestinalis; mucosal ischaemia + bacteria + formula
Hydrops: immune	Anti-D (Rh) antibodies; haemolysis; kernicterus (basal ganglia).
Hydrops: non-immune	>90% of cases now; cardiovascular anomalies (most common cause); Turner 45,X; parvovirus B19; thalassaemia
Potter sequence	Oligohydramnios → pulmonary hypoplasia (lethal) + flattened facies + limb defects.
SIDS	Peak 2–4 months; triple risk model; Back to Sleep reduced incidence >50%; brainstem serotonergic abnormality
Neuroblastoma	Most common extracranial solid tumour; adrenal; MYCN amplification (worst prognosis); ↑VMA/HVA; Homer-Wright rosettes
Wilms tumour	Most common renal tumour in children; triphasic; WT1 (WAGR, Denys-Drash); Beckwith-Wiedemann (IGF2)
Retinoblastoma	RB1 biallelic loss; Flexner-Wintersteiner rosettes; bilateral = germline mutation
SRBCT approach	CD99/TdT first → TdT+ = ALL; CD99+ TdT− = Ewing; then neuroendocrine (neuroblastoma), muscle (RMS), WT1 (Wilms)

Table 11.3: Ultra High-Yield Chapter Summary

Diagnostic thinking: small round blue cells + rosettes + childhood tumour → SRBCT differential (neuroblastoma, Wilms, Ewing, rhabdomyosarcoma, lymphoma)

Diagnostic thinking: abdominal mass + elevated urinary VMA/HVA + N-MYC amplification → neuroblastoma (poor prognosis if N-MYC amplified)

Chapter 12: Ageing and Degenerative Disease

THE BIG PICTURE

Ageing is not merely the passage of time; it is a biological process driven by the progressive accumulation of cellular and molecular damage. The hallmarks of ageing, from telomere attrition to cellular senescence, mitochondrial dysfunction, and stem cell exhaustion, converge to produce the functional decline and increased disease susceptibility that define old age. Degenerative diseases, including Alzheimer disease, osteoporosis, osteoarthritis, and atherosclerosis, are not inevitable consequences of ageing but rather result from the interaction between ageing biology and genetic susceptibility, environmental factors, and cumulative cellular stress. This chapter provides the conceptual framework that underpins the age-related pathology discussed in detail across the systemic pathology chapters.

High-yield topics in this chapter: Hallmarks of ageing (telomere attrition, cellular senescence, SASP, stem cell exhaustion, epigenetic changes, mitochondrial dysfunction); progeroid syndromes (Werner, Hutchinson-Gilford); telomerase in health and disease; mechanisms that counteract ageing; overview of major degenerative diseases.

Every cell carries within it a record of its history. Shortened telomeres mark the number of divisions endured, epigenetic modifications reflect environmental insults accumulated over decades, and damaged mitochondria bear witness to a lifetime of oxidative stress. Ageing is not a single disease but a convergence of molecular processes that, when understood, illuminate the pathogenesis of the most common diseases of modern medicine. For the pathologist, understanding the biology of ageing is essential for interpreting age-related changes in tissue specimens, distinguishing pathology from physiological involution, and appreciating the molecular mechanisms now being targeted by anti-ageing therapeutics.

The Biology of Ageing

Contemporary understanding of ageing is organised around nine interconnected **hallmarks of ageing** (López-Otín et al., initially described in 2013 and expanded to 12 hallmarks in 2023). These hallmarks can be grouped into three categories: primary (causative) hallmarks that generate damage, antagonistic hallmarks that represent responses to damage, and integrative hallmarks that reflect the functional consequences.

Telomere Attrition

Telomeres are repetitive nucleotide sequences (TTAGGG in humans) capping chromosome ends, protected by the shelterin protein complex. With each cell division, 50 to 200 base pairs of telomeric DNA are lost because of the end-replication problem (DNA polymerase cannot fully replicate the 3' end of the lagging strand). When telomeres shorten to a critical length, the shelterin complex is disrupted, exposed

DNA ends activate the DNA damage response (ATM/ATR kinases → p53 → p21), and the cell enters replicative senescence (the Hayflick limit). This mechanism functions as a biological clock limiting the proliferative lifespan of somatic cells.

Telomerase is a ribonucleoprotein enzyme (with a catalytic subunit, TERT, and an RNA template component, TERC) that adds telomeric repeats to chromosome ends, counteracting the end-replication problem. Telomerase is active in germ cells, stem cells, and most cancer cells, but is silenced in the majority of somatic cells. Reactivation of telomerase is one of the hallmarks of cancer (see Chapter 6), enabling unlimited replicative potential. Conversely, inherited mutations in telomere maintenance genes (TERT, TERC, DKC1, RTEL1) cause the **telomeropathies**: a spectrum of premature ageing diseases including dyskeratosis congenita, aplastic anaemia, idiopathic pulmonary fibrosis, and liver cirrhosis (see Volume 1 for bone marrow failure syndromes).

Clinical Pearl

Hayflick limit and the three exceptions. In 1961 Leonard Hayflick observed that normal human fibroblasts in culture divide approximately 40 to 60 times before entering replicative senescence. This ceiling, the Hayflick limit, is set by telomere attrition. Three cell types bypass it by expressing telomerase: germ cells (lifelong telomere maintenance to allow species continuity), stem cells (sufficient telomerase activity to support tissue renewal but not enough to escape senescence entirely), and approximately 90% of cancer cells (reactivated telomerase, often through TERT promoter mutations, granting limitless replicative potential). The clinical mirror image is two-sided: telomerase loss-of-function produces telomeropathies, including dyskeratosis congenita and idiopathic pulmonary fibrosis (see Volume 1); telomerase reactivation drives most human cancers. Both ends of the spectrum are postgraduate-examined.

Cell division → Telomere shortening (50–200 bp/division) → Critical length → Shelterin loss → DDR activation (ATM/p53/p21) → Replicative senescence or apoptosis

Cellular Senescence and the SASP

Cellular senescence is a state of irreversible cell cycle arrest triggered by telomere attrition (replicative senescence), oncogene activation (oncogene-induced senescence, e.g., RAS), DNA damage, oxidative stress, or mitochondrial dysfunction. Senescent cells are characterised by: (1) stable cell cycle arrest mediated by the p53/p21 and p16INK4a/Rb pathways; (2) resistance to apoptosis; (3) morphological changes (enlarged, flattened cells); and (4) senescence-associated beta-galactosidase (SA-β-gal) activity at pH 6.0 (a common laboratory marker).

The most important consequence of senescent cell accumulation is the **senescence-associated secretory phenotype (SASP)**. Senescent cells secrete a complex mixture of pro-inflammatory cytokines (IL-1, IL-6, IL-8), chemokines, growth factors, matrix metalloproteinases, and extracellular vesicles. The SASP has both beneficial and detrimental effects. Acutely, SASP promotes wound healing, tissue remodelling, and tumour suppression (by recruiting immune cells to clear pre-neoplastic senescent cells). Chronically, however, accumulated senescent cells and their SASP create a persistent pro-inflammatory microenvironment ("inflammaging") that promotes tissue dysfunction, fibrosis, and paradoxically, tumorigenesis through paracrine effects on neighbouring cells.

The pathogenesis explains the paradox: cellular senescence is a tumour suppressor mechanism in young organisms (stopping damaged cells from dividing), but the accumulation of senescent cells and their SASP in aged tissues becomes a driver of the very diseases it was designed to prevent.

Clinical Pearl

The senescence paradox is examined as a viva favourite. The same biological process that protects young tissue from cancer drives ageing-related disease in old tissue. In youth, cells with damaged DNA or oncogenic stress are forced into permanent arrest, halting tumour formation. In age, these arrested cells accumulate, secrete the SASP (IL-1, IL-6, IL-8, MMPs), and drive chronic inflammation, fibrosis, and paradoxically tumorigenesis in surrounding tissue. This is antagonistic pleiotropy in cellular biology: a trait selected for early-life benefit becomes detrimental late in life. The therapeutic consequence is the senolytic concept: clearing senescent cells in old tissue removes the SASP-driven damage without losing the tumour-suppressor benefit, because by old age the original protective role has already been served.

Other Hallmarks of Ageing

Mitochondrial dysfunction: Ageing is associated with progressive accumulation of mitochondrial DNA (mtDNA) mutations, decline in electron transport chain efficiency, and increased reactive oxygen species (ROS) production. The "free radical theory of ageing" (Harman, 1956) proposed that cumulative oxidative damage to DNA, proteins, and lipids drives ageing. While this remains an important contributory mechanism, it is now understood that the relationship between ROS and ageing is more nuanced: moderate ROS serve as signalling molecules (hormesis), and antioxidant supplementation trials have not consistently extended lifespan.

Stem cell exhaustion: The regenerative capacity of tissues depends on resident stem cell populations. With ageing, stem cells decline in number and function due to accumulated DNA damage, epigenetic drift, niche deterioration, and SASP-mediated paracrine signalling. This manifests as impaired wound healing, reduced haematopoietic reserve (contributing to anaemia and immunosenescence), decreased intestinal epithelial regeneration, and grey hair (melanocyte stem cell loss).

Epigenetic alterations: Ageing is accompanied by global changes in DNA methylation (both gain and loss at specific loci), histone modifications, and chromatin remodelling. These changes alter gene expression patterns and contribute to cellular dysfunction. The remarkable predictability of age-related DNA methylation changes at specific CpG sites has enabled the development of "epigenetic clocks" (e.g., the Horvath clock), which can estimate biological age from DNA methylation patterns with high accuracy.

Altered intercellular communication: "Inflammaging" is the chronic, sterile, low-grade inflammation that characterises ageing, driven by SASP, gut microbiome changes, and accumulation of damage-associated molecular patterns (DAMPs) from dying cells. Immunosenescence (decline in adaptive immune function, particularly T-cell diversity and function) increases susceptibility to infections and reduces cancer immunosurveillance.

Other hallmarks include genomic instability (accumulation of DNA damage from endogenous and exogenous sources), loss of proteostasis (decline in protein quality control by ubiquitin-proteasome system and autophagy), disabled macroautophagy (impaired clearance of damaged organelles and aggregated proteins), and dysbiosis (age-related changes in gut microbiome composition) (Figure 12.1).

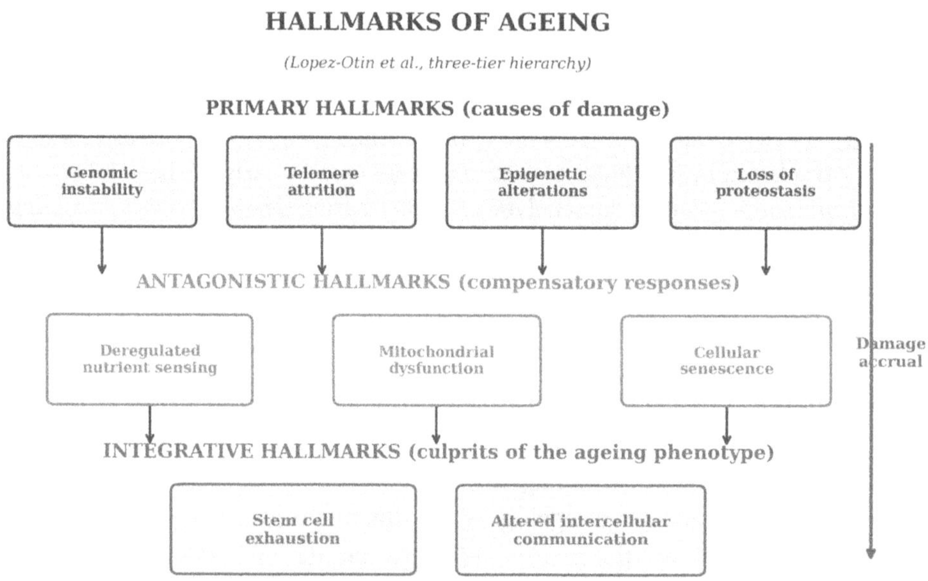

Figure 12.1: The hallmarks of ageing organised in three tiers: primary hallmarks (genomic instability, telomere attrition, epigenetic alterations, loss of proteostasis), antagonistic hallmarks (deregulated nutrient sensing, mitochondrial dysfunction, cellular senescence), and integrative hallmarks (stem cell exhaustion, altered intercellular communication). (Source: Author's original.)

Quick Recall: Biology of Ageing

Telomere attrition: 50–200 bp lost per division; critical shortening → DDR (ATM/p53/p21) → senescence. Telomerase (TERT + TERC) active in germ/stem/cancer cells.

Cellular senescence: Irreversible arrest via p53/p21 and p16INK4a/Rb. SA-β-gal marker.

SASP paradox: Acutely beneficial (wound healing, tumour clearance); chronically detrimental (inflammation, fibrosis, tumorigenesis).

Mitochondrial: mtDNA mutations accumulate; ↑ROS; free radical theory is contributory but not sole mechanism.

Stem cell exhaustion: Impaired wound healing, ↓haematopoietic reserve, immunosenescence, grey hair.

Epigenetic clocks: DNA methylation patterns predict biological age (Horvath clock); epigenetic drift with ageing.

Progeroid Syndromes

Progeroid (premature ageing) syndromes are rare genetic disorders that recapitulate features of normal ageing at an accelerated rate. They provide critical insights into ageing mechanisms.

Syndrome	Gene/Defect	Key Features	Mechanism
Hutchinson-Gilford Progeria	LMNA (lamin A); produces progerin (truncated lamin A)	Onset in infancy; growth failure, alopecia, loss of subcutaneous fat, atherosclerosis; death by 13–15 yrs (MI/stroke)	Progerin disrupts nuclear lamina → nuclear membrane instability, genomic instability, impaired DNA repair, altered gene expression
Werner Syndrome	WRN (RecQ helicase)	"Progeria of adulthood"; onset in 20s; cataracts, greying, skin atrophy, atherosclerosis, diabetes, cancer predisposition; death by 40–50 yrs	Defective DNA repair (especially DSB repair via WRN helicase) → genomic instability, accelerated telomere shortening
Cockayne Syndrome	CSA/CSB (transcription-coupled NER)	Dwarfism, photosensitivity, progressive neurological degeneration, cataracts	Defective repair of transcription-blocking DNA lesions
Ataxia-Telangiectasia	ATM (DNA damage sensor)	Cerebellar ataxia, telangiectasias, immunodeficiency, cancer predisposition (lymphomas, leukaemias)	Defective DDR signalling; impaired cell cycle checkpoint activation

Table 12.1: Progeroid Syndromes

Hutchinson-Gilford progeria syndrome (HGPS) deserves special attention because of its dramatic phenotype and the insights it has provided into normal ageing. The disease is caused by a de novo point mutation in *LMNA* (G608G, C→T), which creates an abnormal splice site producing a truncated lamin A protein called progerin. Progerin accumulates in the nuclear lamina, distorting nuclear morphology, impairing DNA repair, disrupting heterochromatin organisation, and activating NF-κB signalling (contributing to a pro-inflammatory state). Importantly, progerin has been detected at low levels in normal aged cells, suggesting that the same pathogenic mechanism operates in physiological ageing, albeit more slowly. Lonafarnib, a farnesyltransferase inhibitor that prevents progerin from anchoring to the nuclear membrane, was the first FDA-approved treatment for HGPS.

The diagnostic thinking line here is: if premature ageing syndromes recapitulate features of normal ageing, then studying these rare disorders illuminates the fundamental mechanisms that drive ageing in everyone. Progerin in progeria parallels the telomere attrition, genomic instability, and inflammaging of normal ageing.

> **Exam Pitfall: Progeroid Syndromes**
>
> Hutchinson-Gilford progeria (LMNA/progerin) causes accelerated atherosclerosis and cardiovascular death in children, but does NOT increase cancer risk (cells senesce too rapidly). Werner syndrome (WRN helicase) causes BOTH accelerated ageing AND cancer predisposition (sarcomas, thyroid cancer, melanoma). This distinction is exam-relevant.
>
> Do not confuse the progeroid syndromes with the segmental progeria seen in Down syndrome (trisomy 21), which shows accelerated Alzheimer-type neuropathology due to the APP gene (chromosome 21) dosage effect.

Mechanisms That Counteract Ageing

The principal mechanisms are:

1. DNA repair systems: Base excision repair (BER), nucleotide excision repair (NER), mismatch repair (MMR), and homologous recombination (HR) collectively maintain genomic integrity. Their decline with age contributes to mutation accumulation. Progeroid syndromes caused by DNA repair defects (Werner, Cockayne, AT) demonstrate the critical importance of these pathways in counteracting ageing.

2. Autophagy: Macroautophagy is the cellular self-eating mechanism that clears damaged organelles (mitophagy for mitochondria), aggregated proteins, and intracellular debris. Autophagy declines with age, contributing to accumulation of dysfunctional mitochondria and protein aggregates (relevant to Alzheimer and Parkinson disease). Caloric restriction, the most robust intervention known to extend lifespan in multiple organisms, acts in part by upregulating autophagy through AMPK activation and mTOR inhibition.

3. Proteostasis network: The ubiquitin-proteasome system (UPS) and heat shock proteins (chaperones including HSP70, HSP90) maintain protein quality control. Decline in proteostasis with age leads to accumulation of misfolded and aggregated proteins, a central feature of neurodegenerative diseases (amyloid-beta and tau in Alzheimer disease, alpha-synuclein in Parkinson disease).

4. Nutrient sensing pathways: The insulin/IGF-1 signalling pathway, mTOR, AMPK, and sirtuins (SIRT1–7) are key nutrient sensors that regulate cellular metabolism, growth, and stress resistance. Reduced insulin/IGF-1 signalling extends lifespan in model organisms. mTOR inhibition (by rapamycin) and AMPK activation (by metformin) have been shown to extend lifespan in animal models and are under investigation in human clinical trials (e.g., the TAME trial for metformin).

Caloric restriction → ↑AMPK, ↓mTOR, ↑Sirtuins, ↑Autophagy → Improved proteostasis + Reduced inflammation + Enhanced DNA repair → Extended healthspan

Why is caloric restriction effective across species? The answer lies in evolutionary logic. When food is scarce, organisms that divert resources from growth and reproduction toward somatic maintenance and repair survive to reproduce when conditions improve. The molecular mediators of this response, AMPK, sirtuins, and reduced mTOR signalling, are evolutionarily conserved from yeast to humans. Metformin, an AMPK activator used for type 2 diabetes, is now being tested in the TAME (Targeting Aging with Metformin) trial as a potential geroprotective agent in humans. Rapamycin (sirolimus), an mTOR inhibitor, consistently extends lifespan in mice but carries immunosuppressive side effects that limit clinical translation.

5. Antioxidant defences: Superoxide dismutase (SOD), catalase, glutathione peroxidase, and non-enzymatic antioxidants (vitamins C and E, glutathione) neutralise reactive oxygen species. While their decline with age contributes to oxidative damage, supplementation trials with exogenous antioxidants have been largely disappointing, supporting the view that ROS-mediated ageing is more complex than simple oxidative damage accumulation (see Chapter 10 for free radical biology).

Integration: Telomere biology connects to Chapter 1 (cell death and senescence), Chapter 6 (telomerase in cancer), and Volume 1 (telomeropathies/bone marrow failure). DNA repair defects connect to Chapter 8 (genetic disorders). Neurodegenerative diseases are detailed in Chapter 30.

Quick Recall: Mechanisms That Counteract Ageing

Caloric restriction: ↑AMPK, ↓mTOR, ↑sirtuins, ↑autophagy → extended healthspan (conserved yeast to humans). Sirtuins (SIRT1–7): NAD+-dependent deacetylases; SIRT1 stabilises genome, SIRT3 protects mitochondria. mTOR inhibition (rapamycin): extends lifespan in mice; TAME trial testing metformin in humans. Antioxidant defences: SOD, catalase, glutathione peroxidase; exogenous supplementation trials disappointing. Autophagy: clears damaged organelles and aggregated proteins; decline with age contributes to proteotoxicity.

Major Age-Related Degenerative Diseases: Overview

The degenerative diseases of ageing are covered in detail in their respective systemic pathology chapters. This section provides a brief overview of the shared pathological themes, with cross-references.

Disease	Key Pathological Mechanism	Ageing Hallmark(s) Involved	Detailed Coverage
Alzheimer disease	Aβ amyloid plaques + hyperphosphorylated tau (neurofibrillary tangles) → neuronal loss	Loss of proteostasis, inflammaging, epigenetic changes	Chapter 30
Parkinson disease	α-synuclein aggregation (Lewy bodies) in substantia nigra → dopaminergic neuron loss	Loss of proteostasis, mitochondrial dysfunction, impaired	Chapter 30

		autophagy	
Atherosclerosis	Lipid accumulation + chronic inflammation + endothelial dysfunction → plaque formation	Cellular senescence (of endothelial/VSMCs), inflammaging, clonal haematopoiesis	Chapter 13
Osteoporosis	Imbalance: ↑osteoclast resorption > ↓osteoblast formation → reduced bone mass with normal mineralisation	Stem cell exhaustion (MSCs), hormonal decline (oestrogen), inflammaging	Chapter 29
Osteoarthritis	Progressive cartilage degradation + subchondral bone remodelling; chondrocyte senescence	Cellular senescence (chondrocytes), mechanical wear, SASP	Chapter 29
Type 2 diabetes	Insulin resistance + β-cell failure; islet amyloid (IAPP) deposition	Mitochondrial dysfunction, inflammaging, loss of proteostasis	Chapter 27
Age-related macular degeneration	Drusen (lipid-protein deposits) under RPE → RPE atrophy (dry) or choroidal neovascularisation (wet)	Genomic instability, inflammaging, complement dysregulation	Ophthalmology
Benign prostatic hyperplasia	Dihydrotestosterone-driven stromal and glandular hyperplasia	Hormonal changes, altered androgen metabolism	Chapter 24

Table 12.2: Major Age-Related Degenerative Diseases and Their Ageing Hallmarks

A unifying theme across age-related degenerative diseases is the role of **protein aggregation and loss of proteostasis**. Alzheimer disease (amyloid-beta, tau), Parkinson disease (alpha-synuclein), type 2 diabetes (IAPP/amylin), and systemic amyloidosis (transthyretin in senile/wild-type ATTR amyloidosis) all involve the accumulation of misfolded proteins that overwhelm the cell's quality control mechanisms. This convergence is not coincidental; the age-related decline in autophagy, proteasomal function, and chaperone activity creates a permissive environment for protein aggregation pathology.

The Pathologist's Eye: Age-Related Changes vs Disease

The pathologist must distinguish physiological age-related changes from disease. Lipofuscin accumulation ("wear-and-tear pigment") in myocardial and hepatic cells is a normal ageing finding. Mild cerebral cortical atrophy with compensatory ventricular enlargement (hydrocephalus ex vacuo) is normal in the elderly. A few senile (neuritic) plaques and neurofibrillary tangles in the hippocampus may be seen in cognitively intact elderly individuals. The diagnosis of Alzheimer disease requires correlation between the burden of pathology (Braak staging for tangles, CERAD/Thal staging for plaques) and the clinical history of cognitive decline. Pathology without symptoms is not the same as disease.

Quick Recall: Age-Related Diseases

Protein aggregation diseases: Aβ/tau (Alzheimer), α-synuclein (Parkinson), IAPP (T2DM), TTR (senile amyloidosis). All reflect loss of proteostasis.

Inflammaging: Chronic low-grade inflammation driven by SASP + gut dysbiosis + DAMPs; underlies atherosclerosis, T2DM, neurodegeneration.

Lipofuscin: "Wear-and-tear" pigment; undigested lipid-protein residue in lysosomes; marker of ageing, NOT disease.

HGPS: LMNA mutation → progerin; nuclear lamina disruption; atherosclerosis in childhood; NO cancer. Lonafarnib = treatment.

Werner syndrome: WRN helicase; adult-onset; ageing + CANCER predisposition (sarcomas, thyroid ca) (Figure 12.2).

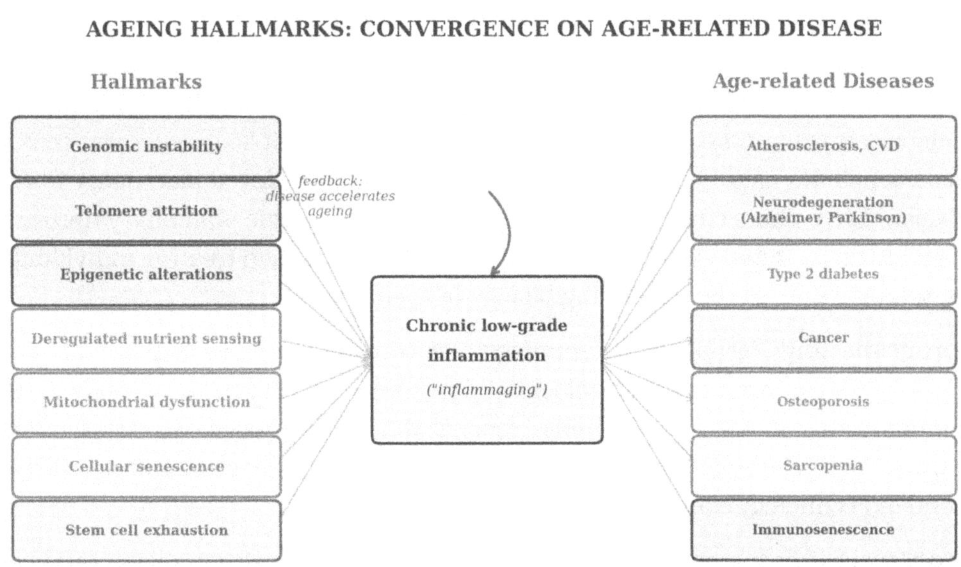

Figure 12.2: Convergence of ageing hallmarks on age-related disease. Telomere attrition, cellular senescence/SASP, mitochondrial dysfunction, loss of proteostasis, and stem cell exhaustion collectively drive Alzheimer disease, atherosclerosis, osteoporosis, and cancer through interconnected feedback loops. (Source: Author's original.)

Integration: Age-related degenerative diseases connect across the systemic chapters: atherosclerosis (Chapter 13), Alzheimer disease and Parkinson disease (Chapter 30), osteoporosis (Chapter 29), osteoarthritis (Chapter 29), type 2 diabetes and metabolic syndrome (Chapter 27), and age-related macular degeneration. The shared hallmarks discussed in this chapter (senescence, mitochondrial dysfunction, loss of proteostasis) provide the mechanistic thread linking these seemingly disparate organ-specific diseases.

Recent Advances

Revised criteria for diagnosis and staging of Alzheimer disease (NIA-AA 2024). The National Institute on Aging and the Alzheimer's Association revised the diagnostic and staging criteria for Alzheimer disease, building on the 2018 research framework and reframing the disease as a biological entity defined by neuropathologic change rather than by clinical syndrome (Jack et al. Alzheimer's & Dementia 2024; 20: 5143–5169; PMID 38934362). The workgroup distinguished early-changing Core 1 biomarkers (amyloid PET, validated cerebrospinal fluid assays, and accurate plasma biomarkers including phosphorylated tau-217) from later-changing Core 2 biomarkers (biofluid and tau PET) that supply prognostic information. An abnormal Core 1 biomarker is sufficient to establish a diagnosis of Alzheimer disease across the clinical continuum, including the asymptomatic phase. An integrated biological and clinical staging scheme accommodates copathologies, cognitive reserve, and resistance, replacing the amyloid–tau–neurodegeneration (A/T/N) research scaffold with a unified biological framework better aligned with the disease-modifying-therapy era. The criteria are now the international reference for Alzheimer-disease diagnosis in clinical care and for trial enrolment.

Senolytics: Senolytic drugs selectively kill senescent cells, removing the source of SASP-driven inflammaging. The prototype combination is dasatinib (a tyrosine kinase inhibitor) plus quercetin (a flavonoid), which targets the anti-apoptotic pathways (BCL-2 family) that keep senescent cells alive. In preclinical models, senolytics have improved cardiovascular function, reduced pulmonary fibrosis, and extended healthspan. Early-phase clinical trials are underway in idiopathic pulmonary fibrosis, diabetic kidney disease, and Alzheimer disease. This is a paradigm shift: rather than treating individual age-related diseases, senolytics target the underlying biology of ageing itself.

Epigenetic reprogramming: Partial reprogramming using transient expression of Yamanaka factors (OCT4, SOX2, KLF4, MYC) can reset epigenetic clocks and restore youthful gene expression patterns in aged cells without inducing pluripotency. In animal models, this has improved tissue regeneration, muscle function, and visual acuity. The clinical translation of epigenetic reprogramming is actively being pursued by several biotechnology companies.

Clonal haematopoiesis of indeterminate potential (CHIP): Age-related somatic mutations in haematopoietic stem cells (commonly in DNMT3A, TET2, ASXL1) lead to clonal expansion without frank malignancy. CHIP is present in over 10% of individuals above age 70 and is associated with a 2- to 4-fold increased risk of cardiovascular disease (through IL-6/NLRP3 inflammasome-mediated vascular inflammation) and a 10-fold increased risk of haematological malignancy. CHIP represents a molecular bridge between ageing, inflammation, and cancer (see Volume 1 for myeloid neoplasm context and Chapter 41 for recent advances).

The key diagnostic clue in distinguishing age-related brain changes from neurodegenerative disease on biopsy or autopsy: sparse neurofibrillary tangles confined to the entorhinal cortex and hippocampus are within the normal ageing spectrum (Braak stage I–II). When tangles and amyloid plaques extend beyond the medial temporal lobe into the neocortex (Braak stage III–VI), the burden exceeds what ageing alone explains and supports a diagnosis of Alzheimer disease. Quantification (NIA-AA criteria) matters more than qualitative presence.

When faced with cortical atrophy on macroscopic examination, the pattern of atrophy narrows the differential: symmetric frontotemporal atrophy with knife-edge gyri suggests frontotemporal lobar degeneration; posterior cortical atrophy with calcarine sparing suggests posterior cortical atrophy variant of Alzheimer disease; and caudate atrophy with ventricular dilatation suggests Huntington disease. Diffuse cortical atrophy without a distinctive regional pattern is non-specific and occurs in both normal ageing and Alzheimer disease.

International Frameworks

Hallmarks of ageing — 2023 update (12 hallmarks). López-Otín and colleagues expanded the original nine hallmarks of ageing (2013) to twelve in the 2023 update: genomic instability, telomere attrition, epigenetic alterations, loss of proteostasis, disabled macroautophagy, deregulated nutrient-sensing, mitochondrial dysfunction, cellular senescence, stem cell exhaustion, altered intercellular communication, chronic inflammation, and dysbiosis. Disabled macroautophagy and dysbiosis are added as discrete hallmarks; chronic inflammation is elevated from a downstream consequence to a primary driver. The hallmarks are interconnected and operationally defined by three criteria: an age-associated manifestation, experimental acceleration of ageing when accentuated, and therapeutic deceleration when targeted. The framework is increasingly used to organise diagnostic and therapeutic stratification in geroscience and age-related disease pathology. Citation: López-Otín C, et al. Cell 2023;186(2):243–278. PMID 36599349.

Ultra High-Yield Chapter Summary

Topic	Must Remember
Telomere attrition	TTAGGG repeats; 50–200 bp lost/division; critical shortening → DDR (ATM/p53/p21) → senescence.
Telomerase	TERT + TERC; active in germ/stem/cancer cells; silenced in somatic cells.
Cellular senescence	Irreversible arrest via p53/p21 and p16INK4a/Rb pathways; SA-β-gal marker; SASP = pro-inflammatory secretome
SASP	IL-1, IL-6, IL-8, MMPs, growth factors; acutely beneficial (wound healing); chronically detrimental (inflammaging, fibrosis, tumorigenesis)

Inflammaging	Chronic sterile inflammation of ageing; driven by SASP + gut dysbiosis + DAMPs + immunosenescence
Free radical theory	Oxidative damage from ROS contributes to ageing; but ROS also serve as signalling molecules (hormesis).
Stem cell exhaustion	Impaired tissue regeneration, immunosenescence, anaemia.
Epigenetic clocks	DNA methylation at specific CpGs predicts biological age (Horvath clock)
HGPS	LMNA → progerin; nuclear lamina disruption; childhood atherosclerosis; NO cancer risk.
Werner syndrome	WRN helicase (RecQ family); adult-onset ageing + cancer predisposition.
Caloric restriction	↑AMPK, ↓mTOR, ↑sirtuins, ↑autophagy → extended lifespan.
Senolytics	Dasatinib + quercetin; kill senescent cells by targeting BCL-2 anti-apoptotic pathways; clinical trials underway
CHIP	DNMT3A/TET2/ASXL1 mutations in HSCs; >10% of >70 yr; ↑2–4× CVD risk, 10× haem malignancy risk
Protein aggregation	Aβ (Alzheimer), α-syn (Parkinson), IAPP (T2DM), TTR (senile amyloidosis); all reflect age-related proteostasis failure
Lipofuscin	Lysosomal lipid-protein residue; marker of ageing (cardiac, hepatic, neuronal); NOT disease

Table 12.3: Ultra High-Yield Chapter Summary

Diagnostic thinking: telomere shortening + senescence markers + mitochondrial dysfunction → cellular ageing (convergence of multiple pathways)

Diagnostic thinking: amyloid plaques + neurofibrillary tangles + cortical atrophy → Alzheimer disease (see also Chapter 30)

PART B

Systemic Pathology

Chapters 13–30

This part of the book covers organ-system-based pathology — cardiovascular, respiratory, head and neck, gastrointestinal, hepatobiliary, renal, genitourinary, gynaecological, breast, endocrine, and musculoskeletal systems. Each chapter integrates general pathology principles from Part A with the distinctive morphology, molecular biology, and clinical correlations of each system.

Chapter 13: Cardiovascular Pathology Part 1: Vessels

THE BIG PICTURE

The vascular system is the common pathway through which virtually all systemic diseases ultimately exert their effects. Atherosclerosis, the most clinically significant vascular disease, is a chronic inflammatory process driven by endothelial dysfunction and lipid accumulation, and its complications (MI, stroke, peripheral vascular disease) account for more deaths than any other disease category worldwide. Vasculitis, a group of disorders classified by vessel size (Chapel Hill 2012), produces characteristic histological patterns that are frequently tested. Aneurysms and dissection represent mechanical failure of the vessel wall.

High-yield topics in this chapter: Atherosclerosis (pathogenesis, risk factors, vulnerable plaque); aneurysms (AAA, thoracic, dissection — Stanford classification); vasculitis (Chapel Hill classification, GCA, Takayasu, PAN, ANCA-associated); hypertensive vascular disease (hyaline vs hyperplastic arteriolosclerosis); vascular tumours (haemangioma, Kaposi sarcoma, angiosarcoma).

Normal Vascular Structure and Function

All blood vessels share a three-layered architecture: the **tunica intima** (endothelium on a thin basement membrane with sparse subendothelial connective tissue), the **tunica media** (smooth muscle cells and elastic laminae), and the **tunica adventitia** (connective tissue with vasa vasorum and nervi vasorum). The internal elastic lamina separates intima from media; the external elastic lamina separates media from adventitia.

Arteries are classified by size and wall composition. **Elastic arteries** (aorta, iliac, carotid) have a media rich in fenestrated elastic lamellae. **Muscular arteries** (coronary, renal, mesenteric) have a predominantly smooth muscle media with well-defined elastic laminae. **Arterioles** are the principal resistance vessels controlling blood pressure. **Capillaries** consist of endothelium and basement membrane alone. **Veins** have thinner walls, contain valves in the extremities, and serve as capacitance vessels (Figure 13.1).

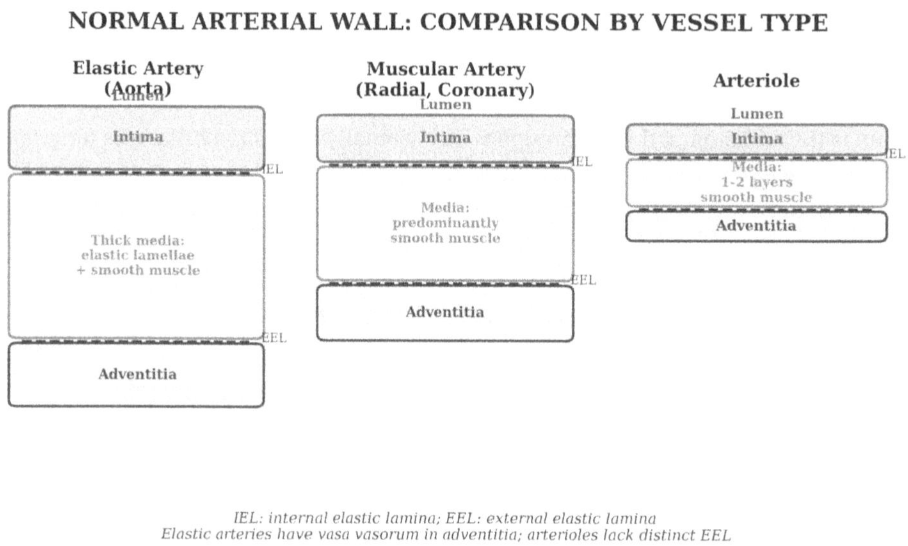

Figure 13.1 : Normal arterial wall layers: elastic artery vs muscular artery vs arteriole

Figure 13.1: Layers of the normal arterial wall: intima (endothelium, subendothelial connective tissue), internal elastic lamina, media (smooth muscle, elastic laminae), external elastic lamina, and adventitia (connective tissue, vasa vasorum), with comparison of elastic artery, muscular artery, and arteriole. (Source: Author's original.)

The endothelium is a dynamic organ that regulates vascular tone (nitric oxide, endothelin), thrombosis (thrombomodulin, prostacyclin), inflammation (adhesion molecules), and permeability. *The key diagnostic clue in vascular pathology is recognising that most major diseases begin with endothelial dysfunction.*

Atherosclerosis

Definition and Epidemiology

Atherosclerosis is a chronic inflammatory disease of large and medium-sized elastic and muscular arteries, characterised by the accumulation of lipids, fibrous tissue, and inflammatory cells in the intima, forming lesions called **atheromatous plaques (atheromas)**. It is the most common and clinically significant form of arteriosclerosis.

Globally, atherosclerosis underlies approximately 50% of all deaths in Western countries. In South Asian populations, cardiovascular disease is the leading cause of mortality and is notable for earlier onset of coronary artery disease (approximately a decade earlier than Western populations), higher prevalence of metabolic syndrome, and a genetic predisposition through elevated lipoprotein(a) levels. The

INTERHEART study demonstrated that nine modifiable risk factors account for over 90% of the population-attributable risk of a first myocardial infarction across all ethnic groups.

Risk Factors

Risk factors for atherosclerosis fall into two categories: **constitutional (non-modifiable)** and **modifiable.** Understanding these is essential for both exam answers and clinical reasoning.

Category	Risk Factor	Mechanism
Constitutional	Age	Cumulative endothelial damage; plaque burden increases with time
Constitutional	Male sex	Oestrogen is protective (premenopausal); risk equalises post-menopause
Constitutional	Genetics/Family history	Familial hypercholesterolaemia (LDLR, PCSK9 mutations); elevated Lp(a); SNPs at 9p21 locus
Major modifiable	Dyslipidaemia	Elevated LDL-C and reduced HDL-C; oxidised LDL drives foam cell formation
Major modifiable	Hypertension	Haemodynamic shear stress damages endothelium at branch points
Major modifiable	Diabetes mellitus	AGE products, oxidative stress, dyslipidaemia, endothelial dysfunction
Major modifiable	Cigarette smoking	Endothelial toxicity, platelet activation, elevated CO reduces O2 carrying capacity, lowers HDL
Additional	Inflammation (CRP)	hsCRP independently predicts risk; statins reduce CRP
Additional	Hyperhomocysteinaemia	Endothelial injury, prothrombotic state
Additional	Metabolic syndrome	Central obesity, insulin resistance, dyslipidaemia, hypertension
Additional	Lipoprotein(a)	Structurally similar to plasminogen; inhibits fibrinolysis; genetically determined

Pathogenesis: The Response-to-Injury Hypothesis

The current understanding of atherogenesis integrates the **response-to-injury hypothesis** with the **chronic inflammatory model.** Atherosclerosis is viewed as a chronic inflammatory response of the arterial wall to endothelial injury. The key steps are as follows.

Endothelial injury/dysfunction → ↑ permeability to lipoproteins → LDL accumulation in intima → LDL oxidation → monocyte recruitment → foam cell formation → smooth muscle migration and proliferation → extracellular matrix deposition → fibrous plaque → plaque complications (rupture, thrombosis)

Endothelial dysfunction is the initiating event. Disturbed laminar flow at arterial branch points, hyperlipidaemia, hypertension, cigarette smoke toxins, and inflammatory mediators all damage endothelial function without necessarily causing denudation. Dysfunctional endothelium shows increased permeability to plasma lipoproteins, upregulated expression of leucocyte adhesion molecules (VCAM-1, ICAM-1), and a shift from an antithrombotic to a prothrombotic phenotype.

Lipid accumulation and oxidation. Low-density lipoproteins (LDL) accumulate in the intima, where they undergo oxidation by reactive oxygen species generated by endothelial cells and macrophages. Oxidised LDL (ox-LDL) is a key driver of atherogenesis: it is chemotactic for monocytes, inhibits macrophage motility (trapping them in the intima), is cytotoxic to endothelium, and stimulates smooth muscle proliferation and cytokine release.

Monocyte recruitment and foam cell formation. Monocytes adhere to activated endothelium via VCAM-1 and ICAM-1, migrate into the intima under the influence of MCP-1 (monocyte chemoattractant protein-1), and differentiate into macrophages. Macrophages ingest ox-LDL via scavenger receptors (SR-A, CD36), which are not downregulated by intracellular cholesterol, leading to massive lipid engorgement and transformation into **foam cells.** Aggregates of foam cells constitute the **fatty streak**, the earliest visible lesion of atherosclerosis.

Smooth muscle cell migration and fibrous cap formation. Growth factors released by activated macrophages and platelets (PDGF, FGF, TGF-β) stimulate smooth muscle cell migration from the media to the intima and their proliferation. These cells synthesise extracellular matrix (collagen, elastin, proteoglycans), forming the **fibrous cap** overlying the lipid core. The balance between matrix synthesis and degradation (by MMPs from activated macrophages) determines plaque stability.

The role of T lymphocytes and immunity. CD4+ T helper cells (Th1 subset) in the plaque secrete IFN-γ, which activates macrophages and inhibits smooth muscle proliferation and collagen synthesis, paradoxically promoting plaque instability. Regulatory T cells (Tregs) may play a protective role. This chronic inflammatory milieu links atherosclerosis to the immune system (see Chapter 5) (Figure 13.2).

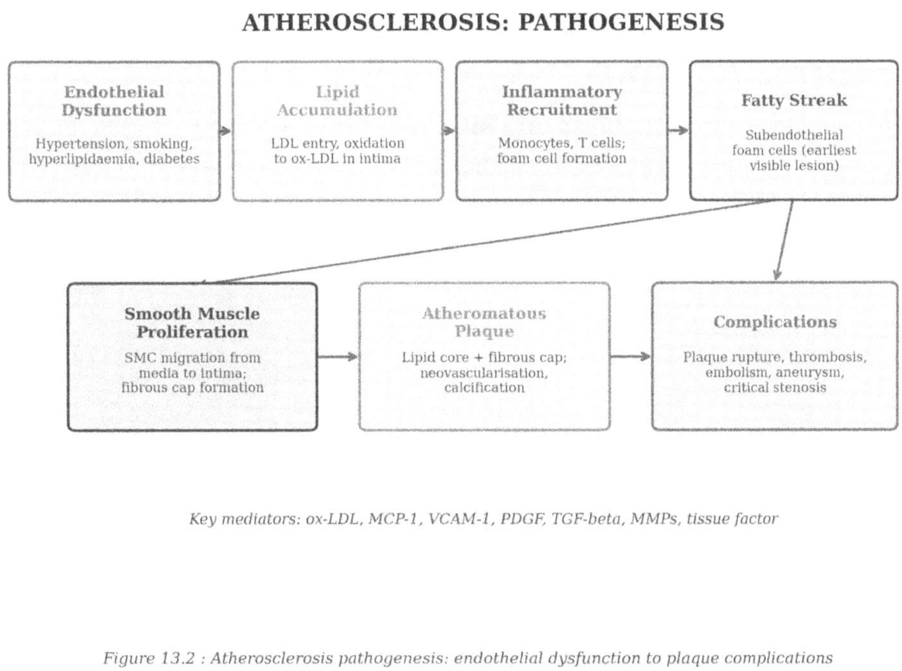

Figure 13.2: Pathogenesis of atherosclerosis. Sequential steps from endothelial dysfunction and LDL oxidation through monocyte recruitment, foam cell formation, fatty streak, smooth muscle cell migration/proliferation, and advanced plaque with lipid core, fibrous cap, neovascularisation, and calcification. (Source: Author's original.)

The pathogenesis explains the morphology: because LDL oxidation drives the inflammatory cascade, reducing LDL with statins not only lowers cholesterol but stabilises plaques by reducing inflammation and MMP activity.

Integration: *The endothelial dysfunction and thrombosis pathways in atherosclerosis connect directly to the coagulation cascade and platelet biology discussed in Volume 1 and the haemodynamic principles covered in Chapter 4.*

Morphology of Atherosclerotic Plaques

The **fatty streak** is the earliest lesion: flat or slightly elevated yellow spots or streaks on the intimal surface, composed of lipid-laden foam cells. Fatty streaks appear in the aorta by age 10 and in coronary arteries by the third decade. They are found in populations worldwide, including those with low atherosclerosis rates, and not all progress to advanced plaques. They are not clinically significant in themselves.

The **atherosclerotic plaque (atheroma)** is the fundamental lesion. It consists of a raised, white-yellow intimal lesion that protrudes into the lumen. The key components are: (1) a **fibrous cap** of smooth muscle cells, collagen, and extracellular matrix facing the lumen; (2) a cellular zone beneath the cap containing macrophages, foam cells, T lymphocytes, and smooth muscle cells; (3) a **necrotic (lipid) core** of cholesterol, cholesterol esters, cellular debris, and foam cells; and (4) a zone of neovascularisation at the plaque periphery.

Plaques preferentially develop at **branch points and areas of disturbed flow**: the proximal left anterior descending coronary artery, carotid bifurcation, abdominal aorta, and iliac arteries. This distribution reflects the role of haemodynamic shear stress in endothelial activation (Figure 13.3).

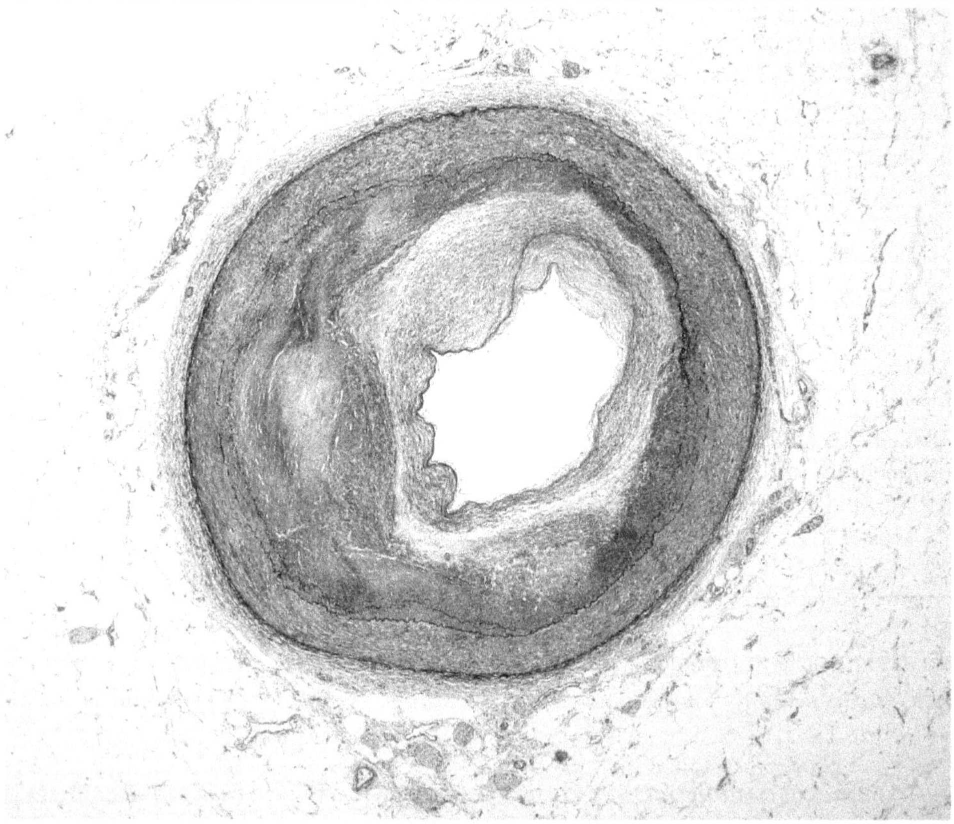

Figure 13.3: Atherosclerosis of the right coronary artery (Movat pentachrome stain, low magnification). Eccentric fibrointimal plaque with marked luminal narrowing. The fibrous cap overlies a lipid-rich necrotic core. (Source: Wikimedia Commons. Public domain.)

Plaque Stability and Complications

The clinical consequences of atherosclerosis depend not only on the degree of luminal narrowing but critically on **plaque stability.** Plaques that cause acute coronary syndromes are often not the most stenotic; rather, they are **vulnerable (unstable) plaques** prone to rupture.

Feature	Stable Plaque	Vulnerable (Unstable) Plaque
Fibrous cap	Thick, intact, collagen-rich	Thin, depleted of collagen
Lipid core	Small	Large (>40% of plaque area)
Inflammatory cells	Fewer macrophages	Many macrophages, T cells at shoulder
MMP activity	Low	High (degrades fibrous cap)
Smooth muscle cells	Abundant	Few (apoptosis from IFN-γ)
Neovascularisation	Minimal	Prominent (prone to intraplaque haemorrhage)
Clinical consequence	Stable angina	Plaque rupture → acute coronary syndrome
Calcification	Dense (protective)	Spotty/microcalcification

Plaque complications include: (1) **plaque rupture**, exposing the thrombogenic lipid core to flowing blood and triggering occlusive or mural thrombus formation; (2) **plaque erosion**, where superficial endothelial loss without deep cap rupture triggers thrombosis (more common in women and smokers); (3) **plaque haemorrhage** from rupture of fragile neovascularisation within the plaque, expanding it acutely; (4) **atherothrombotic embolism**, with cholesterol crystal emboli or thrombus fragments causing distal ischaemia; and (5) **aneurysm formation** due to pressure atrophy of the underlying media.

Clinical Consequences of Atherosclerosis

The clinical manifestations depend on the vascular bed affected, the rate of plaque growth, the degree of stenosis, and the occurrence of acute plaque events.

Vascular Bed	Chronic Consequence	Acute Consequence
Coronary arteries	Stable angina pectoris	Acute MI, sudden cardiac death (see Chapter 14)
Carotid/cerebral arteries	Multi-infarct dementia, TIA	Ischaemic stroke
Aorta	Aneurysm formation	Rupture, dissection, atherothrombotic emboli
Renal arteries	Renovascular hypertension, ischaemic nephropathy	Renal infarction
Mesenteric arteries	Chronic mesenteric ischaemia	Bowel infarction
Lower extremity arteries	Intermittent claudication, chronic	Acute limb ischaemia, gangrene

Vascular Bed	Chronic Consequence	Acute Consequence
	limb ischaemia	

Quick Recall: Atherosclerosis

Definition: Chronic inflammatory disease of large/medium arteries with intimal lipid accumulation, fibrous tissue, and inflammation.

Key pathogenesis: Endothelial injury → LDL oxidation → foam cells → SMC proliferation → fibrous plaque.

Risk factors: Major modifiable: hyperlipidaemia, HTN, DM, smoking. Non-modifiable: age, sex, genetics.

Vulnerable plaque: Thin cap, large lipid core, many macrophages, high MMPs → rupture → thrombosis → acute events.

Aneurysms and Dissection

Definition and Classification

An **aneurysm** is a localised, abnormal dilatation of a blood vessel or the heart wall. Aneurysms are classified by morphology and aetiology.

Classification	Types	Features
By morphology	True aneurysm	Involves all three layers (intima, media, adventitia); wall is thinned but intact. Subtypes: fusiform (circumferential dilatation) and saccular (localised outpouching)
By morphology	False aneurysm (pseudoaneurysm)	Wall defect with contained haematoma communicating with lumen; wall formed by adventitia or perivascular tissue only. Cause: trauma, mycotic infection, anastomotic leak
By aetiology	Atherosclerotic	Most common cause of AAA; media weakened by chronic inflammation
By aetiology	Cystic medial degeneration	Cause of thoracic aortic aneurysms; associated with Marfan, Loeys-Dietz, bicuspid aortic valve (see Chapter 8)
By aetiology	Mycotic	Infected aneurysm (bacterial, not fungal despite the name); from septic emboli or direct bacterial invasion
By aetiology	Syphilitic (luetic)	Obliterative endarteritis of vasa vasorum → medial ischaemia → ascending aortic aneurysm (now rare)

Abdominal Aortic Aneurysm (AAA)

AAA is the most common clinically significant aneurysm. It is defined as a dilatation of the abdominal aorta to greater than 3 cm (normal: approximately 2 cm). AAA occurs predominantly in men over 50 years and is strongly associated with atherosclerosis and smoking. The aneurysm is typically located **infrarenally** (below the renal arteries) and may extend to the iliac bifurcation.

Pathogenesis. Atherosclerotic damage causes chronic inflammation, loss of smooth muscle cells, and degradation of elastic tissue by matrix metalloproteinases (MMP-2, MMP-9), weakening the wall. The infrarenal location reflects the relatively avascular nature of this segment (fewer vasa vasorum) and high wall stress. Genetic predisposition (familial clustering, MMP polymorphisms) contributes (Figure 13.4).

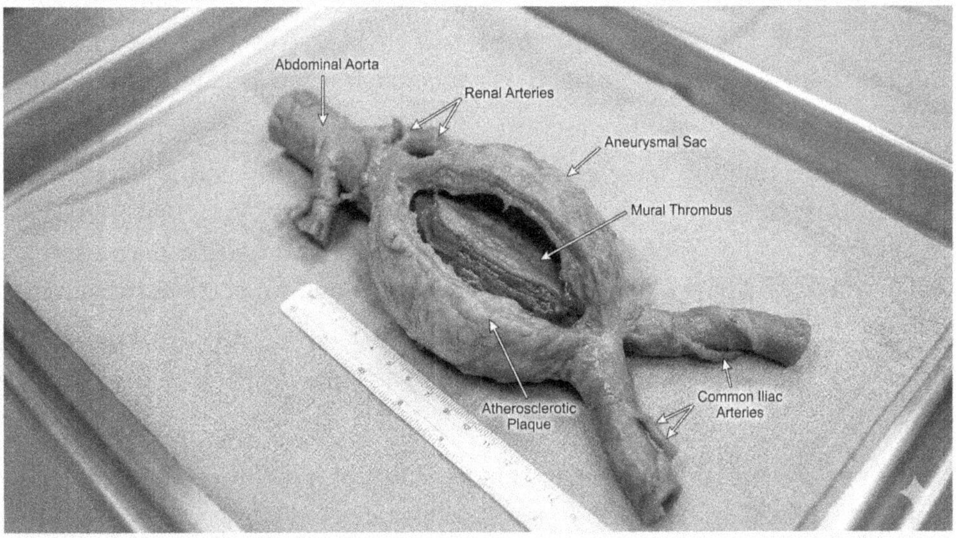

Figure 13.4: Abdominal aortic aneurysm showing fusiform dilatation with mural thrombus and atherosclerotic wall (gross specimen). (Source: Public domain.)

Morphology. AAAs are usually fusiform and may be up to 15 cm or more in diameter. The wall is thinned and composed of atherosclerotic, fibrotic tissue with loss of normal elastic architecture. The lumen typically contains **laminated mural thrombus**, which may fill much of the aneurysm sac. Inflammatory infiltrates (lymphocytes, macrophages) are present in the wall. A variant, the **inflammatory AAA**, shows dense periaortic fibrosis and chronic inflammation, sometimes with retroperitoneal fibrosis.

Complications of AAA

The major complications are: (1) **rupture**, risk increasing sharply above 5 cm diameter (annual risk: <4 cm = <1%; 5-7 cm = 6-11%; >7 cm = 20%+), usually into the retroperitoneum with approximately 80% overall mortality; (2) **thrombosis and embolism** causing distal ischaemia; and (3) **compression of adjacent structures.** Screening with abdominal ultrasound is recommended for men aged 65-75 years who have ever smoked.

Thoracic Aortic Aneurysm

Unlike AAA, thoracic aortic aneurysms are more commonly associated with **cystic medial degeneration**, characterised by loss of smooth muscle cells and degeneration of elastic tissue with accumulation of amorphous extracellular matrix. It is seen in Marfan syndrome (FBN1 mutation, TGF-β dysregulation), Loeys-Dietz syndrome (TGF-β receptor mutations), Ehlers-Danlos type IV (COL3A1), and as a consequence of long-standing hypertension (see Chapter 8). These aneurysms are particularly prone to **aortic dissection.**

Aortic Dissection

Aortic dissection is a life-threatening condition in which blood enters the aortic wall through an intimal tear and dissects along the media, creating a **false lumen.** It should be distinguished from aneurysm, though the two may coexist ("dissecting aneurysm" is a misnomer when used for dissection without pre-existing dilatation).

The Stanford classification is clinically most useful: **Type A** involves the ascending aorta (regardless of origin site; includes DeBakey types I and II) and is a surgical emergency. **Type B** involves only the descending aorta distal to the left subclavian (DeBakey type III) and is usually managed medically. Approximately 65% of tears originate in the ascending aorta within 10 cm of the aortic valve.

Cystic medial degeneration + hypertension → intimal tear → blood enters media → dissection along medial plane → false lumen → ± re-entry or rupture

Risk factors include hypertension (the single most important factor, present in 70%), connective tissue disorders (Marfan, Loeys-Dietz), bicuspid aortic valve, coarctation, and iatrogenic causes (cardiac surgery, catheterisation). Pregnancy in the third trimester is a recognised risk factor in young women.

Complications include rupture into the pericardial sac (cardiac tamponade), haemothorax, coronary artery compromise (MI), aortic regurgitation, and branch artery obstruction (stroke, renal failure, mesenteric ischaemia).

> **Exam Pitfall**
>
> **Dissection vs. aneurysm:** Dissection is a tear through the media creating a false lumen; it does not require pre-existing aneurysmal dilatation. Many dissections occur in aortas of normal or minimally increased diameter. "Dissecting aneurysm" is an outdated misnomer. In exams, distinguish clearly between the two processes.

Why is the ascending aorta the most common site of intimal tear in aortic dissection? The ascending aorta experiences the greatest haemodynamic stress during systole (highest pressure, greatest pulsatile force, and maximal aortic wall motion), making this segment most vulnerable when the media is weakened by cystic degeneration.

Quick Recall: Aneurysms and Dissection

True aneurysm: Involves all 3 wall layers. Fusiform or saccular.

False aneurysm: Wall defect contained by adventitia/perivascular tissue only.

AAA: Infrarenal, atherosclerotic, men >50, rupture risk increases >5 cm. MMP-2/MMP-9.

Thoracic: Cystic medial degeneration. Marfan (FBN1), Loeys-Dietz (TGF-βR), HTN.

Dissection: Stanford A = ascending (surgical); B = descending (medical). #1 risk factor = HTN.

Vasculitis

Vasculitis is inflammation of the vessel wall. It may be **primary (idiopathic)** or **secondary** to infection, autoimmune disease, drugs, or other conditions. The **2012 Revised International Chapel Hill Consensus Conference (CHCC)** classifies vasculitides by the predominant size of vessel affected. This classification is the standard for exam answers (Figure 13.5).

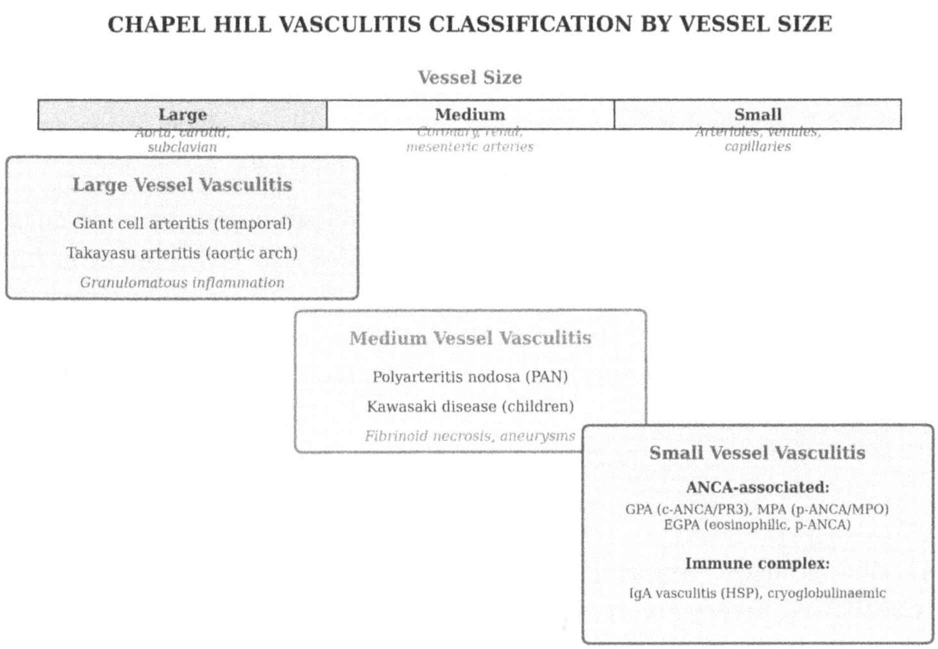

Figure 13.5 : Chapel Hill consensus vasculitis classification by vessel size

Figure 13.5: Chapel Hill Classification of vasculitis by vessel size. Large vessel: giant cell arteritis, Takayasu arteritis. Medium vessel: polyarteritis nodosa, Kawasaki disease. Small vessel: ANCA-associated (GPA, MPA, EGPA) and immune complex (IgA vasculitis, cryoglobulinaemic vasculitis, anti-GBM disease). Variable vessel: Behçet disease, Cogan syndrome. (Source: Author's original.)

Chapel Hill Consensus Classification of Vasculitis (2012 Revised)

Large vessel vasculitis: Giant cell (temporal) arteritis, Takayasu arteritis

Medium vessel vasculitis: Polyarteritis nodosa (PAN), Kawasaki disease

Small vessel vasculitis (ANCA-associated): Granulomatosis with polyangiitis (GPA, formerly Wegener), Microscopic polyangiitis (MPA), Eosinophilic granulomatosis with polyangiitis (EGPA, formerly Churg-Strauss)

Small vessel vasculitis (immune complex): IgA vasculitis (Henoch-Schönlein), Cryoglobulinaemic vasculitis, Anti-GBM disease

Variable vessel vasculitis: Behçet disease, Cogan syndrome

Giant Cell (Temporal) Arteritis

Giant cell arteritis (GCA) is the most common form of vasculitis in adults, affecting patients over 50 years (peak 70-80 years), with a female predominance. It is a **granulomatous inflammation** of large and medium-sized arteries, most characteristically the temporal artery, but also the aorta and its branches (ophthalmic, vertebral arteries).

Pathogenesis involves a T-cell-mediated immune response against an unknown antigen in the vessel wall, with CD4+ Th1 and Th17 cells driving macrophage activation and granuloma formation. IL-6 is a key cytokine (tocilizumab, an anti-IL-6R antibody, is used therapeutically).

Morphology. The temporal artery shows segmental ("skip lesion") involvement with granulomatous inflammation centred on the internal elastic lamina. Multinucleated giant cells, epithelioid histiocytes, lymphocytes, and fibrosis with intimal thickening and luminal narrowing are characteristic. The internal elastic lamina is fragmented and may be engulfed by giant cells. *The distinction from normal age-related intimal fibrosis rests on the presence of granulomatous inflammation with elastic lamina destruction, which is absent in the latter.*

Clinical features include headache, temporal artery tenderness, jaw claudication, and the serious complication of **ophthalmic artery involvement causing sudden, irreversible blindness.** ESR and CRP are markedly elevated. Approximately 40-50% have associated polymyalgia rheumatica. High-dose corticosteroids should be started immediately on clinical suspicion, without waiting for biopsy. Temporal artery biopsy (at least 2-3 cm) is the gold standard but may be negative due to skip lesions.

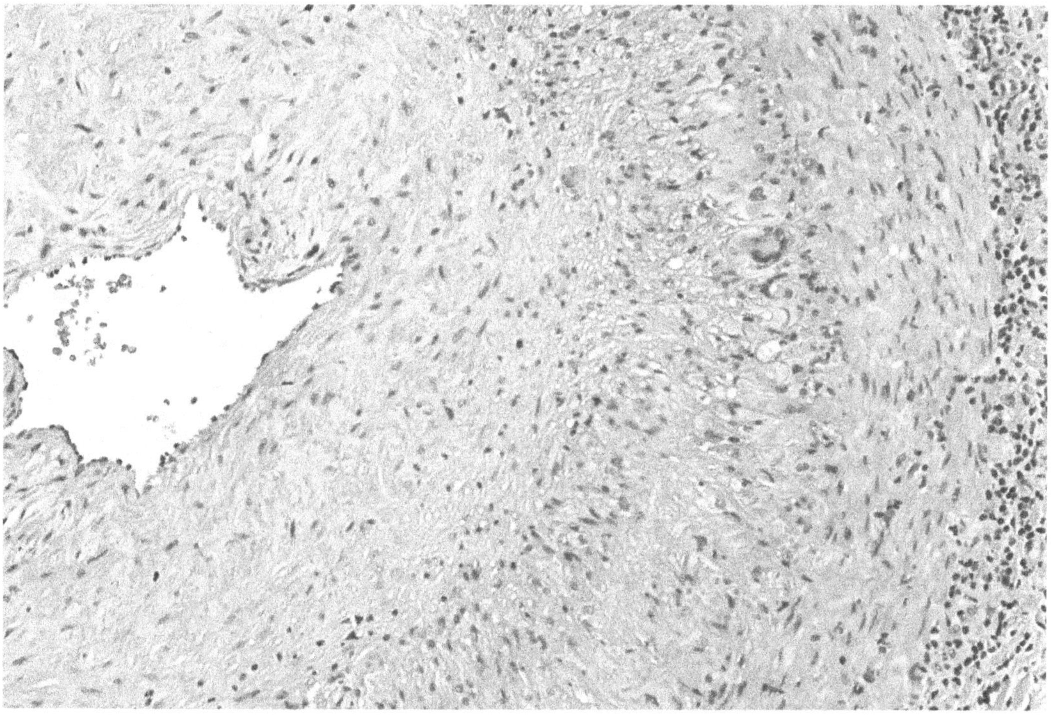

Figure 13.6: Giant cell (temporal) arteritis (H&E, intermediate magnification). Transmural chronic granulomatous inflammation with intimal thickening, fragmented internal elastic lamina, and multinucleated giant cells in the media. (Source: Nephron, Wikimedia Commons, CC BY-SA 3.0.)

Takayasu Arteritis

Takayasu arteritis ("pulseless disease") is a granulomatous vasculitis of large arteries, predominantly the aorta and its major branches. It typically affects young women (15-40 years), with the highest incidence in Asia (Japan, India, Southeast Asia). The pathology is similar to GCA with granulomatous inflammation and elastic lamina destruction, but the distribution is different (aortic arch and branches rather than temporal artery).

The aortic involvement leads to segmental stenosis and wall thickening ("tree-barking"), with resultant upper extremity claudication, absent or diminished pulses (pulseless disease), cerebral ischaemia, hypertension (renal artery stenosis), and aortic regurgitation. *In Asian and Latin American populations, Takayasu arteritis is the most common large vessel vasculitis in young women and should be considered in any young patient presenting with absent pulses, hypertension of unknown cause, or aortic regurgitation.*

Polyarteritis Nodosa (PAN)

PAN is a systemic necrotising vasculitis of **medium-sized muscular arteries**, characterised by **segmental, transmural fibrinoid necrosis** with a mixed inflammatory infiltrate (neutrophils in acute phase, lymphocytes and macrophages in chronic phase). It is **ANCA-negative** (distinguishing it from ANCA-associated small vessel vasculitides). Approximately 30% of cases are associated with hepatitis B infection.

The hallmark is **segmental involvement**: affected and unaffected segments alternate along the vessel, and different stages (acute necrosis, healing, fibrosis) coexist at the same time, reflecting the episodic nature of the disease. Branch points are preferentially involved. The resulting weakening leads to aneurysm formation ("nodosa" refers to the palpable aneurysmal nodules along affected vessels) (Figure 13.7).

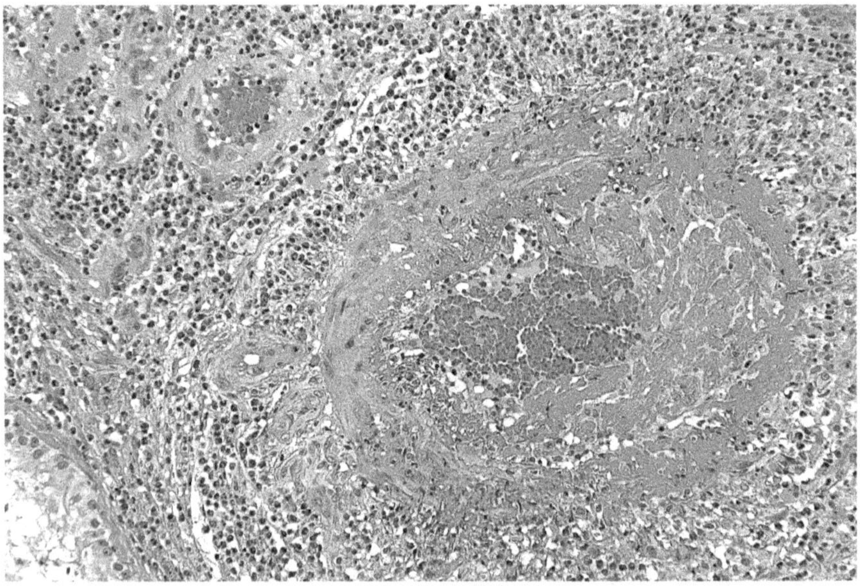

Figure 13.7: Eosinophilic granulomatosis with polyangiitis (Churg–Strauss syndrome). Small vessel showing necrotising vasculitis with prominent eosinophilic infiltrate and extravascular granuloma formation (H&E, high magnification). (Source: Wikimedia Commons, Nephron, CC BY-SA 3.0.)

Clinical features reflect multisystem involvement: renal (hypertension, renal failure, but no glomerulonephritis), gastrointestinal (mesenteric arteritis with abdominal pain, bowel infarction), peripheral neuropathy (mononeuritis multiplex), skin (livedo reticularis, ulcers), and musculoskeletal (myalgia, arthralgia). PAN **does not involve the lungs** (in contrast to ANCA-associated vasculitides). Diagnosis is by biopsy of an affected organ or by angiography showing multiple microaneurysms.

The distinction from microscopic polyangiitis rests on three features: PAN is ANCA-negative, affects medium (not small) vessels, does not involve glomeruli or pulmonary capillaries, and shows fibrinoid necrosis of the full vessel wall.

Kawasaki Disease

Kawasaki disease is an acute, self-limited medium vessel vasculitis of childhood (80% of cases in children under 5 years). Its importance lies in its propensity to cause **coronary artery aneurysms**, which occur in 20-25% of untreated children and are the leading cause of acquired heart disease in children in developed countries. The aetiology remains unknown but is thought to involve an abnormal immune response to an infectious trigger in genetically susceptible individuals.

Clinical features include high spiking fever for at least 5 days, bilateral conjunctival injection, oral mucosal changes (strawberry tongue, lip fissuring), cervical lymphadenopathy, polymorphous rash, and erythema of hands and feet with subsequent desquamation. Treatment with IVIG and aspirin within the first 10 days reduces coronary aneurysm risk to less than 5%.

ANCA-Associated Small Vessel Vasculitis

The three ANCA-associated vasculitides share small vessel necrotising inflammation that is "pauci-immune" (few or no immune complex deposits on immunofluorescence). They are distinguished by the pattern of organ involvement and the ANCA specificity.

Feature	GPA (Wegener)	MPA	EGPA (Churg-Strauss)
ANCA	c-ANCA (PR3)	p-ANCA (MPO)	p-ANCA (MPO) in ~40%
Upper airway	Necrotising granulomas (sinusitis, saddle nose)	No	No
Lung	Necrotising granulomas, cavitation	Pulmonary capillaritis, haemorrhage	Asthma, eosinophilic infiltrates
Kidney	Necrotising crescentic GN (pauci-immune)	Necrotising crescentic GN (pauci-immune)	Less common
Key pathology	Granulomatous vasculitis + necrotising GN	Non-granulomatous necrotising vasculitis	Tissue eosinophilia, granulomas, vasculitis
Distinctive features	Upper airway destruction (saddle nose deformity)	Pulmonary-renal syndrome	Asthma, eosinophilia (>1500/μL), neuropathy

Quick Recall: Vasculitis

Entity	Vessel	Key Histology	Serology	Clinical
Takayasu	Large (aortic arch)	Granulomatous; intimal fibrosis	Elevated ESR; no specific Ab	Young females <40; pulseless disease

GCA	Large (temporal)	Granulomatous + giant cells; fragmented IEL	ESR often >100	Age >50; headache; jaw claudication; visual loss
PAN	Medium (renal, mesenteric)	Fibrinoid necrosis; segmental; all stages coexist	No ANCA; HBsAg+ subset	Spares lungs; microaneurysms; hypertension
Kawasaki	Medium (coronary)	Necrotising; transmural; coronary aneurysm	None specific	Children <5; fever >5 d; coronary aneurysm
GPA	Small (+medium)	Necrotising granulomatous; geographic necrosis	c-ANCA (PR3)	Lung + kidney + upper airway (Wegener triad)
MPA	Small	Pauci-immune necrotising; no granulomas	p-ANCA (MPO)	Lung + kidney; no upper airway (differs from GPA)
EGPA	Small	Eosinophilic + granulomatous + necrotising	p-ANCA (MPO) ~40%	Asthma + eosinophilia + neuropathy
IgA vasculitis	Small (post-capillary)	Leukocytoclastic; IgA on IF	Elevated IgA in some	Children; purpura + arthralgia + GI + nephritis

Vasculitis by Vessel Size

Classification: Chapel Hill 2012: large, medium, small (ANCA-associated and immune complex), variable.

GCA: >50 years, temporal artery, granulomatous, skip lesions, blindness risk. ESR/CRP elevated.

Takayasu: Young women, aortic arch, pulseless disease. Common in Asia.

PAN: Medium vessel, fibrinoid necrosis, ANCA-negative, HBV association, no lung/glomerular involvement.

Kawasaki: Children <5, coronary aneurysms, IVIG treatment.

ANCA: GPA = c-ANCA/PR3 (upper airway + lung + kidney); MPA = p-ANCA/MPO (lung + kidney); EGPA = eosinophilia + asthma.

***Integration:** The renal involvement in vasculitis (crescentic glomerulonephritis in ANCA-associated vasculitides) connects to Chapter 22, while the immunological basis of autoantibody-mediated vessel injury links to Chapter 5.*

Hypertensive Vascular Disease

Hypertension affects approximately a quarter to a third of adults in many populations worldwide and is a major risk factor for atherosclerosis, aortic dissection, stroke, and chronic kidney disease. Two forms of small vessel change are associated with hypertension.

Hyaline arteriolosclerosis is seen in benign (chronic) hypertension and also in diabetes mellitus. There is homogeneous, eosinophilic, acellular thickening of the arteriolar wall due to plasma protein deposition (leakage across damaged endothelium), with luminal narrowing. The renal afferent arterioles are characteristically affected, contributing to nephrosclerosis.

Hyperplastic arteriolosclerosis is the hallmark of **malignant (accelerated) hypertension**. It shows concentric, laminated ("onion-skin") thickening of the arteriolar wall due to smooth muscle cell proliferation and reduplicated basement membrane. In severe cases, **fibrinoid necrosis** of the vessel wall ("necrotising arteriolitis") with red blood cell extravasation is superimposed. These changes are most prominent in renal arterioles.

The Pathologist's Eye

At the microscope, distinguishing hyaline arteriolosclerosis from arteriolar hyalinosis of diabetes can be challenging because both produce eosinophilic wall thickening. **The key clue is distribution:** in hypertension, the changes affect the afferent arteriole predominantly, while in diabetes, both afferent and efferent arterioles are involved. Clinical correlation (BP, HbA1c) is often necessary. Onion-skin hyperplastic change is virtually diagnostic of malignant hypertension.

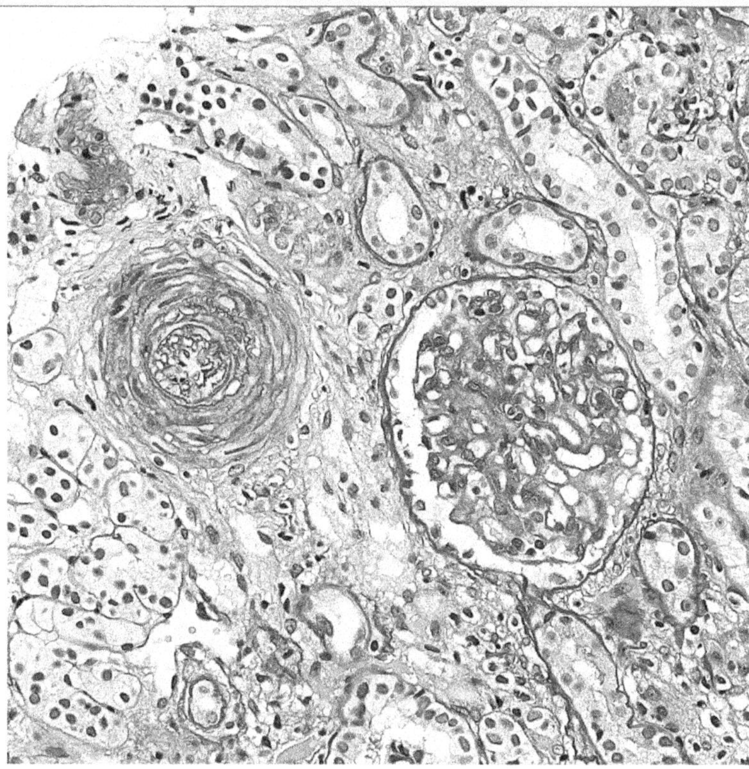

Figure 13.8: Hyperplastic arteriolosclerosis ("onion-skinning") — renal arteriole (PAS stain, high magnification). Concentric, laminated thickening of the arteriolar wall with luminal narrowing, characteristic of malignant hypertension. (Source: Pacolarosa, Wikimedia Commons, CC BY-SA 3.0.)

Venous Diseases

Varicose veins are abnormally dilated, tortuous veins from chronically elevated intraluminal pressure, most commonly affecting lower extremity superficial veins. Risk factors include obesity, prolonged standing, and pregnancy. Complications include stasis dermatitis, chronic venous ulceration (medial malleolus), and superficial thrombophlebitis. Oesophageal varices (portal hypertension, see Chapter 20) and haemorrhoids are important variants. **Deep vein thrombosis (DVT)** and pulmonary thromboembolism are discussed in Chapter 4. Migratory thrombophlebitis (Trousseau sign) is associated with occult visceral malignancy.

Vascular Tumours

Vascular tumours range from benign (haemangiomas) to intermediate (Kaposi sarcoma, haemangioendothelioma) to malignant (angiosarcoma).

Tumour	Behaviour	Key Features
Haemangioma	Benign	Most common vascular tumour. Capillary: skin, lip. Cavernous: liver, brain.
Glomus tumour	Benign	Modified SMCs of glomus body. Subungual, exquisitely painful.
Kaposi sarcoma	Intermediate	HHV-8. Classic, endemic, transplant, AIDS forms. Spindle cells, slit-like spaces.
Angiosarcoma	Malignant	Liver (vinyl chloride, thorotrast, arsenic). Breast (post-radiation). Lymphoedema (Stewart-Treves).

Quick Recall: Vascular Tumours

Haemangioma: Most common; benign; capillary (superficial) or cavernous (deep).

Kaposi sarcoma: HHV-8; slit-like vascular channels; spindle cells; 4 clinical forms.

Angiosarcoma: Malignant; liver (vinyl chloride, thorotrast); breast (post-radiation); lymphoedema (Stewart-Treves).

Diseases of Lymphatics

Lymphangitis is acute inflammation of lymphatic channels, usually secondary to group A streptococcal infection, presenting as red subcutaneous streaks extending proximally. **Lymphoedema** results from obstruction of lymphatic drainage. Primary lymphoedema may be congenital (Milroy disease, VEGFR3 mutation). Secondary causes include surgical excision of lymph nodes, radiation fibrosis, filariasis (Wuchereria bancrofti, the most common cause worldwide and particularly important in tropical regions), and malignant obstruction. Chronic lymphoedema predisposes to lymphangiosarcoma (Stewart-Treves syndrome). Cystic hygroma is a congenital lymphangioma of the posterior triangle of the neck, associated with Turner syndrome.

Recent Advances in Vascular Pathology

EAS consensus — LDL as a causal driver of atherosclerotic cardiovascular disease. A European Atherosclerosis Society consensus statement integrated genetic, epidemiologic, and interventional evidence to establish low-density lipoproteins as causal agents in atherosclerotic cardiovascular disease (Borén et al. European Heart Journal 2020; 41: 2313–2330; PMID 32052833). The statement summarised Mendelian randomisation evidence using LDL-cholesterol-lowering variants in PCSK9, HMGCR, NPC1L1, ATP-citrate lyase, LDLR, and APOB, all of which produce cardiovascular-event reductions concordant with absolute LDL-cholesterol exposure rather than with the molecular target. The retained-particle hypothesis was articulated as the central pathogenic mechanism: apolipoprotein-B-containing lipoproteins traverse the endothelial barrier, are retained in the subendothelial extracellular matrix through proteoglycan binding, and undergo oxidation and aggregation that drives macrophage-mediated foam-cell formation. The statement provided the framework for cardiovascular-event prediction by cumulative LDL exposure (mmol/L · years), rationalising both early intervention and combination lipid-lowering therapy. The consensus is now embedded in ESC/EAS dyslipidaemia guidelines and informs target thresholds for statin, ezetimibe, PCSK9-inhibitor, and inclisiran use.

Clonal haematopoiesis of indeterminate potential (CHIP) and atherosclerosis. A major recent discovery is the association between CHIP (somatic mutations in haematopoietic stem cells, most commonly in TET2 and DNMT3A) and increased cardiovascular risk. TET2-mutant macrophages show enhanced NLRP3 inflammasome activation and IL-1β secretion, promoting plaque inflammation. This finding provides a molecular link between ageing, clonal haematopoiesis, and accelerated atherosclerosis, and has therapeutic implications through IL-1β blockade (canakinumab, as demonstrated in the CANTOS trial).

PCSK9 inhibitors. Proprotein convertase subtilisin/kexin type 9 (PCSK9) promotes degradation of the LDL receptor. Gain-of-function PCSK9 mutations cause familial hypercholesterolaemia, while loss-of-function mutations are associated with very low LDL and reduced cardiovascular risk. Monoclonal antibodies against PCSK9 (evolocumab, alirocumab) and the siRNA inclisiran represent major therapeutic advances for patients with refractory hyperlipidaemia or statin intolerance.

Complement and ANCA vasculitis. The alternative complement pathway, particularly C5a, plays a central role in ANCA-mediated neutrophil activation and vessel injury. Avacopan, an oral C5a receptor antagonist, was approved in 2021 for the treatment of severe ANCA-associated vasculitis as an alternative to high-dose glucocorticoids, representing a paradigm shift in vasculitis management.

Approach to the Histopathology Slide: Vascular Pathology

When presented with a vascular pathology slide in the practical examination, follow a systematic approach.

1. Identify the vessel type. Determine whether you are looking at an artery, vein, or small vessel. Look for the three-layer architecture. An artery has a thicker media with a prominent internal elastic lamina; a vein has a thinner, less well-organised wall.

2. Assess the intima. Is there intimal thickening? If so, is it fibrous (atherosclerosis, intimal fibroplasia), lipid-laden with foam cells and cholesterol clefts (atheroma), or thrombotic? Look for the fibrous cap, lipid/necrotic core, and calcification of atherosclerotic plaques.

3. Assess the media. Is it intact or disrupted? Fibrinoid necrosis (bright eosinophilic, amorphous material replacing the normal medial architecture) suggests vasculitis (PAN) or malignant hypertension. Granulomatous inflammation with giant cells centred on the elastic lamina suggests giant cell arteritis. Loss of elastic tissue with mucoid degeneration suggests cystic medial degeneration.

4. Assess the adventitia. Periadventitial inflammation and fibrosis may be seen in vasculitis or inflammatory aneurysms.

5. Look at the inflammatory infiltrate. Neutrophils suggest acute inflammation (early vasculitis, infected aneurysm). Lymphocytes and macrophages suggest chronic inflammation. Granulomas with giant cells suggest GCA or Takayasu. Eosinophils suggest EGPA or allergic vasculitis.

6. Use special stains. Verhoeff-Van Gieson (VVG) or elastic van Gieson (EVG) stain highlights elastic fibres and is essential for demonstrating elastic lamina disruption in GCA and atherosclerosis. PAS highlights basement membrane reduplication in hypertensive arteriolosclerosis.

Differential Diagnosis of Vascular Pathology

Condition	Key Histology	Distinguishing Feature	Confirmatory Test
Atherosclerosis	Fibrous cap, lipid core, cholesterol clefts, foam cells	Eccentric intimal plaque in medium-large arteries	Clinical + imaging; no biopsy needed routinely
Giant cell arteritis	Granulomatous inflammation of media, intimal fibrosis, fragmented IEL	Temporal artery involvement, age >50, elevated ESR	Temporal artery biopsy (skip lesions — long segment needed)
Takayasu arteritis	Granulomatous inflammation of aortic media, "tree-barking"	Young female, aorta and major branches, pulseless disease	CT/MR angiography; biopsy rarely obtained
Polyarteritis nodosa	Fibrinoid necrosis, transmural neutrophilic inflammation, microaneurysms	Segmental involvement, spares pulmonary arteries, ANCA-negative	Angiography (microaneurysms); biopsy of affected organ
GPA (Wegener)	Necrotising granulomas, vasculitis, geographic necrosis	Upper/lower respiratory + renal involvement	c-ANCA / PR3-ANCA
MPA	Necrotising vasculitis without granulomas, pauci-immune crescentic GN	No granulomas; renal-pulmonary syndrome	p-ANCA / MPO-ANCA
IgA vasculitis (HSP)	Leukocytoclastic vasculitis of small vessels, IgA deposits	Palpable purpura, children, IgA nephropathy pattern	DIF: IgA in vessel walls
Thromboangiitis obliterans	Segmental thrombosis with microabscesses in thrombus,	Young male smoker, extremity claudication	Clinical; biopsy shows inflammation within

	preserved vessel wall		thrombus

The key diagnostic clue on temporal artery biopsy: giant cell arteritis is a segmental (skip) lesion — a negative biopsy does not exclude the diagnosis. The biopsy must be at least 2 cm long, and serial sections should be examined. The diagnostic triad is granulomatous inflammation centred on the internal elastic lamina, fragmentation and duplication of the IEL, and intimal fibrosis with luminal narrowing. Healed arteritis (intimal fibrosis without active inflammation) in the right clinical setting still supports the diagnosis.

When evaluating a vessel biopsy showing fibrinoid necrosis, the size of the involved vessel and the pattern of inflammation determine the diagnosis: medium-sized muscular artery with transmural neutrophilic inflammation and microaneurysms indicates polyarteritis nodosa; small vessel with leukocytoclastic vasculitis and IgA deposits indicates IgA vasculitis; and small vessel with pauci-immune crescentic nephritis on renal biopsy indicates ANCA-associated vasculitis (GPA vs MPA vs EGPA, distinguished by granulomas and eosinophilia).

Ultra High-Yield Chapter Summary

Topic	Must Remember
Atherosclerosis definition	Chronic inflammatory disease of large/medium arteries; intimal lipid + fibrous tissue + inflammation
Response-to-injury	Endothelial dysfunction → LDL oxidation → monocyte recruitment → foam cells → SMC migration → fibrous plaque
Major risk factors	Hyperlipidaemia, HTN, DM, smoking (modifiable); age, male sex, genetics (non-modifiable)
Vulnerable plaque	Thin fibrous cap, large lipid core, many macrophages, high MMP activity → rupture → thrombosis
Fatty streak	Earliest visible lesion; foam cells in intima; present by age 10; not all progress
True vs false aneurysm	True = all 3 layers intact; False = wall defect, contained by adventitia/tissue only
AAA	Infrarenal, atherosclerotic, men >50, rupture risk >5 cm, MMP-2/9, screen with USS
Cystic medial degeneration	Loss of SMC + elastic tissue; Marfan (FBN1), Loeys-Dietz (TGFβR); thoracic aneurysm/dissection
Aortic dissection	Intimal tear → blood in media → false lumen.
GCA	>50 yrs, temporal artery, granulomatous, skip lesions, ↑ESR, risk of blindness.
Takayasu	Young women, aortic arch, pulseless disease.
PAN	Medium vessel, fibrinoid necrosis, ANCA-negative, HBV association,

Topic	Must Remember
	spares lungs/glomeruli
Kawasaki	Children <5, coronary aneurysms (20-25% untreated), IVIG treatment
ANCA vasculitides	GPA = c-ANCA/PR3 (airway + lung + kidney); MPA = p-ANCA/MPO; EGPA = eosinophilia + asthma
Hyaline arteriolosclerosis	Benign HTN, DM. Homogeneous eosinophilic thickening.
Hyperplastic arteriolosclerosis	Malignant HTN.
Angiosarcoma associations	Liver: vinyl chloride, thorotrast, arsenic. Breast: post-radiation.
Kaposi sarcoma	HHV-8; spindle cells; slit-like vascular channels; 4 forms (classic, endemic, transplant, AIDS)
CHIP and CVD	TET2/DNMT3A mutations in HSCs → inflammasome activation → accelerated atherosclerosis
PCSK9 inhibitors	Monoclonal antibodies (evolocumab) and siRNA (inclisiran) for refractory hyperlipidaemia

Cross-References from Chapter 13

Coagulation cascade, platelet biology, Trousseau syndrome → Volume 1. Thromboembolism, DVT, shock → Chapter 4. Autoimmunity, immune complex disease → Chapter 5. Marfan, Ehlers-Danlos, FH → Chapter 8. Filariasis/lymphoedema → Chapter 9. MI, rheumatic heart disease → Chapter 14. Portal hypertension → Chapter 20. Crescentic GN → Chapter 22. VHL syndrome → Chapter 23. CHIP, PCSK9, avacopan → Chapter 41.

Diagnostic thinking: fibrous cap + lipid core + cholesterol clefts + foam cells → atherosclerotic plaque (complicated if haemorrhage/thrombus)

Diagnostic thinking: granulomatous vasculitis + giant cells + temporal artery → giant cell arteritis (vessel size guides classification)

Diagnostic thinking: fibrinoid necrosis + onion-skinning + malignant hypertension → hyperplastic arteriolosclerosis (Figures 13.7–13.10)

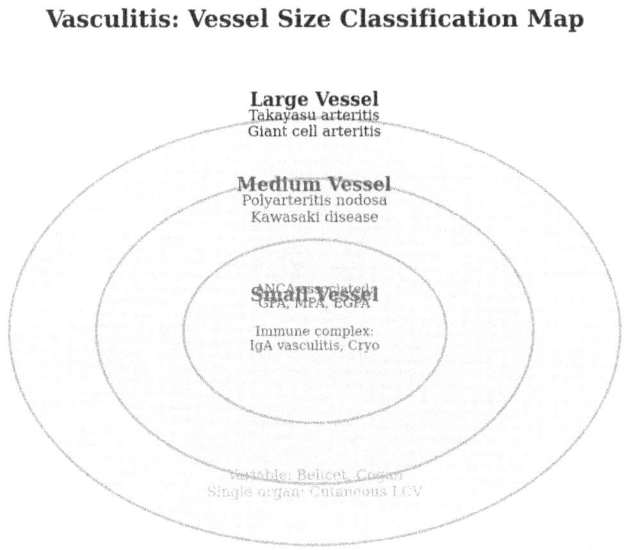

Figure 13.9: Vasculitis: Vessel Size Classification Map. (Source: Author's original.)

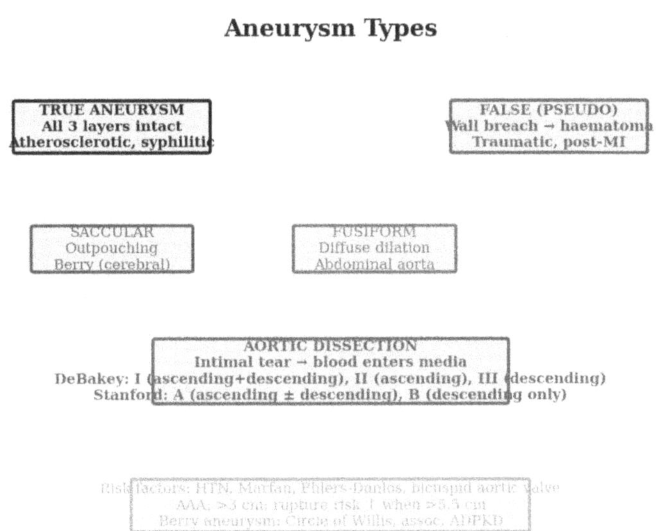

Figure 13.10: Aneurysm Types. (Source: Author's original.)

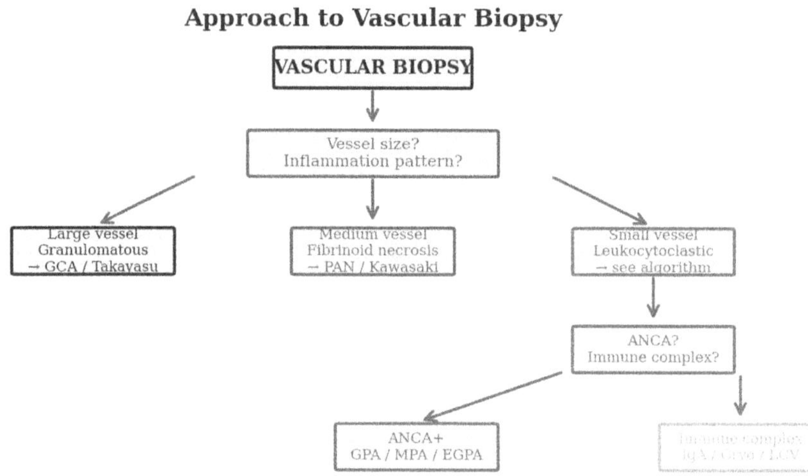

Figure 13.11: Approach to Vascular Biopsy. (Source: Author's original.)

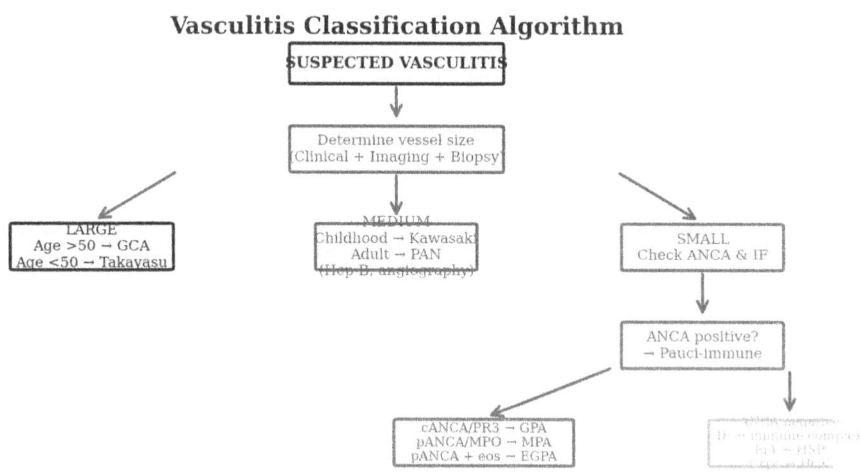

Figure 13.12: Vasculitis Classification Algorithm. (Source: Author's original.)

Chapter 14: Cardiovascular Pathology Part 2: Heart

THE BIG PICTURE

Heart disease remains the leading cause of death worldwide. Ischaemic heart disease, driven by coronary atherosclerosis, accounts for the majority of cardiac deaths. Rheumatic heart disease, though declining globally, persists as a major burden in South Asia and parts of sub-Saharan Africa. Cardiomyopathies, myocarditis, and infective endocarditis round out the spectrum of acquired cardiac pathology. Understanding the morphological evolution of myocardial infarction and the pathological basis of valvular disease is essential for both the examination and the diagnostic bench.

High-yield topics in this chapter: Ischaemic heart disease (MI morphology, complications, reperfusion injury), Rheumatic heart disease (Aschoff body, chronic valvular sequelae), Cardiomyopathies (dilated, hypertrophic, restrictive, arrhythmogenic), Infective endocarditis (acute vs subacute), Congenital heart disease.

The heart beats over 100,000 times a day and pumps approximately 7,000 litres of blood. When this relentless organ fails, it does so through a limited repertoire of pathological responses: ischaemia, inflammation, degeneration, and malformation. The pathologist who understands these four mechanisms can decode virtually any cardiac specimen.

Ischaemic Heart Disease

Ischaemic heart disease (IHD) encompasses a group of syndromes resulting from myocardial ischaemia, an imbalance between coronary blood supply and myocardial oxygen demand. The vast majority of IHD is caused by **coronary atherosclerosis** (see Chapter 13). The clinical syndromes of IHD include stable angina, unstable angina, acute myocardial infarction (MI), chronic IHD with heart failure, and sudden cardiac death.

Angina Pectoris

Angina pectoris is episodic chest pain caused by transient myocardial ischaemia that is insufficient to cause necrosis. Three patterns are recognised. **Stable (typical) angina** is predictable chest pain provoked by exertion or emotional stress and relieved by rest or nitroglycerin; it is caused by fixed atherosclerotic stenosis of >70% of the coronary lumen. **Unstable (crescendo) angina** is increasingly frequent or prolonged angina, occurring at rest or with minimal exertion; it is caused by plaque disruption with superimposed non-occlusive thrombosis and represents an acute coronary syndrome with risk of progression to MI. **Prinzmetal (variant) angina** occurs at rest due to coronary artery vasospasm, often at a site of atherosclerotic plaque; ECG shows transient ST-segment elevation during attacks.

Myocardial Infarction

MI is defined as myocardial necrosis due to prolonged ischaemia. The **universal classification of MI** recognises five types: Type 1 (spontaneous, due to plaque rupture/erosion with thrombosis), Type 2 (supply-demand mismatch without acute coronary thrombosis), Type 3 (MI resulting in death before biomarkers obtained), Types 4a/4b/5 (procedure-related). Type 1 is the classic "heart attack" and the focus of pathological study.

Transmural (STEMI) infarcts involve the full thickness of the ventricular wall in the distribution of a single coronary artery, and are caused by complete thrombotic occlusion. **Subendocardial (NSTEMI) infarcts** involve the inner one-third to one-half of the wall and may be circumferential, reflecting global hypoperfusion; the subendocardium is the most vulnerable zone because it is furthest from the coronary supply and most compressed during systole (Figure 14.1).

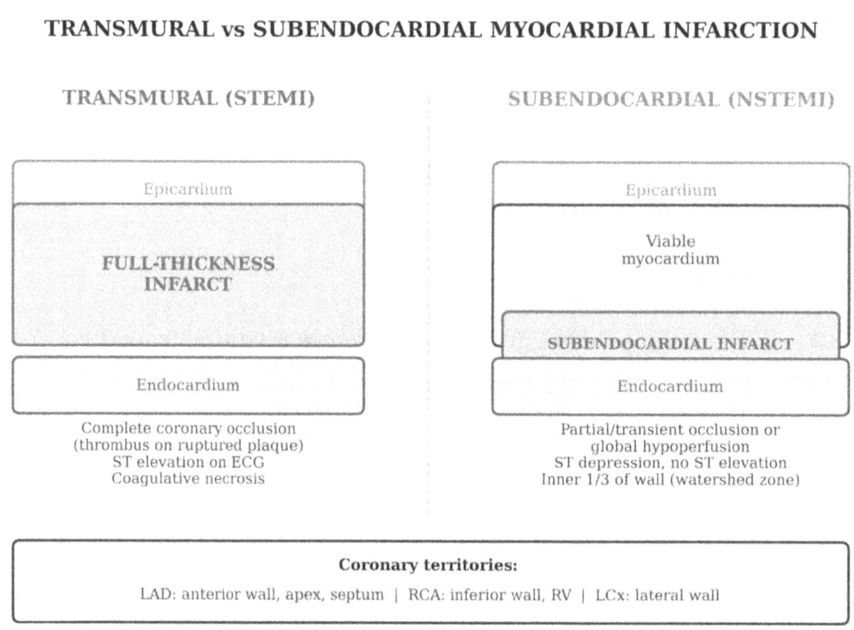

Figure 14.1 : Transmural vs subendocardial myocardial infarction with coronary territories

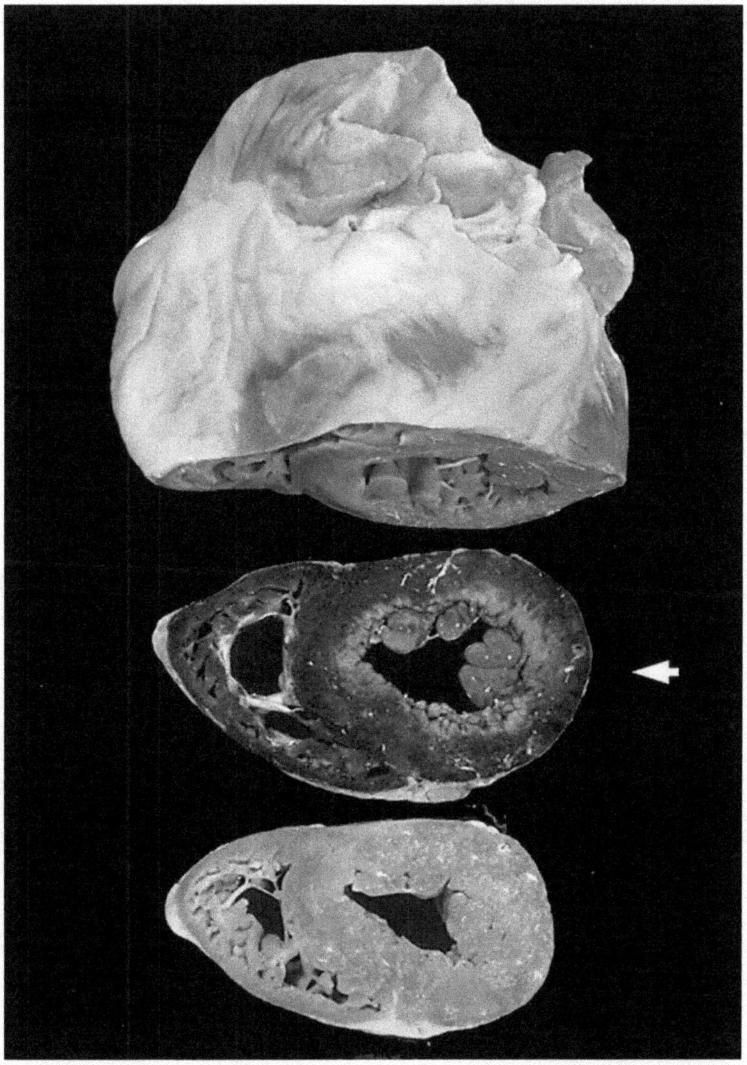

Figure 14.1: Transmural versus subendocardial myocardial infarction. (A) Schematic: transmural infarct (full-thickness, classically in LAD territory — anterior wall, septum, apex) versus circumferential subendocardial infarct (inner one-third of the wall, spares the epicardium); LAD, RCA, and LCx coronary territories indicated. (B) Nitro blue tetrazolium (NBT)-stained myocardium: the bottom heart is a normal control with uniform purple staining; the middle section (white arrow) shows circumferential subendocardial infarction — the unstained (pale) inner rim indicates infarcted tissue that has lost dehydrogenase activity, confirming the subendocardial distribution. (Sources: A — Author's original; B — Katarzyna Michaud et al, on behalf of the Association for European Cardiovascular Pathology (AECVP), Wikimedia Commons, CC BY 3.0.)

Morphological Evolution of Myocardial Infarction

The morphological changes of MI evolve in a predictable temporal sequence that is one of the most frequently tested topics in pathology examinations.

Time	Gross Appearance	Microscopy	Key Feature
0-4 hours	No visible change (may be pale with NBT stain)	No visible change (wavy fibres at periphery)	Reversible injury; wavy fibres from stretching
4-12 hours	Dark mottling (early)	Coagulative necrosis begins; early neutrophilic infiltrate	Loss of nuclei, hypereosinophilic cytoplasm
12-24 hours	Dark mottling	Coagulative necrosis established; heavy neutrophilic infiltrate; contraction band necrosis at margins	Contraction bands (hypercontracted sarcomeres from $Ca2+$ influx)
1-3 days	Yellow-tan centre with hyperaemic border	Coagulative necrosis with neutrophilic infiltrate (peak at 2-3 days)	Maximum neutrophil infiltration
3-7 days	Yellow-tan, softening (maximal softening at 4-7 days)	Macrophage phagocytosis of dead cells; early granulation tissue at margins	DANGER ZONE: wall weakest, risk of rupture
1-3 weeks	Red-grey borders (granulation tissue)	Granulation tissue with neovascularisation, fibroblasts; ongoing macrophage activity	Active repair phase
>3 weeks-months	White scar	Dense collagenous scar (complete by 6-8 weeks)	Mature fibrosis; no regeneration of cardiomyocytes (Figure 14.2)

Time	Gross Appearance	Microscopy	Key Feature

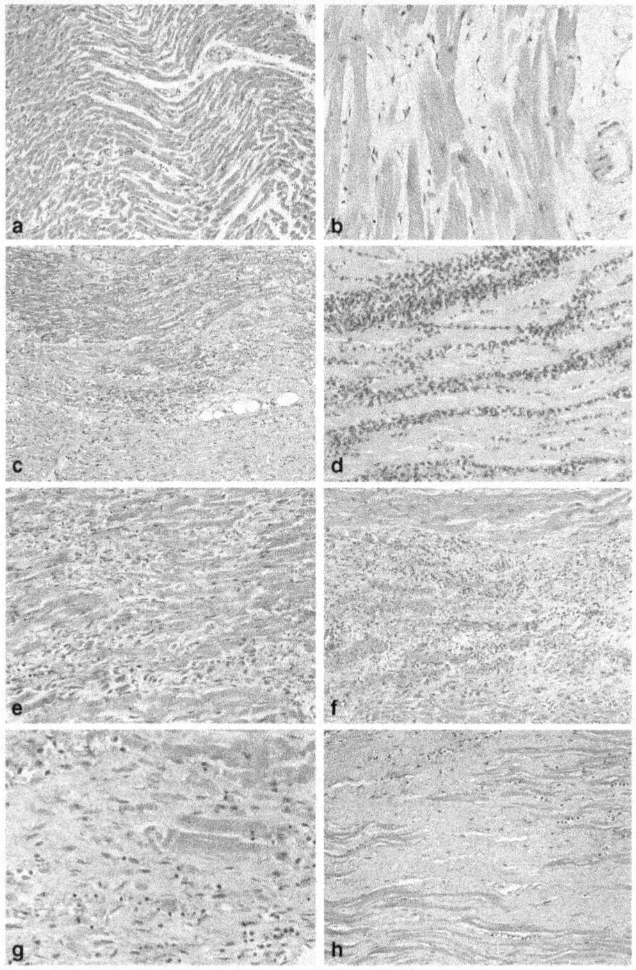

Figure 14.2: Histological features of myocardial infarction at different stages (H&E). (a) Normal myocardium; (b) Coagulative necrosis; (c–d) Neutrophilic infiltration (24–72 hours); (e–f) Macrophage infiltration and granulation tissue; (g) Haemosiderin-laden macrophages; (h) Dense fibrous scar. (Source: Katarzyna Michaud et al, on behalf of the Association for European Cardiovascular Pathology (AECVP), Wikimedia Commons, CC BY 3.0.)

The pathogenesis explains the morphology: because the subendocardium is most vulnerable to ischaemia, infarction begins here and extends as a "wavefront" towards the epicardium over 3-6 hours. Early reperfusion (within the therapeutic window) can salvage the outer zones.

Plaque rupture → thrombosis → coronary occlusion → subendocardial ischaemia → wavefront of necrosis (3-6 hrs) → transmural infarction

Complications of Myocardial Infarction

Essential/Desirable: Diagnostic Criteria — Acute Myocardial Infarction (Pathological)

Essential: Coagulative necrosis of myocardium with contraction band necrosis at margins; wavy fibres in adjacent viable myocardium.

Desirable: Neutrophilic infiltrate (12–24 h onwards); granulation tissue (3–7 d); correlation with coronary artery occlusion at autopsy; TTC negativity in fresh infarct.

Complications are best understood in relation to the temporal evolution of the infarct.

Complication	Timing	Mechanism
Arrhythmia (most common cause of death)	Minutes to hours	Electrical instability of ischaemic myocardium; VF, VT
Cardiogenic shock	Hours to days	Loss of >40% of LV myocardium
Cardiac rupture (free wall)	3-7 days (peak 4-5 days)	Softened necrotic wall; pericardial tamponade; highest risk: first MI, transmural, anterior wall, elderly women
Ventricular septal rupture	3-7 days	Septal necrosis → acute L-to-R shunt
Papillary muscle rupture	3-7 days	Necrosis of papillary muscle → acute severe mitral regurgitation
Mural thrombus / embolism	Days to weeks	Endocardial damage + stasis → thrombus; source of systemic emboli
Pericarditis	2-3 days (fibrinous) or 2-10 weeks (Dressler)	Transmural infarct irritates pericardium; Dressler = autoimmune
Ventricular aneurysm	Weeks to months	Thin scar bulges during systole; site of thrombus, arrhythmia
Heart failure	Acute or chronic	Loss of contractile mass; LV remodelling

Exam Pitfall

Cardiac rupture timing: Rupture occurs at 3-7 days, NOT in the first 24 hours (when the wall is still structurally intact) and NOT after 2-3 weeks (when scar tissue has formed). This is the "danger zone" when the wall is maximally softened by enzymatic digestion of necrotic tissue. Examiners frequently test this temporal window.

Quick Recall: Ischaemic Heart Disease

MI definition: Myocardial necrosis from prolonged ischaemia. Type 1 = plaque rupture + thrombosis.

Wavefront: Begins subendocardially, extends transmurally over 3-6 hours.

Morphology: 0-4h: wavy fibres. 12-24h: coagulative necrosis + neutrophils. 3-7d: softening (rupture risk).

>6wk: white scar.

Rupture window: 3-7 days. Free wall > septum > papillary muscle.

Reperfusion injury: Contraction band necrosis, haemorrhagic infarct, ROS damage, no-reflow.

Reperfusion Injury

Paradoxically, restoration of blood flow to ischaemic myocardium can itself cause additional damage, termed **reperfusion injury.** This is clinically relevant because percutaneous coronary intervention (PCI) and thrombolysis are the standard treatments for STEMI. The mechanisms of reperfusion injury include: (1) generation of reactive oxygen species (ROS) by damaged mitochondria and infiltrating neutrophils; (2) intracellular calcium overload leading to hypercontraction of myofibrils, producing the characteristic **contraction band necrosis** (dense eosinophilic transverse bands of hypercontracted sarcomeres, the histological hallmark of reperfusion); (3) inflammation with complement activation and neutrophil recruitment; and (4) opening of the mitochondrial permeability transition pore (mPTP), causing mitochondrial swelling and cell death.

The **no-reflow phenomenon** occurs when microvascular damage is so severe that blood flow cannot be re-established even after the epicardial coronary artery is reopened. Microvascular obstruction results from endothelial swelling, capillary plugging by neutrophils and platelets, and external compression by oedematous myocytes. Reperfused infarcts are typically haemorrhagic (in contrast to the pale, anaemic appearance of non-reperfused infarcts), because blood leaks through damaged vessels into the necrotic tissue.

Chronic Ischaemic Heart Disease

Chronic IHD (ischaemic cardiomyopathy) develops from progressive myocardial damage due to chronic ischaemia with or without previous infarction. The heart shows diffuse myocardial atrophy, interstitial fibrosis, and multiple areas of healed infarction. These patients present with progressive heart failure. The morphology may overlap with DCM, and clinical correlation with coronary angiography is essential to distinguish the two.

Sudden Cardiac Death

Sudden cardiac death (SCD) is defined as unexpected death from cardiac causes within 1 hour of symptom onset, or unwitnessed death in a person previously seen alive and well within 24 hours. In adults over 35, the most common cause is **coronary artery disease** (acute plaque disruption with or without thrombosis, or chronic arrhythmogenic scar). In young adults and athletes, the major causes are **HCM, ARVC, congenital coronary anomalies, myocarditis, and channelopathies** (long QT, Brugada syndrome). At autopsy, the pathologist must perform meticulous examination of the coronary arteries (serial cross-sections) and systematic sampling of the myocardium to identify the cause.

Rheumatic Heart Disease

Rheumatic heart disease (RHD) is a chronic sequela of **acute rheumatic fever (ARF)**, an immune-mediated multisystem inflammatory disease triggered by pharyngeal infection with group A streptococci (GAS, Streptococcus pyogenes). ARF typically affects children aged 5-15 years. The pathogenesis involves **molecular mimicry**: antibodies and T cells directed against streptococcal M protein cross-react with cardiac antigens (cardiac myosin, laminin, valve glycoproteins), producing a delayed immunological injury to the heart.

GAS pharyngitis → molecular mimicry (M protein vs cardiac antigens) → immune activation → pancarditis (endocarditis, myocarditis, pericarditis) → healing with valve scarring → chronic RHD

Diagnosis of ARF uses the revised Jones criteria (2015 AHA revision), which distinguish low-prevalence from moderate/high-prevalence populations (India falls in the latter category, with a lower threshold for clinical diagnosis).

Jones Criteria	Major Manifestations	Minor Manifestations
Clinical	Carditis (pancarditis), Migratory polyarthritis, Sydenham chorea, Erythema marginatum, Subcutaneous nodules	Arthralgia (or polyarthritis if low-prevalence), Fever (≥38.5°C)
Laboratory		Elevated acute phase reactants (ESR ≥60, CRP ≥3.0), Prolonged PR interval
Diagnosis	2 major OR 1 major + 2 minor	PLUS evidence of preceding GAS infection (positive throat culture, rapid antigen test, or elevated ASO/anti-DNase B titres)

Morphology of acute rheumatic carditis. The hallmark lesion is the **Aschoff body (Aschoff nodule)**, a focus of fibrinoid necrosis surrounded by activated macrophages (Anitschkow cells, "caterpillar cells" with characteristic owl-eye nuclei), multinucleated giant cells (Aschoff giant cells), and T lymphocytes. Aschoff bodies are found in the myocardial interstitium, typically perivascular. Endocarditis manifests as small, sterile, verrucous vegetations along the lines of valve closure (**verrucae**), most commonly on the mitral valve. Pericarditis produces a "bread-and-butter" fibrinous pericarditis (Figure 14.3).

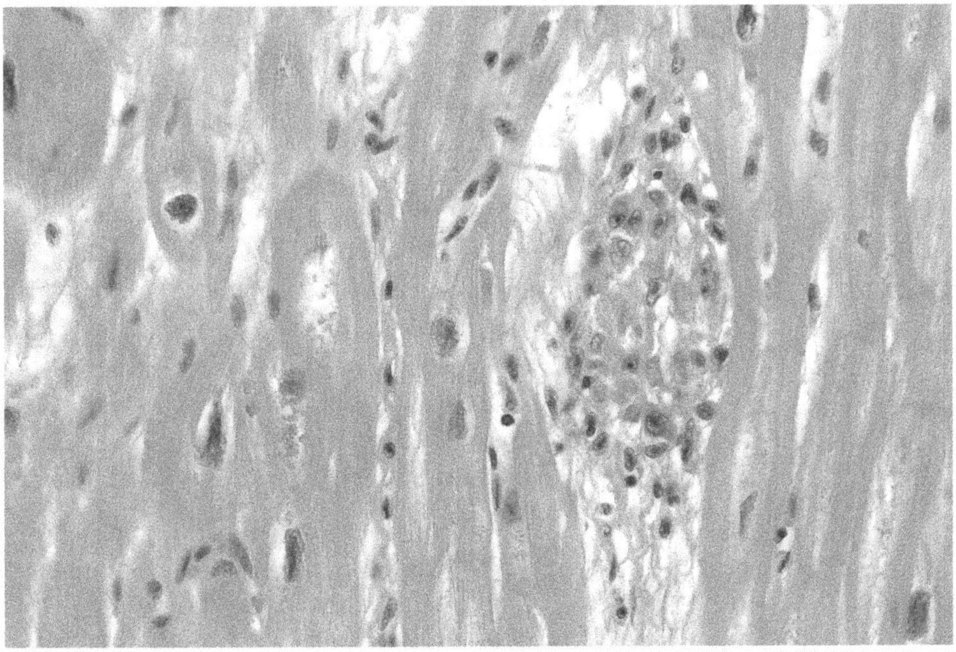

Figure 14.3: Rheumatic myocarditis — Aschoff body (H&E, very high magnification). Fibrinoid change surrounded by Anitschkow cells with characteristic caterpillar/owl-eye chromatin and scattered lymphocytes. (Source: Nephron/Wikimedia Commons, CC BY-SA 3.0.)

Chronic RHD. Recurrent episodes of ARF cause progressive valvular damage. The **mitral valve** is affected in virtually all cases, followed by the aortic valve. Chronic changes include leaflet thickening and fibrosis, commissural fusion, chordal shortening and fusion, and calcification, producing **mitral stenosis** (the classic "fish-mouth" or "buttonhole" orifice). Mitral stenosis leads to left atrial dilatation, atrial fibrillation, and pulmonary venous congestion. Combined mitral stenosis and regurgitation is common. Aortic stenosis develops when the aortic valve is also involved.

Why does rheumatic heart disease cause mitral stenosis rather than regurgitation in its chronic phase? Recurrent inflammation leads to progressive fibrosis and commissural fusion that restricts leaflet opening. While acute carditis causes regurgitation (from valve oedema and dilatation), the chronic scarring, calcification, and chordal fusion progressively narrow the orifice, converting the dominant haemodynamic lesion to stenosis.

Quick Recall: Rheumatic Heart Disease

Trigger: GAS pharyngitis (NOT skin infection). Molecular mimicry: M protein vs cardiac myosin/laminin.

Aschoff body: Fibrinoid necrosis + Anitschkow cells (caterpillar chromatin) + Aschoff giant cells.

Acute: Pancarditis. Verrucous vegetations on mitral valve.

Chronic: Mitral stenosis (fish-mouth orifice). Commissural fusion, chordal shortening.

Jones criteria: Major: carditis, polyarthritis, chorea, erythema marginatum, subcutaneous nodules.

Minor: fever, arthralgia, raised ESR/CRP, prolonged PR.

Infective Endocarditis

Infective endocarditis (IE) is microbial infection of the heart valves or mural endocardium, characterised by **vegetations** composed of organisms, fibrin, platelets, and inflammatory cells. Two clinical forms are recognised. **Acute IE** (Staphylococcus aureus on normal or damaged valves) is a fulminant, destructive infection that rapidly destroys the valve. **Subacute IE** (viridans streptococci, HACEK organisms on previously damaged valves) is an insidious infection that produces smaller, less destructive vegetations.

Feature	Acute IE	Subacute IE
Organism	S. aureus (most common overall)	Viridans streptococci; HACEK group; Enterococcus
Valve	Normal or damaged	Previously damaged (RHD, prosthetic, degenerative)
Vegetation	Large, bulky, destructive	Small, warty
Valve destruction	Severe (ring abscess, perforation)	Minimal
Embolic complications	Septic emboli (brain abscess, mycotic aneurysm)	Non-septic emboli (splenic infarcts); immune complex GN
Clinical course	Days to weeks; fulminant	Weeks to months; insidious
Peripheral signs	Petechiae, Janeway lesions (non-tender)	Osler nodes (tender), splinter haemorrhages, Roth spots

The distinction between IE vegetations and those of rheumatic fever, NBTE, and Libman-Sacks endocarditis rests on culture positivity, vegetation size, and the degree of valve destruction (Figure 14.4).

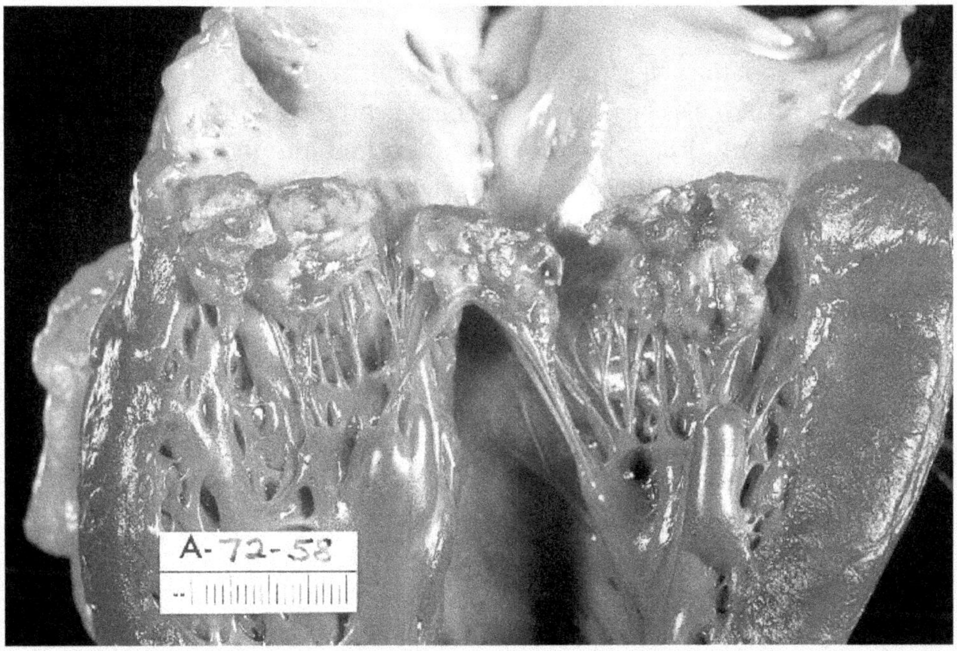

Figure 14.4: Infective endocarditis — gross pathology. Large, friable vegetations on the mitral valve leaflets (Haemophilus parainfluenzae). (Source: CDC/PHIL #851. Public domain.)

Non-Rheumatic Valvular Heart Disease

Calcific aortic stenosis is the most common valvular abnormality requiring surgical intervention in Western countries. It results from "wear and tear" dystrophic calcification of the aortic valve, accelerated by hyperlipidaemia and inflammation (the process shares pathogenetic features with atherosclerosis). Normal trileaflet valves typically become symptomatic in the 7th-8th decade; **bicuspid aortic valves** (present in 1-2% of the population) develop stenosis 1-2 decades earlier due to abnormal haemodynamic stress.

Mitral valve prolapse (MVP) affects 2-3% of the population. The posterior leaflet balloons into the left atrium during systole due to myxomatous degeneration (accumulation of proteoglycans in the spongiosa layer). Most cases are benign with a mid-systolic click and late systolic murmur. Rarely, severe prolapse causes mitral regurgitation requiring surgery. MVP is associated with Marfan syndrome and other connective tissue disorders (see Chapter 8).

Non-bacterial thrombotic endocarditis (NBTE, marantic endocarditis) consists of small, bland, fibrin-platelet vegetations on valve leaflets, typically in hypercoagulable states (mucin-secreting adenocarcinomas, DIC, prolonged debilitating illness). Vegetations are sterile and non-destructive but are a source of systemic thromboembolism. **Libman-Sacks endocarditis** in SLE produces small vegetations on both surfaces of the valve leaflets (see Chapter 5).

Cardiomyopathies

Cardiomyopathies are diseases of the myocardium associated with cardiac dysfunction that are not secondary to ischaemic, valvular, hypertensive, or congenital heart disease. The 2023 ESC classification recognises primary cardiomyopathies based on **morphofunctional phenotype**: dilated (DCM), hypertrophic (HCM), restrictive (RCM), arrhythmogenic right ventricular (ARVC), and non-dilated left ventricular cardiomyopathy. Each phenotype can be genetic or acquired (Figure 14.5).

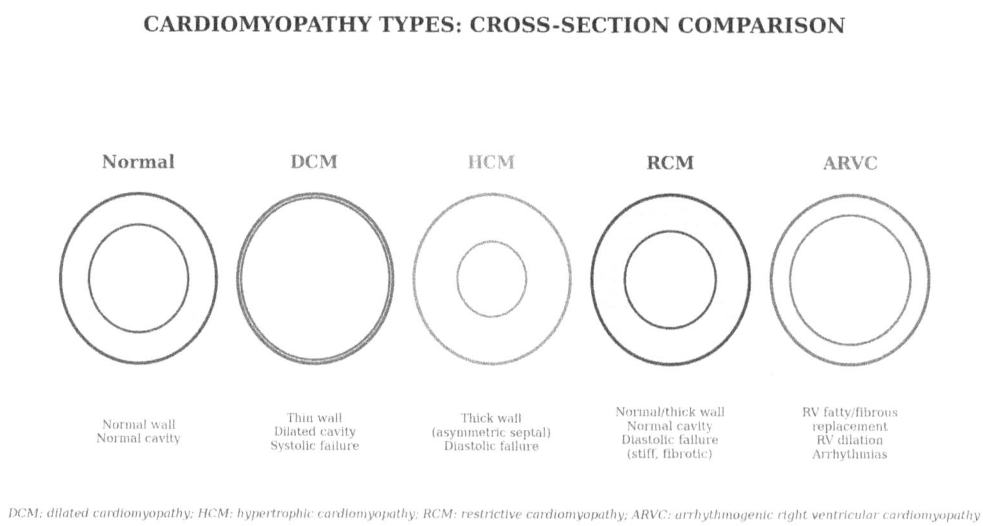

Figure 14.5 : Cardiomyopathy types: cross-section comparison

Figure 14.5: Comparison of the four major cardiomyopathy types: normal heart, dilated cardiomyopathy (dilated chambers, thin walls), hypertrophic cardiomyopathy (asymmetric septal hypertrophy, small LV cavity), restrictive cardiomyopathy (normal size, stiff walls, dilated atria), and arrhythmogenic right ventricular cardiomyopathy (fatty/fibrous replacement of RV myocardium). (Source: Author's original.)

Dilated Cardiomyopathy (DCM)

DCM is characterised by progressive four-chamber dilatation and systolic dysfunction (reduced ejection fraction). It is the most common cardiomyopathy and the most frequent indication for heart transplantation. Approximately 20-35% of cases are familial (autosomal dominant), most commonly due to mutations in **titin (TTN)**, lamin A/C (LMNA), and other cytoskeletal/sarcomeric genes. Acquired causes include myocarditis (post-viral), alcohol, peripartum cardiomyopathy, doxorubicin toxicity, and haemochromatosis.

Morphology. The heart is heavy (often >500 g) with dilated chambers and thin, flabby walls. Mural thrombi are common in the dilated chambers. Microscopically, there is myocyte hypertrophy with nuclear enlargement, interstitial fibrosis, and variable myocyte attenuation. The changes are non-specific (Figure 14.6).

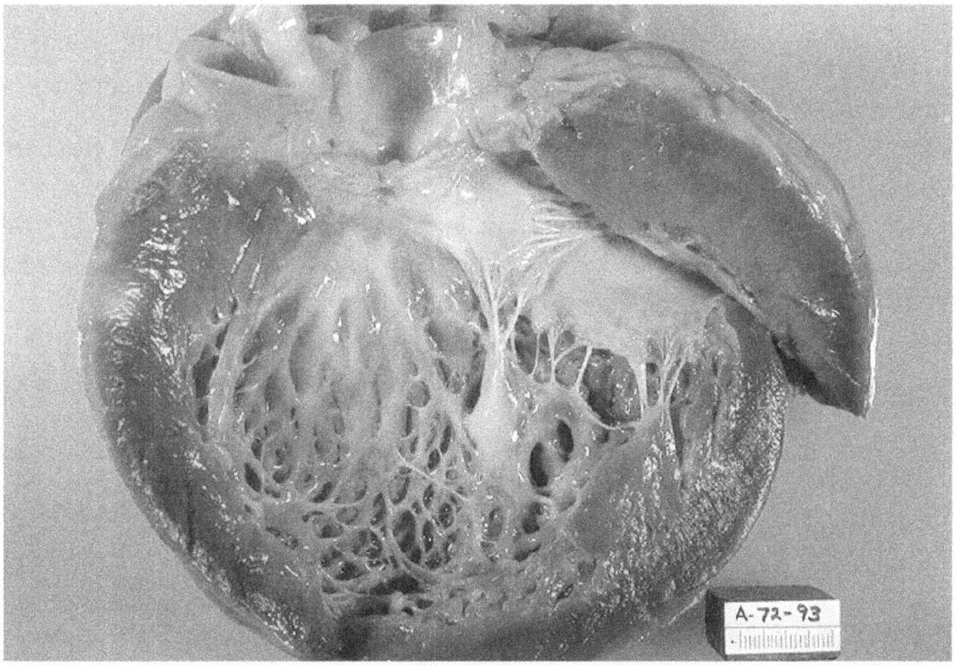

Figure 14.6: Dilated cardiomyopathy (idiopathic) — gross pathology. Four-chamber view showing biventricular dilatation with thinning of the ventricular walls. (Source: CDC/PHIL. Public domain.)

Hypertrophic Cardiomyopathy (HCM)

HCM is characterised by **asymmetric septal hypertrophy** with diastolic dysfunction and a preserved or hyperkinetic ejection fraction. It is the most common cause of **sudden cardiac death in young athletes.** HCM is autosomal dominant with variable penetrance; >70% of genetic cases are caused by mutations in **β-myosin heavy chain (MYH7)** or **cardiac myosin-binding protein C (MYBPC3).** The septum is disproportionately thickened (>1.5:1 septum-to-free-wall ratio), and approximately 25% have dynamic left ventricular outflow tract (LVOT) obstruction, with systolic anterior motion (SAM) of the mitral valve.

Microscopically, the hallmark is **myofibre disarray**: myocytes are arranged in a chaotic, whorled pattern rather than the normal parallel alignment. Interstitial fibrosis and thickened intramural coronary arteries ("small vessel disease") are present. *When faced with unexplained cardiac hypertrophy at autopsy, myofibre disarray on histology points strongly towards HCM, distinguishing it from hypertensive hypertrophy where fibres remain parallel.*

Restrictive Cardiomyopathy (RCM)

RCM is characterised by impaired ventricular filling (diastolic dysfunction) due to decreased myocardial compliance, with preserved systolic function and near-normal ventricular size. The ventricles are stiff.

The key causes are **amyloidosis** (AL or ATTR, see Chapter 5), **endomyocardial fibrosis (EMF)**, **Löffler endocarditis** (eosinophilic endomyocardial disease), radiation fibrosis, sarcoidosis, and storage diseases (haemochromatosis, Fabry disease). Amyloidosis is the most common cause in developed countries. EMF is important in tropical regions including India.

Arrhythmogenic Right Ventricular Cardiomyopathy (ARVC)

ARVC is characterised by progressive replacement of right ventricular myocardium by **fibrofatty tissue**, causing right ventricular dilatation, arrhythmias (VT of RBBB morphology), and sudden death in young adults. It is inherited (autosomal dominant, reduced penetrance), most commonly due to mutations in **desmosomal genes** (plakophilin-2/PKP2, desmoplakin/DSP, desmoglein-2/DSG2). The fibrofatty replacement is best seen in the "triangle of dysplasia" (RV inflow, outflow, and apex). ARVC is the second most common cause of sudden cardiac death in young athletes after HCM.

Feature	DCM	HCM	RCM	ARVC
Chamber size	Dilated (4 chambers)	Normal or small LV	Normal	RV dilated
Wall thickness	Normal or thin	Increased (asymmetric)	Normal	Thin (RV)
Systolic function	Decreased (low EF)	Normal or increased	Normal	Decreased (RV)
Diastolic function	Abnormal	Severely impaired	Severely impaired	Variable
Key pathology	Non-specific changes	Myofibre disarray	Infiltrative (amyloid, fibrosis)	Fibrofatty replacement
Genetics	TTN, LMNA (20-35%)	MYH7, MYBPC3 (>60%)	Rare (desmin, transthyretin)	PKP2, DSP (desmosomal)
Major risk	Heart failure, emboli	Sudden death, LVOT obstruction	Heart failure, AF	VT, sudden death

Quick Recall: Cardiomyopathies

Type	Gross	Histology	Genetics	Clinical
DCM	4-chamber dilation; thin walls; mural thrombi	Myocyte hypertrophy + interstitial fibrosis	TTN (~25%); LMNA, MYH7; viral, alcoholic	Systolic dysfunction; CHF; emboli
HCM	Asymmetric septal hypertrophy; banana LV	Myocyte disarray; interstitial fibrosis	MYH7, MYBPC3; autosomal dominant	Diastolic dysfunction; LVOT obstruction; SCD

Feature	DCM	HCM	RCM	ARVC
RCM	Normal/slight enlargement; rigid walls	Amyloid/endomyocardial fibrosis/iron	TTR (amyloid); HFE (haemochromatosis)	Diastolic dysfunction; low-voltage ECG
ARVC	RV thinning; fibrofatty replacement	Fibrofatty replacement of RV myocardium	PKP2 (plakophilin-2); desmosomal genes	RV arrhythmias; SCD; epsilon waves

Cardiomyopathies — Differential Diagnosis

DCM: Dilated chambers, thin walls, low EF. TTN/LMNA.

HCM: Asymmetric septal hypertrophy, myofibre disarray. MYH7/MYBPC3. #1 cause sudden death in young athletes.

RCM: Stiff ventricles, diastolic dysfunction. Amyloidosis (#1 cause), EMF (tropics), sarcoidosis.

ARVC: RV fibrofatty replacement, desmosomal mutations (PKP2). VT, sudden death.

Integration: *Cardiac amyloidosis in RCM connects to the amyloidosis section of Chapter 5. The genetic basis of HCM (sarcomeric mutations) and ARVC (desmosomal mutations) links to the molecular pathology concepts in Chapter 8.*

Comparative WHO/AHA/ESC Classification of Cardiomyopathies

The AHA 2006 scientific statement and the ESC 2008 position paper together furnish the most widely used clinicopathological classification of cardiomyopathies. The four classical morphological categories — dilated, hypertrophic, restrictive, and arrhythmogenic right ventricular — are defined by dominant ventricular geometry, filling dynamics, and the genetic or acquired substrate. The WHO 2021 working framework integrates these categories with molecular aetiology (sarcomeric, desmosomal, ion-channel, infiltrative) and clinical presentation (heart failure, arrhythmia, sudden death), and explicitly recognises overlap syndromes. A side-by-side view is the form in which the topic is most often asked.

Table 14.1: Comparative Classification of the Four Classical Cardiomyopathies (AHA 2006 / ESC 2008 / WHO 2021 framework)

Feature	DCM	HCM	RCM / ARVC
Ventricular geometry	Dilated LV and often RV; thinned walls; four-chamber enlargement.	Hypertrophied LV, often asymmetric septal hypertrophy; cavity usually small.	RCM: normal chamber size, stiff non-compliant wall. ARVC: RV dilated with fibrofatty replacement.
Filling dynamics	Systolic dysfunction with reduced EF (typically <40	Diastolic dysfunction; dynamic LVOT obstruction	RCM: severe diastolic dysfunction with preserved EF.

Feature	DCM	HCM	RCM / ARVC
	percent).	in HOCM variant.	ARVC: RV systolic dysfunction, ventricular tachycardia.
Genetic basis	Autosomal dominant in 20-35 percent. TTN truncating variants most common; LMNA, MYH7, SCN5A, desmosomal.	Autosomal dominant. Sarcomeric genes dominate: MYBPC3 and MYH7 account for 50-60 percent of clinically diagnosed cases.	RCM: infiltrative causes — transthyretin or AL amyloid, Fabry, haemochromatosis. ARVC: desmosomal — PKP2, DSG2, DSP, DSC2.
Key histology	Myocyte attenuation with variable nuclear enlargement; interstitial and perivascular fibrosis; patchy necrosis if viral or toxic aetiology.	Myocyte hypertrophy with myofibre branching and disarray; interstitial fibrosis; thickened intramural coronaries.	RCM: interstitial amyloid (Congo red apple-green birefringence) or diffuse fibrosis. ARVC: transmural fibrofatty replacement of RV free wall, "triangle of dysplasia".
Prognosis and clinical	Progressive heart failure; 5-year mortality 20-50 percent. SCD risk. Heart transplant is the definitive therapy.	Variable. Sudden cardiac death is the feared complication in young athletes. AF common. ICD for high-risk phenotypes (family history, syncope, massive hypertrophy).	RCM carries the worst prognosis of all classical cardiomyopathies. ARVC is fundamentally a ventricular arrhythmia disease with SCD risk; ICD if high-risk.

Note: In autopsy series from many tertiary centres, dilated cardiomyopathy remains the commonest primary cardiomyopathy, with peripartum and idiopathic aetiologies prominently represented. HCM is a leading cause of sudden cardiac death in young athletes aged under 35; family screening with echocardiography and cascade genetic testing for MYH7 and MYBPC3 variants is standard at major tertiary electrophysiology centres.

Myocarditis

Myocarditis is inflammation of the myocardium causing cardiac dysfunction. The most common cause in the developed world is viral infection (coxsackievirus B, adenovirus, parvovirus B19, SARS-CoV-2). Other causes include autoimmune diseases (giant cell myocarditis, sarcoidosis), drugs (immune checkpoint inhibitors, doxorubicin), hypersensitivity reactions (eosinophilic myocarditis), and parasitic infection (*Trypanosoma cruzi* causing Chagas disease, an important cause of DCM in South America).

Pathogenesis. In viral myocarditis, the virus enters cardiomyocytes (coxsackievirus via the coxsackievirus-adenovirus receptor, CAR; parvovirus B19 via the erythrocyte P antigen on endothelial cells), causing direct cytopathic damage. This is followed by an immune-mediated phase: CD8+ cytotoxic

T cells attack virus-infected and bystander cardiomyocytes, and molecular mimicry between viral and cardiac proteins may perpetuate autoimmune injury even after viral clearance.

Morphology. The Dallas criteria for histological diagnosis require: (1) **myocyte necrosis or degeneration** with (2) an **adjacent inflammatory infiltrate** not typical of an ischaemic event. The infiltrate is predominantly lymphocytic in viral myocarditis. Giant cell myocarditis (idiopathic, aggressive) shows widespread myocyte destruction with multinucleated giant cells, lymphocytes, and eosinophils. Eosinophilic myocarditis shows prominent eosinophilic infiltrates and is often drug-related (hypersensitivity). Many cases of "idiopathic" DCM are thought to represent the end-stage of viral myocarditis.

Pericardial Disease

Acute pericarditis is most commonly viral (coxsackievirus, echovirus) or idiopathic. Uraemic pericarditis, post-MI pericarditis (Dressler syndrome), and tuberculous pericarditis (important in TB-endemic regions) are other significant causes. Morphologically, pericarditis may be serous, fibrinous ("bread-and-butter" appearance), purulent, haemorrhagic, or caseous (TB). **Constrictive pericarditis** results from healing of any form of pericarditis with dense fibrous scarring and calcification, producing a rigid "shell" that restricts diastolic filling. In TB-endemic regions, tuberculosis remains the most common cause of constrictive pericarditis.

The Pathologist's Eye

On an autopsy or surgical specimen, the key distinction is between fibrinous pericarditis (shaggy fibrin strands, no organisms) and purulent pericarditis (thick pus, bacterial colonies on Gram stain). **Caseous pericarditis (granulomas, caseous necrosis, AFB positivity) should raise tuberculosis as the aetiology, particularly in TB-endemic settings.** Haemorrhagic pericarditis suggests malignancy (metastatic carcinoma, commonly lung/breast) or TB.

Congenital Heart Disease

Congenital heart disease (CHD) affects approximately 8-10 per 1,000 live births. CHD is classified haemodynamically into **left-to-right shunts** (acyanotic initially: VSD, ASD, PDA), **right-to-left shunts** (cyanotic: Tetralogy of Fallot, TGA, truncus arteriosus), and **obstructive lesions** (coarctation of aorta, aortic/pulmonary stenosis) (Figure 14.7).

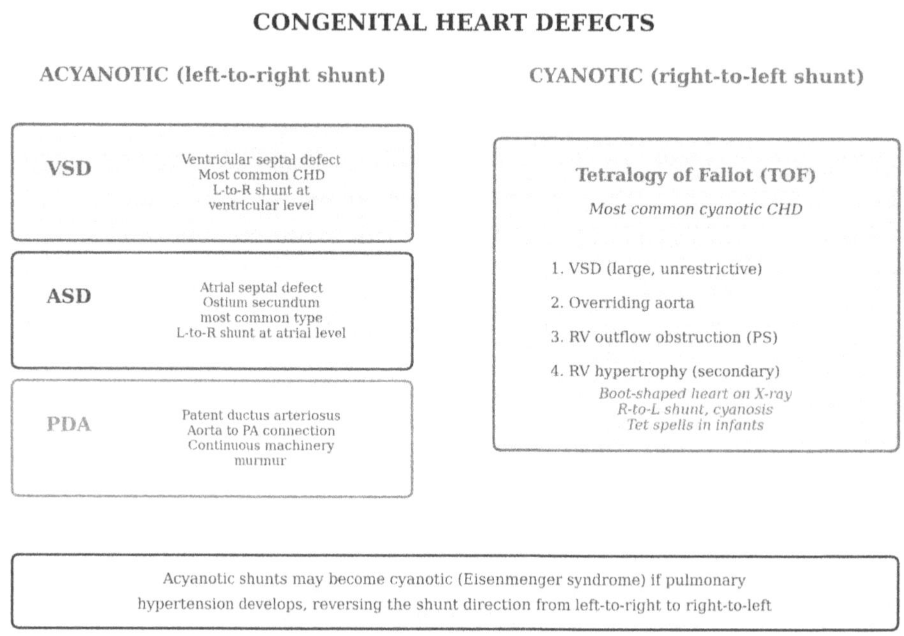

Figure 14.7 : Congenital heart defects: VSD, ASD, PDA, and Tetralogy of Fallot

Figure 14.7: Major congenital heart defects grouped by shunt direction: acyanotic left-to-right shunts (VSD — ventricular septal defect; ASD — atrial septal defect, ostium secundum; PDA — patent ductus arteriosus) and cyanotic right-to-left shunt (Tetralogy of Fallot — VSD, overriding aorta, RV outflow obstruction, RV hypertrophy), with direction of blood flow indicated. (Source: Author's original.)

Defect	Shunt / Lesion	Key Points
VSD	L→R (most common CHD)	Membranous > muscular. Small: spontaneous closure. Large: Eisenmenger syndrome
ASD	L→R	Secundum (fossa ovalis, most common). Primum (associated with MV cleft). Fixed split S2
PDA	L→R (aorta→PA)	Continuous "machinery" murmur. Indomethacin closes; PGE1 keeps open
Tetralogy of Fallot	R→L (most common cyanotic CHD)	VSD + overriding aorta + RV outflow obstruction + RV hypertrophy. Boot-shaped heart
TGA	R→L	Aorta from RV, PA from LV. Incompatible with life without

Defect	Shunt / Lesion	Key Points
		shunt (PDA/ASD/VSD)
Coarctation	Obstruction	Infantile (preductal, Turner) or adult (postductal, rib notching, HTN upper limbs)

Eisenmenger syndrome is the reversal of a left-to-right shunt to right-to-left due to progressive pulmonary vascular disease and irreversible pulmonary hypertension. The sequence is: large shunt → increased pulmonary blood flow → pulmonary arteriolar hypertrophy and intimal fibrosis → fixed pulmonary hypertension → RV pressure exceeds LV → shunt reversal → cyanosis. Once established, the shunt is irreversible and heart-lung transplantation is the only definitive treatment. This is the dreaded late complication of large, unrepaired VSDs, ASDs, and PDAs. Where access to early paediatric cardiac surgery is limited, Eisenmenger physiology is more commonly encountered than in countries with universal early surgical correction.

In settings with limited access to paediatric cardiac surgery, the most common cause of Eisenmenger syndrome remains unrepaired VSD (Figure 14.8).

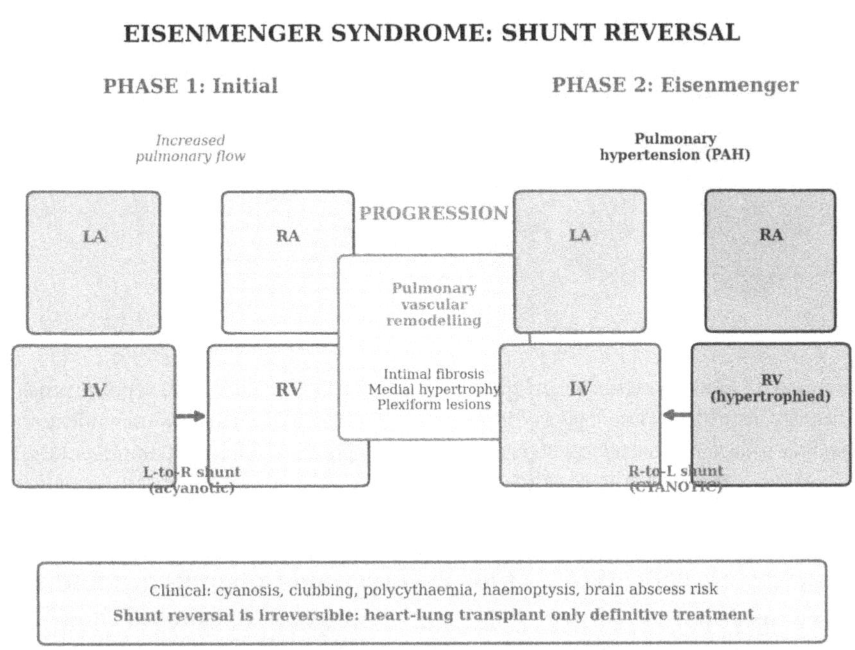

Figure 14.8 : Eisenmenger syndrome: pathophysiology of shunt reversal

Figure 14.8: Pathophysiology of Eisenmenger syndrome. Large VSD with initial left-to-right shunt leading to increased pulmonary flow, pulmonary arteriolar hypertrophy (medial thickening, intimal fibrosis, plexiform lesions), fixed pulmonary hypertension, shunt reversal (right-to-left), and cyanosis. (Source: Author's original.)

Integration: *The pulmonary hypertension and vascular remodelling in Eisenmenger syndrome connect to the pulmonary pathology in Chapter 15, while the genetic basis of CHD (22q11.2 deletion in DiGeorge/TOF, Turner syndrome in coarctation) links to Chapter 8.*

Cardiac Tumours

Primary cardiac tumours are rare. **Cardiac myxoma** is the most common primary tumour in adults: a benign, pedunculated mass typically arising in the left atrium near the fossa ovalis. It presents with a triad of obstructive symptoms (mimicking mitral stenosis), embolic events, and constitutional symptoms (fever, weight loss, elevated ESR from IL-6 secretion). **Rhabdomyoma** is the most common primary cardiac tumour in children, associated with tuberous sclerosis (TSC1/TSC2 mutations). **Metastatic tumours** to the heart are 20-40 times more common than primary tumours, most commonly from lung, breast, and melanoma.

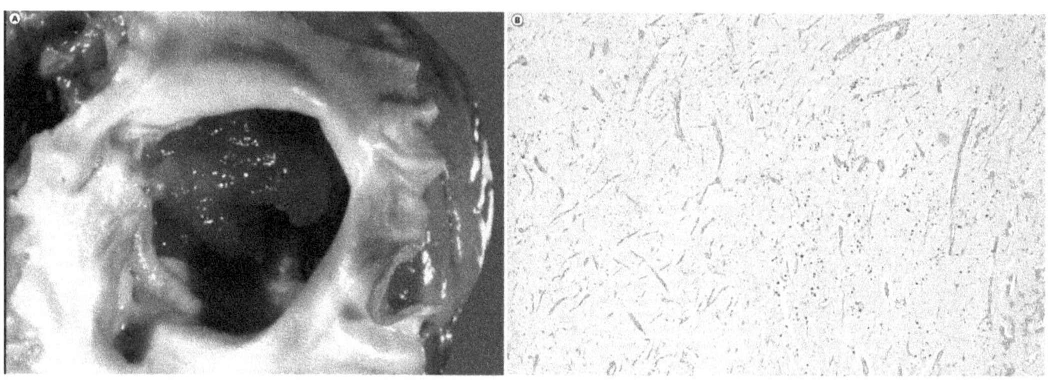

Figure 14.9: Cardiac myxoma. (A) Gross: gelatinous, polypoid mass attached to the interatrial septum, projecting into the left atrium. (Source: Armed Forces Institute of Pathology, Public domain.) (B) Histology (H&E, low magnification): myxoid stroma with scattered stellate cells and hemosiderin deposits. (Source: Nephron, Wikimedia Commons, CC BY-SA 3.0.)

Recent Advances in Cardiac Pathology

ESC 2023 cardiomyopathy classification — morphofunctional phenotypes and the non-dilated left ventricular cardiomyopathy entity. The 2023 European Society of Cardiology guidelines reorganised cardiomyopathy nosology around five morphofunctional phenotypes — hypertrophic, dilated, arrhythmogenic right ventricular, restrictive, and a newly defined non-dilated left ventricular cardiomyopathy — replacing earlier schemes that conflated genetic aetiology with morphology (Arbelo et al. European Heart Journal 2023; 44: 3503–3626; PMID 37622657). Recommendations couple multimodality imaging (echocardiography, cardiac magnetic resonance with native T1/T2 mapping, late gadolinium enhancement) with systematic genetic testing and family screening for first-degree relatives. The non-dilated left ventricular cardiomyopathy phenotype captures patients with non-ischaemic left-ventricular scar or replacement fibrosis without ventricular dilation, a substrate previously labelled "borderline" or "burnt-out" arrhythmogenic cardiomyopathy and now recognised as a sudden-cardiac-death risk category in its own right. Primary-prevention implantable cardioverter-defibrillator decisions are grounded in genotype, family history, late-gadolinium-enhancement burden, and validated calculators (HCM Risk-SCD; ARVC risk score). For the pathologist, the guideline reinforces the importance of the post-mortem molecular autopsy in sudden cardiac death and codifies endomyocardial-biopsy indications in suspected infiltrative or inflammatory cardiomyopathy.

Cardiac MRI and endomyocardial biopsy in myocarditis. Cardiac magnetic resonance imaging with late gadolinium enhancement has become the non-invasive gold standard for diagnosing myocarditis, reducing the need for endomyocardial biopsy. The updated Lake Louise criteria (2018) incorporate T1 mapping and T2 mapping for improved sensitivity. COVID-19-associated myocarditis and mRNA vaccine-associated myocarditis (rare, typically mild and self-limiting) have highlighted the importance of accurate myocarditis diagnosis.

Mavacamten and HCM. Mavacamten, a first-in-class cardiac myosin inhibitor, was approved for obstructive HCM (2022). It reduces the hypercontractility caused by sarcomeric mutations by decreasing the number of actin-myosin cross-bridges, targeting the fundamental molecular defect rather than managing symptoms alone. This represents a paradigm shift from surgical myectomy/alcohol ablation as the only options for drug-refractory obstruction.

Transthyretin cardiac amyloidosis. Recognition of wild-type transthyretin (ATTRwt) cardiac amyloidosis as an underdiagnosed cause of heart failure with preserved ejection fraction (HFpEF) in elderly patients has transformed clinical practice. Tafamidis (a transthyretin stabiliser) reduces mortality and hospitalisations. Technetium-99m pyrophosphate scintigraphy now allows non-invasive diagnosis without biopsy in many cases.

Approach to the Histopathology Slide: Cardiac Pathology

When presented with a cardiac pathology slide, follow this systematic approach.

1. Identify the tissue. Myocardium shows cross-cut and longitudinal cardiomyocytes with central nuclei, intercalated discs, and interstitial capillaries. Valvular tissue shows dense collagenous matrix with an endothelial lining. Pericardium is a serosal membrane with mesothelial cells.

2. Assess the myocytes. Are they normal, hypertrophied (enlarged with box-car nuclei), necrotic (loss of nuclei, hypereosinophilia, contraction bands), or replaced by fibrosis/fat? Coagulative necrosis with neutrophils indicates acute MI. Myofibre disarray indicates HCM. Fibrofatty replacement in the RV indicates ARVC.

3. Assess the interstitium. Is there inflammation (myocarditis: lymphocytic, granulomatous, giant cell, eosinophilic)? Fibrosis (old MI scar, DCM)? Amorphous eosinophilic deposits (amyloid: confirm with Congo red and apple-green birefringence)?

4. If a valve is present. Assess for vegetations (IE: organisms + neutrophils; rheumatic: sterile verrucae; NBTE: bland fibrin), calcification (calcific AS), myxomatous degeneration (MVP), or fibrotic thickening with commissural fusion (chronic RHD).

5. Special stains. Congo red for amyloid (apple-green birefringence under polarised light). Gram stain and tissue culture for IE organisms. Prussian blue for haemochromatosis (iron). PAS for glycogen storage disease.

The key diagnostic clue in endomyocardial biopsy interpretation: when faced with myocyte hypertrophy, interstitial fibrosis, and myocyte disarray, the pattern of disarray matters more than its presence. Myocyte disarray exceeding 20% of the septum in the absence of a haemodynamic cause (aortic stenosis, hypertension) is the histological hallmark of hypertrophic cardiomyopathy. In contrast, the Dallas criteria for myocarditis require an inflammatory infiltrate with associated myocyte necrosis or damage — interstitial infiltrate alone without myocyte injury is borderline myocarditis, not definite.

When evaluating a cardiac valve specimen, the chronological evolution of vegetations narrows the differential: acute vegetations (fibrin-platelet, friable, on previously normal valves) suggest infective endocarditis; small, sterile verrucae along the line of closure suggest rheumatic heart disease (Aschoff bodies in the myocardium confirm it); large, bland vegetations in a patient with malignancy point to non-bacterial thrombotic endocarditis (marantic); and flat, spreading vegetations on both surfaces of the valve with necrosis suggest Libman-Sacks endocarditis of SLE.

Ultra High-Yield Chapter Summary

Topic	Must Remember
MI wavefront	Subendocardial → transmural over 3-6 hours; early reperfusion salvages outer zones
MI morphology timeline	0-4h: wavy fibres. 12-24h: coagulative necrosis + neutrophils. 3-7d: softening. >6wk: scar
Rupture window	3-7 days; free wall > septum > papillary muscle; 1st MI, transmural, anterior, elderly female
Reperfusion injury	Contraction band necrosis, haemorrhagic infarct, ROS, no-reflow phenomenon
Aschoff body	Fibrinoid necrosis + Anitschkow cells (caterpillar chromatin) + Aschoff giant cells
Chronic RHD	Mitral stenosis (fish-mouth); commissural fusion; LA dilatation; AF
Jones criteria	Major: carditis, polyarthritis, chorea, EM, SQ nodules. + evidence of GAS infection
IE: acute vs subacute	Acute: S. aureus, normal valve, destructive.
Calcific AS	Degenerative; bicuspid valve stenoses 1-2 decades earlier; most common valve surgery indication (West)

Topic	Must Remember
MVP	Myxomatous degeneration; 2-3% prevalence; mid-systolic click; Marfan association
DCM	Dilated chambers, low EF, TTN/LMNA. #1 indication for transplant
HCM	Asymmetric septal hypertrophy, myofibre disarray, MYH7/MYBPC3. #1 sudden death young athletes
RCM	Stiff ventricles, amyloidosis #1 cause (West), EMF (tropical).
ARVC	RV fibrofatty replacement, desmosomal mutations (PKP2), triangle of dysplasia
VSD	Most common CHD.
TOF	Most common cyanotic CHD. 4 features.
Eisenmenger	Irreversible reversal of L→R shunt due to pulmonary vascular disease
Cardiac myxoma	Most common primary cardiac tumour in adults.
Mavacamten	Cardiac myosin inhibitor for obstructive HCM; targets fundamental molecular defect
ATTR amyloidosis	Underdiagnosed in elderly HFpEF; Tc-99m PYP scintigraphy; tafamidis treatment

Cross-References from Chapter 14

Coronary atherosclerosis, plaque rupture → Chapter 13. Coagulation, DIC, thromboembolism → Chapter 4 / Volume 1. SLE (Libman-Sacks), amyloidosis, autoimmunity → Chapter 5. Marfan, genetic cardiomyopathies → Chapter 8. COVID-19 myocarditis → Chapter 9. Tuberous sclerosis (rhabdomyoma) → Chapter 30. Constrictive pericarditis (TB, in TB-endemic regions) → Chapter 9. Chagas disease → Chapter 9. ATTR, tafamidis, mavacamten → Chapter 41.

Diagnostic thinking: coagulative necrosis + neutrophilic infiltrate + wavy fibres → acute MI (12–24 hours)

Diagnostic thinking: asymmetric septal hypertrophy + myocyte disarray + sudden death in young athlete → HCM

Diagnostic thinking: vegetations + Duke criteria + positive blood cultures → infective endocarditis (Figures 14.9–14.12)

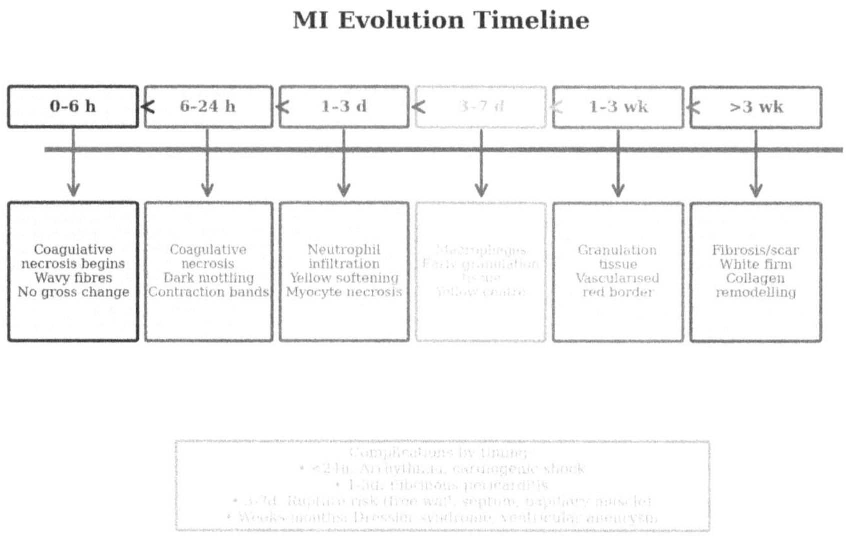

Figure 14.10: MI Evolution Timeline. (Source: Author's original.)

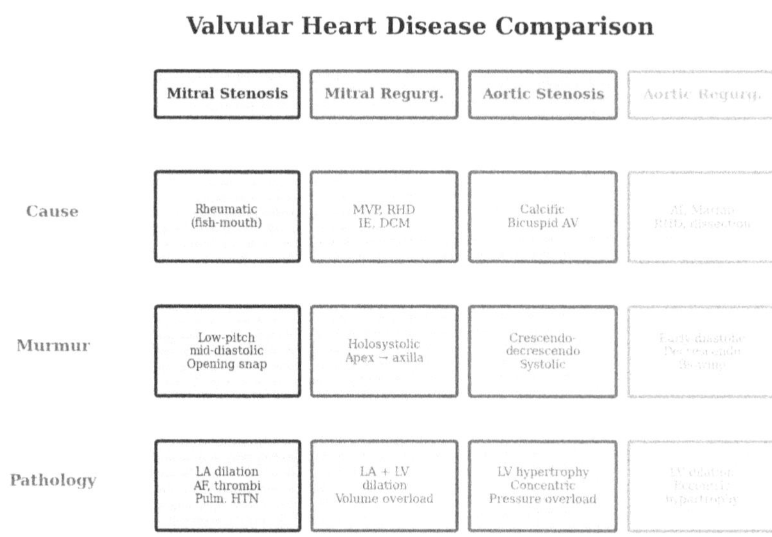

Figure 14.11: Valvular Heart Disease Comparison. (Source: Author's original.)

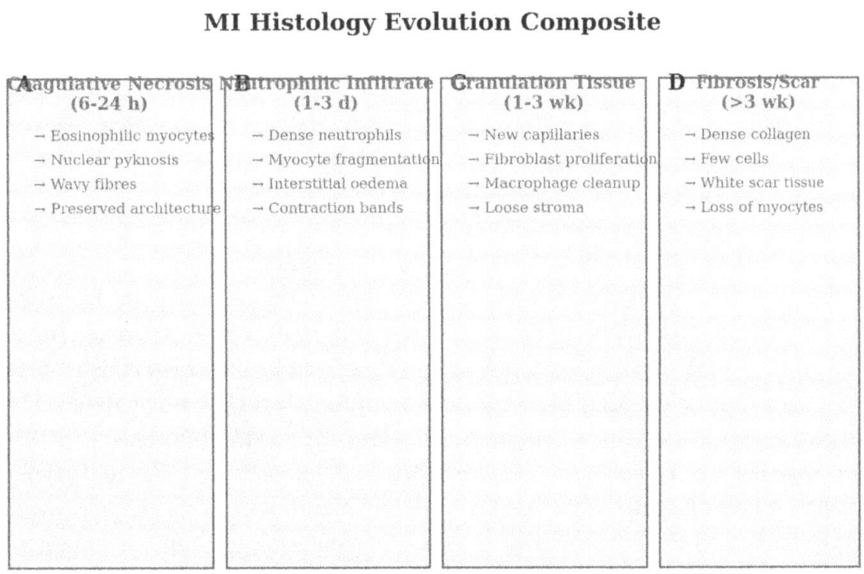

Figure 14.12: MI Histology Evolution Composite. (Source: Author's original.)

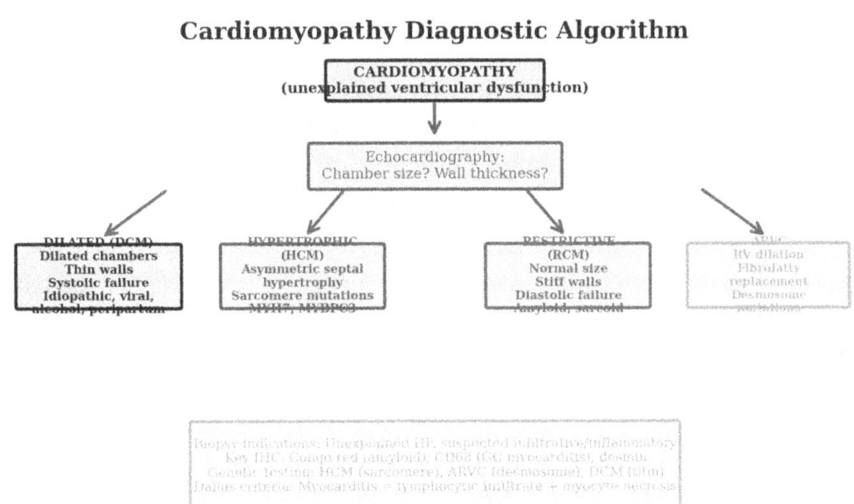

Figure 14.13: Cardiomyopathy Diagnostic Algorithm. (Source: Author's original.)

Chapter 15: Respiratory Pathology Part 1: Obstructive and Restrictive

> **THE BIG PICTURE**
>
> The lung is the interface between the body and the external environment, processing over 10,000 litres of air daily. This unique exposure makes it vulnerable to a vast range of injurious agents, from cigarette smoke and industrial dusts to infectious organisms and autoimmune attack. Obstructive lung diseases (chronic bronchitis, emphysema, asthma, bronchiectasis) are defined by increased resistance to airflow, while restrictive diseases (interstitial lung diseases, pneumoconioses) are defined by reduced lung compliance and total lung capacity. Acute respiratory distress syndrome (ARDS) represents the common endpoint of diverse insults to the alveolar-capillary membrane. Pulmonary hypertension is an increasingly recognised cause of right heart failure with a distinctive vascular pathology. This chapter covers the non-neoplastic, non-infectious diseases of the lung; infections and neoplasms are addressed in Chapter 16.
>
> **High-yield topics in this chapter:** Emphysema (types and pathogenesis); chronic bronchitis; COPD classification, complications, and prognostic indicators; bronchial asthma; bronchiectasis; ARDS/diffuse alveolar damage; usual interstitial pneumonia (UIP)/idiopathic pulmonary fibrosis (IPF); non-specific interstitial pneumonia (NSIP); pneumoconioses (silicosis, asbestosis, coal workers); sarcoidosis; hypersensitivity pneumonitis; pulmonary hypertension.

The lung is simultaneously delicate and resilient: a gas-exchange surface of approximately 70 square metres, thinner than a single sheet of paper at the alveolar-capillary membrane, yet capable of processing thousands of litres of potentially injurious air every day. When this surface is compromised, whether by destruction of alveolar walls (emphysema), chronic airway inflammation (asthma, chronic bronchitis), fibrotic remodelling (interstitial lung diseases), or acute injury (ARDS), the clinical consequences range from chronic breathlessness to rapid respiratory failure. For the pathologist, lung specimens demand pattern recognition: is the process obstructive or restrictive? Airway-centred or parenchymal? Acute or chronic? The answers guide both diagnosis and management.

15.1 Obstructive Lung Diseases

Obstructive lung diseases are characterised by increased resistance to airflow due to partial or complete obstruction of the airways at any level. The hallmark is a reduced FEV1/FVC ratio (forced expiratory volume in 1 second / forced vital capacity) on pulmonary function testing. The four major obstructive diseases are emphysema, chronic bronchitis (together comprising chronic obstructive pulmonary disease, COPD), bronchial asthma, and bronchiectasis.

Emphysema

Emphysema is defined as permanent enlargement of airspaces distal to the terminal bronchioles, accompanied by destruction of alveolar walls without significant fibrosis. It is classified anatomically into four types based on the part of the acinus involved. Centriacinar (centrilobular) emphysema affects the respiratory bronchioles (the central or proximal portion of the acinus), sparing the distal alveolar ducts and sacs. It is the most common type, strongly associated with cigarette smoking, and predominantly affects the upper lobes. Panacinar (panlobular) emphysema involves the entire acinus uniformly, from respiratory bronchiole to terminal alveolus. It is classically associated with alpha-1 antitrypsin (AAT) deficiency and predominantly affects the lower lobes. Distal acinar (paraseptal) emphysema involves the distal acinus (alveolar ducts and sacs) adjacent to the pleura and interlobular septa. It can cause spontaneous pneumothorax in young adults. Irregular (paracicatricial) emphysema involves the acinus irregularly, adjacent to scars and fibrotic foci; it is common but rarely clinically significant.

Cigarette smoke → recruitment of neutrophils and macrophages → release of elastase, MMP-9, MMP-12 → destruction of alveolar walls → loss of elastic recoil → airspace enlargement → expiratory airflow obstruction

The protease-antiprotease imbalance hypothesis is the central pathogenetic mechanism. Cigarette smoke recruits neutrophils and macrophages to the lung, which release serine proteases (neutrophil elastase) and matrix metalloproteinases (MMP-9 from macrophages, MMP-12). Simultaneously, smoke inactivates alpha-1 antitrypsin (the principal anti-elastase) through oxidation of a critical methionine residue. The resulting imbalance between protease activity and antiprotease protection leads to progressive destruction of elastic fibres and alveolar walls. In AAT deficiency (an autosomal codominant condition, most commonly the PiZZ phenotype), the baseline antiprotease level is critically low, making the lung exquisitely vulnerable to even normal levels of protease activity. An additional oxidant-antioxidant imbalance plays a synergistic role: reactive oxygen species from cigarette smoke and activated inflammatory cells directly damage alveolar walls and further inactivate antiproteases.

Grossly, emphysematous lungs are voluminous and pale, with enlarged airspaces visible to the naked eye (especially in panacinar disease). The lungs fail to deflate normally when the thorax is opened at autopsy. Microscopically, there is destruction and fenestration of alveolar walls with enlargement of airspaces. In centriacinar emphysema, the destruction is centred on the respiratory bronchioles with relative sparing of the distal alveolar sacs. In advanced disease, there is loss of the capillary bed within the destroyed walls, contributing to pulmonary hypertension and cor pulmonale.

Integration: Alpha-1 antitrypsin deficiency (PiZZ phenotype, liver disease with PAS-positive globules) is discussed in Chapter 8 (Genetic Disorders) and Chapter 20 (Hepatobiliary Pathology). The relationship between smoking and lung carcinogenesis is covered in Chapter 16 and Chapter 10 (Figure 15.1).

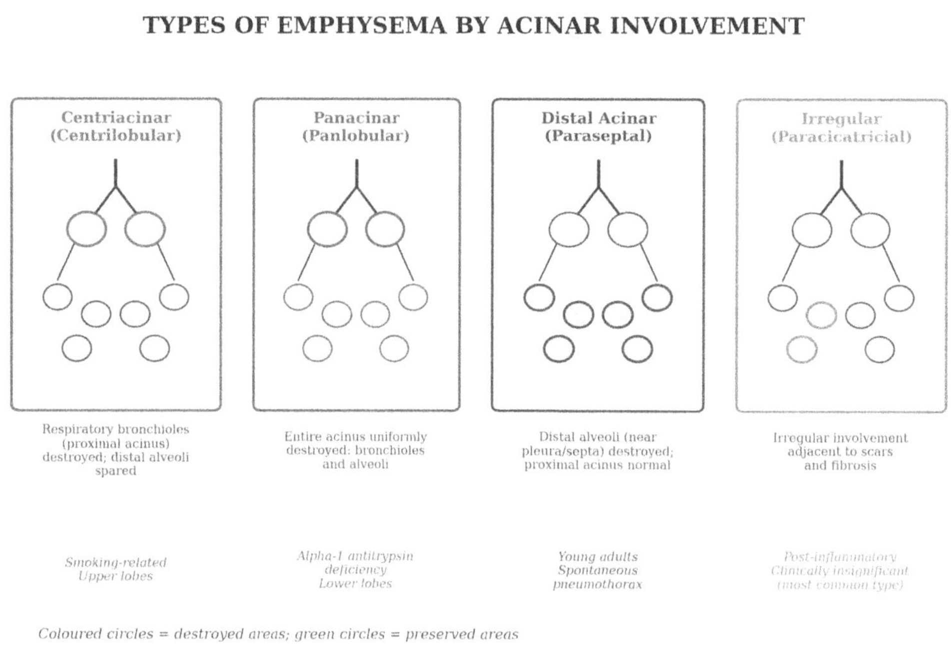

Figure 15.1 : Types of emphysema by pattern of acinar involvement

Figure 15.1: Types of emphysema by acinar involvement: centriacinar (proximal acinus, upper lobes, smoking-related), panacinar (entire acinus, lower lobes, α1-antitrypsin deficiency), distal acinar (peripheral/subpleural, pneumothorax risk), and irregular (adjacent to scars). (Source: Author's original.)

Type	Acinar Involvement	Location	Association	Clinical Significance
Centriacinar (centrilobular)	Proximal (respiratory bronchioles)	Upper lobes	Cigarette smoking	Most common; COPD
Panacinar (panlobular)	Entire acinus	Lower lobes (diffuse)	AAT deficiency (PiZZ)	Severe, early-onset
Distal acinar (paraseptal)	Distal (alveolar ducts/sacs)	Subpleural, along septa	Young adults	Spontaneous pneumothorax; bullae
Irregular (paracicatricial)	Irregular, adjacent to scars	Variable	Scarring/fibrosis	Common; usually asymptomatic

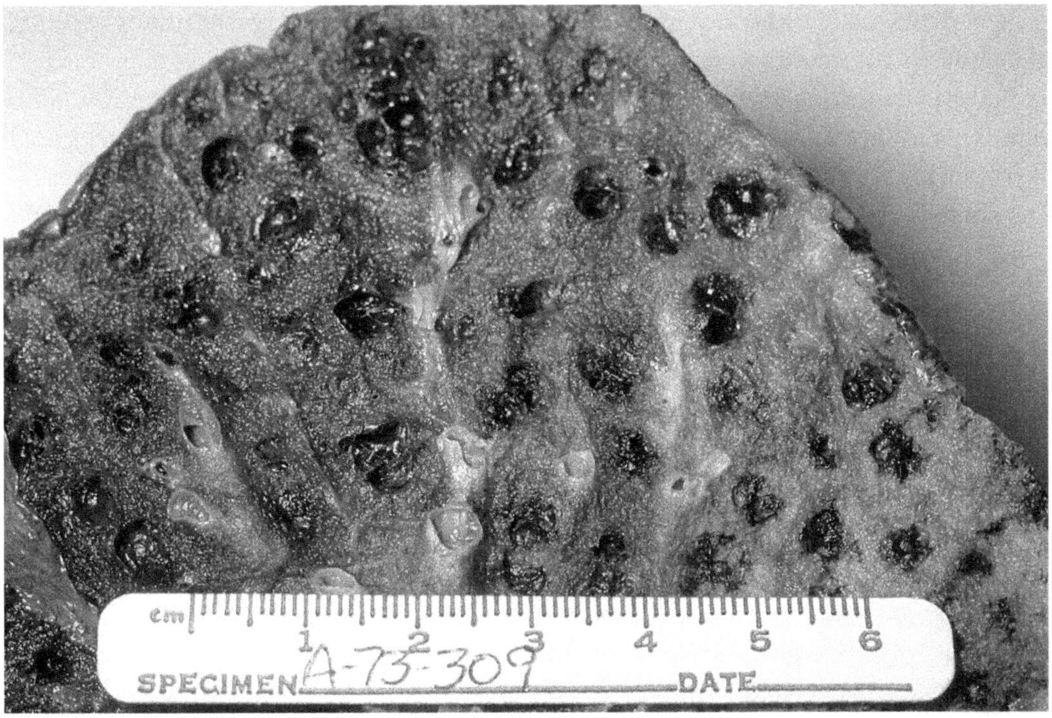

Figure 15.2: Centriacinar (centrilobular) emphysema — gross specimen. Upper-lobe-predominant destruction of respiratory bronchioles with enlarged airspaces centrally within the acinus. (Source: Dr. Edwin P. Ewing Jr., CDC/PHIL. Public domain.)

Chronic Bronchitis

Chronic bronchitis is defined clinically as a persistent productive cough for at least 3 months in at least 2 consecutive years, in the absence of other identifiable causes. Pathologically, the hallmark is hypertrophy and hyperplasia of the submucosal mucous glands in the bronchi, quantified by the Reid index (ratio of gland thickness to total bronchial wall thickness; normal less than 0.4, increased to more than 0.5 in chronic bronchitis). There is also goblet cell metaplasia in the small airways (bronchioles, which normally lack goblet cells), mucous plugging, chronic inflammation of the bronchial walls, and squamous metaplasia of the bronchial epithelium.

The pathogenesis involves chronic irritation from cigarette smoke (the dominant factor), air pollution, and recurrent infections. The sequence begins with mucous gland hypertrophy and goblet cell metaplasia in response to chronic irritation, leading to excessive mucus production and impaired mucociliary clearance. This creates a fertile environment for recurrent bacterial infections, which in turn perpetuate inflammation and further damage the airway epithelium. Small airway disease (chronic bronchiolitis with peribronchiolar fibrosis and goblet cell metaplasia of bronchiolar epithelium) is the critical component responsible for airflow obstruction in chronic bronchitis, rather than the large airway mucous gland changes.

Bronchial Asthma

Asthma is a chronic inflammatory disorder of the airways characterised by reversible bronchospasm, airway inflammation, and airway hyperresponsiveness to diverse stimuli. Atopic (extrinsic, allergic) asthma is the most common form, mediated by a type I (IgE-mediated) hypersensitivity reaction. Inhaled allergens are processed by dendritic cells, which activate Th2 lymphocytes to produce IL-4 (promotes IgE class-switching in B cells), IL-5 (recruits and activates eosinophils), and IL-13 (stimulates mucus secretion and smooth muscle hyperresponsiveness). Non-atopic asthma may be triggered by infections (especially viral), cold air, exercise, or drugs (aspirin-exacerbated respiratory disease, caused by COX-1 inhibition and shunting of arachidonic acid metabolism toward the leukotriene pathway).

Histologically, the asthmatic airway shows: bronchial smooth muscle hypertrophy and hyperplasia; subbasement membrane fibrosis (thickening of the reticular basement membrane); oedema and chronic inflammatory infiltrate (eosinophils, mast cells, lymphocytes) in the bronchial wall; goblet cell hyperplasia with mucous plugging; and shedding of the surface epithelium. Curschmann spirals (mucous casts of small airways), Charcot-Leyden crystals (crystallised eosinophil membrane protein, galectin-10), and Creola bodies (clusters of shed epithelial cells) may be found in the sputum.

Allergen → Th2 activation → IL-4 (IgE), IL-5 (eosinophils), IL-13 (mucus, hyperresponsiveness) → mast cell degranulation (immediate phase) → eosinophilic inflammation (late phase) → airway remodelling

Exam Pitfall

The reticular basement membrane thickening in asthma is NOT true basement membrane thickening. It is subepithelial fibrosis (deposition of collagen types III and V below the true basement membrane). This distinction is frequently tested (Figure 15.3).

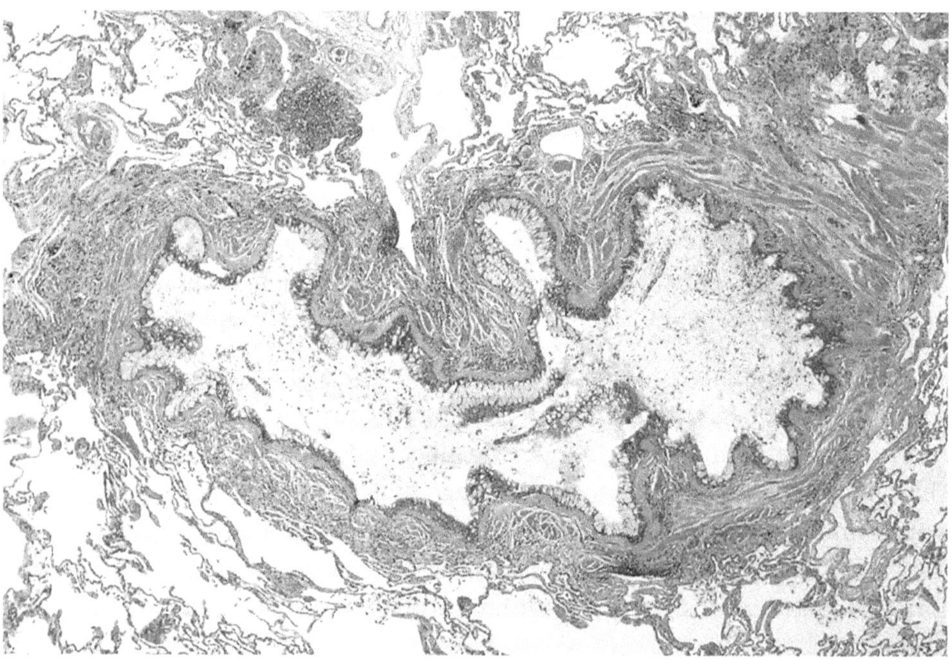

Figure 15.3: Bronchial asthma (H&E, low magnification). Smooth muscle hypertrophy, goblet cell hyperplasia, mucous plugging, basement membrane thickening, and peribronchial inflammation. (Source: Yale Rosen, Wikimedia Commons, CC BY-SA 2.0.)

Status asthmaticus refers to a severe, prolonged asthma attack that does not respond to standard bronchodilator therapy and is a medical emergency. At autopsy, the lungs are hyperinflated and fail to deflate when the thorax is opened. The airways are occluded by thick, tenacious mucous plugs containing Curschmann spirals and Charcot-Leyden crystals, and the bronchial walls show the full spectrum of asthmatic changes.

Bronchiectasis

Bronchiectasis is permanent dilation of bronchi and bronchioles caused by destruction of the muscular and elastic components of the bronchial wall, usually as a consequence of chronic necrotising infection. Predisposing conditions include cystic fibrosis (the most common genetic cause in Western populations), primary ciliary dyskinesia (Kartagener syndrome: bronchiectasis, situs inversus, sinusitis), post-infectious (severe childhood pneumonia, tuberculosis, measles), bronchial obstruction (tumour, foreign body), and immunodeficiency states. In TB-endemic regions, post-tubercular bronchiectasis remains the most important cause. Morphologically, affected airways are dilated (cylindrical, varicose, or saccular types), with destruction of the wall, chronic inflammatory infiltrate, fibrosis, and often squamous metaplasia of the lining epithelium. Clinically, patients present with chronic cough, copious foul-smelling sputum, recurrent infections, haemoptysis, and, in advanced cases, cor pulmonale. Secondary (AA) amyloidosis is a rare but recognised complication of longstanding bronchiectasis.

Why does emphysema cause airflow obstruction when the problem is destruction of alveolar walls, not narrowing of airways? Because alveolar walls provide radial traction that holds small airways open during expiration. When alveolar walls are destroyed, this traction is lost, and small airways collapse during expiration, trapping air. Additionally, loss of elastic recoil means the driving pressure for expiratory airflow is reduced. The combination of airway collapse and reduced elastic recoil produces the characteristic expiratory airflow limitation.

Feature	Emphysema	Chronic Bronchitis	Asthma	Bronchiectasis
Definition	Airspace enlargement + wall destruction	Productive cough 3mo/2yr	Reversible bronchospasm + airway hyperresponsiveness	Permanent airway dilation
Key pathology	Alveolar wall destruction; no fibrosis	Mucous gland hypertrophy (Reid index >0.5); goblet cell metaplasia	Smooth muscle hypertrophy; subbasement membrane fibrosis; eosinophils	Wall destruction; chronic inflammation; fibrosis
Primary site	Acinus (alveoli)	Bronchi and bronchioles	Bronchi (medium airways)	Bronchi and bronchioles
Reversibility	Irreversible	Partly reversible (inflammation)	Reversible (early); remodelling (late)	Irreversible

Smoking association	Strong (centriacinar)	Strong	Weak	Indirect (infection susceptibility)
Key complication	Pneumothorax (paraseptal); cor pulmonale	Recurrent infections; cor pulmonale	Status asthmaticus; airway remodelling	Haemoptysis; abscess; amyloidosis; cor pulmonale

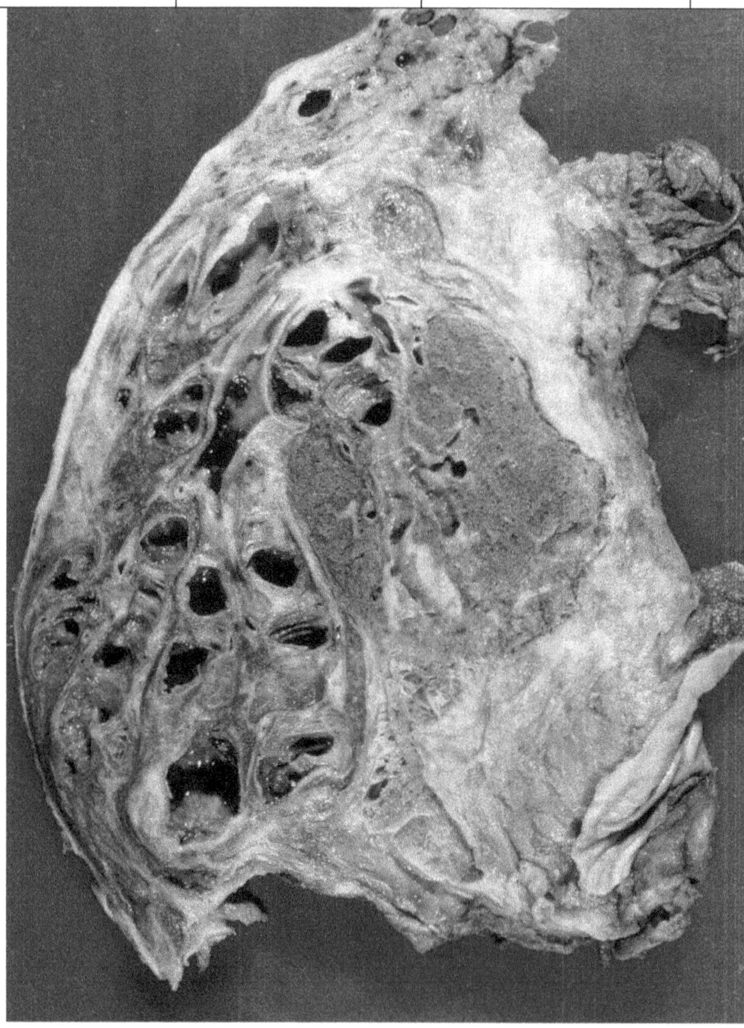

Figure 15.4: Bronchiectasis — gross specimen. Permanent dilatation of bronchi with thickened walls and surrounding fibrosis. Dilated airways visible as irregular cavities on cut section. (Source: Yale Rosen, Wikimedia Commons, CC BY-SA 2.0.)

COPD: The Integrated Clinical-Pathological Entity

Chronic obstructive pulmonary disease (COPD) is not a single disease but a clinical syndrome encompassing emphysema and chronic bronchitis, which coexist in most patients to varying degrees. COPD is defined by persistent airflow limitation that is not fully reversible, progressive, and associated with an enhanced chronic inflammatory response to noxious particles or gases. The Global Initiative for Chronic Obstructive Lung Disease (GOLD) classification stratifies severity based on post-bronchodilator

FEV1 as a percentage of predicted: GOLD 1 (mild, FEV1 80% or more predicted), GOLD 2 (moderate, 50 to less than 80%), GOLD 3 (severe, 30 to less than 50%), and GOLD 4 (very severe, less than 30%). The revised GOLD ABE assessment combines spirometric grade with symptom burden and exacerbation history for management decisions.

The pathology of COPD involves the entire lung. Large airway disease (mucous gland hypertrophy, goblet cell hyperplasia, squamous metaplasia) produces the chronic bronchitis phenotype. Small airway disease (chronic bronchiolitis with peribronchiolar fibrosis, goblet cell metaplasia, mucous plugging of membranous bronchioles) is the major site of airflow obstruction and correlates best with decline in FEV1. Parenchymal destruction (emphysema) adds loss of elastic recoil and small airway collapse. Pulmonary vascular remodelling (medial hypertrophy of small pulmonary arteries due to chronic hypoxia) leads to pulmonary hypertension and cor pulmonale. These four pathological domains coexist in individual patients in varying proportions.

The classical clinical phenotypes, though an oversimplification, remain useful for understanding the pathophysiology. The "pink puffer" (predominantly emphysema) maintains relatively normal blood gases through increased work of breathing (tachypnoea, pursed-lip breathing, barrel chest, use of accessory muscles), with mild hypoxaemia and normal or low $PaCO_2$. The "blue bloater" (predominantly chronic bronchitis) develops significant hypoxaemia and hypercapnia early, with cyanosis, peripheral oedema from cor pulmonale, and secondary polycythaemia (erythropoietin-mediated response to chronic hypoxia). Most patients are mixed phenotypes.

The pathogenesis explains the morphology: because chronic inflammation in small airways produces peribronchiolar fibrosis and luminal narrowing, and because emphysematous destruction of alveolar walls removes the radial traction that normally holds these small airways open, the combination produces the progressive, irreversible airflow limitation that defines COPD.

Complications of COPD include acute exacerbations (triggered by bacterial or viral infections, air pollution), progressive respiratory failure (type II with hypercapnia), cor pulmonale (right ventricular hypertrophy and dilation secondary to pulmonary hypertension from chronic hypoxic vasoconstriction), secondary polycythaemia (due to chronic hypoxaemia-driven erythropoietin production), spontaneous pneumothorax (rupture of bullae, especially in paraseptal emphysema), and increased susceptibility to lung carcinoma. Barrel chest (increased anteroposterior diameter from hyperinflation), flattened diaphragms on imaging, and bullae visible on CT are characteristic radiological findings.

Prognostic indicators in COPD include FEV1 (the single most important predictor; decline rate and absolute value correlate with mortality), the BODE index (Body mass index, airflow Obstruction by FEV1, Dyspnoea by mMRC scale, Exercise capacity by 6-minute walk test; a multidimensional score validated to predict mortality better than FEV1 alone), frequency and severity of acute exacerbations (two or more moderate exacerbations or one hospitalisation per year defines the "frequent exacerbator" phenotype with worse prognosis), $PaCO_2$ (chronic hypercapnia indicates advanced disease), pulmonary hypertension (cor pulmonale predicts poor outcome), and nutritional status (low BMI is an independent risk factor for mortality in advanced COPD).

Quick Recall: Obstructive Lung Diseases and COPD

Emphysema: Centriacinar (smoking, upper lobes) vs panacinar (AAT deficiency, lower lobes). Protease-antiprotease imbalance.

Chronic bronchitis: Clinical definition (3 months, 2 years). Reid index >0.5.

COPD: GOLD 1-4 by FEV1. Four pathological domains: large airway, small airway (main site of obstruction), parenchymal destruction, vascular remodelling.

Asthma: Reversible bronchospasm. Th2-mediated (IL-4, IL-5, IL-13). Smooth muscle hypertrophy, subbasement membrane fibrosis, eosinophils.

Bronchiectasis: Permanent airway dilation. CF (#1 genetic cause in West), post-TB, Kartagener, obstruction.

15.2 Restrictive (Interstitial) Lung Diseases

Restrictive lung diseases are characterised by reduced lung compliance, decreased total lung capacity (TLC), and a normal or increased FEV1/FVC ratio (because both FEV1 and FVC are proportionally reduced). Most restrictive diseases are interstitial lung diseases (ILDs), a heterogeneous group affecting the pulmonary interstitium (alveolar walls, perivascular and perilymphatic tissue). The interstitial lung diseases are classified by aetiology (known cause: pneumoconioses, drug-induced, radiation, connective tissue disease-associated) or as idiopathic interstitial pneumonias (IIPs) when no cause is identified.

Idiopathic Pulmonary Fibrosis (IPF) / Usual Interstitial Pneumonia (UIP)

UIP is a histological pattern; when it occurs in the absence of an identifiable cause, the clinical entity is called idiopathic pulmonary fibrosis (IPF). IPF is the most common and most lethal of the IIPs, with a median survival of 3 to 5 years. It typically presents in older males (over 50 years) with gradually progressive dyspnoea and non-productive cough. High-resolution CT shows a characteristic pattern of basal-predominant, peripheral, reticular opacities with honeycombing and traction bronchiectasis.

Histologically, UIP is defined by two cardinal features: temporal heterogeneity (areas of dense fibrosis and honeycombing coexist with areas of normal or near-normal lung) and spatial heterogeneity (the fibrosis is patchy, predominantly subpleural and paraseptal, worse in the lower lobes). Fibroblastic foci (collections of immature myofibroblasts and loose connective tissue at the leading edge of fibrosis) are the hallmark of active disease. Honeycombing (cystically dilated airspaces lined by metaplastic bronchiolar epithelium, surrounded by dense fibrosis) represents the end stage. Inflammation is minimal, distinguishing UIP from NSIP.

The distinction from NSIP rests on three features: UIP shows temporal heterogeneity (different ages of fibrosis side by side), fibroblastic foci, and honeycombing; NSIP shows temporal homogeneity (fibrosis of the same age throughout), no honeycombing, and a better prognosis (Figure 15.5).

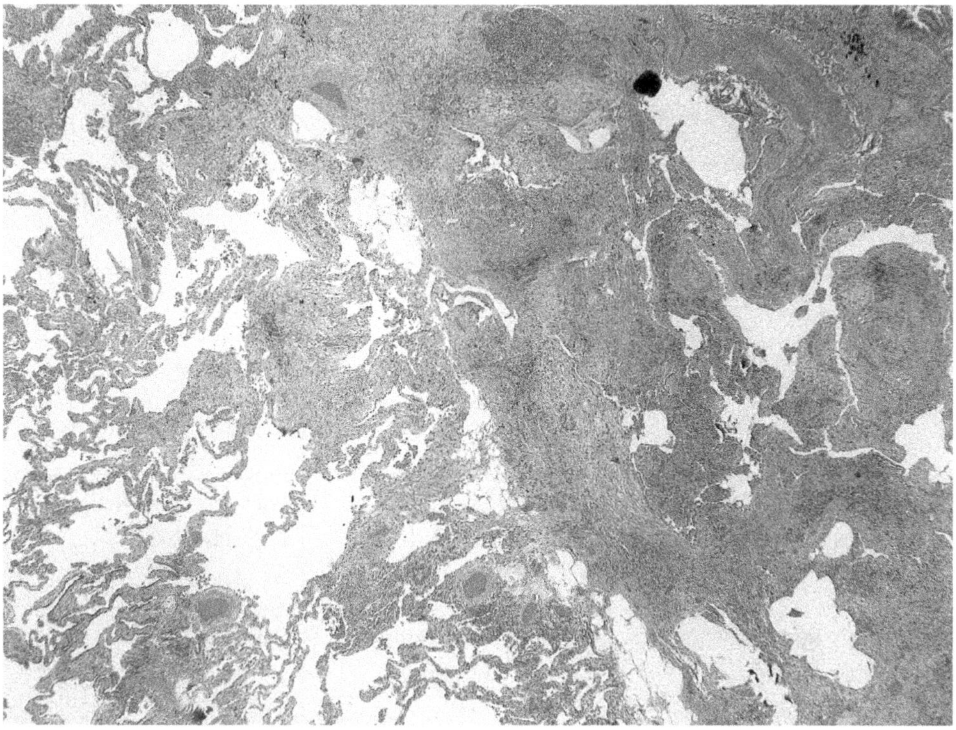

Figure 15.5: Usual interstitial pneumonia (UIP) pattern (H&E, low magnification). Spatial heterogeneity with alternating areas of dense subpleural fibrosis, fibroblastic foci, and relatively preserved alveolar architecture. (Source: Yale Rosen, Wikimedia Commons, CC BY-SA 2.0.)

Non-Specific Interstitial Pneumonia (NSIP)

NSIP is a distinct histological pattern characterised by temporally homogeneous (uniform age) interstitial inflammation and/or fibrosis. It may be cellular (predominantly lymphoplasmacytic inflammation) or fibrotic (predominantly fibrosis), or mixed. Unlike UIP, the fibrosis in NSIP is of the same age throughout, without fibroblastic foci or honeycombing. NSIP may be idiopathic or secondary to connective tissue disease (the most common association), drug reactions, or hypersensitivity pneumonitis. The prognosis is substantially better than UIP/IPF, with a 5-year survival exceeding 80% for cellular NSIP.

Other Interstitial Pneumonias

Cryptogenic organising pneumonia (COP) is the idiopathic form of organising pneumonia. Histologically, it shows intraluminal plugs of granulation tissue (Masson bodies) within alveolar ducts and alveoli, with preservation of the underlying lung architecture. It responds well to corticosteroids. Respiratory bronchiolitis-interstitial lung disease (RB-ILD) and desquamative interstitial pneumonia (DIP) represent a spectrum of smoking-related ILD. RB-ILD shows pigmented ("smoker's") macrophages in respiratory bronchioles, while DIP shows diffuse filling of alveoli by pigmented macrophages with mild fibrosis. Lymphoid interstitial pneumonia (LIP) shows dense lymphoplasmacytic interstitial infiltrate, associated with Sjogren syndrome, HIV, and CVID. Acute interstitial pneumonia (AIP) shows DAD pattern histologically and represents idiopathic ARDS with high mortality.

IIP Pattern	Key Histology	Distribution	Prognosis	Key Association
UIP / IPF	Temporal heterogeneity, fibroblastic foci, honeycombing, minimal inflammation	Subpleural, basal	Poor (median 3–5 yr)	Idiopathic; also CTD, chronic HP
NSIP	Temporally homogeneous inflammation/fibrosis; no honeycombing	Diffuse	Good (>80% 5-yr cellular)	CTD (most common), drugs, HP
COP	Intraluminal organising plugs (Masson bodies), preserved architecture	Patchy, peribronchovascular	Excellent (steroid-responsive)	Post-infection, drugs, CTD, idiopathic
DIP	Diffuse alveolar filling by pigmented macrophages; mild fibrosis	Diffuse, lower lobes	Good (stop smoking)	Smoking
RB-ILD	Pigmented macrophages in respiratory bronchioles	Bronchiolocentric	Good (stop smoking)	Smoking
LIP	Dense lymphoplasmacytic interstitial infiltrate	Diffuse	Variable	Sjogren, HIV, CVID
AIP	DAD pattern (hyaline membranes, organising phase)	Diffuse	Poor (>50% mortality)	Idiopathic (= idiopathic ARDS)

Quick Recall: Interstitial Lung Diseases

Pattern	Distribution	Key Histology	Temporal	Prognosis
UIP	Peripheral, basal	Patchy fibrosis + fibroblast foci; honeycombing	Heterogeneous (old + new)	Poor; 3-5 yr; IPF; steroid-resistant
NSIP	Diffuse, lower lobes	Uniform inflammation +/- fibrosis; preserved architecture	Homogeneous	Better; steroid-responsive
OP	Patchy, peribronchial	Masson bodies (intraluminal granulation tissue plugs)	Uniform	Good; steroid-responsive; formerly

				BOOP
DIP	Diffuse, lower lobes	Pigmented macrophages filling alveoli	Uniform	Good with smoking cessation
LIP	Diffuse	Dense lymphoid infiltrate; germinal centres	Uniform	Variable; Sjogren, HIV; lymphoma risk

ILD Patterns — Differential Diagnosis

UIP/IPF: Temporal + spatial heterogeneity, fibroblastic foci, honeycombing, minimal inflammation. Worst prognosis.
NSIP: Temporal homogeneity, no honeycombing. CTD association.
COP: Masson bodies (intraluminal organising plugs). Steroid-responsive.
DIP/RB-ILD: Smoking-related. Pigmented macrophages.

15.3 Pneumoconioses

Pneumoconioses are non-neoplastic lung diseases caused by inhalation of mineral dusts, organic dusts, or chemical fumes in occupational or environmental settings. The type of disease depends on the type of dust, the dose and duration of exposure, and host susceptibility factors. Particles of 1 to 5 micrometres in diameter are the most dangerous because they reach the terminal airways and alveoli. Particles larger than 10 micrometres are filtered by the nose and upper airways; particles smaller than 0.5 micrometres remain in suspension and are exhaled. The pathogenicity of a dust depends on its ability to activate macrophages and trigger fibrosis (silica, asbestos) versus its relative inertness (carbon/coal dust in small quantities).

Silicosis

Silicosis is caused by inhalation of crystalline silica (quartz). Occupational exposure occurs in mining, sandblasting, stone cutting, and glass manufacturing. Inhaled silica particles are engulfed by macrophages, which are then killed by the cytotoxic effects of silica (it disrupts phagolysosomal membranes and activates the NLRP3 inflammasome, releasing IL-1β and IL-18). Released particles are re-engulfed in a cycle of macrophage death and inflammation. The hallmark lesion is the silicotic nodule: a well-circumscribed, concentrically layered nodule of whorled collagen fibres ("onion-skin" pattern) with a central zone of hyalinisation, surrounded by macrophages and fibroblasts. Silica is birefringent under polarised light.

Simple silicosis (multiple small nodules, predominantly in the upper lobes and hilar lymph nodes) may progress to progressive massive fibrosis (PMF) or complicated silicosis (coalescent nodules forming large fibrotic masses greater than 2 cm). Accelerated silicosis develops within 5 to 10 years of heavy exposure, and acute silicosis (silicoproteinosis) presents within weeks to months of massive exposure with alveolar filling by PAS-positive lipoproteinaceous material similar to pulmonary alveolar proteinosis. Silicosis increases susceptibility to tuberculosis (silico-tuberculosis) and is associated with an increased risk of lung cancer. Eggshell calcification of hilar lymph nodes is a characteristic radiological finding.

Asbestosis and Asbestos-Related Diseases

Asbestos comprises a group of silicate mineral fibres (serpentine: chrysotile; amphibole: crocidolite, amosite, tremolite). Asbestosis refers specifically to interstitial pulmonary fibrosis caused by asbestos exposure. The fibrosis begins in the lower lobes around respiratory bronchioles and progresses to involve the alveolar walls. The hallmark is the asbestos body (ferruginous body): a golden-brown, dumbbell-shaped structure formed by iron and protein coating of an asbestos fibre, highlighted by Perl Prussian blue stain. Asbestos exposure also causes pleural plaques (the most common asbestos-related finding; well-circumscribed plaques of dense, acellular, hyalinised collagen on the parietal pleura, often calcified, especially on the diaphragmatic surface), pleural effusions, mesothelioma (see Chapter 16), and increased risk of lung carcinoma (especially in smokers, where the risk is multiplicative).

Ferruginous (asbestos) body: See Figure 10.4 (Chapter 10, Environmental Pathology) for photomicrograph.

Coal Workers' Pneumoconiosis

Coal workers' pneumoconiosis (CWP) is caused by inhalation of coal dust. Simple CWP is characterised by coal macules (aggregates of carbon-laden macrophages around respiratory bronchioles) and coal nodules (macules with additional collagen deposition), with associated focal emphysema. Simple CWP is usually asymptomatic. Complicated CWP (progressive massive fibrosis) presents as large, densely fibrotic masses, usually in the upper lobes, which may undergo central necrosis. Mixed-dust pneumoconiosis is common because coal miners are often co-exposed to silica. Caplan syndrome refers to the coexistence of coal workers' pneumoconiosis (or silicosis) with rheumatoid arthritis, characterised by rapidly developing large rheumatoid nodules in the lung.

Pneumoconiosis	Causative Agent	Key Histology	Distribution	Complications
Silicosis	Crystalline silica (quartz)	Whorled collagen nodules (onion-skin); birefringent particles	Upper lobes, hilar LN	TB, PMF, lung cancer
Asbestosis	Asbestos fibres (amphibole > serpentine)	Interstitial fibrosis + asbestos (ferruginous) bodies	Lower lobes	Mesothelioma, lung cancer, pleural plaques
CWP	Coal dust	Coal macules/nodules around bronchioles; focal emphysema	Upper lobes	PMF, Caplan syndrome (RA + CWP)
Berylliosis	Beryllium	Non-caseating granulomas (identical to sarcoidosis)	Diffuse	Progressive fibrosis

15.4 Sarcoidosis

Sarcoidosis is a systemic granulomatous disease of unknown aetiology characterised by non-caseating (non-necrotising) granulomas in multiple organs, most commonly the lungs and hilar lymph nodes. It is a diagnosis of exclusion; infection (especially tuberculosis and fungal disease) must be ruled out. The granulomas follow a lymphangitic distribution in the lung (along bronchovascular bundles, interlobular septa, and pleura), a feature that distinguishes sarcoidosis from hypersensitivity pneumonitis (which is airway-centred). The granulomas are "tight," well-formed, composed of epithelioid macrophages and multinucleated giant cells with scant surrounding lymphocytic inflammation. Schaumann bodies (laminated calcium-protein concretions) and asteroid bodies (star-shaped inclusions within giant cells) may be seen but are not specific.

With progression, the granulomas may coalesce and undergo hyalinisation and fibrosis. Systemic manifestations include bilateral hilar lymphadenopathy (the most common radiographic finding), skin lesions (erythema nodosum, lupus pernio), uveitis, hepatic granulomas, hypercalcaemia (due to 1-alpha hydroxylase activity in macrophages converting 25-hydroxyvitamin D to 1,25-dihydroxyvitamin D), and elevated serum ACE levels. Kveim-Siltzbach test (intradermal injection of sarcoid tissue extract producing a granulomatous reaction at 4-6 weeks) is of historical interest but no longer used.

When faced with non-caseating granulomas in a lung biopsy, the first question to ask is: have we excluded infection? Request AFB and GMS stains on every case. Sarcoidosis is a diagnosis of exclusion.

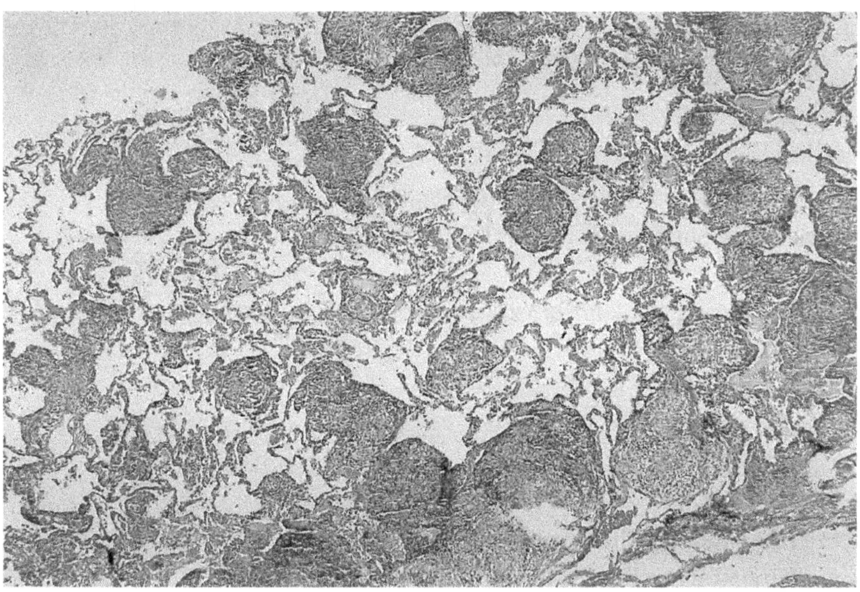

Figure 15.6: Pulmonary sarcoidosis — non-caseating granulomas (H&E, low magnification). Multiple compact, well-formed epithelioid granulomas distributed along bronchovascular bundles and interlobular septa in the alveolar parenchyma. (Source: Author's original.)

Stage	Radiographic Finding	Prognosis

0	Normal chest radiograph	N/A
I	Bilateral hilar lymphadenopathy alone	Best; >60% spontaneous remission
II	Hilar lymphadenopathy + pulmonary infiltrates	Moderate; remission in ~50%
III	Pulmonary infiltrates without hilar lymphadenopathy	Guarded
IV	Advanced pulmonary fibrosis	Worst; irreversible

15.5 Hypersensitivity Pneumonitis

Hypersensitivity pneumonitis (HP, also called extrinsic allergic alveolitis) is an immunologically mediated inflammatory lung disease caused by repeated inhalation of organic antigens or low-molecular-weight chemicals. Common forms include farmer's lung (thermophilic actinomycetes in mouldy hay), bird fancier's lung (avian proteins in droppings and feathers), and humidifier lung. The histological triad of HP is: (1) airway-centred (peribronchiolar) chronic interstitial inflammation, (2) poorly formed, non-necrotising granulomas or isolated giant cells ("loose granulomas"), and (3) organising pneumonia (Masson bodies). In chronic HP, fibrosis may develop with a UIP-like or NSIP-like pattern, creating diagnostic difficulty. The 2020 ATS/JRS/ALAT clinical practice guideline reclassified HP into non-fibrotic HP (acute and subacute, generally good prognosis) and fibrotic HP (chronic, prognosis depends on extent of fibrosis and UIP-like pattern).

Quick Recall: Pneumoconioses, Sarcoidosis, HP

Silicosis: Whorled collagen nodules, birefringent. Upper lobes. TB risk.

Asbestosis: Lower lobe fibrosis + ferruginous bodies (Perl+). Pleural plaques.

Sarcoidosis: Non-caseating granulomas, lymphangitic distribution. Bilateral hilar LAD. Hypercalcaemia (1-alpha hydroxylase).

HP triad: Peribronchiolar inflammation + loose granulomas + organising pneumonia. Airway-centred (vs lymphangitic in sarcoidosis).

15.6 Acute Respiratory Distress Syndrome (ARDS) / Diffuse Alveolar Damage (DAD)

ARDS is a clinical syndrome of acute respiratory failure characterised by bilateral pulmonary infiltrates and severe hypoxaemia not fully explained by cardiac failure. The Berlin definition (2012) grades ARDS by severity based on the PaO2/FiO2 ratio: mild (200 to 300 mmHg), moderate (100 to 200 mmHg), and severe (less than 100 mmHg), all with bilateral opacities on imaging within 7 days of a known clinical insult and not fully explained by cardiac failure or fluid overload. Diffuse alveolar damage (DAD) is the histological pattern underlying most cases of ARDS, though not all patients with clinical ARDS have DAD on biopsy (other patterns include organising pneumonia and diffuse alveolar haemorrhage).

DAD may be triggered by diverse insults including sepsis (the most common cause), severe pneumonia (including COVID-19), aspiration, trauma, pancreatitis, inhalation injury, and drug toxicity. When no cause is identified, the condition is termed acute interstitial pneumonia (AIP), which is essentially idiopathic ARDS.

The pathogenesis involves damage to the alveolar epithelium and/or capillary endothelium, leading to increased permeability of the alveolar-capillary barrier, flooding of alveoli with protein-rich oedema fluid, and activation of the coagulation cascade. Pro-inflammatory cytokines (TNF-α, IL-1, IL-6, IL-8) recruit neutrophils that release reactive oxygen species and proteases, amplifying tissue damage. Surfactant dysfunction (damage to type II pneumocytes) causes alveolar collapse and further impairs gas exchange.

DAD evolves through two phases. The exudative (acute) phase (days 1 to 7) is characterised by interstitial and intra-alveolar oedema, fibrin deposition, and hyaline membranes (eosinophilic, glassy membranes composed of fibrin and necrotic epithelial cell debris lining the alveolar surfaces). Capillary congestion, haemorrhage, and alveolar epithelial necrosis (type I pneumocyte damage) are also present. The organising (proliferative) phase (after 1 to 2 weeks) shows type II pneumocyte hyperplasia (attempting to regenerate the alveolar lining), fibroblast proliferation within the alveolar walls and airspaces, and progressive interstitial fibrosis. Outcome is variable: some patients recover completely, while others develop progressive fibrosis leading to chronic ventilator dependence.

Insult (sepsis, pneumonia, trauma) → endothelial/epithelial damage → increased permeability → protein-rich oedema + fibrin → hyaline membranes (exudative phase) → type II pneumocyte hyperplasia + fibroblast proliferation (organising phase) (Figure 15.7)

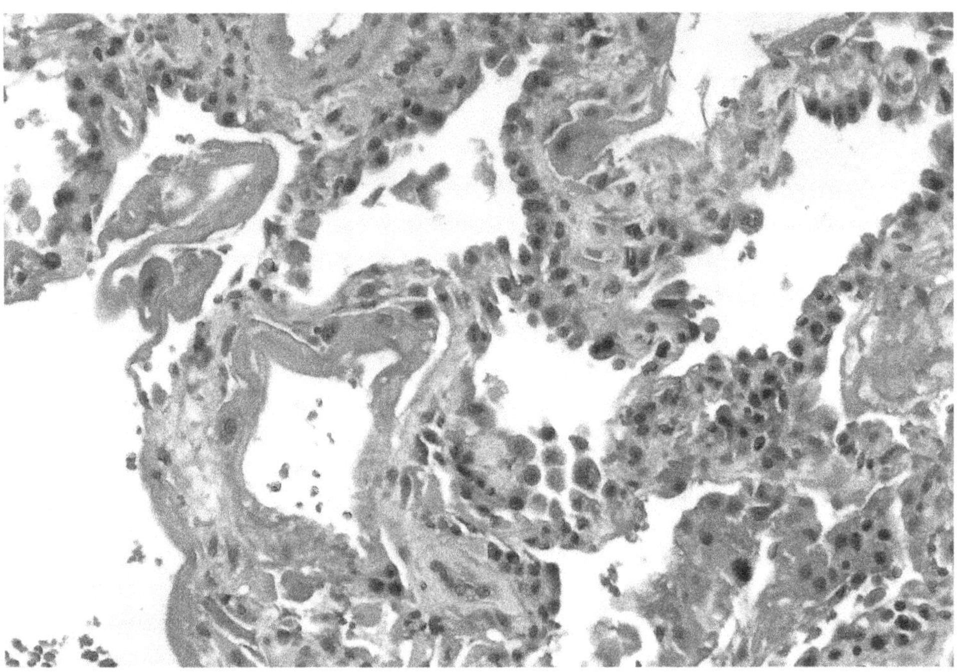

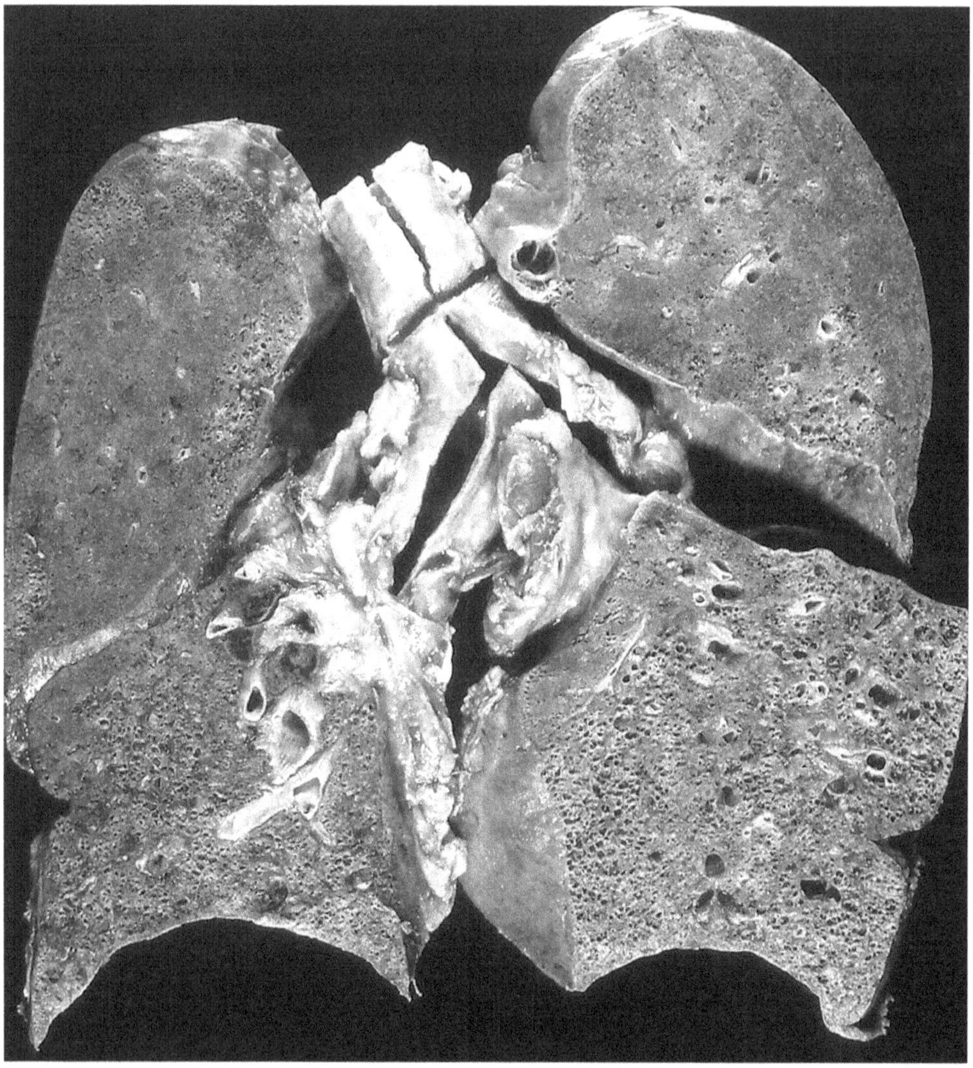

Figure 15.7: Diffuse alveolar damage (DAD) / acute respiratory distress syndrome (ARDS). (A) Histology (H&E, high magnification): prominent hyaline membranes lining alveolar surfaces with interstitial oedema and type II pneumocyte hyperplasia — exudative phase. (B) Gross specimen: bilateral heavy, beefy-red consolidated lungs with rigid parenchyma — the characteristic 'wet lung' appearance of ARDS. (Source: Yale Rosen, Wikimedia Commons, CC BY-SA 2.0; both panels from the same series.)

Integration: Neonatal respiratory distress syndrome (hyaline membrane disease of the newborn) shares the histological feature of hyaline membranes but results from surfactant deficiency rather than alveolar-capillary damage (see Chapter 11). The role of sepsis and shock in triggering ARDS is discussed in Chapter 4. COVID-19 DAD with microvascular thrombosis is covered in Chapter 16.

15.7 Pulmonary Hypertension

Pulmonary hypertension (PH) is defined as a mean pulmonary arterial pressure (mPAP) exceeding 20 mmHg at rest (revised from the previous threshold of 25 mmHg by the 6th World Symposium on Pulmonary Hypertension, 2018). It is a haemodynamic state, not a single disease, and the underlying cause determines treatment and prognosis.

Group	Category	Examples	Pathophysiology
1	Pulmonary arterial hypertension (PAH)	Idiopathic, heritable (BMPR2 mutation), drug-induced, CTD-associated, HIV, portal HTN, CHD	Precapillary; pulmonary vascular remodelling
2	PH due to left heart disease	HFrEF, HFpEF, valvular disease	Postcapillary; elevated LA pressure; most common cause overall
3	PH due to chronic lung disease/hypoxia	COPD, ILD (IPF), sleep-disordered breathing, chronic altitude	Hypoxic vasoconstriction; vascular remodelling
4	Chronic thromboembolic PH (CTEPH)	Organised thrombi in pulmonary arteries	Mechanical obstruction + secondary vasculopathy; potentially curable (endarterectomy)
5	Multifactorial/unclear mechanisms	Haematological (myeloproliferative), sarcoidosis, metabolic	Mixed mechanisms

The vascular pathology of pulmonary hypertension progresses through a predictable sequence. Early changes include medial hypertrophy of muscular pulmonary arteries (smooth muscle hyperplasia and hypertrophy) and muscularisation of normally non-muscular arterioles. As the disease progresses, concentric laminar intimal fibrosis ("onion-skin" pattern) develops, narrowing the lumen. In severe Group 1 PAH, plexiform lesions form: complex, glomeruloid-like tufts of proliferating endothelial-lined channels that are pathognomonic of severe PAH. These plexiform lesions are monoclonal endothelial proliferations, suggesting a neoplastic-like component to the pathogenesis. Necrotising arteritis and fibrinoid necrosis may be seen in the most advanced stages. Thrombosis in situ commonly complicates the vascular changes. The end result is right ventricular hypertrophy and eventually right heart failure (cor pulmonale).

Heritable PAH (Group 1) is most commonly caused by loss-of-function mutations in the BMPR2 gene (bone morphogenetic protein receptor type 2), a member of the TGF-β superfamily signalling pathway that normally inhibits smooth muscle proliferation and promotes apoptosis. BMPR2 mutations are found in approximately 70% of familial PAH and 10 to 20% of apparently sporadic idiopathic PAH. Additional genetic contributors include ACVRL1 (ALK1), ENG, SMAD9, and, more recently, TBX4 and SOX17. The incomplete penetrance of BMPR2 mutations (approximately 20%) suggests a "two-hit" model requiring additional environmental or genetic triggers (Figure 15.8).

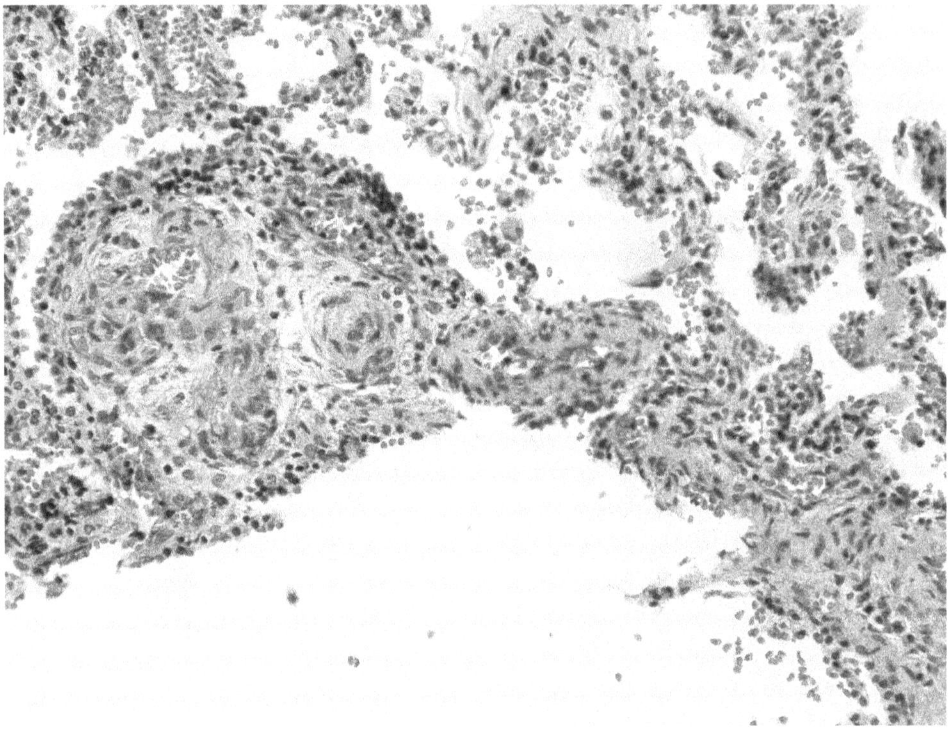

Figure 15.8: Pulmonary hypertension — plexiform lesion (H&E, high magnification). Angiomatoid/plexiform proliferation of endothelial channels within a muscular pulmonary artery. (Source: Yale Rosen, Wikimedia Commons, CC BY-SA 2.0.)

This finding, when seen alongside a history of recurrent pulmonary emboli, points strongly towards chronic thromboembolic pulmonary hypertension (CTEPH, Group 4), which is the only potentially curable form of PH through surgical pulmonary endarterectomy. Organised, recanalized thrombi with fibrous webs and bands in the major pulmonary arteries are the pathological hallmark.

Quick Recall: ARDS and Pulmonary Hypertension

ARDS Berlin criteria: Acute onset (<7 days), bilateral opacities, not cardiac, PaO2/FiO2: mild 200–300, moderate 100–200, severe <100.

DAD phases: Exudative (hyaline membranes, oedema, necrosis) → Organising (type II hyperplasia, fibroblast proliferation, fibrosis).

PH Groups: 1 (PAH, BMPR2), 2 (left heart, most common), 3 (lung disease/hypoxia), 4 (CTEPH, curable), 5 (multifactorial).

PH vascular changes: Medial hypertrophy → intimal fibrosis → plexiform lesions (pathognomonic of Group 1) → cor pulmonale.

15.8 Pulmonary Alveolar Proteinosis and Other Conditions

Pulmonary alveolar proteinosis (PAP) is characterised by accumulation of surfactant-like, PAS-positive, proteinaceous material within alveoli. The most common form (autoimmune PAP, approximately 90%)

is caused by autoantibodies against GM-CSF, which impair macrophage function and surfactant clearance. Secondary PAP can occur with haematopoietic disorders, immunodeficiency, or heavy dust exposure (especially silica). Congenital PAP results from mutations in surfactant protein genes (SP-B, SP-C) or the GM-CSF receptor. The histological differential diagnosis includes Pneumocystis jirovecii pneumonia (foamy, PAS-positive alveolar exudate), which must be excluded with GMS stain, especially in immunocompromised patients. CT shows a characteristic "crazy-paving" pattern (ground-glass opacity with superimposed interlobular septal thickening). Treatment for autoimmune PAP is whole-lung lavage; inhaled GM-CSF is an emerging alternative.

Eosinophilic pneumonias are a group of conditions characterised by prominent eosinophilic infiltration of the lung. Chronic eosinophilic pneumonia shows peripheral ("photographic negative of pulmonary oedema") consolidation on imaging, responds dramatically to corticosteroids, and should be distinguished from eosinophilic granulomatosis with polyangiitis (EGPA, formerly Churg-Strauss syndrome), which additionally involves vasculitis, asthma, and extrapulmonary organ involvement.

The Pathologist's Eye: Airspace vs Interstitial Pattern Recognition on Lung Biopsy

The first decision at the microscope when evaluating a lung biopsy is whether the dominant pattern is airspace or interstitial. Airspace disease fills alveolar spaces with exudate (pneumonia), oedema fluid, blood (haemorrhage), or organised fibrin (organising pneumonia), while the alveolar walls remain relatively thin. Interstitial disease, by contrast, thickens alveolar septa with inflammation, fibrosis, or neoplastic infiltration, while airspaces remain patent (though may be compressed). The practical approach: examine at low power and ask whether the alveolar architecture is preserved or obliterated. If alveolar walls are identifiable but thickened, the pattern is interstitial; if airspaces are filled and walls are obscured, the pattern is airspace-dominant. Mixed patterns are common (DAD shows both hyaline membranes lining alveolar walls and oedema filling airspaces), but identifying the dominant pattern immediately narrows the differential. UIP shows patchy interstitial fibrosis with temporal heterogeneity; NSIP shows uniform interstitial inflammation and fibrosis; organising pneumonia fills airspaces with Masson bodies; DAD shows diffuse hyaline membranes.

15.9 Recent Advances in Pulmonary Pathology

ATS/ERS/JRS/ALAT 2022 guideline — IPF update and the formal definition of progressive pulmonary fibrosis. The 2022 American Thoracic Society / European Respiratory Society / Japanese Respiratory Society / Asociación Latinoamericana de Tórax clinical practice guideline updated the diagnostic and management framework for idiopathic pulmonary fibrosis and introduced a formal definition of progressive pulmonary fibrosis applicable to interstitial lung diseases other than IPF (Raghu et al. American Journal of Respiratory and Critical Care Medicine 2022; 205: e18–e47; PMID 35486072). Radiological and histopathological criteria for IPF were refined: the high-resolution CT pattern of usual interstitial pneumonia is supported by basal-predominant subpleural reticulation, honeycombing, and traction bronchiectasis, while the histopathological pattern is defined by patchy interstitial fibrosis with temporal heterogeneity, fibroblastic foci, and architectural distortion. The guideline issued a conditional recommendation for transbronchial lung cryobiopsy as an acceptable alternative to surgical lung biopsy in centres with appropriate multidisciplinary expertise. Progressive pulmonary fibrosis was defined as at least two of three criteria — worsening respiratory symptoms, radiological progression, and physiological decline in forced vital capacity or diffusion capacity — within the preceding twelve months in a patient with an interstitial lung disease other than IPF, with a conditional recommendation for nintedanib that extended the antifibrotic indication beyond IPF and aligned with the INBUILD evidence already discussed in this chapter.

Nintedanib and pirfenidone, the two approved antifibrotic agents for IPF, have demonstrated ability to slow the decline in lung function (FVC) but do not reverse established fibrosis. The INBUILD trial (2019) extended the indication for nintedanib to progressive fibrosing ILDs beyond IPF (including chronic HP, CTD-ILD, and unclassifiable ILD). These trials have shifted the paradigm from disease-specific treatment to a phenotype-based "progressive pulmonary fibrosis" (PPF) approach, formalised in the 2022 ATS/ERS/JRS/ALAT guidelines. PPF is defined as at least two of three criteria (worsening symptoms, radiological progression, and physiological decline) occurring within a 12-month period despite standard management, in any fibrosing ILD other than IPF.

In ARDS, the COVID-19 pandemic generated vast pathological data. Post-mortem studies confirmed DAD as the predominant pattern in fatal COVID-19, with additional findings of extensive microvascular thrombosis (immunothrombosis), endotheliitis, and prominent type II pneumocyte hyperplasia with viral cytopathic changes. These observations supported the use of corticosteroids (dexamethasone, RECOVERY trial) and anticoagulation in severe COVID-19.

Multidisciplinary discussion (MDD) involving the pulmonologist, radiologist, and pathologist is now considered the gold standard for diagnosis of interstitial lung diseases. The 2022 ATS/ERS/JRS/ALAT clinical practice guideline for IPF formalised the MDD approach, including the role of genomic classifiers (e.g., Envisia) as ancillary tools for classifying UIP pattern from transbronchial biopsies. Cryobiopsy has emerged as a viable alternative to surgical lung biopsy for ILD diagnosis, with comparable diagnostic yield and lower morbidity. In pulmonary hypertension, sotatercept (an activin receptor IIA-Fc fusion protein that rebalances pro- and anti-proliferative signalling) showed significant haemodynamic improvement in the STELLAR trial (2023) for Group 1 PAH, representing the first new mechanism of action in over a decade.

15.10 Approach to the Histopathology Slide: Non-Neoplastic Lung

When examining a lung biopsy or resection for non-neoplastic disease, adopt a pattern-based approach. At low power, determine the dominant pattern: (1) Airspace filling (oedema, haemorrhage, proteinaceous material, organising plugs); (2) Interstitial thickening (inflammation, fibrosis, or both); (3) Nodular pattern (granulomas, pneumoconiotic nodules); (4) Near-normal (emphysema, subtle bronchiolitis). Then refine the diagnosis using the following questions.

For fibrosis: is it temporally heterogeneous (UIP) or homogeneous (NSIP)? Is there honeycombing (UIP)? Are fibroblastic foci present (UIP)? Is it subpleural (UIP) or diffuse? For granulomas: are they well-formed and tight (sarcoidosis) or loose and airway-centred (HP)? Is there necrosis (infection, GPA)? Always request AFB and GMS stains. For airspace filling: are there hyaline membranes (DAD)? Organising plugs (COP)? Pigmented macrophages (DIP/RB-ILD)? Eosinophils (eosinophilic pneumonia)?

PAS-positive material (PAP, Pneumocystis)? For pneumoconiosis: is there birefringent material under polarised light (silica)? Ferruginous bodies (asbestos)?

The Pathologist's Eye

Three critical reflexes for lung biopsies: (1) Always polarise: silica, foreign material (aspiration), and even endogenous calcium oxalate in sarcoidosis giant cells are revealed by polarised light. (2) Always get bug stains (AFB, GMS) when granulomas are present, regardless of how "classic" the sarcoidosis looks. (3) In a UIP-pattern biopsy, always check for asbestos bodies (iron stain) and look for features of chronic HP (granulomas, peribronchiolar inflammation) before accepting a diagnosis of IPF. The aetiology changes the treatment: an IPF patient gets antifibrotics; a chronic HP patient needs antigen avoidance first (Figure 15.9).

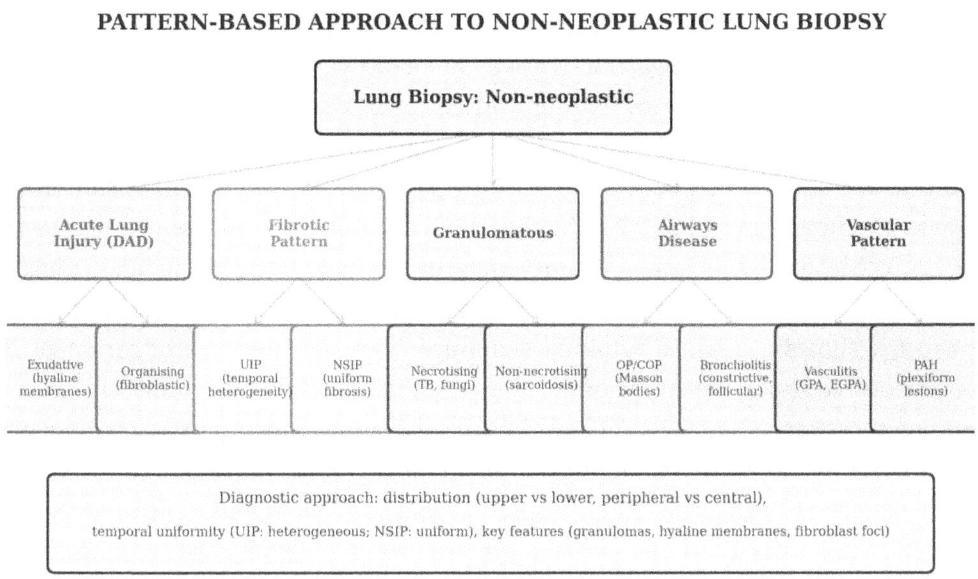

Figure 15.8 : Pattern-based approach to non-neoplastic lung biopsy interpretation

Figure 15.9: Pattern-based approach to non-neoplastic lung biopsy interpretation. Decision tree branching from dominant pattern (airspace filling, interstitial, nodular, near-normal) to specific diagnoses with key histological discriminators and ancillary tests at each branch point. (Source: Author's original.)

International Frameworks

International frameworks for obstructive and interstitial lung disease — GOLD, GINA, and the ATS/ERS classification of idiopathic interstitial pneumonias. Respiratory pathology in postgraduate examinations is structured around three international frameworks that the FRCPath candidate must integrate with morphology. The Global Initiative for Chronic Obstructive Lung Disease (GOLD) report stratifies chronic obstructive pulmonary disease by post-bronchodilator spirometry (FEV1/FVC less than 0.70 confirms airflow obstruction; GOLD grades 1 to 4 by FEV1 percent predicted) and combines this with symptom burden (Modified Medical Research Council dyspnoea or COPD Assessment Test) and exacerbation history, with the GOLD 2023 report consolidating the historical ABCD assessment groups into ABE — collapsing the high-symptom groups while flagging the exacerbator phenotype as a distinct treatment indication. The pathologist's responsibilities are limited but specific: recognising centriacinar versus panacinar emphysema patterns on lobectomy or autopsy specimen, identifying alpha-1 antitrypsin deficiency where panacinar lower-lobe emphysema raises the index of suspicion (PAS-D-resistant globules in hepatocytes), and distinguishing cigarette-related small airway disease from the inflammatory infiltrate of asthma. The Global Initiative for Asthma (GINA) report classifies asthma by control level (well controlled, partly controlled, uncontrolled) and by severity (mild, moderate, severe), with the recent shift from the symptom-driven short-acting beta-2 agonist-only paradigm to inhaled corticosteroid-formoterol as preferred reliever therapy in steps 1 and 2 reflecting the recognition that all asthma deaths begin with inflammation. Histopathologically, asthma is characterised by basement membrane thickening, goblet cell hyperplasia, smooth muscle hypertrophy, and eosinophilic inflammation in T2-high disease; T2-low (neutrophilic) asthma shows a distinct cytokine signature. The ATS/ERS classification of idiopathic interstitial pneumonias recognises seven major entities — idiopathic pulmonary fibrosis (with the usual interstitial pneumonia pattern of patchy subpleural fibrosis, fibroblast foci, microscopic honeycombing, and temporal heterogeneity), nonspecific interstitial pneumonia (uniform interstitial inflammation and fibrosis without architectural distortion), cryptogenic organising pneumonia (intra-alveolar plugs of granulation tissue), acute interstitial pneumonia (organising diffuse alveolar damage), respiratory bronchiolitis-interstitial lung disease and desquamative interstitial pneumonia (smoking-related, with peribronchiolar pigmented macrophages), and lymphoid interstitial pneumonia — alongside rare entities including pleuroparenchymal fibroelastosis. The framework is operationalised through a multidisciplinary team approach in which the radiologist's HRCT pattern, the pathologist's biopsy interpretation, and the clinician's history are integrated, replacing the historical primacy of histology alone. The 2018 ATS/ERS/JRS/ALAT clinical practice guideline for idiopathic pulmonary fibrosis formalises this with HRCT pattern categories — typical UIP, probable UIP, indeterminate for UIP, and alternative diagnosis — that determine whether a surgical lung biopsy is required for definitive diagnosis. Citation: Travis WD, Costabel U, Hansell DM, et al; ATS/ERS Committee on Idiopathic Interstitial Pneumonias. An official American Thoracic Society/European Respiratory Society statement: update of the international multidisciplinary classification of the idiopathic interstitial pneumonias. Am J Respir Crit Care Med 2013; 188: 733–748. PMID 24032382.

Ultra High-Yield Chapter Summary

Topic	Must Remember
Centriacinar emphysema	Smoking, upper lobes, proximal acinus destruction
Panacinar emphysema	AAT deficiency (PiZZ), lower lobes, entire acinus
Protease-antiprotease	Neutrophil elastase + MMP vs AAT; smoke oxidises AAT
Chronic bronchitis	Clinical definition (3mo/2yr); Reid index >0.5; goblet cell metaplasia
COPD prognostic indicators	FEV1 (most important), BODE index, exacerbation frequency, PaCO2, BMI
COPD complications	Cor pulmonale, secondary polycythaemia, pneumothorax, respiratory failure, lung cancer
Asthma histology	Smooth muscle hypertrophy, subbasement membrane fibrosis, eosinophils, goblet cell hyperplasia
Th2 cytokines in asthma	IL-4 (IgE), IL-5 (eosinophils), IL-13 (mucus + hyperresponsiveness)
Bronchiectasis causes	CF (#1 genetic in West), post-TB, Kartagener, obstruction, immunodeficiency
UIP/IPF	Temporal + spatial heterogeneity, fibroblastic foci, honeycombing, subpleural, poor prognosis
NSIP	Temporal homogeneity, no honeycombing, CTD association, good prognosis
COP	Masson bodies (organising plugs), steroid-responsive
Silicosis	Whorled collagen nodules (onion-skin), birefringent, upper lobes, TB risk
Asbestosis	Lower lobe fibrosis, ferruginous bodies (Perl+), pleural plaques, mesothelioma risk
Sarcoidosis	Non-caseating granulomas, lymphangitic, bilateral hilar LAD, hypercalcaemia, exclude infection
HP triad	Peribronchiolar inflammation + loose granulomas + organising pneumonia
ARDS Berlin criteria	Acute <7 days, bilateral opacities, non-cardiac, PaO2/FiO2 ratio grades severity
DAD exudative phase	Hyaline membranes, oedema, type I pneumocyte necrosis
DAD organising phase	Type II pneumocyte hyperplasia, fibroblast proliferation, interstitial fibrosis

Pulmonary HTN groups	1 (PAH, BMPR2), 2 (left heart, commonest), 3 (lung disease), 4 (CTEPH, curable), 5 (misc)
Plexiform lesions	Pathognomonic of severe Group 1 PAH; monoclonal endothelial proliferations
PAP	PAS-positive alveolar proteinaceous material; anti-GM-CSF antibodies; crazy-paving CT; exclude PCP
Antifibrotics for IPF	Nintedanib, pirfenidone (slow FVC decline, do not reverse fibrosis); PPF concept extends to other ILDs

Cross-References from Chapter 15

Pulmonary hypertension, right heart failure, cor pulmonale → Chapter 14. Vasculitis involving the lung (GPA, EGPA, MPA) → Chapter 13. Pulmonary infections (TB, fungal, viral, COVID-19) → Chapters 6 and 9. Lung neoplasms, bronchogenic carcinoma, mesothelioma, carcinoid → Chapter 16. Autoimmune ILD (RA, SLE, systemic sclerosis, IgG4-related disease) → Chapter 5. α1-antitrypsin deficiency, cystic fibrosis (CFTR), familial pulmonary fibrosis (BMPR2, TERT) → Chapter 8. Haemosiderin-laden macrophages, pulmonary haemorrhage syndromes, iron metabolism → Volume 1. ARDS, shock lung, fat embolism, pulmonary thromboembolism → Chapter 4. Pirfenidone, nintedanib, mepolizumab, dupilumab → Chapter 41.

Diagnostic thinking: temporal heterogeneity + fibroblastic foci + honeycombing → UIP pattern (IPF clinically)

Diagnostic thinking: mucus plugging + eosinophils + Charcot-Leyden crystals + smooth muscle hypertrophy → asthma

Diagnostic thinking: non-caseating granulomas + asteroid bodies + bilateral hilar LAP → sarcoidosis (exclude TB first in TB-endemic regions) (Figures 15.8–15.10)

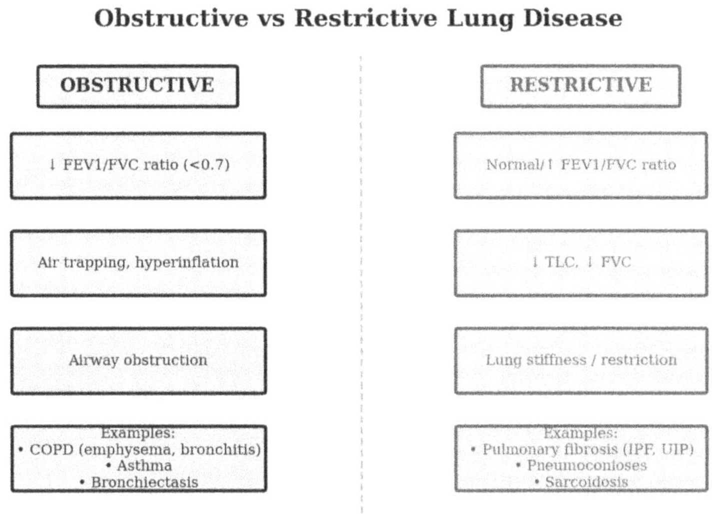

Figure 15.10: Obstructive vs Restrictive Lung Disease. (Source: Author's original.)

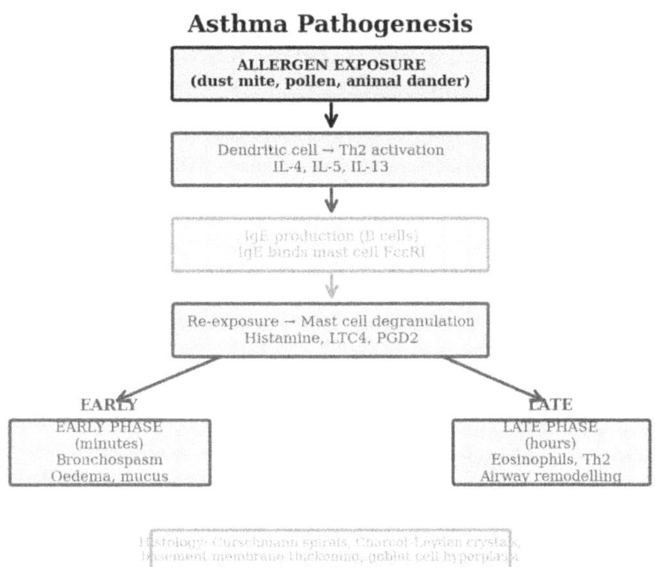

Figure 15.11: Asthma Pathogenesis. (Source: Author's original.)

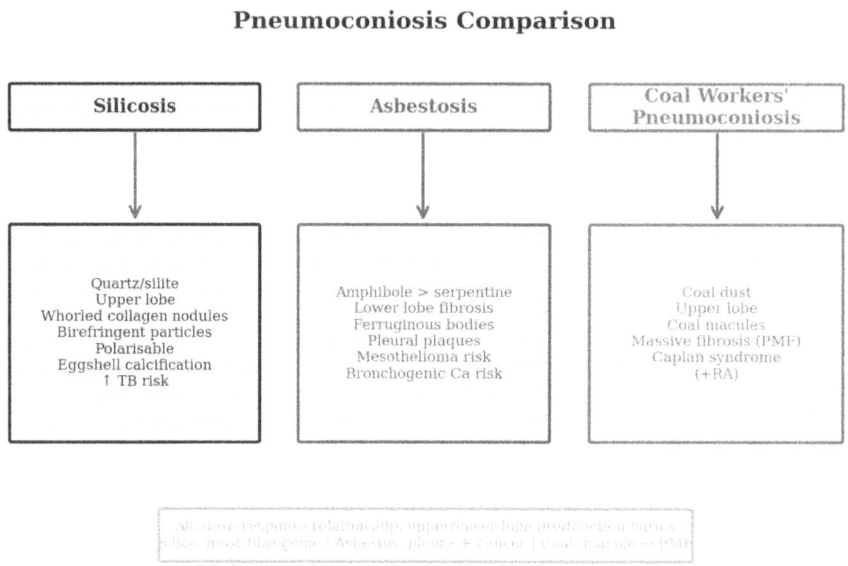

Figure 15.12: Pneumoconiosis Comparison. (Source: Author's original.)

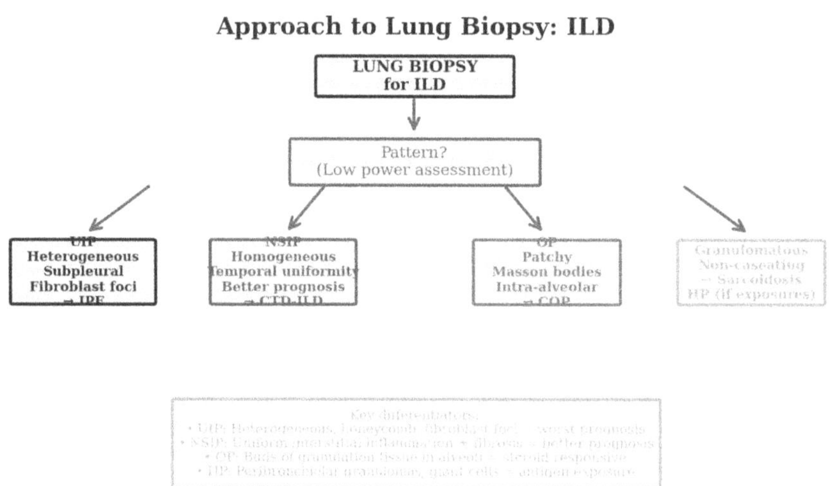

Figure 15.13: Approach to Lung Biopsy: ILD. (Source: Author's original.)

Chapter 16: Respiratory Pathology Part 2: Infections and Neoplasms

THE BIG PICTURE

Lung cancer is the leading cause of cancer-related death worldwide and, in many populations, the most common malignancy in men. For the pathologist, accurate histological typing, molecular profiling, and PD-L1 assessment of lung carcinoma are now inseparable from the diagnostic act, as they directly determine treatment. This chapter covers pulmonary infections (community-acquired pneumonia, atypical pneumonia, opportunistic infections in the immunocompromised host, and COVID-19-associated diffuse alveolar damage) and lung neoplasms (adenocarcinoma, squamous cell carcinoma, small cell carcinoma, large cell neuroendocrine carcinoma, carcinoid tumours, and mesothelioma). The WHO 5th Edition classification of lung tumours and the molecular landscape of lung adenocarcinoma are essential exam topics.

High-yield topics in this chapter: WHO 5th Edition classification of lung tumours; adenocarcinoma subtypes, grading, and STAS; squamous cell carcinoma; small cell carcinoma vs large cell neuroendocrine carcinoma; carcinoid tumours and DIPNECH; IHC panel for lung carcinoma typing (TTF-1, p40, Napsin A); molecular targets (EGFR, ALK, ROS1, KRAS, PD-L1); mesothelioma vs adenocarcinoma; community-acquired and atypical pneumonias; opportunistic pulmonary infections; COVID-19 pulmonary pathology.

Lung cancer kills more people each year than breast, colon, and prostate cancers combined. Yet the past two decades have witnessed a revolution: what was once treated as a monolithic disease is now stratified by histological subtype, molecular driver, and immune checkpoint status, with each stratum dictating a specific therapeutic strategy. Simultaneously, the pathologist must recognise and characterise the diverse pulmonary infections that remain a leading cause of morbidity and mortality, particularly in the immunocompromised host. This chapter demands integration of morphology, immunohistochemistry, and molecular pathology at every turn.

16.1 Pulmonary Infections

Pulmonary infections are classified by the pattern of involvement: bronchopneumonia (patchy consolidation centred on bronchioles and adjacent alveoli, usually caused by Staphylococcus, Streptococcus, Haemophilus, or Gram-negative organisms), lobar pneumonia (confluent consolidation of an entire lobe, classically caused by Streptococcus pneumoniae), and interstitial (atypical) pneumonia (diffuse interstitial inflammation with lymphocytic infiltrate and minimal alveolar exudate, caused by Mycoplasma pneumoniae, respiratory viruses, Chlamydophila, and Legionella).

The morphological pattern depends on the organism, host immune status, and the route of infection. Community-acquired pneumonia (CAP) is most commonly caused by Streptococcus pneumoniae (pneumococcus). Lobar pneumonia progresses through four classic stages: congestion (first 24 hours: vascular engorgement, serous exudate), red hepatisation (days 2 to 3: massive fibrinopurulent exudate filling alveoli with neutrophils, red blood cells, and fibrin), grey hepatisation (days 4 to 8: progressive degradation of red cells, persistent fibrinopurulent exudate), and resolution (enzymatic digestion and resorption of the exudate). Complications include abscess formation, empyema, and organisation (organising pneumonia).

Congestion (vascular engorgement) → Red hepatisation (fibrin + RBCs + neutrophils) → Grey hepatisation (degraded RBCs, persistent fibrin) → Resolution (enzymatic digestion)

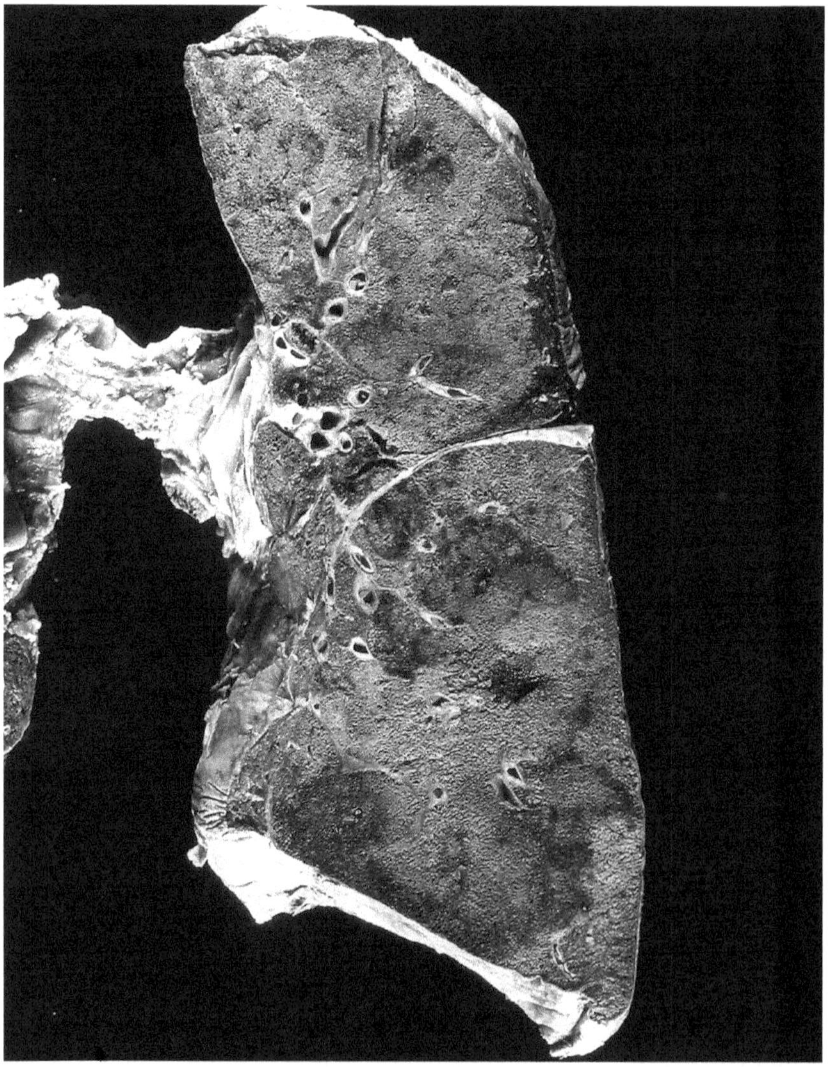

Figure 16.1: Lobar pneumonia — gross specimen. Uniform consolidation of an entire lobe, contrasting with the patchy bronchocentric pattern of bronchopneumonia (Figure 16.2). (Source: Yale Rosen, Wikimedia Commons, CC BY-SA 2.0.)

Pattern	Distribution	Common Organisms	Histology
Lobar pneumonia	Entire lobe	S. pneumoniae (most	Intra-alveolar

	(confluent)	common), Klebsiella	fibrinopurulent exudate; four stages
Bronchopneumonia	Patchy, bronchiole-centred	Staph aureus, Strep, H. influenzae, GNR	Patchy neutrophilic infiltrate centred on bronchioles
Interstitial (atypical)	Diffuse interstitial	Mycoplasma, viruses (RSV, influenza), Chlamydophila, Legionella	Interstitial lymphocytic infiltrate; minimal alveolar exudate
Lung abscess	Localised cavity	Anaerobes, Staph aureus, Klebsiella	Suppurative necrosis with cavity formation

Pulmonary Infections in the Immunocompromised Host

The immunocompromised patient (HIV/AIDS, organ transplant recipients, patients on immunosuppressive therapy including checkpoint inhibitors) is susceptible to opportunistic infections that rarely cause disease in immunocompetent individuals. The pattern of infection often points to the nature of the immune defect: T-cell deficiency (HIV, transplant) predisposes to Pneumocystis, CMV, and mycobacteria; neutropenia predisposes to invasive fungal infections (Aspergillus, Mucor); and humoral deficiency predisposes to encapsulated bacteria.

The key diagnostic clue in this setting is: the morphological pattern combined with clinical context often narrows the differential to a short list of organisms. Foamy eosinophilic alveolar exudate in an HIV patient is Pneumocystis until proved otherwise; angioinvasive septate hyphae in a neutropenic patient is Aspergillus until proved otherwise.

Pneumocystis jirovecii pneumonia (PCP) causes a diffuse, bilateral interstitial pneumonia that is the defining opportunistic infection of advanced HIV (CD4 count below 200 cells/µL). The histological hallmark is foamy, eosinophilic alveolar exudate resembling pulmonary alveolar proteinosis. The organisms are not visible on H&E; cyst forms are demonstrable on GMS (Grocott methenamine silver) stain as crushed ping-pong ball or cup-shaped structures, and trophozoites are seen on Giemsa. Bronchoalveolar lavage (BAL) is the standard diagnostic specimen; sensitivity exceeds 95% with appropriate staining. PCP prophylaxis (trimethoprim-sulfamethoxazole) is standard for CD4 below 200 or prior PCP episode.

Cytomegalovirus (CMV) pneumonitis produces characteristic enlarged cells ("cytomegalic" cells) with large basophilic intranuclear inclusions ("owl-eye" appearance) surrounded by a clear halo and smaller cytoplasmic granular inclusions. CMV pneumonitis occurs predominantly in transplant recipients and can be confirmed by IHC or in situ hybridisation.

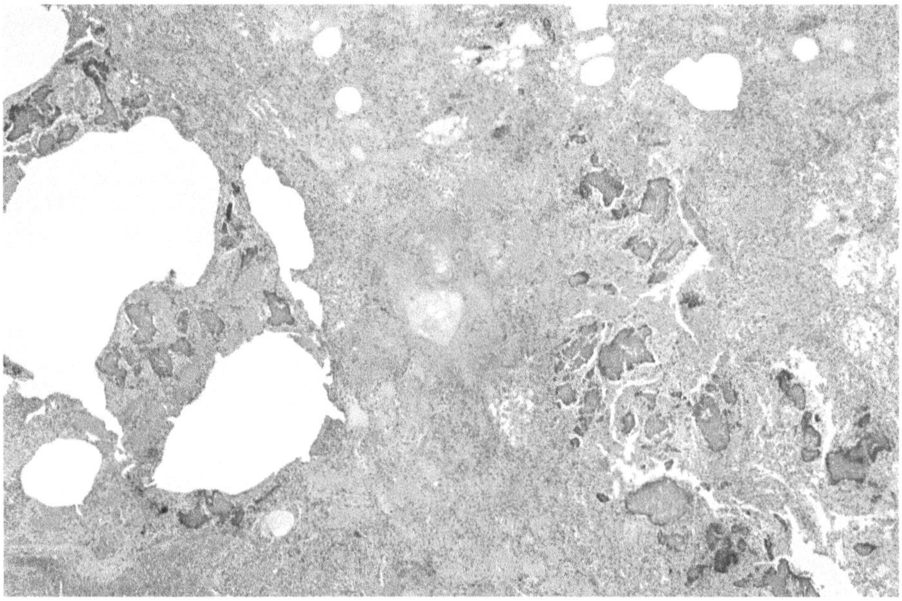

Figure 16.2: Bronchopneumonia — gross specimen. Patchy areas of consolidation centred on bronchi with intervening aerated lung, contrasting with the uniform consolidation of lobar pneumonia (Figure 16.1). (Source: Yale Rosen, Wikimedia Commons, CC BY-SA 2.0.)

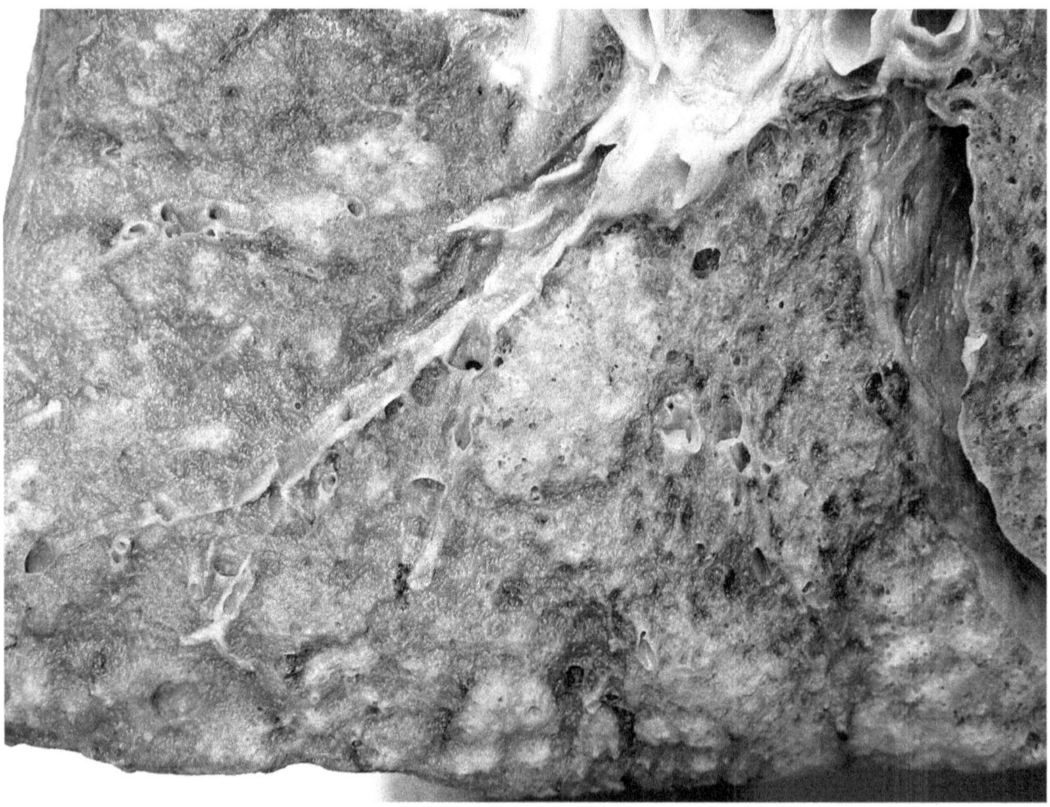

Figure 16.3: Pneumocystis jirovecii pneumonia (H&E). Alveoli filled with characteristic foamy eosinophilic

exudate. (Source: Wellcome Collection, CC BY 4.0.)

Aspergillus species cause a spectrum of pulmonary disease determined by the host immune status. Allergic bronchopulmonary aspergillosis (ABPA) occurs in atopic individuals and patients with cystic fibrosis; it is a type I and III hypersensitivity reaction characterised by mucoid impaction of bronchi, eosinophilia, elevated IgE, and proximal bronchiectasis. Aspergilloma ("fungus ball") develops in pre-existing pulmonary cavities (most commonly from healed tuberculosis, an important association in TB-endemic regions); it consists of a tangled mass of Aspergillus hyphae, fibrin, and debris within a cavity and may cause haemoptysis. Invasive (angioinvasive) aspergillosis is the most serious form, occurring in severely immunocompromised patients (prolonged neutropenia, HSCT); septate hyphae with acute-angle (approximately 45-degree) dichotomous branching invade blood vessel walls, causing thrombosis and haemorrhagic infarction. On imaging, the halo sign (ground-glass opacity surrounding a nodule) is characteristic early; the air-crescent sign appears during recovery.

Mucormycosis (caused by Rhizopus, Mucor, and related genera) shows broad, ribbon-like, pauciseptate hyphae with irregular (wide-angle) branching and prominent angioinvasion. It is classically associated with diabetic ketoacidosis and surged across South Asia during the COVID-19 second wave (mucormycosis associated with corticosteroid use and uncontrolled hyperglycaemia). The rhinocerebral form (see Chapter 17) is the most common presentation in this context.

Form	Host	Pathology	Morphology/Diagnosis
ABPA	Atopic, cystic fibrosis	Type I + III hypersensitivity	Mucoid impaction, eosinophilia, raised IgE, proximal bronchiectasis
Aspergilloma	Pre-existing cavity (healed TB)	Fungus ball in cavity	Tangled hyphae + fibrin + debris; haemoptysis; no tissue invasion
Chronic pulmonary	Mild immunosuppression, COPD	Slowly progressive cavitary disease	Cavity with wall thickening; Aspergillus in cavity wall
Invasive angioinvasive	Severe neutropenia, HSCT	Vascular invasion, thrombosis, infarction	Septate hyphae with 45° branching; halo sign on CT; GMS/PAS stain

COVID-19 Pulmonary Pathology

SARS-CoV-2 infection causes a spectrum of pulmonary injury. The dominant histological pattern in fatal COVID-19 is diffuse alveolar damage (DAD), identical to DAD from other causes (see Chapter 15), progressing through an exudative phase (hyaline membranes, oedema, fibrin, type II pneumocyte hyperplasia) and an organising phase (interstitial fibroblast proliferation, squamous metaplasia of alveolar epithelium). Distinctive features described in COVID-19 autopsy studies include microvascular thrombosis (small vessel fibrin thrombi, more prominent than in other causes of DAD), endothelialitis (viral infection of endothelial cells with lymphocytic infiltration), and megakaryocytes in pulmonary capillaries. Superimposed bronchopneumonia is common in prolonged cases.

Internationally, autopsy studies from multiple international centres during the 2020 and 2021 waves confirmed DAD as the predominant pattern, with a high frequency of secondary bacterial and fungal infections (mucormycosis, aspergillosis) attributable to corticosteroid therapy and comorbidities. COVID-19-associated pulmonary aspergillosis (CAPA) and COVID-19-associated mucormycosis (CAM) emerged as significant pathological entities, particularly across South Asia.

SARS-CoV-2 → ACE2 receptor binding → type II pneumocyte injury → DAD (exudative → organising) + microvascular thrombosis + endothelialitis

Integration: *Pulmonary tuberculosis, leprosy, and other granulomatous infections are discussed in Chapter 9 (Infectious Disease Pathology). ARDS and DAD pathogenesis are covered in Chapter 15. Rhinocerebral mucormycosis is discussed in Chapter 17 (Head and Neck Pathology).*

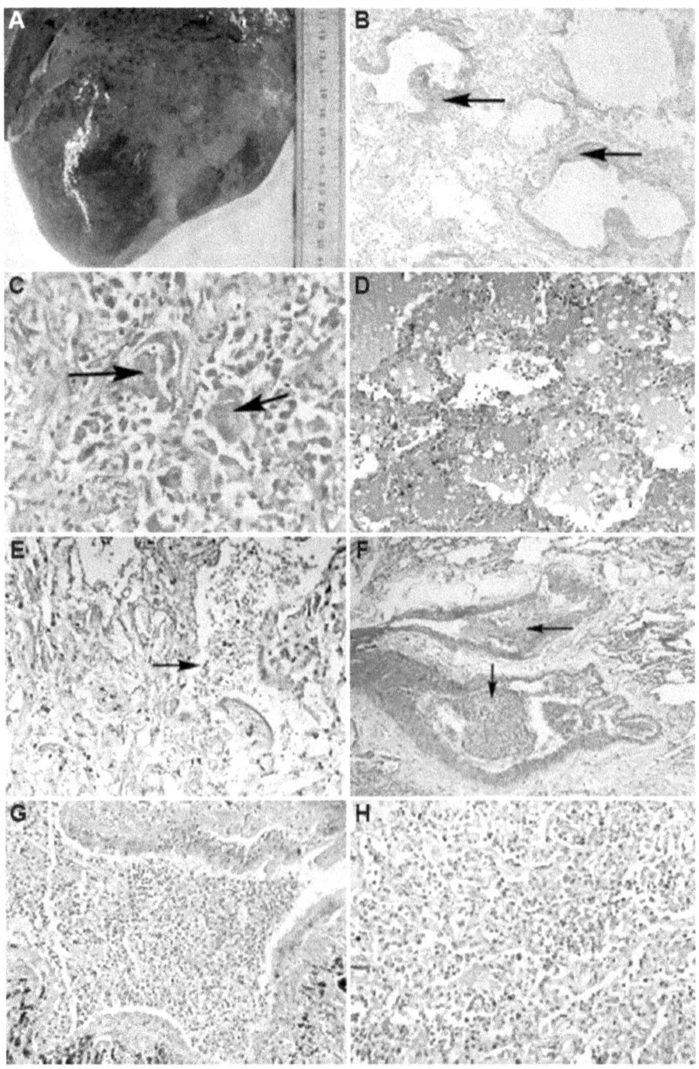

Figure 16.4: COVID-19 lung pathology composite (H&E). Diffuse alveolar damage with hyaline membranes, type II pneumocyte hyperplasia, and microvascular thrombi. (Source: Indian J Med Res, CC BY 4.0.)

Quick Recall: Pulmonary Infections

Lobar pneumonia: S. pneumoniae. Four stages: congestion → red hepatisation → grey hepatisation → resolution.

Bronchopneumonia: Patchy, bronchiole-centred. Staph, Strep, Haemophilus, GNR.

Atypical pneumonia: Interstitial pattern, lymphocytic. Mycoplasma, viruses, Chlamydophila.

Pneumocystis: Foamy alveolar exudate. GMS+ cyst forms (crushed cup). CD4 <200.

Aspergillus spectrum: ABPA (atopy) → aspergilloma (cavity) → invasive angioinvasive (neutropenia). Septate, 45° branching.

Mucormycosis: Broad, ribbon-like, pauciseptate, irregular branching. Angioinvasive.

COVID-19 lung: DAD + microvascular thrombosis + endothelialitis. Secondary mucormycosis/aspergillosis especially noted across South Asia.

16.2 Lung Neoplasms: Overview and Classification

Lung cancer is classified histologically into non-small cell lung carcinoma (NSCLC, approximately 85%) and small cell lung carcinoma (SCLC, approximately 15%). NSCLC is further divided into adenocarcinoma (the most common subtype, approximately 40–50%), squamous cell carcinoma (approximately 25–30%), and large cell carcinoma (approximately 5–10%). Neuroendocrine tumours of the lung range from the low-grade typical carcinoid through atypical carcinoid to the high-grade small cell and large cell neuroendocrine carcinomas. The WHO 5th Edition (2021) classification refines the subtypes of adenocarcinoma, introduces a formal grading system for resected non-mucinous adenocarcinoma, and recognises the importance of molecular subtyping for therapeutic decision-making.

Cigarette smoking is the dominant risk factor, responsible for approximately 85% of lung cancers. Squamous cell carcinoma and small cell carcinoma have the strongest association with smoking. Adenocarcinoma, while also related to smoking, is the most common type in never-smokers and in women, and is the type most frequently associated with actionable molecular targets (EGFR, ALK, ROS1). Other risk factors include asbestos exposure (synergistic with smoking, multiplicative risk), radiation, radon, air pollution, and pulmonary fibrosis ("scar carcinoma" arising in areas of fibrosis, especially UIP).

WHO 5th Edition Classification of Lung Tumours (2021) — Selected Key Categories

Epithelial tumours, malignant:

Adenocarcinoma: Lepidic, acinar, papillary, micropapillary, solid, invasive mucinous, colloid, fetal, enteric

Preinvasive: Atypical adenomatous hyperplasia (AAH), Adenocarcinoma in situ (AIS; non-mucinous,

mucinous)
Minimally invasive adenocarcinoma (MIA; non-mucinous, mucinous)
Squamous cell carcinoma: Keratinising, non-keratinising, basaloid
Preinvasive: Squamous cell carcinoma in situ
Large cell carcinoma
Adenosquamous carcinoma
Sarcomatoid carcinomas: Pleomorphic, spindle cell, giant cell, carcinosarcoma, pulmonary blastoma

Neuroendocrine tumours:

Small cell carcinoma (combined small cell carcinoma)
Large cell neuroendocrine carcinoma (combined LCNEC)
Typical carcinoid; Atypical carcinoid
Preinvasive: Diffuse idiopathic pulmonary neuroendocrine cell hyperplasia (DIPNECH)

New entities (WHO 2021):

Thoracic SMARCA4-deficient undifferentiated tumour
NUT carcinoma of the lung
Adenocarcinoma grading system (Grade 1/2/3 for resected non-mucinous adenocarcinoma)

Adenocarcinoma

Pulmonary adenocarcinoma is the most common type of lung cancer worldwide. It typically arises in the peripheral lung. The WHO classification recognises a spectrum from preinvasive lesions (atypical adenomatous hyperplasia, AAH; adenocarcinoma in situ, AIS) through minimally invasive adenocarcinoma (MIA, invasion ≤5 mm) to invasive adenocarcinoma. AIS and MIA have nearly 100% 5-year survival after complete resection. AAH is a small (usually less than 5 mm), discrete focus of atypical pneumocyte proliferation along alveolar walls; it is the adenoma-carcinoma sequence equivalent in the lung. AIS is a lesion of 3 cm or less with pure lepidic growth and no invasion, lymphovascular invasion, or STAS. MIA is a small (≤3 cm), predominantly lepidic adenocarcinoma with an invasive component of 5 mm or less.

Adenocarcinoma Spectrum	Size/Invasion	Pattern	Prognosis
AAH (preinvasive)	Usually <5 mm	Atypical pneumocyte proliferation along alveolar walls	Precursor; no treatment needed
AIS (preinvasive)	≤3 cm; no invasion	Pure lepidic; no invasion, no LVI, no STAS	~100% 5-yr survival
MIA	≤3 cm; invasion ≤5 mm	Predominantly lepidic; small invasive component	~100% 5-yr survival
Invasive	Any size; invasion	Lepidic, acinar, papillary,	Variable by grade and

adenocarcinoma	>5 mm	micropapillary, solid	stage

Invasive adenocarcinoma is subtyped by the predominant growth pattern: lepidic (non-mucinous cells growing along pre-existing alveolar walls, formerly called "bronchioloalveolar carcinoma"; the most favourable invasive pattern), acinar (gland-forming), papillary (papillae with fibrovascular cores), micropapillary (papillary tufts without fibrovascular cores, floating in airspaces; aggressive), and solid (sheets of cells without glandular or papillary architecture; mucin stain required to confirm adenocarcinoma). All patterns should be reported with their percentages in 5% increments, as the predominant pattern determines the grade.

The WHO 5th Edition grading system for resected non-mucinous adenocarcinoma is based on the predominant pattern: Grade 1 (well-differentiated; lepidic-predominant with less than 20% high-grade pattern), Grade 2 (moderately differentiated; acinar or papillary-predominant with less than 20% high-grade pattern), Grade 3 (poorly differentiated; any tumour with 20% or more high-grade pattern, defined as solid, micropapillary, cribriform, or complex glandular pattern). This grading system has been validated as an independent prognostic factor, with Grade 3 tumours having significantly worse disease-free survival. There is no established grading system for invasive mucinous adenocarcinoma or SCC.

Variants include invasive mucinous adenocarcinoma (formerly mucinous bronchioloalveolar carcinoma; tall columnar cells with abundant apical mucin, lepidic growth; often TTF-1 negative, KRAS mutant), colloid adenocarcinoma, fetal adenocarcinoma, and enteric adenocarcinoma.

Spread through air spaces (STAS) is defined as tumour cells within airspaces beyond the edge of the main tumour. Three morphological patterns of STAS are described: micropapillary clusters, solid nests, and single cells. Its presence excludes a diagnosis of AIS or MIA, is associated with increased recurrence after limited resection (wedge), and should be reported on all resection specimens. *The distinction from artefactual displacement ("knife effect") during grossing rests on the observation that STAS cells are found in airspaces distant from the cut surface, while artefactual cells cluster along the knife track.*

Squamous Cell Carcinoma

Squamous cell carcinoma (SCC) is strongly associated with smoking and typically arises centrally in the major bronchi, often preceded by a multistep sequence of squamous metaplasia, dysplasia, and carcinoma in situ. Histologically, it shows keratinisation, keratin pearls, and/or intercellular bridges. The WHO classifies SCC into keratinising (most common; overt keratinisation and/or pearls), non-keratinising (recognised by IHC: p40+, TTF-1 negative), and basaloid (peripheral palisading of tumour cell nests; aggressive). IHC: positive for p40 (most specific squamous marker), p63, and CK5/6; negative for TTF-1 and Napsin A. SCC is associated with paraneoplastic hypercalcaemia (PTHrP secretion), cavitation on imaging (due to central necrosis), and Pancoast syndrome (superior sulcus tumours invading the brachial plexus).

Neuroendocrine Tumours of the Lung

The lung is the second most common site (after the GI tract) for neuroendocrine tumours. The WHO classification recognises a four-tier spectrum: typical carcinoid (low-grade), atypical carcinoid (intermediate-grade), large cell neuroendocrine carcinoma (LCNEC; high-grade), and small cell carcinoma (high-grade). Diffuse idiopathic pulmonary neuroendocrine cell hyperplasia (DIPNECH) is the recognised preinvasive neuroendocrine proliferation, and carcinoid tumourlets (less than 5 mm) represent the earliest step in neuroendocrine tumour progression.

Typical carcinoid is a low-grade neuroendocrine tumour characterised by fewer than 2 mitoses per 2 mm^2 and no necrosis. It typically presents as a central, well-circumscribed endobronchial mass in younger patients (mean age approximately 50 years). Histologically, it shows organoid, trabecular, or insular architecture with uniform cells displaying finely granular "salt-and-pepper" chromatin. Carcinoid syndrome is rare with pulmonary carcinoids (more common with intestinal carcinoids and hepatic metastases; see Chapter 27). Five-year survival exceeds 90%.

Atypical carcinoid is intermediate-grade (2–10 mitoses per 2 mm^2 and/or punctate foci of necrosis). It has a higher rate of lymph node metastasis and worse prognosis than typical carcinoid (5-year survival approximately 60–70%).

Small cell carcinoma (SCLC) is a high-grade neuroendocrine carcinoma with the strongest association with heavy smoking. It is typically central and hilar, often presenting with bulky mediastinal lymphadenopathy. Histologically, the cells are small (smaller than three resting lymphocytes), with scant cytoplasm, finely granular ("salt-and-pepper") chromatin, nuclear moulding, absent or inconspicuous nucleoli, high mitotic rate (more than 10 mitoses per 2 mm^2, often more than 60), extensive necrosis, and the Azzopardi effect (DNA encrustation of blood vessel walls). IHC shows positivity for neuroendocrine markers (synaptophysin, chromogranin, CD56, INSM1) and cytokeratin (dot-like perinuclear pattern). Ki-67 is characteristically very high (often approaching 100%). Molecularly, RB1 and TP53 are nearly universally inactivated (more than 90%). Paraneoplastic syndromes are common, including SIADH (hyponatraemia), ectopic ACTH (Cushing syndrome), and Lambert-Eaton myasthenic syndrome. SCLC is treated primarily with chemotherapy and radiation (not surgery); immune checkpoint inhibitors (atezolizumab, durvalumab) are now added to first-line chemotherapy.

Large cell neuroendocrine carcinoma (LCNEC) is a high-grade neuroendocrine tumour with features of non-small cell carcinoma cytologically (large cell size, vesicular chromatin, prominent nucleoli, abundant cytoplasm) but neuroendocrine architecture (organoid nesting, palisading, rosettes, trabeculae). It requires demonstration of at least one neuroendocrine marker by IHC (other than NSE) and has more than 10 mitoses per 2 mm^2 with necrosis. It has a similarly poor prognosis to SCLC.

The distinction from small cell carcinoma rests on three features: LCNEC cells are larger (more than three lymphocytes), have vesicular (open) chromatin with prominent nucleoli, and show more abundant cytoplasm. Small cell carcinoma shows finely granular ("salt-and-pepper") chromatin, nuclear moulding, and inconspicuous nucleoli. This distinction matters because SCLC is treated with platinum-etoposide chemotherapy, while LCNEC management remains debated (NSCLC-type or SCLC-type regimens).

Feature	Small Cell Carcinoma	Large Cell Neuroendocrine Carcinoma
Cell size	<3 resting lymphocytes	>3 resting lymphocytes
Cytoplasm	Scant	Moderate to abundant
Chromatin	Finely granular (salt-and-pepper)	Vesicular (open)
Nucleoli	Absent or inconspicuous	Prominent
Nuclear moulding	Characteristic	Usually absent
Mitotic rate	>10/2mm^2 (often >60)	>10/2mm^2
Necrosis	Extensive	Present (often geographic)
Azzopardi effect	Characteristic	Uncommon
Ki-67	~80–100%	~40–80%
RB1/TP53 loss	>90%	Variable (~40–70%)
Treatment	Platinum-etoposide + ICI	Debated (NSCLC vs SCLC regimen)

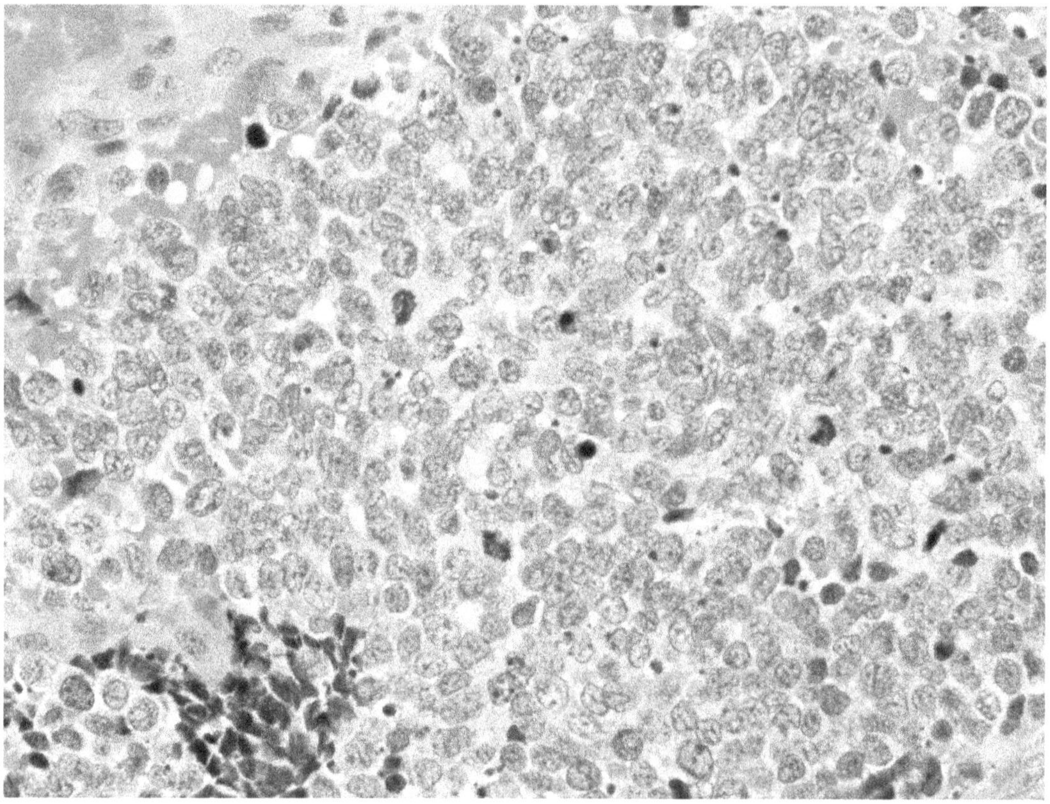

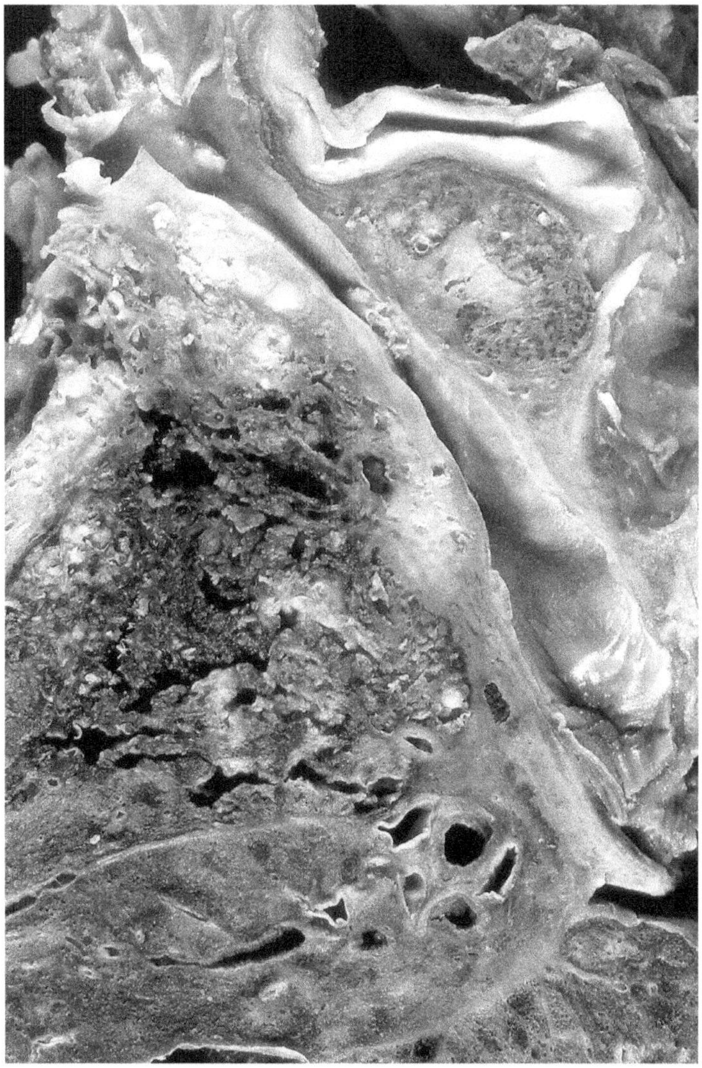

Figure 16.5: Small cell lung carcinoma. (A) Histology (H&E, medium magnification): sheets of small blue cells with scant cytoplasm, salt-and-pepper chromatin, nuclear moulding, and extensive necrosis. (B) Gross specimen: central tumour invading and obstructing the superior vena cava — a classic clinical complication of SCLC. (Source: Yale Rosen, Wikimedia Commons, CC BY-SA 2.0; two panels from the same series.)

Why does crush artefact make it difficult to diagnose small cell carcinoma on bronchial biopsies, and what is the solution? Small cell carcinoma is notorious for crush artefact because the cells are fragile with scant cytoplasm and high nuclear-to-cytoplasmic ratio. Crushed cells appear as smeared basophilic streaks. The solution is to rely on IHC (cytokeratin, Ki-67, synaptophysin) and to identify even small areas of preserved morphology. A high Ki-67 (≥80%) on crushed tissue supports SCLC.

Tumour	Location	Key Histology	IHC	Molecula	Prognosis

				r	
Adenocarcinoma	Peripheral	Glands, papillae, lepidic, solid + mucin	TTF-1+, Napsin A+, CK7+	EGFR, KRAS, ALK, ROS1, BRAF	Variable by grade/stage
Squamous cell ca	Central	Keratinisation, pearls, intercellular bridges	p40+, CK5/6+; TTF-1−	FGFR1 amp, PIK3CA	Moderate
Small cell ca	Central, hilar	Small cells, moulding, salt-pepper, necrosis, Azzopardi	Synapto+, CgA+, CD56+, INSM1+; Ki-67 ~100%	RB1 + TP53 loss (>90%)	Poor
LCNEC	Peripheral	NE architecture + NSCLC cytology; high mitoses, necrosis	≥1 NE marker+	Variable (TP53, RB1, STK11)	Poor
Typical carcinoid	Central	Organoid/trabecular; <2 mitoses/2mm^2; no necrosis	NE markers+; Ki-67 low	MEN1 (some)	Excellent (>90% 5-yr)
Atypical carcinoid	Central/peripheral	Carcinoid morphology; 2–10 mitoses/2mm^2 and/or necrosis	NE markers+; Ki-67 intermediate	Variable	Intermediate (~60–70%)

Exam Pitfall

Never perform neuroendocrine IHC stains on a lung tumour unless there is morphological evidence of neuroendocrine differentiation (organoid nesting, rosettes, salt-and-pepper chromatin). Incidental neuroendocrine marker positivity in a conventional adenocarcinoma or SCC does not change treatment or prognosis. The IHC panel for typing a poorly differentiated NSCLC should start with one adenocarcinoma marker (TTF-1) and one squamous marker (p40).

Quick Recall: Lung Carcinoma Typing by IHC

Adenocarcinoma: TTF-1+, Napsin A+, CK7+. p40−, CK5/6−.

Squamous cell: p40+ (most specific), CK5/6+, p63+. TTF-1−, Napsin A−.

Minimal IHC panel: TTF-1 + p40. If both negative: cytokeratin to confirm carcinoma → NSCLC-NOS.

Mucinous adenocarcinoma: TTF-1 may be negative. CK20+, CDX2+ possible.

NE tumours: Synaptophysin, chromogranin, CD56, INSM1. Only if NE morphology present.
SCLC vs LCNEC: Cell size, chromatin pattern, nucleoli, and Ki-67 distinguish. Both high-grade NE.

IHC Panel: Lung Carcinoma Subtyping on Small Biopsy

Marker	Interpretation
TTF-1	Adenocarcinoma (sensitivity ~80%); also positive in SCLC (~85%)
Napsin A	Adenocarcinoma (more specific than TTF-1; negative in SCLC)
p40	Squamous cell carcinoma (most specific squamous marker)
CK5/6	Squamous cell carcinoma (less specific than p40)
Synaptophysin	Neuroendocrine differentiation; use only if NE morphology present
Chromogranin A	Neuroendocrine differentiation; more specific than Syn
Ki-67	Proliferation index; >80% supports SCLC; helps grade carcinoids

16.3 Molecular Targets and Predictive Biomarkers

Molecular testing is mandatory for all advanced non-squamous NSCLC (and should be considered in SCC with atypical features or in never-smokers). The major actionable targets include EGFR activating mutations (exon 19 deletions and exon 21 L858R point mutation, together accounting for approximately 85% of EGFR mutations; treated with EGFR tyrosine kinase inhibitors such as osimertinib), ALK gene rearrangements (most commonly EML4-ALK fusion; approximately 5% of adenocarcinomas; treated with alectinib, lorlatinib), ROS1 rearrangements (approximately 1–2%; treated with crizotinib, entrectinib), KRAS G12C mutation (approximately 13%; treated with sotorasib, adagrasib), BRAF V600E mutation (approximately 2–3%; treated with dabrafenib + trametinib), MET exon 14 skipping mutations, RET fusions, and NTRK fusions (tumour-agnostic indication for larotrectinib, entrectinib). HER2 mutations (approximately 2–3%) are now also targetable with trastuzumab deruxtecan.

PD-L1 immunohistochemistry (using the 22C3 antibody for pembrolizumab eligibility) is required for all advanced NSCLC. A tumour proportion score (TPS) of 50% or greater qualifies for first-line single-agent pembrolizumab; TPS 1–49% qualifies for pembrolizumab in combination with chemotherapy. Tumour mutational burden (TMB) is emerging as an additional biomarker for immunotherapy response. The distinction between companion diagnostics (22C3 for pembrolizumab, SP142 for atezolizumab with specific scoring algorithms) and laboratory-developed tests is an important practical consideration.

Adenocarcinoma diagnosis → reflex molecular testing (EGFR, ALK, ROS1, KRAS, BRAF, MET, RET, NTRK, HER2) + PD-L1 IHC → targeted therapy or immunotherapy selection

Target	Frequency in Adenoca	Patient Profile	Testing Method	Targeted Therapy
EGFR mutation	10–20% Caucasian; 35–45% Asian; 25–30% Indian	Never/light smokers, women, East Asian	Sequencing (NGS), PCR	Osimertinib (first-line)
ALK rearrangement	~5%	Young, never-smokers	FISH, IHC (D5F3), NGS	Alectinib, lorlatinib
ROS1 rearrangement	1–2%	Young, never-smokers	FISH, NGS	Crizotinib, entrectinib
KRAS G12C	~13%	Smokers	NGS	Sotorasib, adagrasib
BRAF V600E	2–3%	Variable	NGS, IHC (VE1)	Dabrafenib + trametinib
MET exon 14 skip	~3%	Older patients	NGS, RNA-based assays	Capmatinib, tepotinib
RET fusion	1–2%	Never-smokers	NGS, FISH	Selpercatinib, pralsetinib
HER2 mutation	2–3%	Never-smokers, women	NGS	Trastuzumab deruxtecan
NTRK fusion	<1%	Variable	NGS, IHC (pan-TRK)	Larotrectinib, entrectinib
PD-L1 (not mutation)	Variable expression	All NSCLC	IHC (22C3 for pembro)	Pembrolizumab (≥50% TPS: mono; 1–49%: + chemo)

The Pathologist's Eye

Tissue stewardship is critical in lung cancer diagnosis. Approximately 70% of lung cancers are diagnosed on small biopsies or cytology, not resections. The pathologist must: (1) Use the minimal IHC panel (TTF-1 + p40) to conserve tissue for molecular testing. (2) Avoid unnecessary IHC (no NE markers without NE morphology). (3) Prioritise sections with the highest tumour cellularity for molecular testing (ideally more than 20% tumour cells). (4) Report histological subtype using the WHO terminology ("non-small cell carcinoma, favour adenocarcinoma" on biopsy; specific subtype on resection). (5) Always assess for pleural invasion (request elastin/EVG stain) and STAS on resection specimens, as both impact staging and management. (6) When tissue is insufficient for molecular testing, request liquid biopsy (ctDNA) as an alternative.

Quick Recall: Molecular Targets in Lung Adenocarcinoma

EGFR: Exon 19 del + L858R (85% of mutations). Osimertinib first-line.

ALK: EML4-ALK fusion. 5% of adeno. Young, never-smokers.

KRAS G12C: 13% of adeno. Smokers. Sotorasib, adagrasib.

PD-L1: 22C3 antibody. TPS ≥50%: pembrolizumab monotherapy.

Reflex testing: All advanced non-squamous NSCLC. NGS preferred.

Essential/Desirable: Diagnostic Criteria -- Small Cell Lung Carcinoma

Essential: Small cells with scant cytoplasm, nuclear moulding, salt-and-pepper chromatin, high mitotic rate (>10/2 mm2), extensive necrosis, Azzopardi effect.

Desirable: CgA+, Syn+, Ki-67 >80%, TTF-1+ (~85%); RB1/TP53 loss; exclude Merkel cell (CK20+) and lymphoma (CD45+).

Essential/Desirable: Diagnostic Criteria -- Lung Adenocarcinoma

Essential: Invasive glandular/lepidic/acinar/papillary/micropapillary/solid pattern with TTF-1+ or Napsin A+; invasion beyond basement membrane (excludes AIS/MIA).

Desirable: Mucin positivity (AB/PAS+); EGFR/KRAS/ALK/ROS1 molecular profile; PD-L1 TPS; STAS assessment on resection.

16.4 Malignant Mesothelioma

Malignant mesothelioma is a primary malignancy of the pleural (or, less commonly, peritoneal) mesothelial lining, strongly associated with asbestos exposure (especially amphibole fibres such as crocidolite and amosite). The latency period between asbestos exposure and mesothelioma development is typically 25 to 45 years. Grossly, mesothelioma encases the lung as a thick, firm, white rind, often with pleural effusion. The three histological subtypes are epithelioid (most common, approximately 60%, best prognosis), sarcomatoid (worst prognosis), and biphasic (mixed).

Epithelioid mesothelioma shows tubulopapillary, solid, or trabecular patterns of bland to mildly atypical cuboidal cells. The nuclear grading system (based on nuclear atypia and mitotic count) provides prognostic stratification within the epithelioid subtype. Sarcomatoid mesothelioma shows spindle cell morphology with varying degrees of atypia and may be difficult to distinguish from other spindle cell neoplasms. Desmoplastic mesothelioma (a subtype of sarcomatoid) is characterised by dense collagenous stroma and can mimic reactive pleural fibrosis.

The key diagnostic clue in this setting is: distinguishing mesothelioma from adenocarcinoma on the one hand, and from reactive mesothelial proliferation on the other. The IHC panel and ancillary markers serve these two distinct purposes.

Marker	Mesothelioma	Adenocarcinoma (lung)

Calretinin	Positive (nuclear + cytoplasmic)	Negative
CK5/6	Positive	Negative
WT-1	Positive (nuclear)	Negative
D2-40	Positive	Negative
GATA3	Positive	Negative
TTF-1	Negative	Positive
Napsin A	Negative	Positive
CEA (monoclonal)	Negative	Positive
Claudin-4	Negative	Positive
BerEP4	Negative	Positive
BAP1 loss	Present (malignant)	Retained
CDKN2A (p16) FISH deletion	Present (malignant)	Absent

A panel of at least two mesothelial and two carcinoma markers is recommended. Loss of BAP1 nuclear expression by IHC (or detection of BAP1 mutation) and homozygous deletion of CDKN2A (p16) by FISH are used to distinguish malignant mesothelioma from reactive mesothelial proliferations. MTAP IHC (loss correlates with CDKN2A deletion) is emerging as a cheaper surrogate for FISH. Germline BAP1 mutations define a familial cancer predisposition syndrome (BAP1 tumour predisposition syndrome) with increased risk of mesothelioma, uveal melanoma, and renal cell carcinoma.

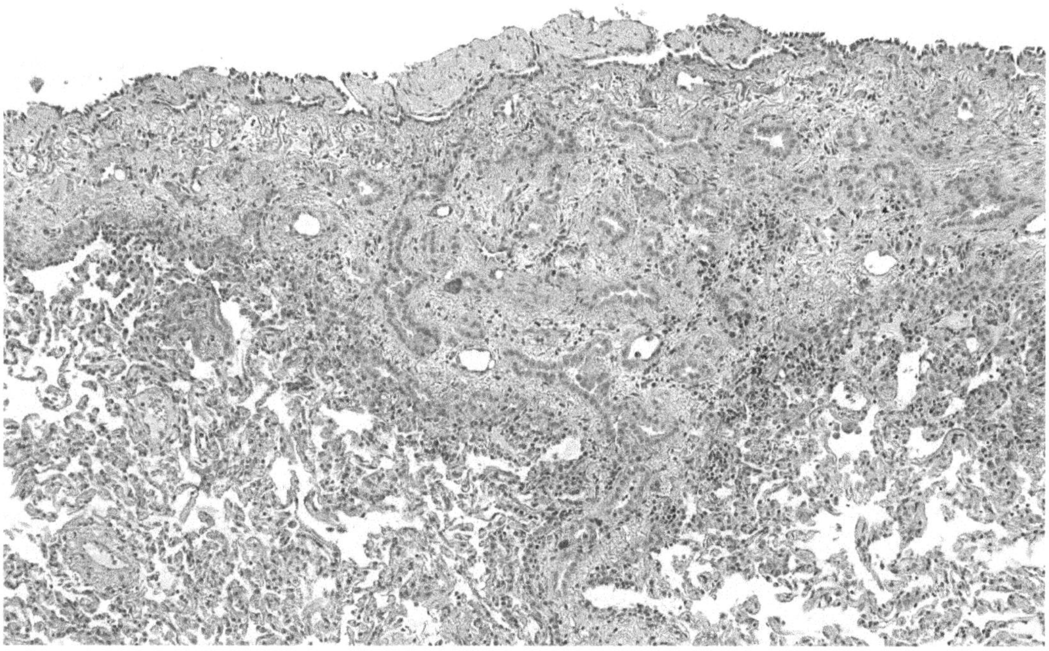

Figure 16.6: Epithelioid mesothelioma — tubulopapillary pattern with bland cuboidal cells (H&E, intermediate magnification). (Source: Nephron, Wikimedia Commons, CC BY-SA 3.0.)

Quick Recall: Mesothelioma

Mesothelial markers: Calretinin, CK5/6, WT-1, D2-40. All positive in mesothelioma, negative in adenocarcinoma.

Adenocarcinoma markers: TTF-1, Napsin A, CEA, Claudin-4, BerEP4. Positive in adenocarcinoma, negative in mesothelioma.

Malignant vs reactive: BAP1 loss (IHC) or CDKN2A/p16 deletion (FISH/MTAP IHC) = malignant.

Asbestos: Amphibole fibres (crocidolite > amosite). Latency 25–45 years.

Exam Pitfall

Desmoplastic mesothelioma can closely mimic reactive pleural fibrosis, making it one of the most difficult diagnoses in surgical pathology. Features favouring malignancy include bland necrosis (necrosis in a paucicellular collagenous area), frankly sarcomatoid foci, and invasion into adipose tissue or lung parenchyma. BAP1 loss by IHC and CDKN2A homozygous deletion by FISH (or MTAP loss as a surrogate) are the critical ancillary tests. In reactive mesothelial proliferations, BAP1 is retained and CDKN2A is intact.

16.5 Other Pulmonary and Pleural Tumours

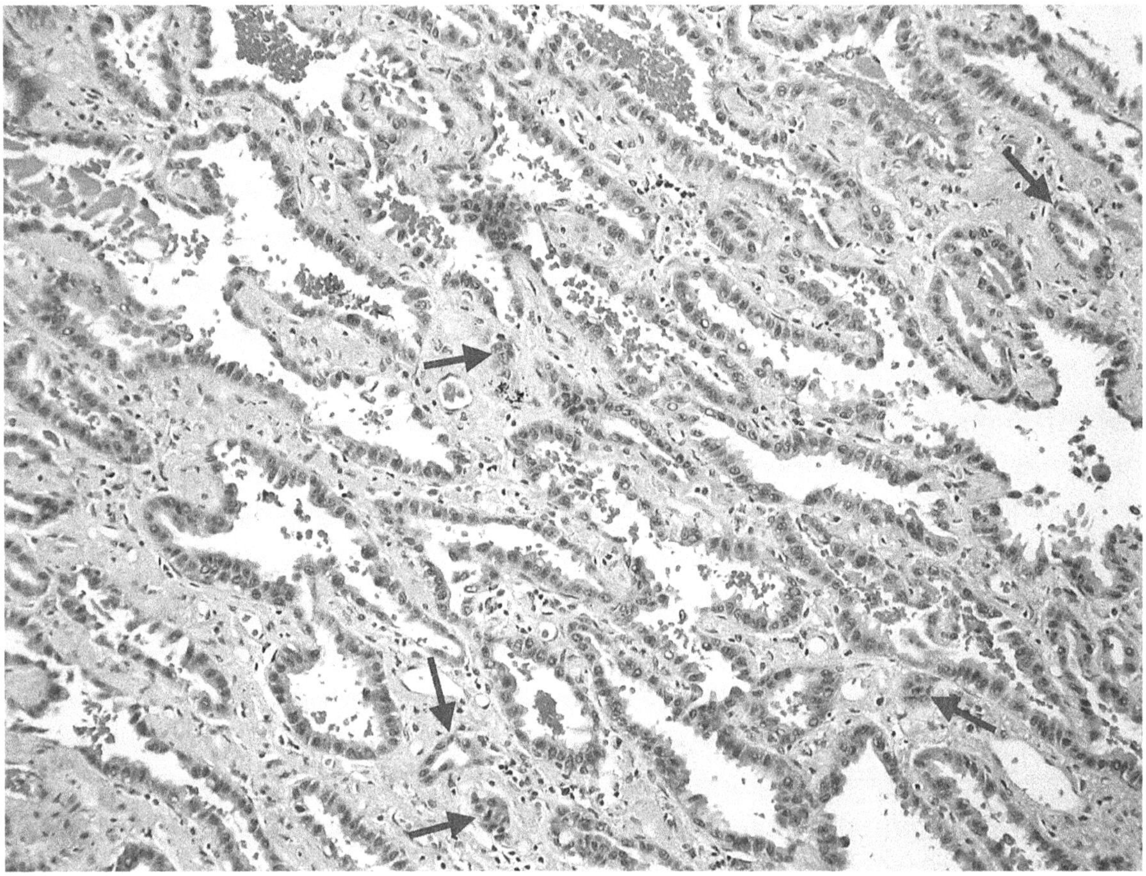

Figure 16.7: Lepidic pattern adenocarcinoma — neoplastic cells growing along pre-existing alveolar walls without stromal invasion (H&E, ×100). (Source: Yale Rosen, Wikimedia Commons, CC BY-SA 2.0.)

Pulmonary hamartoma is the most common benign lung tumour. It is a well-circumscribed peripheral nodule composed of varying proportions of cartilage, fat, fibromyxoid tissue, and entrapped respiratory epithelium ("coin lesion" on imaging). HMGA2 fusions are characteristic. On FNAC, the finding of fibromyxoid stroma admixed with benign epithelial sheets is diagnostic.

Solitary fibrous tumour of the pleura shows a "patternless pattern" of bland spindle cells with collagenised stroma and staghorn (haemangiopericytoma-like) vessels; STAT6 nuclear positivity (reflecting NAB2-STAT6 fusion) is diagnostic. CD34 is positive in most cases but is less specific than STAT6.

Lymphangioleiomyomatosis (LAM) is a rare, diffuse, cystic lung disease occurring almost exclusively in young women, associated with tuberous sclerosis (TSC2 mutations); the proliferating cells co-express smooth muscle markers (SMA) and melanocytic markers (HMB-45). **Inflammatory myofibroblastic tumour (IMT)** shows bland spindle cells with a prominent lymphoplasmacytic infiltrate; ALK rearrangement is present in approximately 50% of cases and is targetable with crizotinib.

Integration: *Metastatic tumours to the lung are common and must always be considered in the differential of a pulmonary nodule. IHC panels to distinguish primary lung adenocarcinoma from metastatic carcinoma are discussed in Chapter 36 (Immunohistochemistry in Diagnostic Pathology). Molecular fusions and targeted therapy principles are covered in Chapter 37 and Chapter 41.*

The Pathologist's Eye: Distinguishing Lung Carcinoma Subtypes on Small Biopsy and Cytology

On small biopsy or cytology, the critical first distinction is adenocarcinoma vs squamous cell carcinoma, as this determines eligibility for molecular testing and targeted therapy. Morphological clues: squamous differentiation shows keratinisation (bright eosinophilic cytoplasm, keratin pearls) and intercellular bridges; glandular differentiation shows acinar or papillary architecture and intracytoplasmic mucin vacuoles. When morphology alone is insufficient (poorly differentiated tumours), a limited IHC panel resolves most cases: TTF-1 positive and p40 negative favours adenocarcinoma; p40 positive and TTF-1 negative favours squamous cell carcinoma. CK7 and napsin A support adenocarcinoma; CK5/6 supports squamous differentiation. The panel should be kept to a minimum (TTF-1 and p40 suffice in most cases) to preserve tissue for molecular testing. Avoid the diagnosis of NSCC-NOS whenever possible; it should represent fewer than 5% of cases when IHC is applied. Small cell carcinoma (neuroendocrine markers positive, Ki-67 >80%) must be excluded first, as its treatment is entirely different.

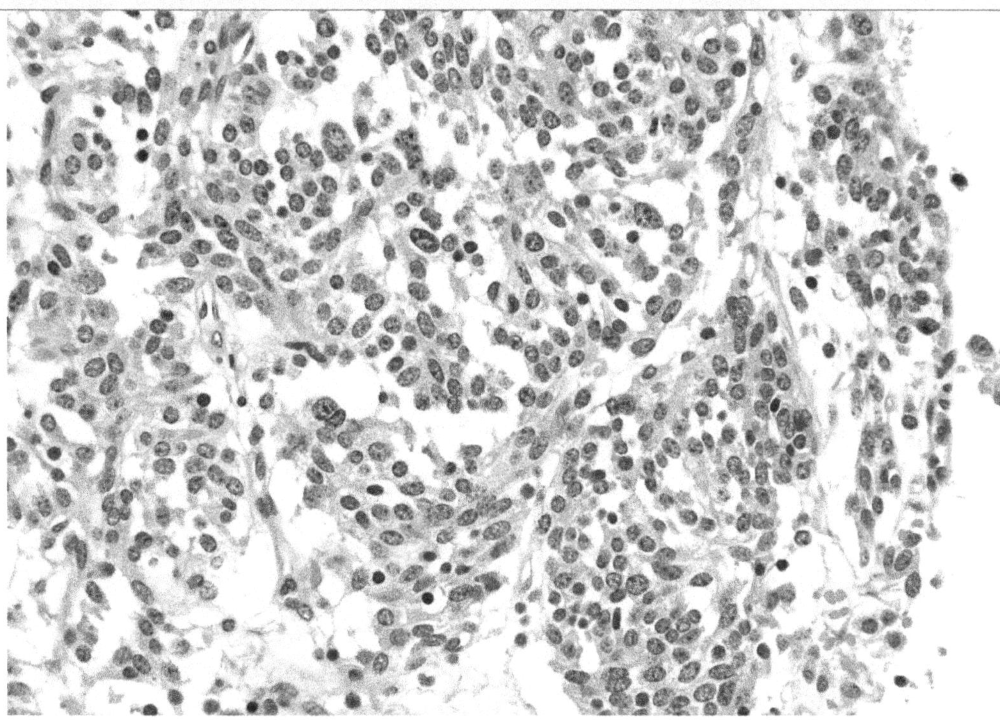

Figure 16.8: Typical carcinoid tumour of lung (H&E, very high magnification). Nests of uniform neuroendocrine cells with salt-and-pepper chromatin, moderate cytoplasm, and absent necrosis. Mitotic rate <2 per 10 HPF. (Source: Nephron, Wikimedia Commons, CC BY-SA 3.0.)

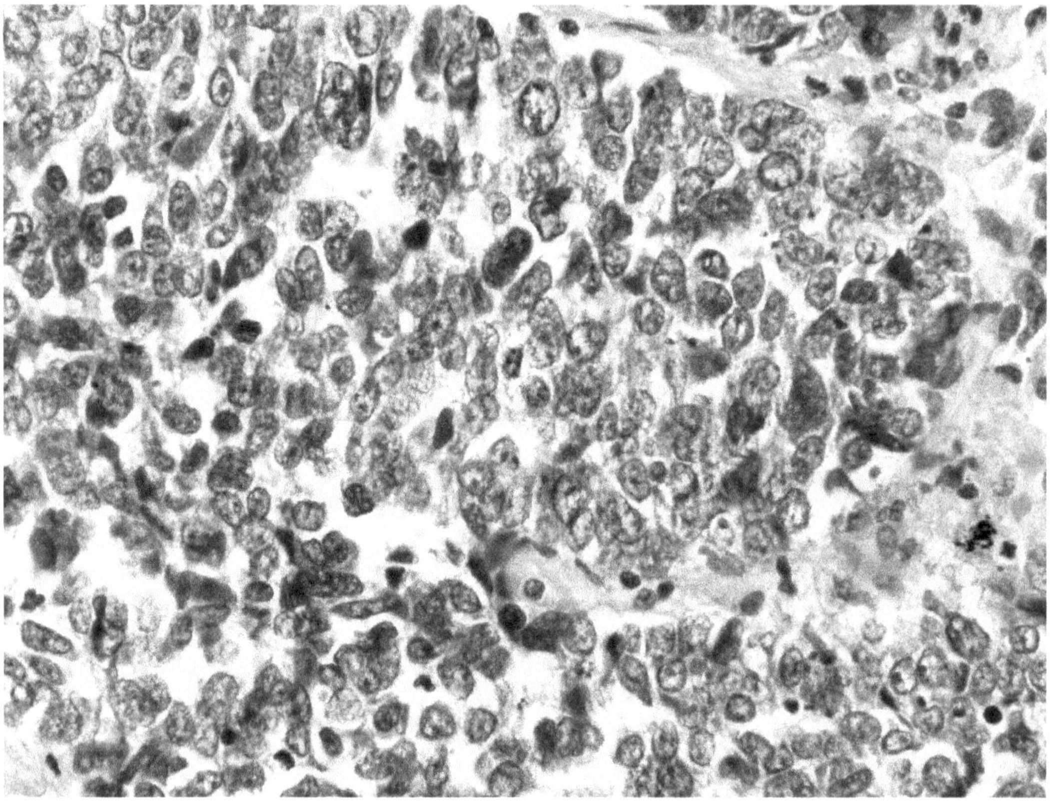

Figure 16.9: Large cell neuroendocrine carcinoma (H&E, high magnification). Sheets of large polygonal cells with moderate eosinophilic cytoplasm, vesicular chromatin, and prominent nucleoli — distinguishing LCNEC from small cell carcinoma, which has scant cytoplasm, dense chromatin, and inconspicuous nucleoli. Neuroendocrine immunophenotype (synaptophysin, chromogranin, CD56) and high mitotic rate (>10/2 mm^2) confirm the diagnosis per WHO 5th Edition. (Source: Yale Rosen, Wikimedia Commons, CC BY-SA 2.0.)

16.6 Recent Advances in Lung Cancer

KEYNOTE-024 — pembrolizumab versus platinum doublet in PD-L1-high non-small-cell lung cancer. KEYNOTE-024 established programmed death-ligand 1 immunohistochemistry as a predictive biomarker that directly determines first-line systemic therapy in advanced non-small-cell lung cancer (Reck et al. New England Journal of Medicine 2016; 375: 1823–1833; PMID 27718847). In an open-label phase 3 trial, 305 previously untreated patients with metastatic non-small-cell lung cancer, no sensitising EGFR or ALK alterations, and PD-L1 expression on at least 50% of tumour cells were randomised to pembrolizumab monotherapy or platinum-doublet chemotherapy. Median progression-free survival was 10.3 months with pembrolizumab versus 6.0 months with chemotherapy (hazard ratio 0.50; 95% CI 0.37–0.68; P<0.001), and grade 3 or higher treatment-related adverse events were less frequent in the pembrolizumab arm. The trial validated the 22C3 pharmDx companion diagnostic, the tumour-proportion-score reporting metric, and the 50% cut-point now embedded in NCCN, ESMO, and IASLC pathology recommendations. For the surgical pathologist the implication is that adequate tumour sampling and reflex PD-L1 immunohistochemistry should be prioritised on advanced-stage non-small-cell lung cancer biopsies, with TPS reported in the required intervals (negative; 1–49%; ≥50%) to permit treatment selection between pembrolizumab monotherapy, pembrolizumab plus chemotherapy, and other regimens.

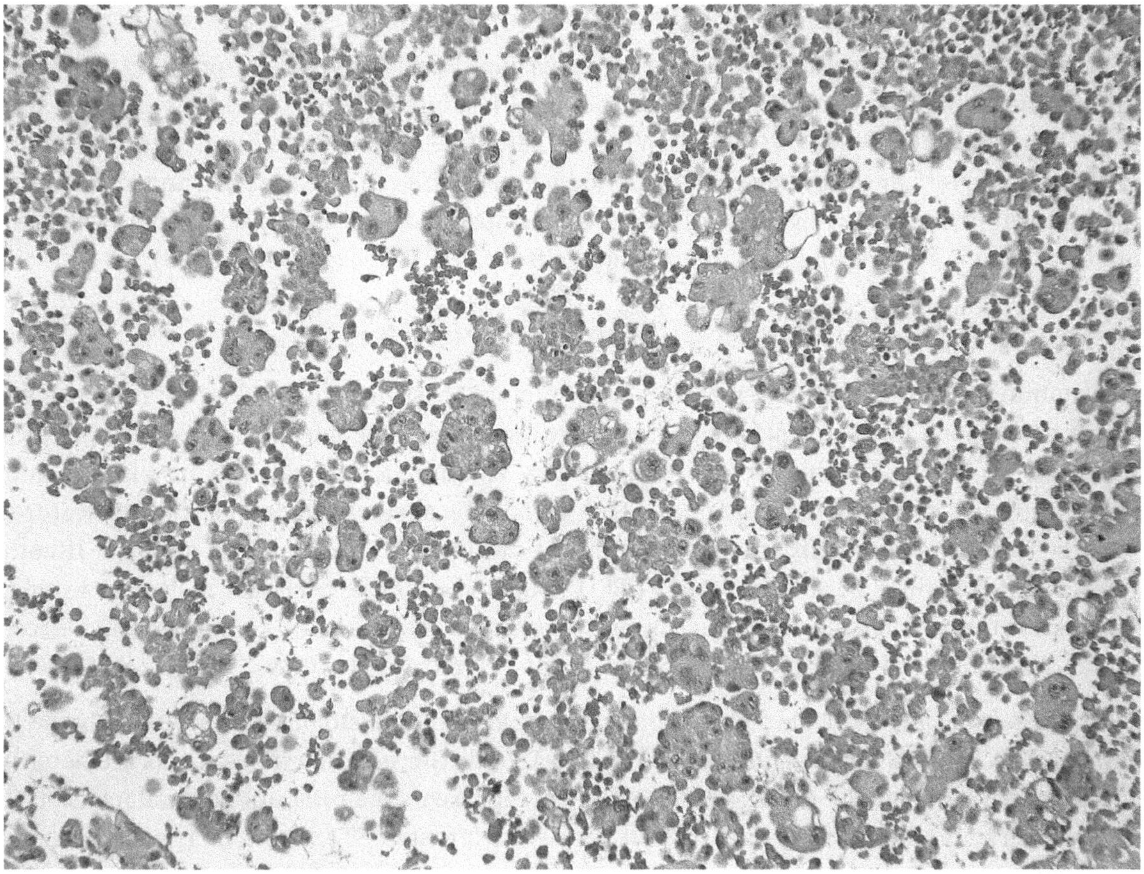

Figure 16.10: Micropapillary pattern — small papillary tufts without fibrovascular cores floating in airspaces (H&E, ×200). (Source: Yale Rosen, Wikimedia Commons, CC BY-SA 2.0.)

The introduction of osimertinib (a third-generation EGFR TKI active against both sensitising mutations and the T790M resistance mutation) as first-line therapy for EGFR-mutant NSCLC (FLAURA trial) has significantly improved progression-free and overall survival. KRAS G12C, long considered "undruggable," now has approved inhibitors (sotorasib, adagrasib), representing a major therapeutic advance. Amivantamab, a bispecific antibody targeting EGFR and MET, and the antibody-drug conjugate trastuzumab deruxtecan (for HER2-mutant NSCLC) are expanding the targeted therapy repertoire. Perioperative combination strategies (osimertinib adjuvant therapy, ADAURA trial) have shown remarkable improvement in disease-free survival for resected EGFR-mutant NSCLC.

Immune checkpoint inhibitor (ICI) therapy, particularly anti-PD-1 (pembrolizumab, nivolumab) and anti-PD-L1 (atezolizumab, durvalumab) antibodies, has become standard of care in advanced NSCLC without actionable driver mutations. More recently, neoadjuvant chemoimmunotherapy (nivolumab + chemotherapy, CheckMate 816 trial) followed by surgery has shown significant improvement in pathological complete response and event-free survival in resectable NSCLC, bringing the pathologist into the centre of response assessment. The pathological complete response (pCR) rate and major pathological response (MPR, ≤10% residual viable tumour) are now standard endpoints that pathologists must assess on resection specimens using systematic tumour bed sampling.

Liquid biopsy (circulating tumour DNA, ctDNA) is increasingly used for molecular profiling when tissue is insufficient, for monitoring treatment response (minimal residual disease), and for detecting resistance mutations (such as EGFR T790M, C797S). The WHO 5th Edition (2021) has introduced the adenocarcinoma grading system and recognised thoracic SMARCA4-deficient undifferentiated tumour and NUT carcinoma as new entities. Artificial intelligence (AI)-assisted histopathological analysis is being evaluated for automated tumour subtyping and mutation prediction from H&E slides (see Chapter 38).

16.7 Approach to the Histopathology Slide: Lung Neoplasms

When examining a lung biopsy or resection with a tumour, first determine whether the neoplasm is primary or metastatic. Clinical history (known primary elsewhere) and morphology (patterns atypical for primary lung cancer) guide this. For a primary lung carcinoma, identify the histological subtype morphologically if possible (keratinisation for SCC, glands for adenocarcinoma, small cell features for SCLC). If the tumour is poorly differentiated, apply the minimal IHC panel: TTF-1 and p40. If both are negative and cytokeratin is positive, report as NSCLC-NOS and conserve tissue for molecular testing. For neuroendocrine tumours, classify by grade: carcinoid (typical vs atypical based on mitoses and necrosis) vs high-grade NEC (small cell vs LCNEC based on cell size and cytological features).

On resection specimens, report the following mandatory elements: histological type and subtype (with percentages of each growth pattern for adenocarcinoma), grade (for non-mucinous adenocarcinoma using WHO 2021 system), tumour size (invasive component size for part-solid tumours), pleural invasion (PL0–PL3, with elastin stain), lymphovascular invasion, perineural invasion, STAS (with morphological pattern), margin status, and lymph node status. Ensure adequate tissue is triaged for molecular testing. For neoadjuvant-treated specimens, assess and report percentage of residual viable tumour, necrosis, and stroma (for MPR/pCR assessment).

Pleural invasion is graded as PL0 (tumour within the lung parenchyma or invades only the visceral pleural connective tissue without penetrating the elastic layer), PL1 (invasion beyond the elastic layer), PL2 (invasion to the visceral pleural surface), and PL3 (invasion into the parietal pleura or chest wall). PL1 and PL2 upstage the tumour to at least T2a regardless of size. Elastin staining (Verhoeff-Van Gieson or Miller) is recommended when invasion beyond the elastic layer is uncertain on H&E. This is a commonly tested topic, as examiners expect knowledge of both the grading and its staging implications.

Cytological diagnosis of bronchogenic carcinoma relies on bronchial brushings, bronchial washings, and bronchoalveolar lavage (BAL) for central lesions, and CT-guided FNAC or EBUS-guided TBNA for peripheral or mediastinal lesions. On cytology, adenocarcinoma shows three-dimensional clusters and acinar arrangements with vacuolated cytoplasm and eccentric nuclei; SCC shows dense orangeophilic cytoplasm, sharp cell borders, and nuclear hyperchromasia (on Papanicolaou stain); SCLC shows fragile cells with nuclear moulding and crush artefact. Cell block preparation from cytology specimens is essential for IHC and molecular testing (Figure 16.11).

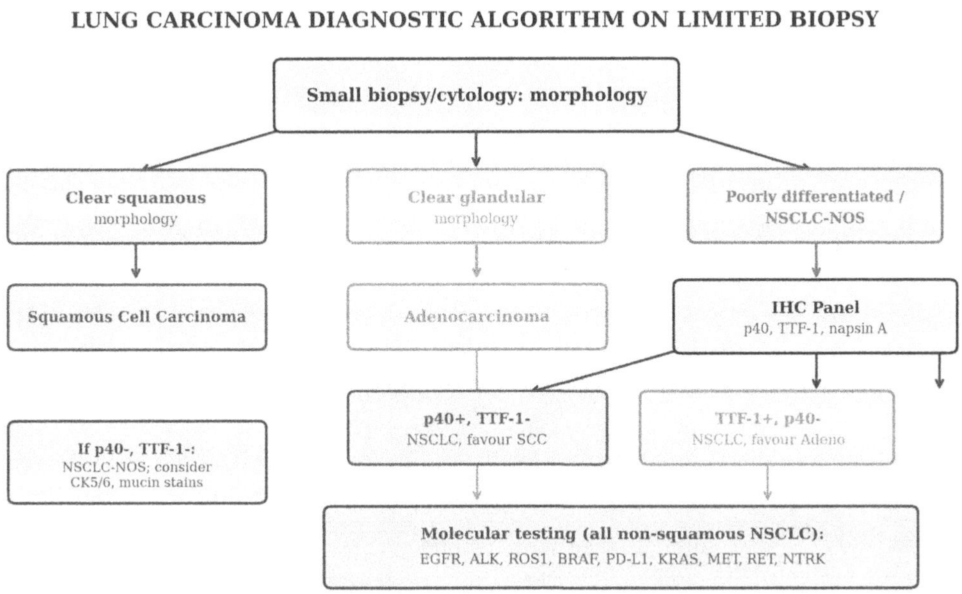

Figure 16.10 : Lung carcinoma diagnostic algorithm on limited biopsy (TTF-1/p40 panel)

Figure 16.11: Diagnostic algorithm for lung carcinoma on limited biopsy. Morphology assessment directs to squamous cell carcinoma or adenocarcinoma if clear; poorly differentiated tumours require TTF-1/p40 immunohistochemistry panel for classification as NSCLC-favour adenocarcinoma, NSCLC-favour squamous, or NSCLC-NOS. Neuroendocrine morphology triggers NE markers with grading by mitotic count and necrosis. (Source: Author's original.)

International Frameworks

IASLC Lung Cancer Staging Project, 8th edition (2017). The 8th edition TNM, derived from a multinational cohort of 94,708 cases assembled by the IASLC Staging and Prognostic Factors Committee, refined T descriptors by introducing 1-cm increments for T1 (T1a ≤1 cm, T1b >1–2 cm, T1c >2–3 cm) and reclassified tumours >5–7 cm as T3 and >7 cm as T4. Lobar atelectasis or pneumonitis is now T2 (previously T2/T3). M descriptors were stratified into M1a (intrathoracic), M1b (single extrathoracic), and M1c (multiple extrathoracic). The reporting implication is that pathologists must record the largest invasive dimension (excluding lepidic component) on resection specimens, since size cut-offs drive stage migration that in turn determines adjuvant therapy decisions. Citation: Goldstraw P, et al. J Thorac Oncol 2016;11(1):39–51. PMID 26762738.

IASLC Pathology Committee adenocarcinoma grading (2020). A three-tier grading system for invasive non-mucinous pulmonary adenocarcinoma was validated across 796 cases in training, validation, and test cohorts (combined AUC 0.69–0.79 for recurrence-free and overall survival). Grade 1 is lepidic-predominant tumour with no or <20% high-grade pattern; Grade 2 is acinar- or papillary-predominant tumour with no or <20% high-grade pattern; Grade 3 is any tumour with ≥20% high-grade pattern (solid, micropapillary, or complex glandular). Interobserver agreement was substantial ($\kappa = 0.617$). Reporting requirement: pathologists must quantify each pattern in 5% increments and combine the predominant pattern with the proportion of any high-grade component to assign grade. Citation: Moreira AL, et al. J Thorac Oncol 2020;15(10):1599–1610. PMID 32562873.

Ultra High-Yield Chapter Summary

Topic	Must Remember
Lobar pneumonia stages	Congestion → red hepatisation → grey hepatisation → resolution
Atypical pneumonia	Interstitial pattern, lymphocytic.
Pneumocystis	Foamy PAS+ alveolar exudate; GMS+ cysts (crushed cup); CD4 <200; BAL diagnostic
Aspergillus spectrum	ABPA (atopy) → aspergilloma (cavity, post-TB in endemic regions) → invasive angioinvasive (neutropenia).
COVID-19 lung pathology	DAD + microvascular thrombosis + endothelialitis; secondary mucormycosis/aspergillosis (notable across South Asia)
Most common lung cancer	Adenocarcinoma (~40–50%). SCC is #2.
Adenocarcinoma IHC	TTF-1+, Napsin A+. p40–.
SCC IHC	p40+ (most specific), CK5/6+. TTF-1–.
Minimal IHC panel	TTF-1 + p40 (conserve tissue for molecular testing)
WHO adeno grading (2021)	G1: lepidic; G2: acinar/papillary; G3: ≥20% high-grade pattern (solid, micropapillary, cribriform)
STAS	Spread through air spaces. Excludes AIS/MIA.
SCLC features	Small cells, moulding, salt-pepper, necrosis, Azzopardi; Ki-67 ~100%; RB1+TP53 loss
SCLC vs LCNEC	Cell size, chromatin (granular vs vesicular), nucleoli (absent vs prominent).
SCLC paraneoplastic	SIADH, ectopic ACTH (Cushing), Lambert-Eaton
Carcinoid grading	Typical: <2 mitoses, no necrosis.

EGFR mutations	Exon 19 del + L858R (85%); osimertinib first-line; 25–30% in South Asian adenocarcinoma
ALK rearrangement	EML4-ALK; 5% of adeno; young, never-smokers; alectinib, lorlatinib
KRAS G12C	13% adeno; sotorasib, adagrasib; smokers; formerly undruggable
PD-L1 testing	22C3 antibody; TPS ≥50%: pembrolizumab monotherapy; TPS 1–49%: pembro + chemo
Mesothelioma IHC	Calretinin, CK5/6, WT-1, D2-40 (positive); TTF-1, CEA, Claudin-4, BerEP4 (negative)
Mesothelioma vs reactive	BAP1 loss + CDKN2A/p16 FISH deletion (or MTAP loss) → malignant
Pulmonary hamartoma	Most common benign lung tumour; cartilage + fat + epithelium; HMGA2 fusion; coin lesion
Neoadjuvant response	pCR and MPR (≤10% viable tumour) are standard pathological endpoints post-chemoimmunotherapy

Cross-References from Chapter 16

Tuberculosis, fungal pneumonia, viral pneumonias, parasitic lung infections → Chapters 6 and 9. Non-neoplastic lung disease, pneumoconioses, ILD, pulmonary hypertension → Chapter 15. Coronary atherosclerosis and cardiac metastases → Chapters 13 and 14. Paraneoplastic syndromes (SIADH, ectopic ACTH, Lambert-Eaton, hypercalcaemia) → Chapters 5 and 29. Neuroendocrine tumour grading and classification → Chapters 19 and 29. Metastatic disease pathways, sentinel lymph node biology → Chapter 4. TNM staging principles, grading and staging frameworks → Chapter 3. Molecular diagnostics (EGFR, ALK, ROS1, BRAF, MET, RET, NTRK, KRAS G12C), NGS, liquid biopsy, PD-L1 theranostics → Chapter 42. FNAC, EBUS-TBNA, ROSE, cytology–histology correlation → Chapter 40. Osimertinib, alectinib, crizotinib, lorlatinib, sotorasib, pembrolizumab → Chapter 41.

Diagnostic thinking: TTF-1+/Napsin A+ + glandular morphology → lung adenocarcinoma

Diagnostic thinking: p40+/CK5/6+ + keratinisation → lung squamous cell carcinoma

Diagnostic thinking: salt-and-pepper chromatin + high mitotic rate + extensive necrosis + Ki-67 >80% → small cell lung carcinoma (Figures 16.4–16.7)

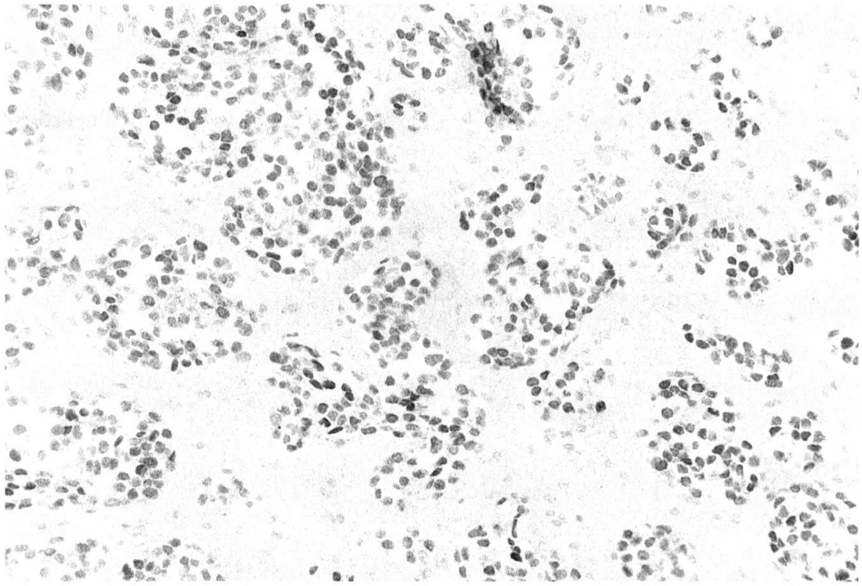

Figure 16.12: Lung adenocarcinoma — glandular architecture with TTF-1 positivity (IHC, high magnification). (Source: Nephron, Wikimedia Commons, CC BY-SA 3.0.)

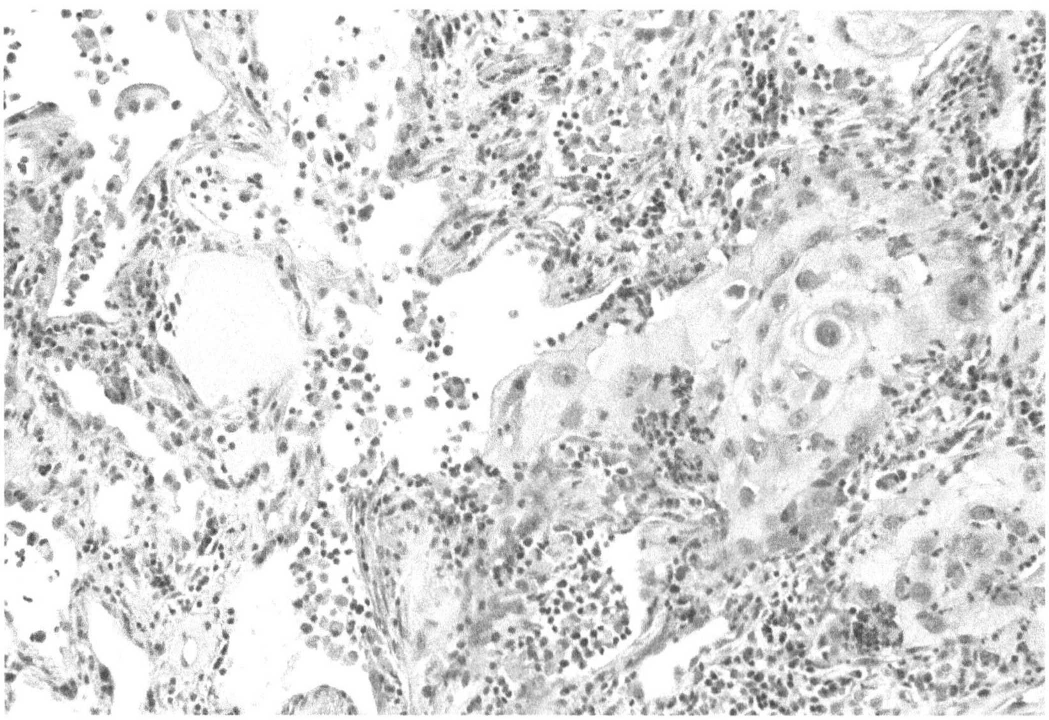

Figure 16.13: Lung squamous cell carcinoma (H&E, intermediate magnification). Keratinising squamous differentiation with keratin pearls, intercellular bridges, and eosinophilic cytoplasm. (Source: Nephron, Wikimedia Commons, CC BY-SA 3.0.)

Chapter 17: Head and Neck Pathology

THE BIG PICTURE

The head and neck region encompasses the oral cavity, major and minor salivary glands, the sinonasal and nasopharyngeal tracts, the oropharynx and larynx, the thyroid and parathyroid glands, and the odontogenic apparatus of the jaws. Head and neck pathology is dominated by squamous-lineage lesions (from potentially malignant disorders of the oral mucosa to invasive squamous cell carcinoma and its variants) and a characteristic family of salivary gland neoplasms in which recognition rests on morphology augmented by immunohistochemistry and an expanding set of molecular signatures. Across South Asia, oral submucous fibrosis and oral squamous cell carcinoma driven by tobacco and areca nut exposure constitute one of the heaviest disease burdens the surgical pathologist will encounter. The pathologist's task is to distinguish dysplasia from invasion, separate architecturally mimicking salivary gland tumours using biphasic patterns and myoepithelial markers, and recognise the molecular hallmarks that now define entities such as adenoid cystic carcinoma (MYB/MYBL1), mucoepidermoid carcinoma (MAML2), secretory carcinoma (ETV6–NTRK3), and polymorphous adenocarcinoma (PRKD). Thyroid pathology adds a layer of nuclear-feature-based diagnosis in which morphology alone decides between benign and malignant labels for a majority of follicular-derived lesions.

High-yield topics in this chapter: Oral potentially malignant disorders and oral squamous cell carcinoma (including WPOI scoring and the verrucous variant); salivary gland benign and malignant neoplasms with their diagnostic immunohistochemical panels and defining molecular fusions; nasopharyngeal carcinoma and EBER-based diagnosis of WHO type III undifferentiated tumours; sinonasal papillomas; odontogenic cysts and tumours (ameloblastoma, odontogenic keratocyst); papillary and medullary thyroid carcinoma with their nuclear and stromal hallmarks; approach to salivary gland biopsy and head-and-neck tumour IHC classification.

Oral Cavity Lesions

The oral cavity is lined by stratified squamous epithelium of varying thickness and keratinisation. The most important pathological processes in this region are premalignant mucosal disorders and squamous cell carcinoma, both of which carry enormous public health significance across South Asia.

Oral Potentially Malignant Disorders

The WHO recognises several oral potentially malignant disorders (OPMDs), of which **leukoplakia, erythroplakia, and oral submucous fibrosis (OSMF)** are the most clinically significant. Leukoplakia is a clinical term for a white patch that cannot be characterised clinically or pathologically as any other disease. It is found in 0.5 to 3% of the population, with malignant transformation rates of 3 to 5%. Erythroplakia, a red velvety patch, carries a much higher risk, with up to 50% showing severe dysplasia or carcinoma in situ on biopsy.

The key diagnostic clue in oral biopsy interpretation is the degree and pattern of epithelial dysplasia, which remains the single most important predictor of malignant transformation.

Histologically, oral epithelial dysplasia is graded as mild (confined to the lower third of the epithelium), moderate (extending to the middle third), or severe (more than two-thirds involvement). The WHO 5th Edition recognises a binary grading system as an alternative: low-grade dysplasia (mild) versus high-grade dysplasia (moderate and severe combined), which has better interobserver reproducibility.

Areca nut → Arecoline → Fibroblast activation → ↑Collagen I/III synthesis + ↓Collagenase → Submucosal fibrosis → Epithelial atrophy → Dysplasia → SCC

ORAL SQUAMOUS CELL CARCINOMA (OSCC)

Definition: Malignant neoplasm of squamous epithelium of the oral mucosa. Most common malignancy of the oral cavity; in South Asia accounts for a substantial proportion of all cancers.

Etiology/Risk factors: Tobacco (smoked and smokeless), areca nut, alcohol. Strongest synergy: tobacco + alcohol. Most common subsites: buccal mucosa and lateral border of tongue.

Pathogenesis: Tobacco/areca nut exposure → Chronic mucosal irritation → Epithelial dysplasia (mild → moderate → severe) → Carcinoma in situ → Invasive SCC

Grading: Broder system (well/moderately/poorly differentiated) or, more importantly, **worst pattern of invasion (WPOI) score**: WPOI 5 (tumour satellites >1 mm from main tumour mass) = significantly worse prognosis, may warrant adjuvant therapy even in early-stage disease.

Microscopy: Nests and cords of malignant squamous cells with **keratinisation, intercellular bridges, and keratin pearl formation**. Nuclear pleomorphism, increased mitotic activity, invasive growth with desmoplastic stromal response. Adverse prognostic features: perineural invasion, lymphovascular invasion.

Key DDx: Verrucous carcinoma (pushing deep margins, no conventional invasion, excellent prognosis) vs conventional SCC (infiltrative margins, worse prognosis). Adequate sampling mandatory to exclude hybrid/conventional SCC components in verrucous lesions.

Exam yield: ★★★ HIGH — OSCC histology, WPOI scoring, and the verrucous vs conventional SCC distinction are perennial exam favourites.

Verrucous carcinoma is a distinct, low-grade variant of SCC that presents as a broad-based, warty, exophytic growth. It has a pushing border without conventional stromal invasion, and is associated with smokeless tobacco. Hybrid or conventional SCC components must be excluded on adequate sampling, as the prognosis changes markedly.

Quick Recall: Oral Cavity Lesions

Leukoplakia: Clinical diagnosis; 3-5% malignant transformation; biopsy to assess dysplasia grade.

Erythroplakia: Red patch; up to 50% show severe dysplasia or carcinoma in situ.

OSMF: Areca nut; submucosal fibrosis; 7-13% malignant transformation; highest prevalence in South Asia.

OSCC grading: WPOI score 5 (tumour satellites >1 mm from main mass) = worst prognosis.
Verrucous carcinoma: Pushing borders, no conventional invasion; smokeless tobacco association.

Salivary Gland Pathology

The major salivary glands (parotid, submandibular, sublingual) and the hundreds of minor salivary glands scattered throughout the oral cavity, pharynx, and sinonasal tract give rise to a remarkably diverse group of tumours. The WHO 5th Edition classification recognises over 30 histological types. Two general rules help guide diagnosis: first, the smaller the gland, the more likely a tumour is malignant; second, many salivary neoplasms are defined by recurrent molecular alterations that are increasingly essential for diagnosis.

Integration: Salivary gland IHC panels use myoepithelial markers (p63, p40, SMA, calponin, S100) extensively; principles of myoepithelial biology connect to Chapter 36 (Immunohistochemistry). Molecular fusions (PLAG1, MAML2, MYB) connect to Chapter 37 (Molecular Pathology).

Benign Tumours

PLEOMORPHIC ADENOMA (PA)

Definition: Most common salivary gland tumour (~60% of all salivary neoplasms). Benign mixed tumour with epithelial and mesenchymal-like components.

Components: (1) Epithelial ductal structures, (2) myoepithelial cells (spindled, plasmacytoid, or epithelioid), (3) mesenchymal-like stroma (myxoid, chondroid, fibrous, or osseous). Cytologically bland despite architectural pleomorphism.

Gross: Well-circumscribed; encapsulation variable. Pseudopodia and satellite nodules at capsular margin explain local recurrence after incomplete excision.

Microscopy: Three intermingled components blending seamlessly. Key diagnostic feature: **chondromyxoid stroma admixed with epithelial and myoepithelial elements**

Molecular: PLAG1 or HMGA2 gene fusions in the vast majority; diagnostically useful.

FNA: Classic metachromatic fibrillary stroma ('troll hair' on Diff-Quik) with admixed epithelial and myoepithelial cells (Figures 17.1–17.2).

Complications: Carcinoma ex PA arises in longstanding/recurrent PA (risk ~10% at 15 years). Usually high-grade (salivary duct ca., adenocarcinoma NOS, myoepithelial ca.). Prognosis depends on invasion: intracapsular (excellent), minimally invasive (<1.5 mm beyond capsule, good), frankly invasive (poor).

Exam yield: ★★★ HIGH — PA morphology, PLAG1 fusion, FNA features, and carcinoma ex PA are perennial exam topics.

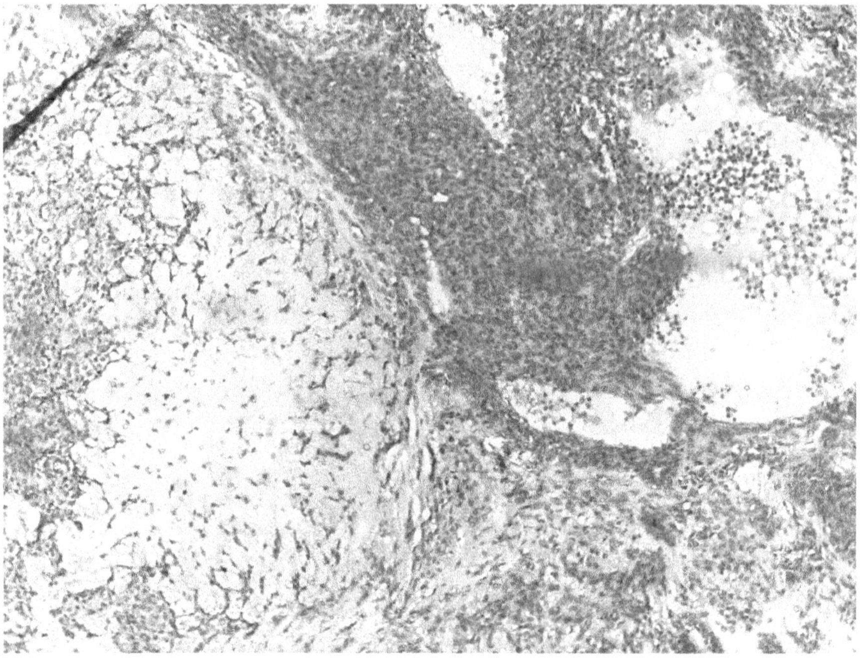

Figure 17.1: Pleomorphic adenoma of the salivary gland. Biphasic tumour showing epithelial ductal structures admixed with myoepithelial cells in a chondromyxoid stroma. Note the characteristic blending of epithelial and mesenchymal-like elements. H&E, 10×. (Source: Calicut Medical College, Wikimedia Commons, CC BY-SA 4.0.)

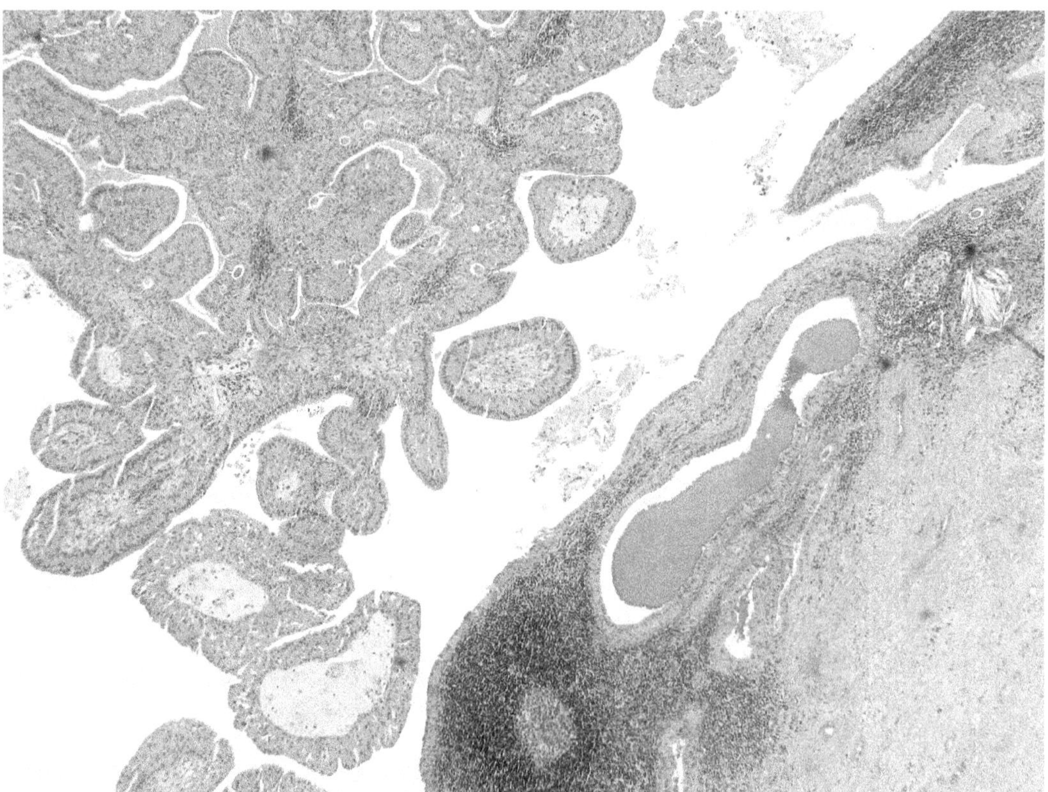

Figure 17.2: Warthin tumour (papillary cystadenoma lymphomatosum). Bilayered oncocytic epithelium lining papillary and cystic spaces, supported by a dense lymphoid stroma with germinal centres. H&E. (Source: Nephron, Wikimedia Commons, CC BY-SA 3.0.)

Prognosis of carcinoma ex PA depends on invasion extent: intracapsular (excellent), minimally invasive (<1.5 mm beyond capsule, good), or frankly invasive (poor). The carcinomatous component is usually salivary duct carcinoma, adenocarcinoma NOS, or myoepithelial carcinoma.

WARTHIN TUMOUR

Definition: Second most common benign salivary tumour. Arises almost exclusively in the parotid gland.

Etiology: Strong association with smoking. Can be bilateral or multifocal.

Microscopy: Bilayered oncocytic epithelium lining papillary and cystic spaces, supported by a lymphoid stroma with germinal centres

FNA: Thick, dark 'motor oil' fluid with oncocytes in flat sheets and polymorphous lymphoid background (Figure 17.2).

Exam yield: ★★ MODERATE — Bilateral parotid swelling + oncocytic epithelium + lymphoid stroma = classic viva slide.

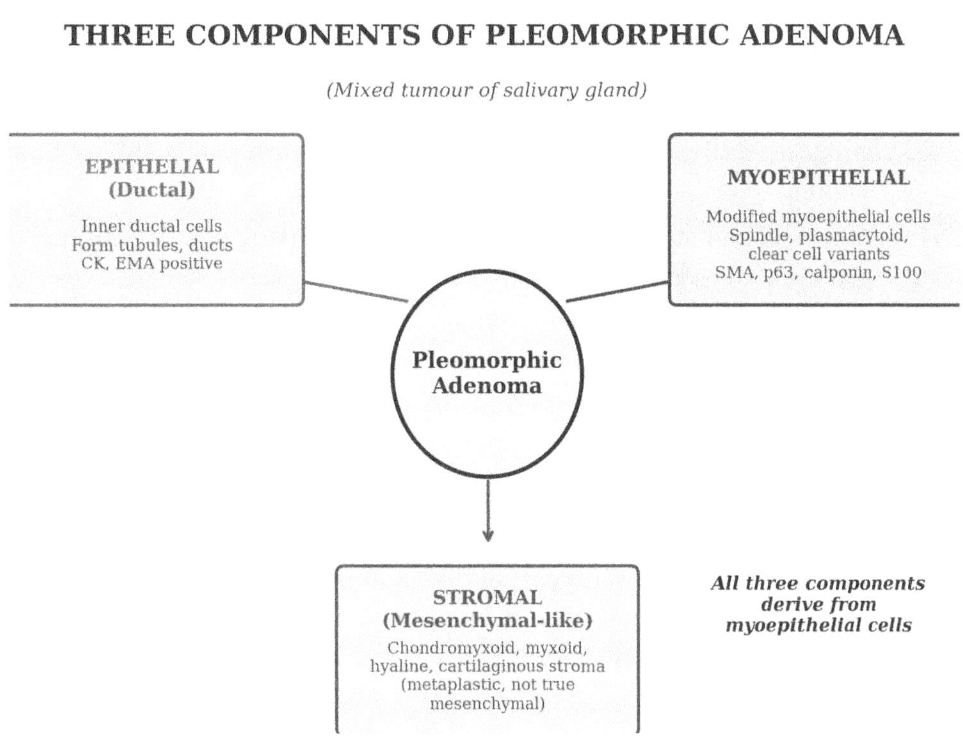

Figure 17.3: Three components of pleomorphic adenoma: epithelial ducts, myoepithelial cells (spindled/plasmacytoid), and stromal matrix (myxoid/chondroid), with capsular encapsulation and pseudopodia. (Source: Author's original.)

BASAL CELL ADENOMA

Definition: Well-circumscribed, encapsulated benign tumour, usually parotid. Composed of basaloid cells with peripheral palisading.

Patterns: Solid, trabecular, membranous, or tubular. Lacks chondromyxoid stroma (distinguishes from PA).

Molecular: CTNNB1 mutations with nuclear beta-catenin expression on IHC. Membranous subtype associated with dermal cylindromas (Brooke-Spiegler syndrome, CYLD1 mutations).

Exam yield: ★★ MODERATE — Distinguish from PA (no chondromyxoid stroma) and from basal cell adenocarcinoma (BCA is encapsulated, bland).

Inflammatory and Non-Neoplastic Conditions

SJÖGREN SYNDROME

Definition: Chronic systemic autoimmune disease characterised by lymphocytic infiltration of exocrine glands, producing keratoconjunctivitis sicca (dry eyes) and xerostomia (dry mouth). Predominantly affects older women.

Serology: Anti-Ro/SSA and anti-La/SSB autoantibodies.

Pathogenesis: Autoimmune T-cell attack on exocrine glands → Lymphocytic infiltration → Acinar destruction → Sicca symptoms → Risk of MALT lymphoma

Biopsy: Labial minor salivary gland biopsy: **focus score >1 focus (cluster of ≥50 lymphocytes) per 4 mm^2 of glandular tissue**

Microscopy: Progressive lymphocytic infiltration, acinar atrophy, and characteristic lymphoepithelial lesions (LELs) — lymphocytes infiltrate and destroy ductal epithelium, forming epimyoepithelial islands.

Complications: 15–20-fold increased risk of extranodal marginal zone lymphoma (MALT lymphoma) of salivary gland. Any persistent enlargement should be investigated with IHC to confirm polyclonality.

Exam yield: ★★★ HIGH — Sjögren focus score, LELs, anti-Ro/SSA, and MALT lymphoma risk are classic exam topics.

IgG4-related sialadenitis (Küttner tumour) is part of the multiorgan IgG4-related disease spectrum. It presents as firm, tumefactive swelling, usually of the submandibular gland. Histologically, it shows a dense lymphoplasmacytic infiltrate, storiform fibrosis, obliterative phlebitis, and increased IgG4-positive plasma cells (more than 100 per high-power field). Preserved lobular architecture with extensive fibrosis and florid germinal centre formation are typical. Serum IgG4 is often elevated. *The distinction from lymphoma rests on the preservation of lobular architecture, polyclonal plasma cells, and the characteristic storiform fibrosis pattern.*

Other non-neoplastic conditions include **sialadenosis**, a bilateral, painless salivary gland enlargement associated with systemic conditions such as diabetes mellitus, alcoholism, malnutrition, and eating disorders. It results from autonomic neuropathy causing acinar cell hypertrophy. Histologically, the acinar cells are enlarged but otherwise unremarkable. **Necrotising sialometaplasia** is a self-limited, benign condition typically affecting the palatal minor salivary glands, caused by ischaemic necrosis. It is a classic mimic of squamous cell carcinoma on biopsy; the lobular architecture is preserved, the squamous metaplasia has smooth, rounded contours, and there is associated coagulative necrosis of acini and inflammation. Recognising the lobular pattern prevents misdiagnosis.

Exam Pitfall: Necrotising Sialometaplasia vs SCC

Necrotising sialometaplasia of the palatal minor salivary glands can closely mimic squamous cell carcinoma due to the presence of squamous metaplasia, cellular atypia (reactive), and tissue necrosis. The three features that distinguish it from SCC are: (1) preservation of lobular architecture (SCC destroys it), (2) smooth, rounded contours of the squamous nests (SCC shows infiltrative, irregular margins), and (3) associated inflammation and acinar coagulative necrosis (SCC shows desmoplastic reaction). Awareness of this entity prevents unnecessary radical surgery.

Quick Recall: Non-Neoplastic Salivary Gland Disease

Sjögren syndrome: Autoimmune; anti-Ro/SSA, anti-La/SSB; focus score >1; MALT lymphoma risk.

IgG4-related sialadenitis: Dense lymphoplasmacytic infiltrate + storiform fibrosis + obliterative phlebitis; IgG4+ >100/HPF.

Necrotising sialometaplasia: Ischaemic; palate; lobular pattern preserved; mimic of SCC.

Sialadenosis: Bilateral enlargement; diabetes/alcoholism; acinar hypertrophy; non-neoplastic.

Malignant Tumours

MUCOEPIDERMOID CARCINOMA (MEC)

Definition: Most common salivary gland malignancy. Contains three cell types: mucin-secreting cells, squamoid cells, and intermediate cells.

Grading: Based on proportion of cystic vs solid, cytological atypia, mitotic rate, perineural invasion, and necrosis. Low-grade: predominantly cystic, abundant mucinous cells, excellent prognosis. High-grade: solid, squamoid/intermediate predominant, atypia, necrosis, poor prognosis.

Microscopy: Admixture of mucous cells (pale vacuolated cytoplasm), intermediate cells, and epidermoid (squamoid) cells

Molecular: MAML2 rearrangements (usually CRTC1::MAML2 fusion) in the majority; virtually diagnostic. Presence correlates with favourable outcome (Figure 17.4).

Exam yield: ★★★ HIGH — Three cell types, grading system, and MAML2 rearrangement are core exam topics.

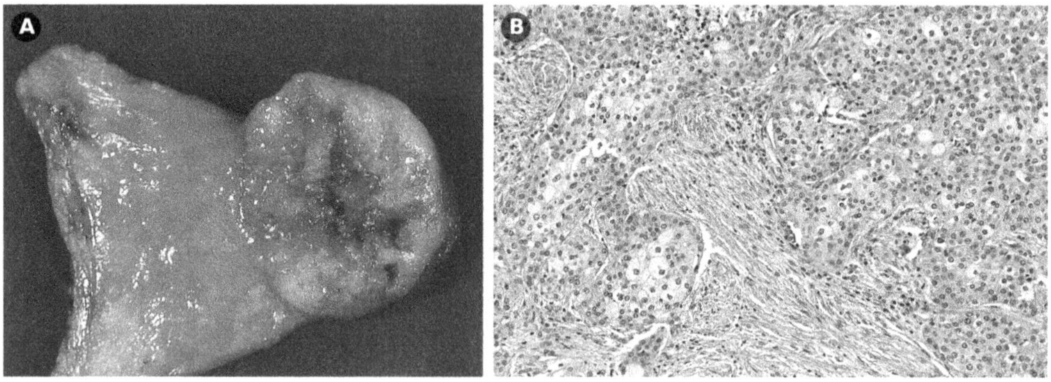

Figure 17.4: Mucoepidermoid carcinoma of the salivary gland. (A) Gross specimen: well-circumscribed, partially cystic tumour with a tan-white cut surface and focal haemorrhage. (Source: Yale Rosen, Wikimedia Commons, CC BY-SA 2.0.) (B) H&E, high magnification: admixture of mucous cells (with pale, vacuolated cytoplasm), intermediate cells, and epidermoid (squamoid) cells. (Source: Nephron, Wikimedia Commons, CC BY-SA 3.0.)

ADENOID CYSTIC CARCINOMA (AdCC)

Definition: Prototypical salivary malignancy characterised by relentless perineural invasion. Biphasic: myoepithelial cells + ductal cells.

Microscopy: Three growth patterns: **cribriform (classic 'Swiss cheese' with pseudocystic spaces containing basophilic mucoid/hyaline material), tubular (best prognosis), and solid (worst prognosis, >30% solid)**

Key DDx: Distinguished from other basaloid salivary tumours by: (1) biphasic nature (myoepithelial + ductal), (2) cribriform architecture with mucoid pseudocysts, (3) characteristic perineural invasion.

Molecular: MYB::NFIB or MYBL1::NFIB fusions (~60%).

Prognosis: Adequate 5-year survival but poor long-term survival due to persistent local recurrence and late distant metastases (lung, 10–15 years post-diagnosis). The 5-year vs 15-year survival discrepancy is a classic viva question.

Exam yield: ★★★ HIGH — Cribriform pattern, perineural invasion, MYB fusion, and late metastasis are heavily tested.

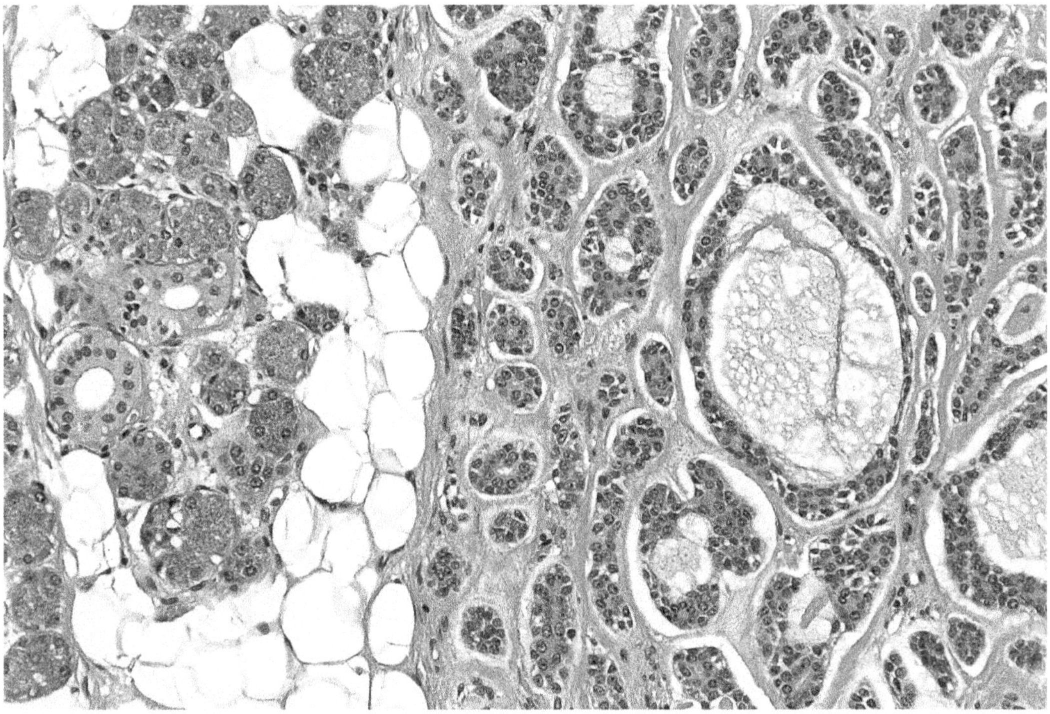

Figure 17.5: Adenoid cystic carcinoma of the salivary gland. Cribriform ("Swiss cheese") architecture with pseudocystic spaces containing basement membrane-like mucoid material, surrounded by biphasic basaloid tumour cells (H&E, high mag). (Source: Nephron, Wikimedia Commons, CC BY-SA 3.0.)

ACINIC CELL CARCINOMA

Acinic cell carcinoma is a low-grade malignancy composed of cells resembling serous acinar cells with basophilic, PAS-D positive zymogen granules. Architecture varies from solid to cystic or follicular. Usually arises in the parotid. Molecular: NR4A3 translocations. IHC: DOG1 positive (membranous/canalicular), SOX10 positive.

Exam yield: ★★ MODERATE — DOG1 positivity, NR4A3 translocation, and zymogen granules are key exam identifiers.

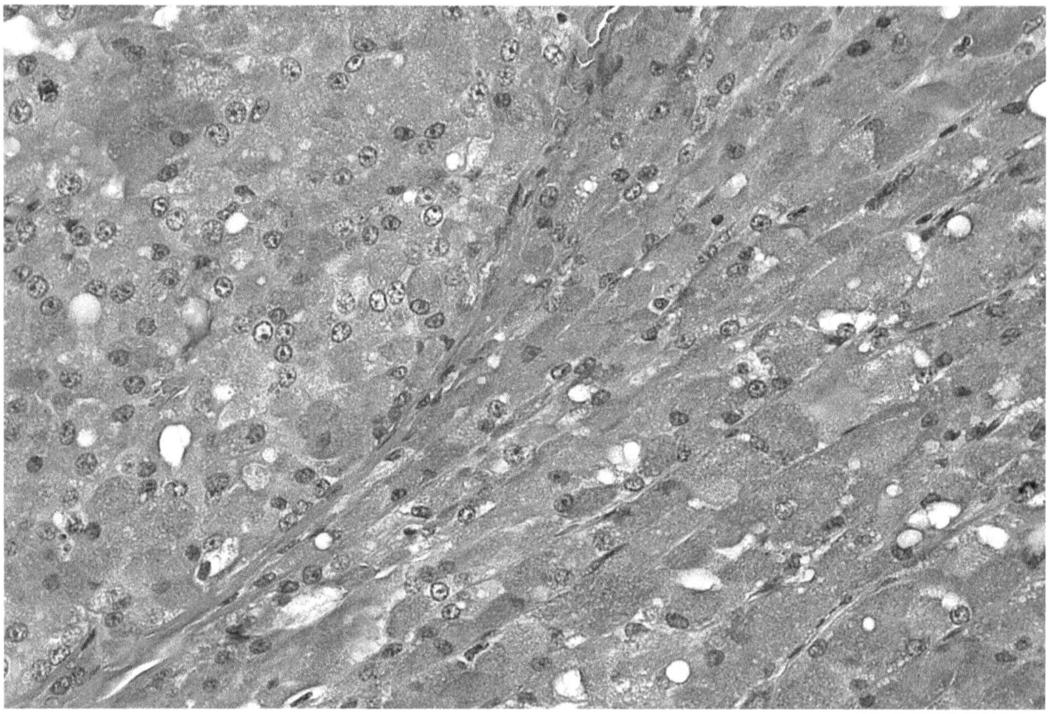

Figure 17.6: Acinic cell carcinoma of the salivary gland. Solid and microcystic architecture composed of cells resembling serous acinar cells, with basophilic granular cytoplasm containing PAS-D positive zymogen granules. DOG1 shows membranous/canalicular positivity; NR4A3 rearrangement is the defining molecular event (H&E, high mag). (Source: Nephron, Wikimedia Commons, CC BY-SA 3.0.)

SECRETORY CARCINOMA

Secretory carcinoma (formerly mammary analogue secretory carcinoma) is an indolent malignancy defined by the **ETV6::NTRK3 fusion**. Morphology shows tubular, papillary, and cystic growth with eosinophilic, bubbly, vacuolated cytoplasm and characteristic luminal eosinophilic secretions. IHC: S100 positive, mammaglobin positive, PanTRK positive; p63/p40 negative.

Exam yield: ★★ MODERATE — ETV6::NTRK3 fusion defines this entity; PanTRK IHC is the screening test.

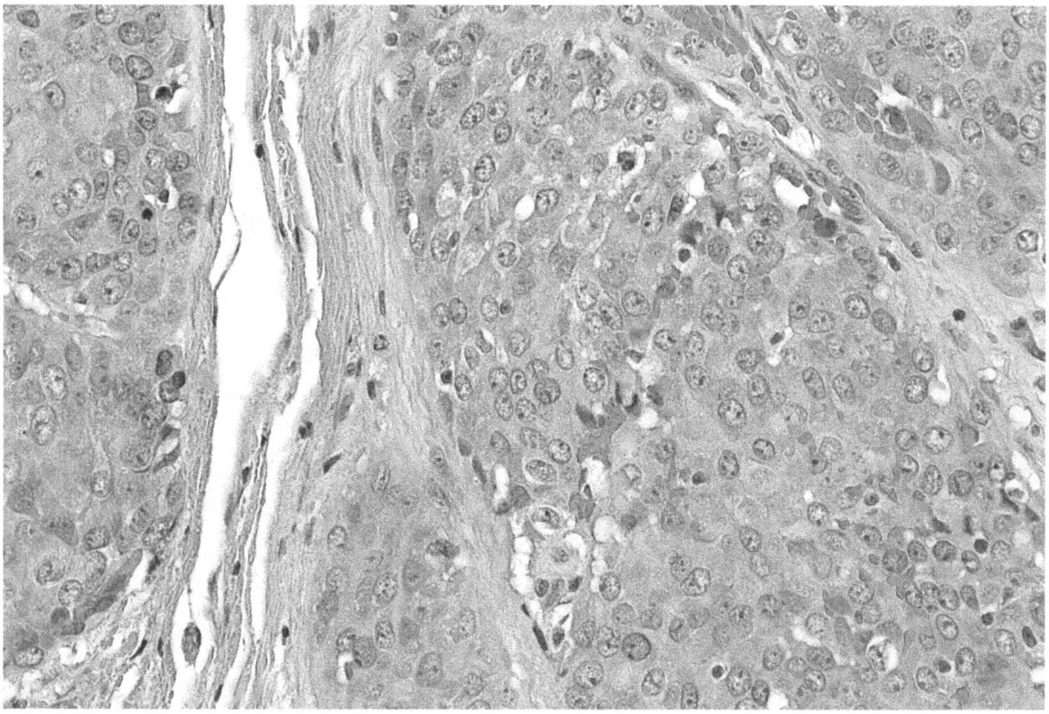

Figure 17.7: Secretory carcinoma of the salivary gland (formerly mammary analogue secretory carcinoma). Tubular, papillary, and microcystic growth with eosinophilic, bubbly, vacuolated cytoplasm and characteristic luminal eosinophilic secretions. Defined by the ETV6::NTRK3 fusion; IHC shows S100, mammaglobin, and PanTRK positivity (H&E, high mag). (Source: Nephron, Wikimedia Commons, CC BY-SA 4.0.)

POLYMORPHOUS ADENOCARCINOMA

Polymorphous adenocarcinoma (formerly PLGA) is a low-grade carcinoma arising exclusively in minor salivary glands, most often the palate. It shows monomorphic, bland cells with remarkable architectural diversity ('polymorphous') including concentric whorling, tubular, cribriform, and single-file patterns. Significant perineural invasion. Molecular: PRKD mutations/fusions. IHC: S100 strongly positive.

Exam yield: ★★ MODERATE — Minor salivary gland (palate) + architectural polymorphism + bland cells = polymorphous adenocarcinoma.

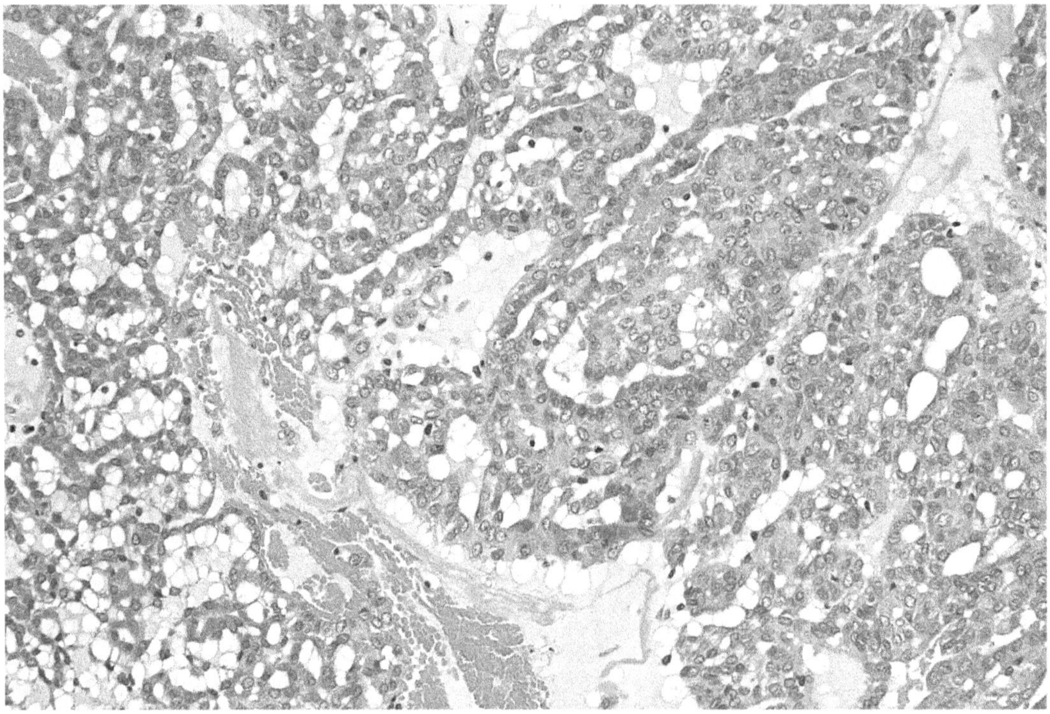

Figure 17.8: Polymorphous adenocarcinoma (formerly PLGA) of minor salivary gland origin. Monomorphic, bland cells displaying remarkable architectural diversity including concentric whorling, tubular, cribriform, and single-file patterns. Perineural invasion is characteristic; S100 is strongly positive and PRKD mutations/fusions define the molecular profile (H&E, high mag). (Source: Nephron, Wikimedia Commons, CC BY-SA 3.0.)

SALIVARY DUCT CARCINOMA

Salivary duct carcinoma is a high-grade malignancy morphologically resembling high-grade invasive ductal carcinoma of the breast. It shows cribriform, papillary, and solid patterns with comedo necrosis, marked pleomorphism, and frequent apocrine differentiation. IHC: AR strongly positive, HER2 amplified in approximately 30%. This tumour commonly arises as the carcinomatous component in carcinoma ex pleomorphic adenoma.

Exam yield: ★★ MODERATE — Resembles breast IDC; AR+, HER2 amplified in ~30%; arises in carcinoma ex PA.

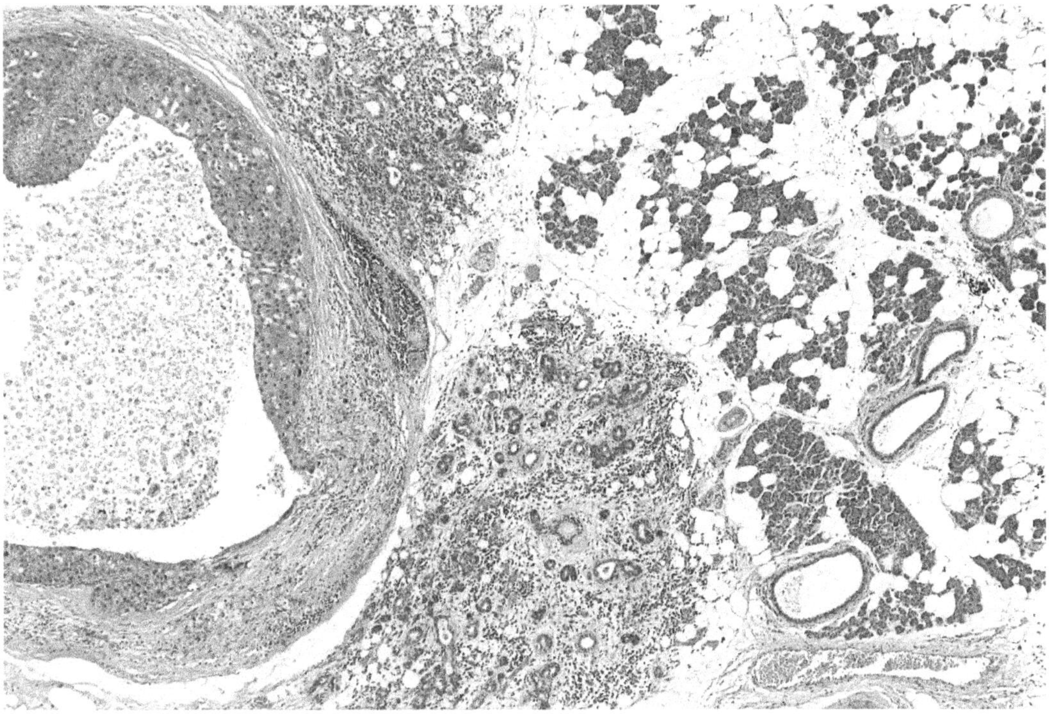

Figure 17.9: Salivary duct carcinoma. High-grade malignancy morphologically resembling high-grade invasive ductal carcinoma of the breast, showing cribriform and solid patterns with comedo-type necrosis, marked pleomorphism, and apocrine differentiation. Androgen receptor (AR) is strongly positive and HER2 is amplified in approximately 30% of cases. Frequently arises as the carcinomatous component of carcinoma ex pleomorphic adenoma (H&E, low mag). (Source: Nephron, Wikimedia Commons, CC BY-SA 3.0.)

Exam Pitfall: Epithelial/Myoepithelial Tumour Overlap

Multiple salivary tumours show both epithelial and myoepithelial components (PA, AdCC, epithelial-myoepithelial carcinoma, polymorphous adenocarcinoma). The key to differential diagnosis lies in recognising the stromal character (chondromyxoid in PA; mucoid pseudocysts in AdCC; clear cell myoepithelium around ducts in EMC), growth pattern (polymorphous architecture in polymorphous adenocarcinoma), and molecular signature (PLAG1 for PA; MYB for AdCC; MAML2 for MEC). Never rely on a single IHC marker; use a panel-based approach.

WHO 5th Edition Classification: Major Salivary Gland Tumours (Selected)

Benign: Pleomorphic adenoma, Warthin tumour, Basal cell adenoma, Oncocytoma, Cystadenoma, Myoepithelioma, Sclerosing polycystic adenoma

Malignant: Mucoepidermoid carcinoma, Adenoid cystic carcinoma, Acinic cell carcinoma, Secretory carcinoma, Polymorphous adenocarcinoma, Salivary duct carcinoma, Epithelial-myoepithelial carcinoma, Myoepithelial carcinoma, Basal cell adenocarcinoma, Intraductal carcinoma, Carcinoma ex pleomorphic adenoma, Hyalinizing clear cell carcinoma

Tumour	Key Morphology	IHC	Molecular

Pleomorphic adenoma	Mixed epithelial + myoepithelial + stroma	CK+, SMA+, S100+, GFAP+	PLAG1 or HMGA2 fusions
Mucoepidermoid ca.	Mucous + squamoid + intermediate cells	p63+, PAS-D+ (mucin), S100−	MAML2 rearrangement
Adenoid cystic ca.	Cribriform/tubular/solid; biphasic	p40+ (myoepithelial), CD117+ (ductal)	MYB or MYBL1::NFIB fusion
Acinic cell ca.	Serous acinar cells, zymogen granules	DOG1+, SOX10+, PAS-D+	NR4A3 translocation
Secretory ca.	Tubular/papillary/cystic, eosinophilic secretions	S100+, mammaglobin+, PanTRK+	ETV6::NTRK3 fusion
Polymorphous adenoca.	Bland cells, polymorphous patterns, PNI	S100+ (strong), p63+, p40−	PRKD mutations/fusions
Salivary duct ca.	High-grade, comedo necrosis, apocrine	AR+, HER2 (30%), CK7+	TP53, PIK3CA, HRAS

A viva hook to consider: Why does adenoid cystic carcinoma have such a discrepancy between 5-year and 15-year survival? The answer lies in its relentless perineural invasion and indolent but persistent growth. Many patients achieve local control initially, but skip metastases along nerve sheaths and late haematogenous lung metastases (often 10 to 15 years after diagnosis) ultimately determine long-term outcome.

Quick Recall: Salivary Gland Tumours

DDx: Salivary Gland Tumours

Entity	Key Features
Pleomorphic adenoma	Biphasic (epithelial + myoepithelial); chondromyxoid

	stroma; PLAG1 rearrangement; most common salivary tumour
Warthin tumour	Bilayered oncocytic epithelium; lymphoid stroma with GCs; parotid; smokers; bilateral/multifocal
Mucoepidermoid carcinoma	Mucous, intermediate, epidermoid cells; MAML2 rearrangement; grading determines prognosis
Adenoid cystic carcinoma	Cribriform/ tubular/solid; mucoid pseudocysts; perineural invasion; MYB/MYBL1 fusion; late distant metastases
Acinic cell carcinoma	Serous acinar differentiation; PAS+ zymogen granules; DOG1+; NR4A3 rearrangement

IHC Panel: Salivary Gland Tumours

Marker	Interpretation
DOG1	Acinic cell carcinoma (highly sensitive and specific)
CD117 (KIT)	Adenoid cystic carcinoma (luminal cells); also positive in PDAC
p63/p40	Myoepithelial differentiation; basal cells in many salivary tumours
S100	Myoepithelial cells; also melanoma -- use panel
SOX10	Myoepithelial; secretory carcinoma; melanoma marker -- context critical

MYB	Adenoid cystic carcinoma (nuclear; IHC surrogate for MYB fusion)
MAML2 FISH	Mucoepidermoid carcinoma; positive predicts favourable outcome

Most common benign: Pleomorphic adenoma (PLAG1/HMGA2 fusions).
Most common malignant: Mucoepidermoid carcinoma (MAML2 rearrangement).
Perineural invasion hallmark: Adenoid cystic carcinoma (MYB::NFIB fusion).
NTRK fusion tumour: Secretory carcinoma (ETV6::NTRK3); PanTRK IHC positive.
Rule of the gland: Smaller gland = higher proportion of malignant tumours.
FNA pearl: PA shows metachromatic fibrillary stroma; Warthin yields 'motor oil' fluid.

OROPHARYNGEAL SQUAMOUS CELL CARCINOMA

Oropharyngeal squamous cell carcinoma (OPSCC) arises from the palatine and lingual tonsils, base of tongue, soft palate, and posterior pharyngeal wall. The WHO 5th Edition recognises two biologically and clinically distinct entities: HPV-associated OPSCC and HPV-independent OPSCC. This dichotomy has fundamentally changed staging, prognosis, and management, and is one of the most consequential recent shifts in head and neck pathology.

HPV-associated OPSCC: Driven predominantly by HPV 16 (greater than 90 percent), with HPV 18, 31, and 33 accounting for most of the remainder. The tumour arises in the reticulated crypt epithelium of the palatine or lingual tonsil, where the basement membrane is discontinuous and HPV readily infects basal cells. Classical risk factors (tobacco, alcohol) are less prominent; sexual transmission is the principal exposure route. Patients are typically younger (40–60 years), male, non-smokers or light smokers, and present with small (often occult) primary tumours accompanied by a large, often cystic cervical lymph node metastasis.

Morphology: Non-keratinising squamous cell carcinoma with sheets and nests of basaloid cells showing hyperchromatic nuclei, scant cytoplasm, indistinct cell borders, minimal keratinisation, and a "pushing" rather than infiltrative invasion pattern. Apoptotic bodies and comedo-type necrosis are frequent. Prominent lymphoid stroma is characteristic. Variants include basaloid, papillary, adenosquamous, and lymphoepithelial-like patterns. Nodal metastases are often cystic and may be misinterpreted as branchial cleft cysts in adults over 40 — a recurring diagnostic pitfall (compare with branchial cleft cyst in the neck masses section).

HPV testing: p16 immunohistochemistry is the accepted screening surrogate, with strong, diffuse nuclear AND cytoplasmic block staining in at least 70 percent of tumour cells (sensitivity greater than 95 percent; specificity approximately 85–90 percent for oropharyngeal primary tumours). Confirmation by HPV DNA ISH, HPV RNA ISH (detecting E6/E7 transcripts — the most specific method), or PCR is recommended in non-oropharyngeal sites, in equivocal p16 staining, and in rare non-oropharyngeal sites. Per the 2018 CAP guideline, p16 IHC alone is sufficient for diagnostic classification in oropharyngeal primary tumours.

HPV-independent OPSCC: Shows conventional keratinising morphology, typically in older patients with heavy tobacco/alcohol use. p53 mutations are common; p16 is negative (patchy or absent staining). Prognosis is substantially worse than HPV-associated disease, stage for stage.

AJCC 8th Edition staging: The 8th Edition introduced completely separate TNM staging systems for p16-positive and p16-negative OPSCC — a departure unprecedented in other head and neck sites. The p16-positive system uses a simplified framework (for example, up to four ipsilateral nodes all ≤ 6 cm qualify as cN1), reflecting the markedly better prognosis. Three-year overall survival is approximately 80–85 percent for HPV-associated OPSCC versus 50–60 percent for HPV-independent disease.

Therapeutic implications: The favourable biology of HPV-associated OPSCC has driven multiple de-escalation trials (RTOG 1016, De-ESCALaTE, PATHOS) testing reduced-intensity chemoradiotherapy or transoral robotic surgery with tailored adjuvant therapy. To date, no de-escalated regimen has proven non-inferior to standard therapy; concurrent cisplatin-based chemoradiotherapy remains the standard of care for locally advanced disease.

Key diagnostic finding: Non-keratinising basaloid SCC at a tonsillar or base-of-tongue site, with a cystic cervical nodal metastasis and p16 block positivity, is diagnostic of HPV-associated oropharyngeal squamous cell carcinoma.

Exam yield: ★★★ HIGH — Increasingly tested in international postgraduate examinations; the HPV-associated versus HPV-independent dichotomy, AJCC 8th Edition dual staging, and p16 IHC interpretation are examined most frequently.

NASOPHARYNGEAL CARCINOMA (NPC)

Definition: Malignant epithelial neoplasm of the nasopharynx with a strong EBV association and distinctive geographic distribution.

Etiology: EBV (virtually 100% of non-keratinising subtypes). Endemic in southern China, Southeast Asia. Risk factors: EBV, salted fish consumption, HLA haplotypes, genetic susceptibility.

Pathogenesis: EBV latent infection of nasopharyngeal epithelium → LMP1 activation of NF-κB → Immune evasion + proliferation → Malignant transformation

WHO classification: Keratinising SCC (associated with smoking/alcohol, non-endemic); non-keratinising SCC (differentiated and undifferentiated subtypes; EBV-driven; endemic). The undifferentiated subtype (formerly "lymphoepithelioma") is the most common.

Microscopy: Undifferentiated subtype: **syncytial sheets of large tumour cells with vesicular nuclei, prominent nucleoli, and indistinct cell borders**, infiltrated by abundant reactive lymphocytes (lymphoepithelioma pattern). May mimic lymphoma on biopsy.

IHC/Molecular: CK+ (AE1/AE3, CK5/6); p63+; EBER ISH positive (gold standard for EBV confirmation). Plasma EBV DNA for screening and treatment monitoring.

Treatment: Radiosensitive. Concurrent chemoradiotherapy is standard. PD-L1 checkpoint inhibitors emerging in recurrent/metastatic setting.

Exam yield: ★★★ HIGH — NPC WHO classification, EBV association, and EBER ISH are classic viva questions.

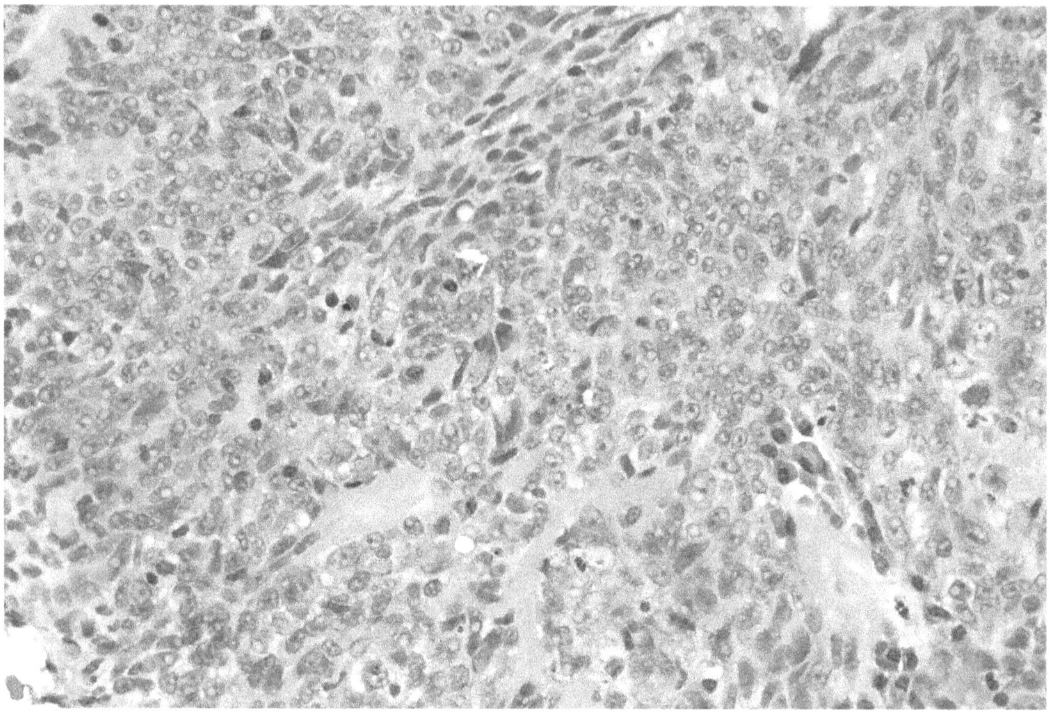

Figure 17.10A: Nasopharyngeal carcinoma, undifferentiated (WHO type III). Syncytial sheets of large tumour cells with vesicular nuclei and prominent nucleoli, admixed with abundant reactive lymphocytes (H&E, high mag). (Source: Nephron, Wikimedia Commons, CC BY-SA 4.0.)

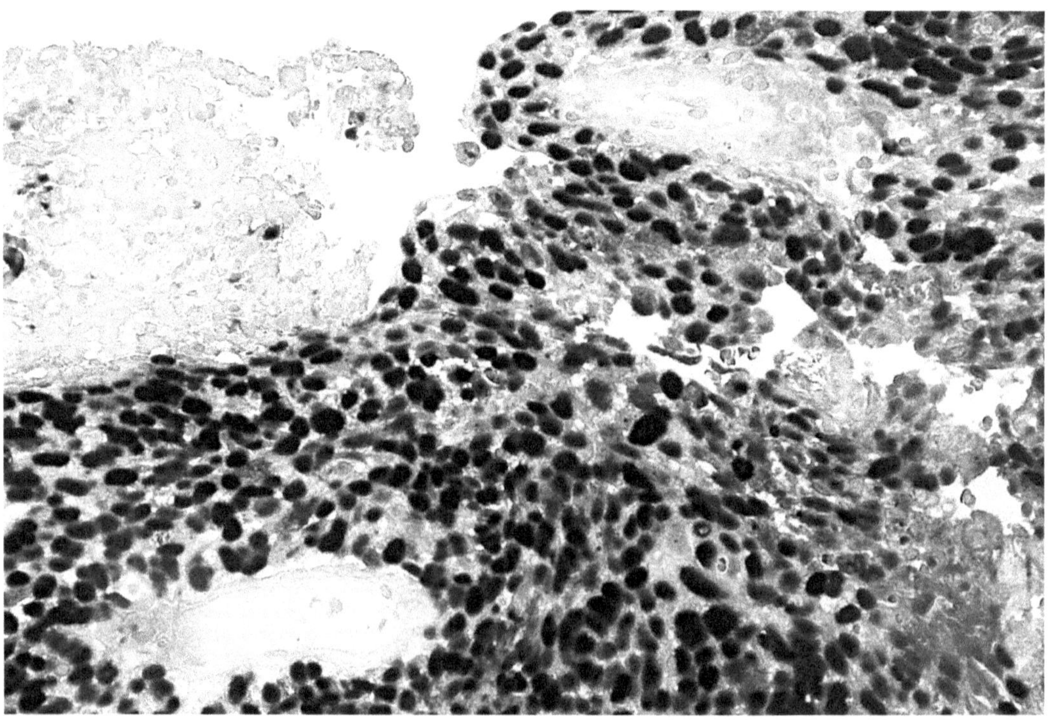

Figure 17.10B: Nasopharyngeal carcinoma (same case). EBER in-situ hybridisation shows strong diffuse nuclear

positivity in tumour cells, confirming EBV association. (Source: Nephron, Wikimedia Commons, CC BY-SA 4.0.)

Quick Recall: Nasopharyngeal Carcinoma

EBV association: Non-keratinising subtypes are virtually all EBER positive.

Diagnosis: EBER ISH on tissue biopsy; plasma EBV DNA for screening/monitoring.

Morphology: Syncytial tumour cells + dense lymphoplasmacytic infiltrate.

Treatment: Radiosensitive; concurrent chemoradiation is standard of care.

Sinonasal Pathology

The sinonasal tract gives rise to a wide spectrum of benign and malignant neoplasms, many of which have been recently reclassified in the WHO 5th Edition based on molecular findings.

Sinonasal Papillomas

SINONASAL (SCHNEIDERIAN) PAPILLOMAS

Definition: Benign epithelial neoplasms arising from the Schneiderian (respiratory) mucosa of the sinonasal tract. Three types with distinct molecular drivers.

Classification: Exophytic (septal; KRAS mutations) | Inverted (lateral wall; most common; EGFR mutations; 5–15% SCC transformation risk) | Oncocytic (KRAS mutations; eosinophilic columnar cells with intraepithelial microabscesses).

Microscopy (Inverted): Ribbon-like endophytic (inverted) growth of thickened Schneiderian epithelium into the underlying stroma

Key features: No stromal invasion (distinguishes from SCC). Transmission-type mucous glands within epithelium. Neutrophilic microabscesses in oncocytic type.

Management: Complete excision (endoscopic medial maxillectomy for inverted type). Recurrence if incompletely excised. Long-term surveillance for SCC transformation.

Exam yield: ★★ MODERATE — Inverted papilloma morphology, EGFR mutations, and SCC transformation risk are commonly asked.

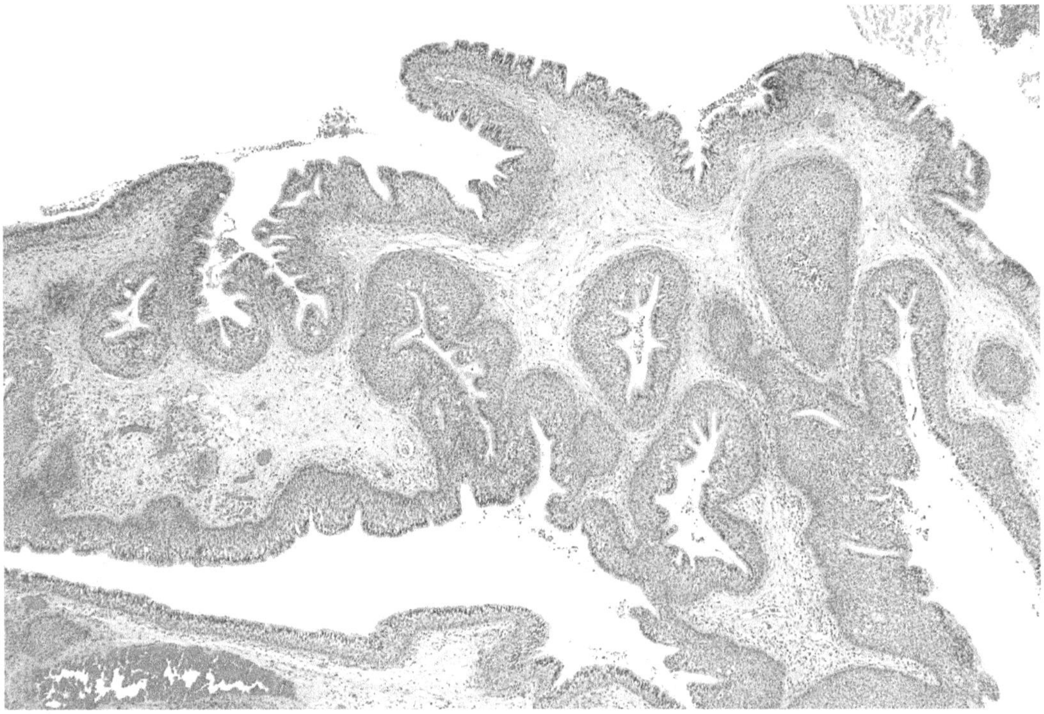

Figure 17.11: Inverted sinonasal papilloma: ribbon-like endophytic growth with intraepithelial neutrophils (H&E, ×40) (Source: Nephron, Wikimedia Commons, CC BY-SA 3.0.)

Sinonasal Malignancies

SCC is the most common sinonasal malignancy, associated with tobacco, occupational exposures, and in some cases HPV or inverted papilloma. Several newly defined entities with specific molecular signatures are now recognised:

Sinonasal undifferentiated carcinoma (SNUC) is a high-grade carcinoma without squamous, glandular, or neuroendocrine differentiation (a diagnosis of exclusion). IDH2 R172 mutations are frequently found. **NUT carcinoma** shows poorly differentiated cells with 'abrupt keratinisation' and is defined by NUTM1 rearrangements (NUT IHC positive). **SWI/SNF-deficient sinonasal carcinoma** is characterised by loss of INI-1 (SMARCB1) or BRG1 (SMARCA4) expression; aggressive behaviour. **HPV-related multiphenotypic sinonasal carcinoma** shows adenoid cystic-like morphology with myoepithelial differentiation but is driven by high-risk HPV (especially type 33) rather than MYB fusions.

Olfactory neuroblastoma (esthesioneuroblastoma) is a malignant neuroectodermal tumour arising from the olfactory mucosa of the cribriform plate. It shows lobulated nests of small round blue cells with fibrillary neuropil and Homer-Wright rosettes. Sustentacular cells at the periphery of nests are highlighted by S100 (sustentacular pattern). IHC: synaptophysin and chromogranin positive; cytokeratin negative or focal. Graded by the Hyams system (I to IV based on architecture, mitotic activity, nuclear pleomorphism, necrosis, and neuropil).

Marker	SCC	SNUC	NUT Ca.	NPC	Olfactory NB	Ewing

CK	+	+	+	+	−/focal	±
p40/p63	+	−	±	+	−	−
Synaptophysin	−	−	−	−	+	±
NUT	−	−	+	−	−	−
INI-1	Intact	Intact	Intact	Intact	Intact	Intact
EBER	−	−	−	+	−	−
CD99	−	−	−	−	−	+(memb.)
S100	−	−	−	−	+(sust.)	−

Table 17.1: IHC panel for sinonasal small round blue cell/undifferentiated tumour differential diagnosis.

Quick Recall: Sinonasal Lesions

Inverted papilloma: Lateral wall; endophytic growth; EGFR mutations; 5-15% SCC risk.

SNUC: Diagnosis of exclusion; IDH2 R172 mutations; aggressive.

NUT carcinoma: NUTM1 fusions; NUT IHC positive; poor prognosis.

Olfactory neuroblastoma: Cribriform plate; neuropil; S100 sustentacular pattern; Hyams grading.

SWI/SNF-deficient: Loss of INI-1 or BRG1; SMARCB1/SMARCA4 inactivation.

Laryngeal Pathology

The larynx is predominantly affected by squamous cell carcinoma, which accounts for over 95% of laryngeal malignancies. Risk factors include smoking, alcohol, and their synergistic effect. Laryngeal SCC may arise in the supraglottis, glottis (most common, earliest symptoms due to hoarseness), or subglottis. Glottic carcinomas have the best prognosis because of early detection and limited lymphatic drainage.

Laryngeal squamous papilloma (recurrent respiratory papillomatosis) is a benign HPV-driven (types 6 and 11) proliferation that presents as exophytic papillary masses, most commonly in children (juvenile-onset) or young adults (adult-onset). Histology shows papillary fronds with fibrovascular cores covered by bland, maturing squamous epithelium. Koilocytic change may be present. Malignant transformation is rare but can occur, particularly with HPV-11.

Integration: The squamous metaplasia-dysplasia-carcinoma sequence in the larynx parallels the oral cavity and cervical SCC pathways discussed in Chapter 25 (Female Genital Tract). HPV biology and carcinogenesis connect to Chapter 6 (Neoplasia Part 1) and Chapter 9 (Infectious Disease Pathology).

Odontogenic Cysts and Tumours

The jaw bones harbour a unique group of cysts and tumours derived from the epithelial, mesenchymal, and ectomesenchymal remnants of tooth development. Although most are benign, some are locally aggressive with high recurrence rates, and clinical-radiographic correlation is essential for accurate diagnosis.

Odontogenic Cysts

Radicular (periapical) cyst is the most common odontogenic cyst, arising from the proliferating epithelial rests of Malassez following pulp necrosis (usually from dental caries). It is found at the apex of a nonvital tooth, typically in the maxilla. Histology shows a fibrous wall with non-keratinising hyperplastic squamous epithelium ('arcading pattern'), chronic inflammation, cholesterol clefts with foreign-body giant cells, foamy macrophages, and sometimes Rushton hyaline bodies.

Dentigerous (follicular) cyst is the most common developmental odontogenic cyst, arising by fluid accumulation between the reduced enamel epithelium and the crown of an unerupted tooth. Most commonly affects impacted mandibular third molars. Lined by thin, non-keratinising squamous epithelium.

ODONTOGENIC KERATOCYST (OKC)

Definition: Developmental odontogenic cyst with aggressive local behaviour and high recurrence rate. Reclassified from keratocystic odontogenic tumour back to OKC in WHO 2022.

Microscopy: Thin, uniform parakeratinised stratified squamous lining (6–8 cell layers) with **corrugated (wavy) parakeratinised surface and palisaded columnar basal layer**

Key features: No rete ridges. Daughter cysts and satellite cysts in wall explain recurrence. Luminal desquamated keratin.

Molecular: PTCH1 mutations (Hedgehog pathway). Multiple OKCs = Gorlin syndrome (nevoid basal cell carcinoma syndrome).

Key DDx: OKC vs orthokeratinised odontogenic cyst: OKC has parakeratinised surface + palisaded basal layer + PTCH1 mutations; orthokeratinised variant is non-aggressive, no Gorlin association.

Exam yield: ★★★ HIGH — OKC lining features, PTCH1/Gorlin association, and recurrence are very frequently tested.

Odontogenic Tumours

Ameloblastoma is the most common odontogenic tumour (excluding odontomas). It typically arises in the posterior mandible and presents as a multilocular radiolucency. The classic (conventional) type is a solid or multicystic intraosseous tumour showing follicular islands of epithelium with peripheral columnar cells showing nuclear palisading and reverse polarity ('piano key' arrangement), surrounding loosely arranged stellate reticulum-like cells that may undergo cystic degeneration. Other patterns include plexiform, desmoplastic, granular, acanthomatous, and basaloid. Molecular: BRAF V600E is the most common mutation, with MAPK pathway activation. Treatment is wide local excision due to high recurrence with simple curettage. IHC: SOX10 negative (distinguishes from basaloid salivary gland tumours).

The unicystic variant presents as a single cystic cavity, often in younger patients, associated with an impacted tooth. It has a better prognosis and may be treated more conservatively. Odontomas (compound and complex) are the most common odontogenic tumours overall; they are hamartomatous malformations containing dental hard tissues and are treated by simple excision.

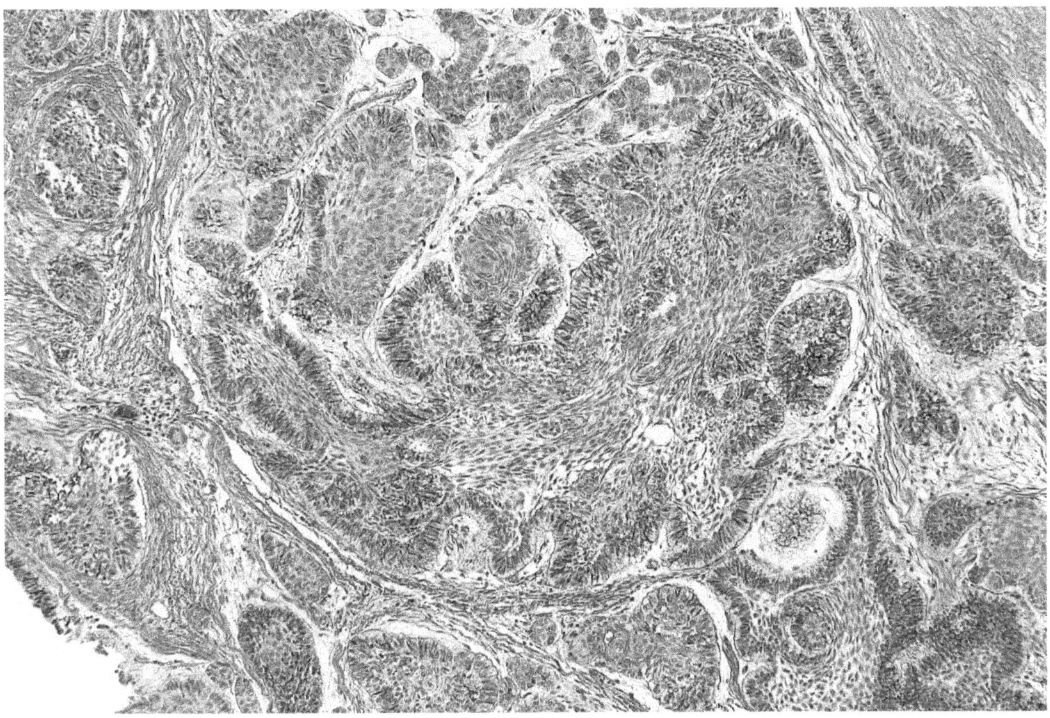

Figure 17.12: Ameloblastoma (follicular pattern). Islands of odontogenic epithelium in fibrous stroma with peripheral columnar ameloblast-like cells showing reverse nuclear polarity, surrounding central stellate reticulum-like cells (H&E, intermediate mag). (Source: Nephron, Wikimedia Commons, CC BY-SA 3.0.)

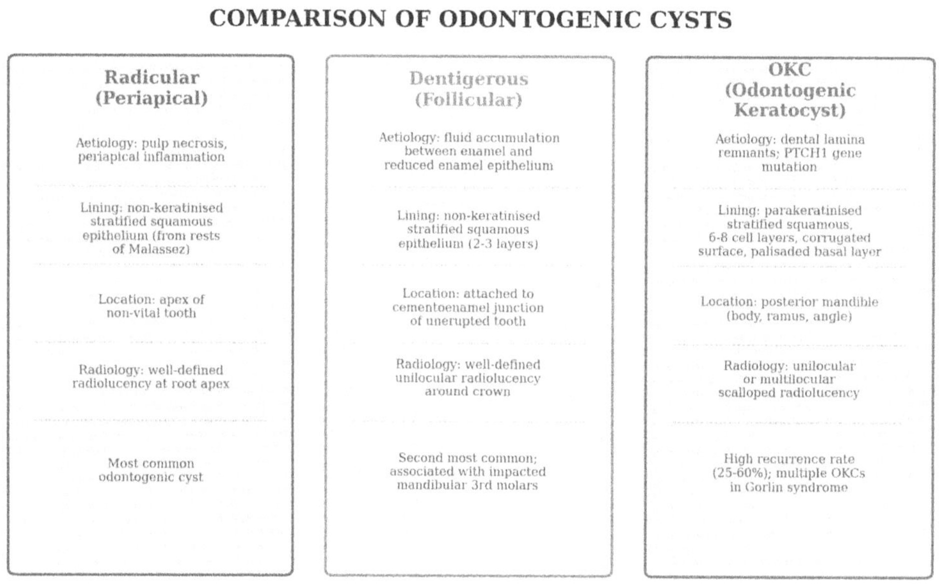

Figure 17.13: Comparison of odontogenic cysts: radicular cyst (at apex of non-vital tooth), dentigerous cyst (enveloping unerupted crown), and odontogenic keratocyst (parakeratinised lining with basal palisading). (Source: Author's original.)

The Pathologist's Eye: Odontogenic Cyst Lining

When examining a jaw cyst, the lining epithelium is the single most important diagnostic clue. A thin, regular parakeratinised lining with palisading basal cells and a corrugated surface is virtually pathognomonic of OKC. Do not confuse it with the orthokeratinised odontogenic cyst (which has a granular layer and flat basal cells, lacks the corrugated surface, and has a much lower recurrence rate). Inflamed OKCs lose their characteristic lining and may be misdiagnosed as radicular cysts, so always examine the least inflamed areas.

Quick Recall: Odontogenic Cysts and Tumours

Most common jaw cyst: Radicular (periapical) cyst; nonvital tooth apex.

Most common developmental cyst: Dentigerous cyst; unerupted tooth crown.

OKC: Parakeratinised, corrugated, basal palisading; PTCH1 mutations; 25% recurrence.

Gorlin syndrome: Multiple OKCs + basal cell carcinomas; germline PTCH1 mutation.

Most common odontogenic tumour: Odontoma (hamartoma); ameloblastoma if excluding odontomas.

Ameloblastoma: Posterior mandible; BRAF V600E; wide excision required.

Developmental Cysts of the Neck

Thyroglossal duct cyst is the most common congenital neck mass, arising from persistence of the thyroglossal duct along the midline path of thyroid descent. It presents as a painless midline mass, often attached to the hyoid bone. Histology shows a cyst lined by respiratory or squamous epithelium with thyroid follicular tissue in the wall. Treatment is the Sistrunk procedure (excision of the cyst, the central portion of the hyoid bone, and the tract to the foramen caecum).

Branchial cleft cyst arises from remnants of the branchial apparatus, presenting as a lateral neck mass, usually anterior to the sternocleidomastoid muscle. Lined by squamous epithelium with abundant lymphoid tissue (often with germinal centres) in the wall. *In any patient older than 40 years with a lateral cystic neck mass, the most important differential is cystic metastatic squamous cell carcinoma (from an oropharyngeal primary), not a branchial cleft cyst.* A thorough clinical and radiological workup is mandatory before labelling any lateral cystic neck mass as 'branchial cleft cyst' in older adults.

Special Tumours of the Head and Neck

Nasopharyngeal (juvenile) angiofibroma is a locally aggressive, richly vascular fibrovascular neoplasm that occurs almost exclusively in adolescent boys. Patients typically present with unilateral nasal obstruction and recurrent epistaxis. Histologically, it shows irregular, variably sized blood vessels (many thin-walled and dilated, some with smooth muscle) set within a variably cellular fibrous stroma. The vessels lack a complete muscular wall, which explains the torrential bleeding that can complicate biopsy. IHC: nuclear beta-catenin positive, androgen receptor (AR) positive. Treatment involves preoperative embolisation followed by surgical excision. Despite benign histology, it can be locally destructive with extension into the infratemporal fossa and orbit.

Paraganglioma of the head and neck arises from the paraganglia associated with cranial nerves and vessels. The carotid body tumour (at the carotid bifurcation) is the most common; others include the jugulotympanic (glomus jugulare, middle ear), vagal, and laryngeal paragangliomas. Histologically, these tumours show the classic 'Zellballen' pattern: nests of chief cells (positive for synaptophysin and chromogranin) surrounded by sustentacular cells (S100 positive). Most are benign and sporadic, but approximately 10 to 40% are familial (SDH gene mutations, particularly SDHB, SDHC, SDHD). *Paragangliomas of the carotid body are reported more frequently in populations residing at high altitude, where chronic hypoxia drives paraganglia hyperplasia.* Malignancy in paraganglioma is defined by metastasis, not by histological features.

FNAC of Salivary Gland Tumours: Diagnostic Approach and Pitfalls

Fine needle aspiration cytology (FNAC) plays a central role in the preoperative assessment of salivary gland masses. The Milan System for Reporting Salivary Gland Cytopathology (MSRSGC) provides a standardised, risk-stratified reporting framework analogous to the Bethesda system for thyroid cytology.

Milan Category	Description	Risk of Malignancy

I	Non-diagnostic	25%
II	Non-neoplastic	10%
III	Atypia of undetermined significance	20%
IVA	Benign neoplasm	<5%
IVB	Salivary gland neoplasm of uncertain malignant potential	35%
V	Suspicious for malignancy	60%
VI	Malignant	90%

Table 17.2: Milan System for Reporting Salivary Gland Cytopathology.

Key cytological features for common tumours include the following. Pleomorphic adenoma shows metachromatic, fibrillary stroma ('troll hair' on Diff-Quik), epithelial cells in cohesive clusters, and scattered myoepithelial cells; the stroma is the diagnostic hallmark. Warthin tumour yields abundant thin, dark ('motor oil') cyst fluid with oncocytes in flat sheets and a polymorphous lymphoid background. Mucoepidermoid carcinoma shows mucin-secreting cells (confirmed with mucicarmine or PAS-D), intermediate cells, and sometimes squamoid cells; low-grade tumours may be mistakenly classified as mucoceles. Adenoid cystic carcinoma classically shows hyaline globules of basement membrane material with small basaloid cells and myoepithelial cells ('stromal exclusion' pattern on Diff-Quik); the distinction from basal cell adenoma on FNA can be difficult.

The Pathologist's Eye: FNAC Pitfalls in Salivary Gland Tumours

1. Pleomorphic adenoma with minimal stroma (cellular PA) can mimic basaloid malignancies. Look carefully for even small amounts of metachromatic stroma on Diff-Quik.
2. Low-grade mucoepidermoid carcinoma can be cystic and bland, resembling a mucocele or salivary duct cyst. Always stain for mucin (PAS-D or mucicarmine) if cyst fluid contains epithelial cells.
3. Warthin tumour with extensive squamous metaplasia (due to prior FNA or infarction) can mimic SCC metastasis. Clinical correlation (parotid mass, smoking history, bilateral presentation) is essential.
4. Adenoid cystic carcinoma vs basal cell adenoma: both are basaloid. AdCC shows infiltrative margins with perineural invasion on excision, but on FNA the hyaline globules and 'stromal exclusion' pattern favour AdCC.
5. Acinic cell carcinoma may be mistaken for normal serous acinar tissue on FNA. Key: look for architectural abnormality (solid sheets, vacuolated cytoplasm variants) and clinical mass.

Quick Recall: FNAC of Salivary Gland Tumours

Milan System: 6-tier system (I-VI); Category IVA = benign neoplasm (<5% ROM); Category VI = malignant (90% ROM).

PA on FNA: Metachromatic fibrillary stroma = diagnostic hallmark.
MEC pitfall: Low-grade cystic MEC mimics mucocele; stain for mucin.
AdCC on FNA: Hyaline globules + basaloid cells + stromal exclusion pattern.
Warthin on FNA: Motor oil fluid + oncocytes + lymphocytes.

Recent Advances

CAP 2018 guideline — high-risk HPV testing in head and neck carcinomas. The 2018 College of American Pathologists guideline established evidence-based recommendations for high-risk human papillomavirus testing in head and neck carcinomas, with binding implications for the surgical-pathology report (Lewis et al. Archives of Pathology and Laboratory Medicine 2018; 142: 559–597; PMID 29251996). The systematic review supporting the guideline addressed six key questions and produced two principal recommendations. First, every newly diagnosed oropharyngeal squamous cell carcinoma should undergo high-risk HPV testing, performed either on the primary tumour or on a cervical nodal metastasis, using p16 immunohistochemistry interpreted with a 70% nuclear and cytoplasmic staining cut-off as the surrogate marker. Second, routine HPV testing of non-squamous oropharyngeal carcinomas and of non-oropharyngeal head-and-neck carcinomas was not recommended, because of the lower prevalence of true HPV-driven disease and the substantial risk of false-positive p16 staining outside the oropharynx. The guideline also addressed cytological samples (HPV testing on fine-needle-aspiration cell blocks is acceptable), the handling of locoregional and distant recurrence specimens, and reporting language (tumours are reported as "HPV positive" or "p16 positive" rather than as a generic "HPV-related"). For the pathologist the protocol harmonises HPV reporting across institutions and supports the AJCC 8 separate staging algorithm for p16-positive oropharyngeal cancer covered earlier in this chapter.

Molecular reclassification of salivary gland tumours. The WHO 5th Edition has incorporated molecular diagnostics into the classification framework. Several tumours are now defined by recurrent gene fusions: secretory carcinoma (ETV6::NTRK3), hyalinizing clear cell carcinoma (EWSR1::ATF1), and intraductal carcinoma subtypes (NCOA4::RET, TRIM33::RET). PLAG1 immunohistochemistry is emerging as a practical surrogate for PLAG1 FISH in confirming pleomorphic adenoma. The recognition of NTRK-fused tumours has direct therapeutic implications, as TRK inhibitors (larotrectinib, entrectinib) show high response rates in secretory carcinoma.

Sinonasal tumour redefinition. Multiple new entities have been formally codified in the WHO 5th Edition based on molecular signatures: SWI/SNF-deficient sinonasal carcinoma (SMARCB1/SMARCA4 loss), NUT carcinoma (NUTM1 fusions), HPV-related multiphenotypic sinonasal carcinoma (high-risk HPV with myoepithelial differentiation), and biphenotypic sinonasal sarcoma (PAX3::MAML3 fusion). These molecular definitions have improved diagnostic reproducibility and opened avenues for targeted therapies.

Liquid biopsy in head and neck SCC. Circulating tumour DNA (ctDNA) and plasma EBV DNA are being investigated as non-invasive biomarkers. Plasma EBV DNA is already established for NPC screening, treatment monitoring, and recurrence detection in endemic regions. For OSCC, ctDNA-based detection of

TP53 mutations post-surgery can identify minimal residual disease and predict relapse before clinical or radiological evidence, though this remains largely investigational.

Approach to the Histopathology Slide

When presented with a head and neck histopathology slide, adopt a systematic approach:

Step 1: Identify the tissue and site. Recognise the epithelial lining (squamous, respiratory, salivary), the presence of salivary gland tissue, bone (odontogenic lesion), or lymphoid tissue (neck mass). Minor salivary glands in the palate, floor of mouth, or lip are a frequent source of biopsy specimens.

Step 2: Determine the nature of the lesion. Is it inflammatory (chronic sialadenitis, mucous retention cyst), cystic (odontogenic cyst, developmental neck cyst), or neoplastic? For neoplasms, identify whether it is epithelial, mesenchymal, neuroendocrine, or lymphoid.

Step 3: For salivary gland tumours, assess three features: (a) is there a dual population (epithelial and myoepithelial)? (b) What is the stromal character (myxochondroid in PA, none in MEC, mucoid pseudocysts in AdCC)? (c) Is it encapsulated (PA, BCA) or infiltrative (AdCC, polymorphous adenocarcinoma)?

Step 4: For squamous lesions, assess the degree of dysplasia (mild/moderate/severe or low/high grade) and look for invasion. In invasive SCC, assess the pattern of invasion, perineural invasion, and keratinisation pattern (keratinising, non-keratinising, verrucous).

Step 5: For jaw lesions, examine the cyst lining carefully. Parakeratinised with basal palisading = OKC. Ameloblastomatous epithelium with reverse polarity = ameloblastoma or calcifying odontogenic cyst.

Step 6: Apply IHC judiciously. For undifferentiated sinonasal tumours, the panel must include CK (epithelial), p40 (squamous), synaptophysin/chromogranin (neuroendocrine), NUT, INI-1, EBER, S100, CD99, and CD45. For salivary tumours, myoepithelial markers (p63, SMA, S100) and specific markers (DOG1 for acinic cell, PanTRK for secretory carcinoma) guide diagnosis.

International Frameworks

AJCC 8th edition Head and Neck staging (2017). The 8th edition introduced a separate staging algorithm for high-risk HPV-associated (p16-positive) oropharyngeal squamous cell carcinoma, distinguishing it from HPV-negative oropharyngeal cancer because of its substantially better prognosis at equivalent anatomical extent. Other major modifications include the addition of extranodal extension to the N category for all non-viral and non-mucosal-melanoma sites, incorporation of depth of invasion (DOI) into oral cavity T staging (T1 ≤5 mm, T2 >5 to ≤10 mm, T3 >10 mm or >4 cm), the relocation of cutaneous head-and-neck malignancies to a dedicated chapter, and division of pharyngeal staging into nasopharynx, oropharynx, and hypopharynx chapters. Reporting implication: histopathology reports for oropharyngeal SCC must include p16 immunohistochemistry status (block staining ≥70% accepted as surrogate for high-risk HPV), and oral cavity reports must include DOI measured from the basement membrane of adjacent normal mucosa to the deepest point of invasion. Citation: Lydiatt WM, et al. CA Cancer J Clin 2017;67(2):122–137. PMID 28128848.

Ultra High-Yield Chapter Summary

Topic	Must Remember
OSMF	Areca nut; submucosal fibrosis; 7-13% malignant transformation; highest prevalence in South Asia
Oral SCC	Buccal mucosa and tongue most common in South Asia; WPOI-5 = worst prognosis; verrucous ca. has pushing borders
Pleomorphic adenoma	Most common salivary tumour; mixed (ductal + myoepithelial + stroma); PLAG1/HMGA2 fusions
Mucoepidermoid ca.	Most common salivary malignancy; mucous + squamoid + intermediate cells; MAML2 rearrangement
Adenoid cystic ca.	Cribriform/tubular/solid; perineural invasion hallmark; MYB::NFIB fusion; poor long-term survival
Secretory carcinoma	ETV6::NTRK3 fusion; PanTRK+; S100+, mammaglobin+; TRK inhibitor responsive
Warthin tumour	Parotid; bilayered oncocytic epithelium + lymphoid stroma; smoking association
Nasopharyngeal ca.	EBV-driven (EBER+); non-keratinising undifferentiated most common;

	radiosensitive
Inverted papilloma	Endophytic; lateral nasal wall; EGFR mutations; 5-15% SCC risk
Olfactory neuroblastoma	Cribriform plate; neuropil; S100 sustentacular pattern; Hyams grading
SNUC	Dx of exclusion; IDH2 R172 mutation; aggressive
NUT carcinoma	NUTM1 fusion; NUT IHC+; abrupt keratinisation; very poor prognosis
Radicular cyst	Most common jaw cyst; nonvital tooth apex; arcading squamous epithelium + cholesterol clefts
OKC	Parakeratinised, corrugated surface, basal palisading; PTCH1 mutations; Gorlin syndrome if multiple
Ameloblastoma	Most common odontogenic tumour (excl. odontomas); posterior mandible; BRAF V600E; wide excision
Thyroglossal duct cyst	Midline neck; attached to hyoid; thyroid tissue in wall; Sistrunk procedure
Branchial cleft cyst	Lateral neck; squamous lining + lymphoid tissue; exclude cystic SCC metastasis in older adults
Salivary gland IHC	Myoepithelial markers (p63, SMA, S100); DOG1 for acinic cell; PanTRK for secretory ca.

Diagnostic thinking: biphasic epithelial-myoepithelial pattern + chondromyxoid stroma → pleomorphic adenoma

Diagnostic thinking: cribriform/tubular pattern + perineural invasion + MYB-NFIB fusion → adenoid cystic carcinoma

Diagnostic thinking: Orphan Annie eye nuclei + psammoma bodies + papillary architecture → papillary thyroid carcinoma (Figure 17.14A)

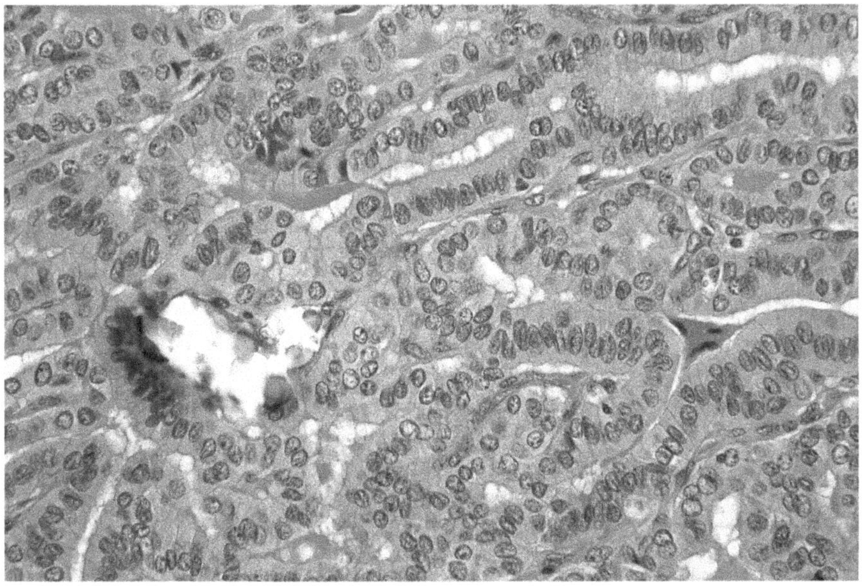

Figure 17.14A: Papillary thyroid carcinoma (Tall cell variant): Nuclear grooves and irregular nuclear membranes (H&E, high mag). (Source: Nephron, Wikimedia Commons, CC BY-SA 3.0.)

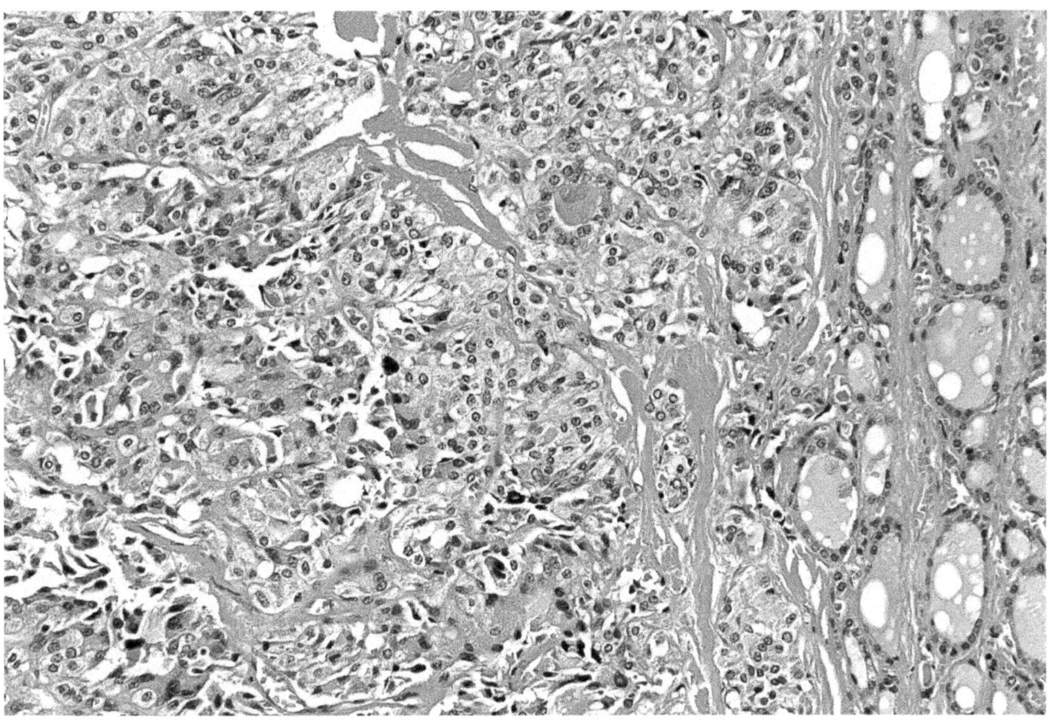

Figure 17.14B: Medullary thyroid carcinoma. Nests and trabeculae of tumour cells with amphophilic granular cytoplasm and salt-and-pepper chromatin, set in an amyloid stroma. H&E, intermediate magnification. (Source: Nephron, Wikimedia Commons, CC BY-SA 3.0.)

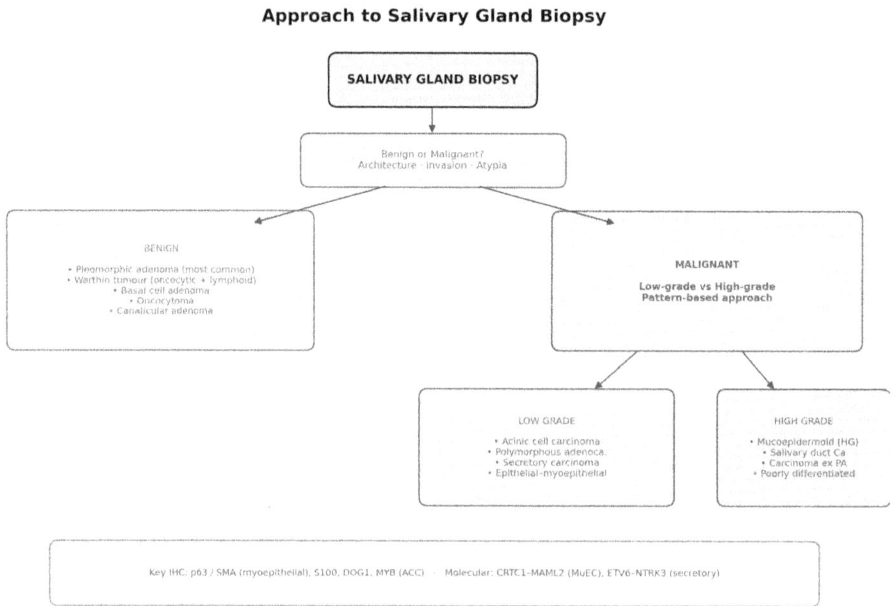

Figure 17.15: Approach to Salivary Gland Biopsy. (Source: Author's original.)

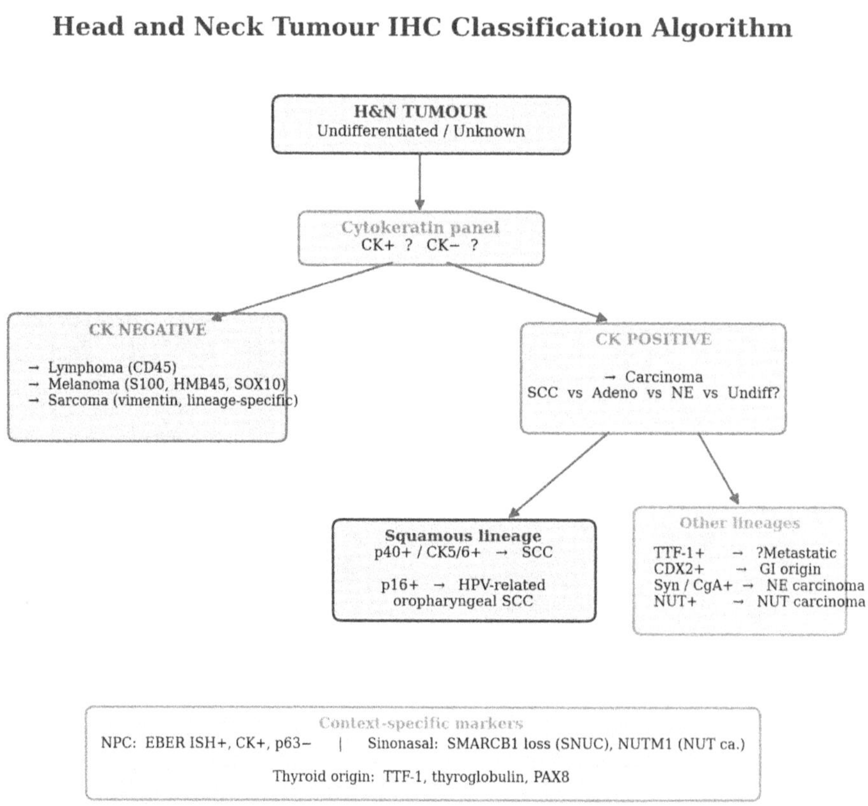

Figure 17.16: Head and Neck Tumour IHC Classification Algorithm. (Source: Author's original.)

Chapter 18: Gastrointestinal Pathology Part 1: Upper GI

THE BIG PICTURE

The upper gastrointestinal tract, comprising the oesophagus, stomach, and duodenum, is a common source of endoscopic biopsies in clinical practice. The pathologist's role in interpreting these biopsies extends well beyond simple diagnosis: accurate grading of Barrett oesophagus dysplasia determines surveillance intervals and treatment, classification of gastritis guides H. pylori eradication, recognition of autoimmune gastritis prevents missed pernicious anaemia and neuroendocrine tumour risk, and molecular subtyping of gastric carcinoma directs targeted therapy (HER2, MSI, EBV). In South Asia and the wider Asian oesophageal cancer belt, squamous cell carcinoma remains the predominant oesophageal malignancy, while gastric carcinoma presents at a younger age and more advanced stage than in Western populations.

High-yield topics in this chapter: Barrett oesophagus (definition, pathogenesis, dysplasia grading, p53 IHC); H. pylori-associated gastric disease; chronic gastritis classification (autoimmune vs environmental); gastric carcinoma (morphological subtypes, molecular classification, HER2 testing); gastrointestinal stromal tumour (KIT/PDGFRA, risk stratification); celiac disease (Marsh grading); gastric neuroendocrine tumours (types I-III).

No organ system generates more biopsy specimens in a pathologist's daily practice than the gastrointestinal tract. The oesophageal and gastric mucosa, constantly exposed to acid, bile, dietary carcinogens, and infectious agents, display a rich repertoire of metaplastic, inflammatory, and neoplastic responses that the diagnostic pathologist must navigate with precision. This chapter covers the upper GI tract: from the squamocolumnar junction of the oesophagus to the duodenum, encompassing the diseases most frequently examined in university and board examinations.

WHO Classification: Upper GI Tumours (5th Ed, 2019) -- Selected

Oesophageal: Squamous cell carcinoma (keratinising, non-keratinising, basaloid); adenocarcinoma (arising in Barrett); NEC; mixed NE-non-NE.

Gastric epithelial: Tubular, papillary, poorly cohesive (including signet ring cell), mucinous, mixed; gastric carcinoma with lymphoid stroma; hepatoid carcinoma.

Gastric mesenchymal: GIST (KIT/PDGFRA); leiomyoma; schwannoma; glomus tumour.

Gastric NE: Type I (autoimmune gastritis-associated, G1); Type II (Zollinger-Ellison/MEN1); Type III (sporadic, aggressive).

Oesophageal Pathology (Figure 18.1)

Oesophagitis

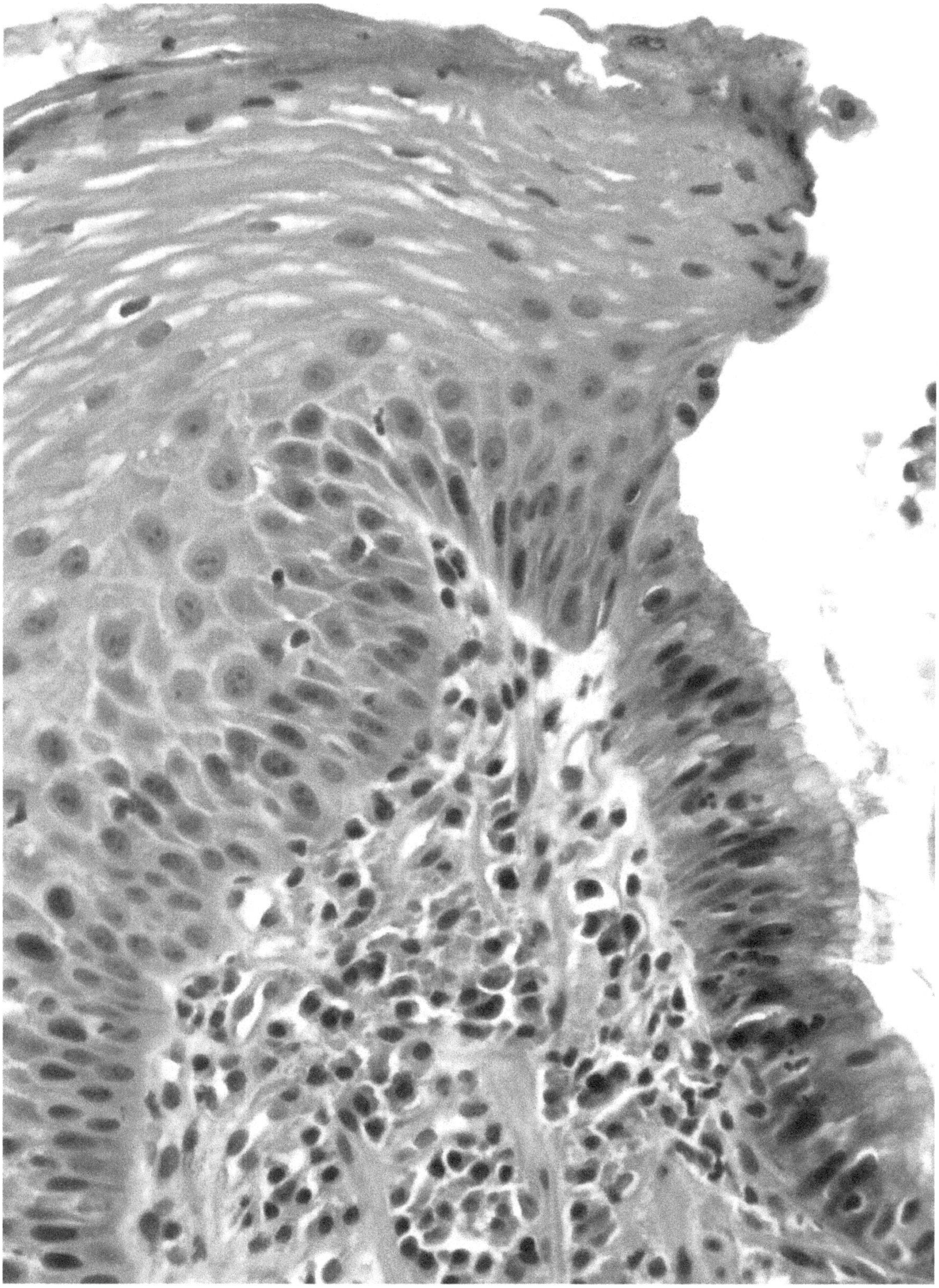

Figure 18.1: Reflux oesophagitis: basal cell hyperplasia, papillary elongation, and scattered eosinophils (H&E, ×200) (Source: Mikael Häggström, Wikimedia Commons, CC0.)

Gastro-oesophageal reflux disease (GERD) is the most common oesophageal disorder globally. Histologically, reflux oesophagitis shows basal cell hyperplasia (exceeding 15% of epithelial thickness), elongation of vascular papillae (reaching the upper third of the epithelium), scattered intraepithelial eosinophils (usually fewer than 15 per high-power field), intercellular oedema (spongiosis), and dilated intercellular spaces. These changes are most prominent in the distal oesophagus near the gastro-oesophageal junction (GEJ).

Eosinophilic oesophagitis (EoE) is a clinico-pathological diagnosis characterised by oesophageal dysfunction (dysphagia, food impaction in adults; feeding difficulty in children) and a dense eosinophilic infiltrate (typically more than 15 eosinophils per HPF, often more than 20/HPF) with eosinophilic microabscesses and degranulation. Unlike GERD, the eosinophilic infiltrate is often diffuse or worse proximally. EoE is associated with the 'atopic triad' (allergies, asthma, eczema). Endoscopically, the oesophagus shows rings, furrows, and 'trachealization.'

Infectious oesophagitis occurs primarily in immunocompromised patients. **Candida** causes pseudomembranous plaques with hyphae and pseudohyphae (highlighted by PAS-D and GMS stains). **HSV** produces multinucleated squamous epithelial cells with ground-glass nuclei, nuclear moulding, and margination of chromatin ('3 Ms': moulding, multinucleation, margination); the viral cytopathic changes are found at the ulcer edge in squamous cells. **CMV** produces large, deeply basophilic intranuclear inclusions ('owl's eye') and smaller cytoplasmic inclusions in endothelial and stromal cells (mesenchymal, not epithelial) at the ulcer base. *The key diagnostic clue distinguishing HSV from CMV oesophagitis is the cell type affected: HSV infects squamous epithelial cells (ulcer edge), while CMV infects mesenchymal and endothelial cells (ulcer base).*

BARRETT OESOPHAGUS

Definition: Replacement of normal squamous epithelium of the distal oesophagus by columnar epithelium with goblet cells (intestinal metaplasia), extending ≥1 cm above gastric folds (ACG/AGA criteria).

Etiology: Complication of chronic GERD. Risk factors: obesity, male sex, smoking, Caucasian ethnicity.

Pathogenesis: Chronic acid reflux → Squamous mucosal injury → Intestinal metaplasia (goblet cells) → Low-grade dysplasia → High-grade dysplasia → Oesophageal adenocarcinoma

Microscopy: Non-dysplastic Barrett shows 'the four lines' of preserved cell polarity: apical mucin cap, base of mucin cap, cytoplasm, basal row of nuclei. **Goblet cells (intestinal metaplasia) replacing squamous epithelium**

Risk: Annual progression to adenocarcinoma ~0.5% per year in non-dysplastic Barrett (Figure 18.2).

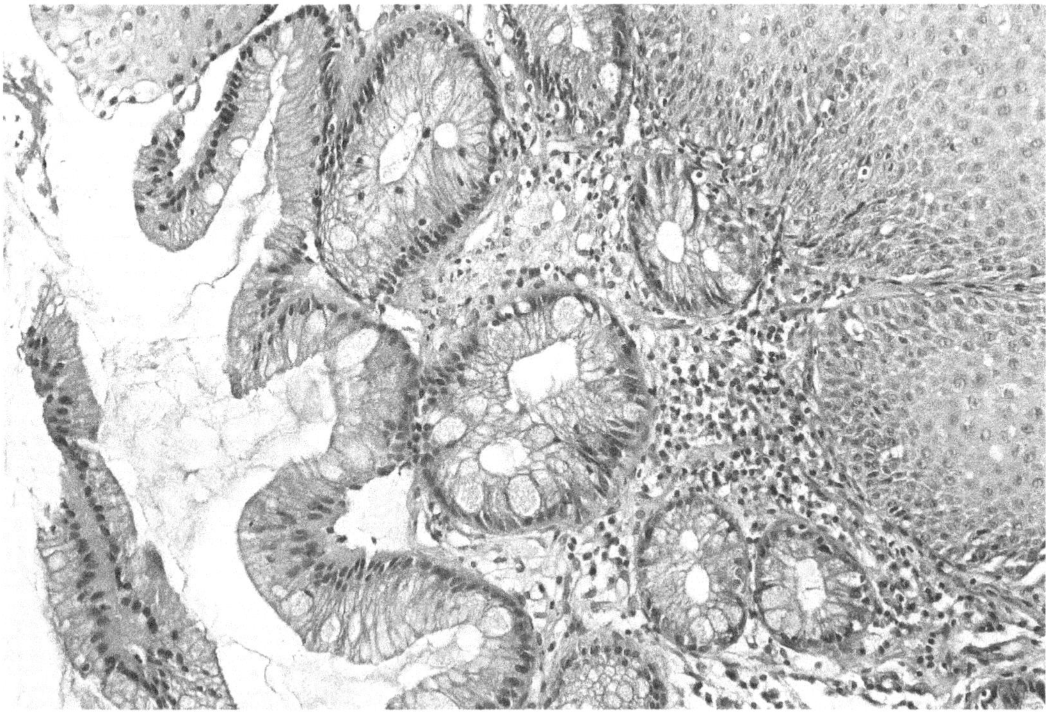

Figure 18.2: Barrett oesophagus (H&E). Intestinal metaplasia with mucin-secreting goblet cells (right) replacing normal stratified squamous epithelium (left) at the gastro-oesophageal junction. (Source: CoRus13, Wikimedia Commons, CC BY-SA 4.0.)

Chronic GERD → Columnar metaplasia → Intestinal metaplasia (goblet cells) → Low-grade dysplasia → TP53 mutation → High-grade dysplasia → Chromosomal instability → Adenocarcinoma

Histologically, two types of intestinal metaplasia are recognised. Complete (type I) intestinal metaplasia shows absorptive cells (with a brush border) interspersed with goblet cells, closely resembling small intestinal mucosa. Incomplete (type II) intestinal metaplasia shows goblet cells interspersed with foveolar-type (gastric) cells rather than absorptive cells; this pattern, more common at the GEJ, carries a higher dysplasia risk.

Dysplasia grading in Barrett oesophagus is one of the most consequential diagnoses in GI pathology. Barrett without dysplasia shows 'the four lines' of preserved cell polarity: apical mucin cap, base of mucin cap, cytoplasm, and basal row of nuclei. **Low-grade dysplasia (LGD)** shows adenoma-like changes: pencillate, hyperchromatic, pseudostratified nuclei that extend to the surface epithelium but retain basal orientation, with loss of the four-line pattern but nuclei remaining in the lower half of the cell. **High-grade dysplasia (HGD)** shows marked nuclear hyperchromasia and pleomorphism, loss of nuclear polarity (nuclei reaching the cell apex), rounded irregular nuclei, no surface maturation, and complex architecture (cribriform, back-to-back glands). The distinction between HGD and intramucosal carcinoma rests on the presence of single cells or irregular glands invading the lamina propria.

p53 immunohistochemistry has emerged as a critical adjunct to H&E morphology in Barrett dysplasia assessment. An aberrant p53 staining pattern (strong, diffuse overexpression in every nucleus, or complete absence ['null' pattern]) indicates TP53 mutation and supports a diagnosis of dysplasia. Wild-type (patchy, variable intensity) staining favours a reactive/non-dysplastic interpretation. The 2019 BSG guidelines recommend p53 IHC on all Barrett biopsies where dysplasia is considered.

Exam Pitfall: Barrett Dysplasia Grading

Inflammation can mimic dysplasia in Barrett oesophagus. In the setting of active inflammation (oesophagitis), the category 'indefinite for dysplasia' should be used, the patient treated with proton pump inhibitor therapy, and biopsies repeated in 3 to 6 months when inflammation has resolved. Never diagnose LGD or HGD in the presence of significant acute inflammation, as reactive atypia can closely mimic dysplastic changes. p53 IHC can help in equivocal cases.

Quick Recall: Barrett Oesophagus

Essential/Desirable: Diagnostic Criteria -- Barrett Oesophagus

Essential: Columnar mucosa extending >=1 cm above gastric folds (endoscopic) with goblet cells (intestinal metaplasia) on biopsy.

Desirable: AB/PAS+ goblet cells confirming intestinal-type mucin; p53 IHC (aberrant pattern supports dysplasia); CDX2+ columnar epithelium.

Definition: Columnar epithelium with goblet cells (intestinal metaplasia) ≥1 cm above gastric folds.

Malignant progression: Metaplasia → LGD → HGD → Adenocarcinoma; ~0.5%/year without dysplasia.

The four lines: Mucin cap → base of cap → cytoplasm → basal nuclei = preserved polarity = no dysplasia.

p53 IHC: Aberrant (overexpression or null pattern) = TP53 mutation = supports dysplasia.

Management: No dysplasia: 3-5 yr surveillance; LGD: mucosal ablation; HGD: ablation or EMR.

Oesophageal Neoplasms

Two major types of oesophageal carcinoma account for over 95% of cases. **Squamous cell carcinoma (SCC)** is the predominant type in the 'Asian oesophageal cancer belt,' linked to tobacco (smoked and chewed), alcohol, very hot beverages, and dietary factors (nitrosamines). It arises in the middle third of the oesophagus (most common site) through a squamous dysplasia-carcinoma sequence. Histologically, it shows keratinisation, intercellular bridges, and nuclear pleomorphism. Subtypes include verrucous (well-differentiated, pushing borders, minimal atypia) and spindle cell (sarcomatoid) carcinoma. Molecular: TP53 mutations are nearly universal; CDKN2A loss and CCND1 amplification are common.

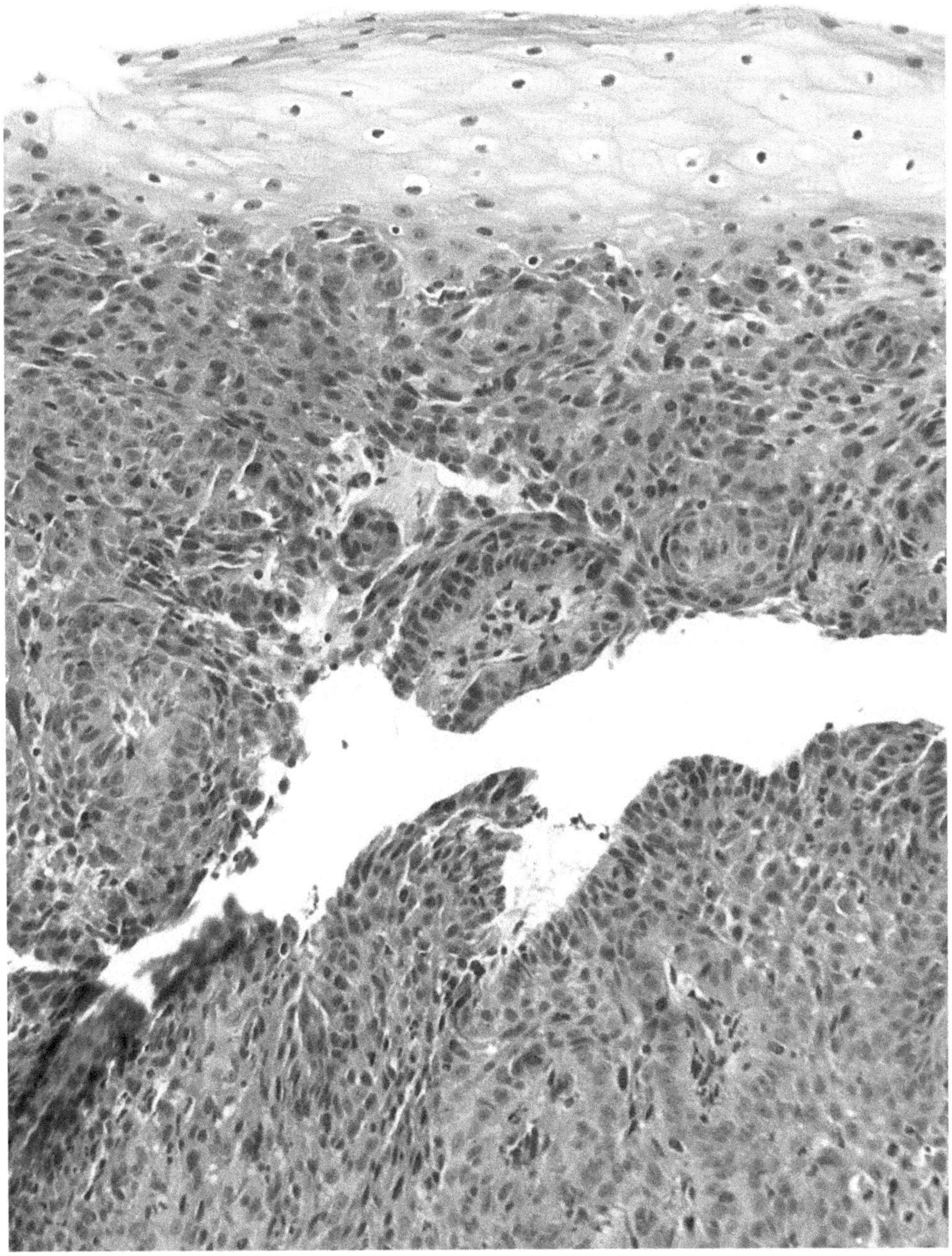

Figure 18.3: Oesophageal squamous cell carcinoma. Invasive keratinising nests of malignant squamous epithelium beneath intact surface epithelium, with central keratin pearl formation and stromal desmoplasia (H&E, intermediate mag). (Source: Nephron, Wikimedia Commons, CC BY-SA 3.0.)

Adenocarcinoma arises in the distal oesophagus and GEJ, almost exclusively in the setting of Barrett oesophagus. It is the predominant type in Western countries and its incidence is rising. Morphology ranges from well-formed glands to poorly cohesive (signet ring) patterns. Staging follows the AJCC 8th Edition TNM system; tumours with epicentre within 2 cm of the GEJ are staged as oesophageal carcinomas. Key predictive biomarkers include HER2 (tested by IHC and FISH; HER2-targeted therapy with trastuzumab for advanced disease) and PD-L1 (for immune checkpoint inhibitor eligibility).

Integration: The metaplasia-dysplasia-carcinoma sequence in Barrett oesophagus is a classic example of multistep carcinogenesis discussed in Chapter 6 (Neoplasia Part 1). Barrett metaplasia was introduced in Chapter 1 (Cell Injury, Adaptation). Oesophageal SCC carcinogenesis connects to environmental and nutritional factors in Chapter 10.

Gastric Pathology

Gastritis: Classification and Pathogenesis

Gastritis is classified into two major categories based on aetiology and topography. **H. pylori gastritis** (environmental, antral-predominant) is the most common form globally. **Autoimmune gastritis** (body-predominant) is less common but has important implications for pernicious anaemia and gastric neuroendocrine tumour development. The Updated Sydney System (1996) remains the standard for reporting gastric biopsies, grading five parameters: chronic inflammation, activity (neutrophilic), atrophy, intestinal metaplasia, and H. pylori density, with separate assessment of antral and corpus mucosa.

Helicobacter pylori is a Gram-negative, microaerophilic, spiral bacterium that colonises the gastric mucosa in approximately 50% of the world's population. In low- and middle-income settings, seroprevalence may exceed 70%. The bacterium produces urease (which neutralises gastric acid), CagA (injected into epithelial cells via a type IV secretion system, activating oncogenic signalling pathways), and VacA (induces epithelial cell vacuolation and apoptosis). CagA-positive strains carry a significantly higher risk of gastric carcinoma.

H. pylori colonisation → Chronic active gastritis → Mucosal atrophy → Intestinal metaplasia → Dysplasia → Gastric adenocarcinoma (Correa cascade)

Histologically, H. pylori gastritis shows a superficial band of lymphoplasmacytic inflammation with active neutrophilic infiltration ('activity'), prominent lymphoid follicles with germinal centres (a hallmark), and the organisms are visible as curved bacilli on the mucosal surface and in gastric pits, best seen at high magnification. Giemsa stain and immunohistochemistry for H. pylori improve detection in cases with low organism density. H. pylori is associated with peptic ulcer disease (duodenal more than gastric), gastric adenocarcinoma (WHO class I carcinogen), and extranodal marginal zone lymphoma (MALT lymphoma).

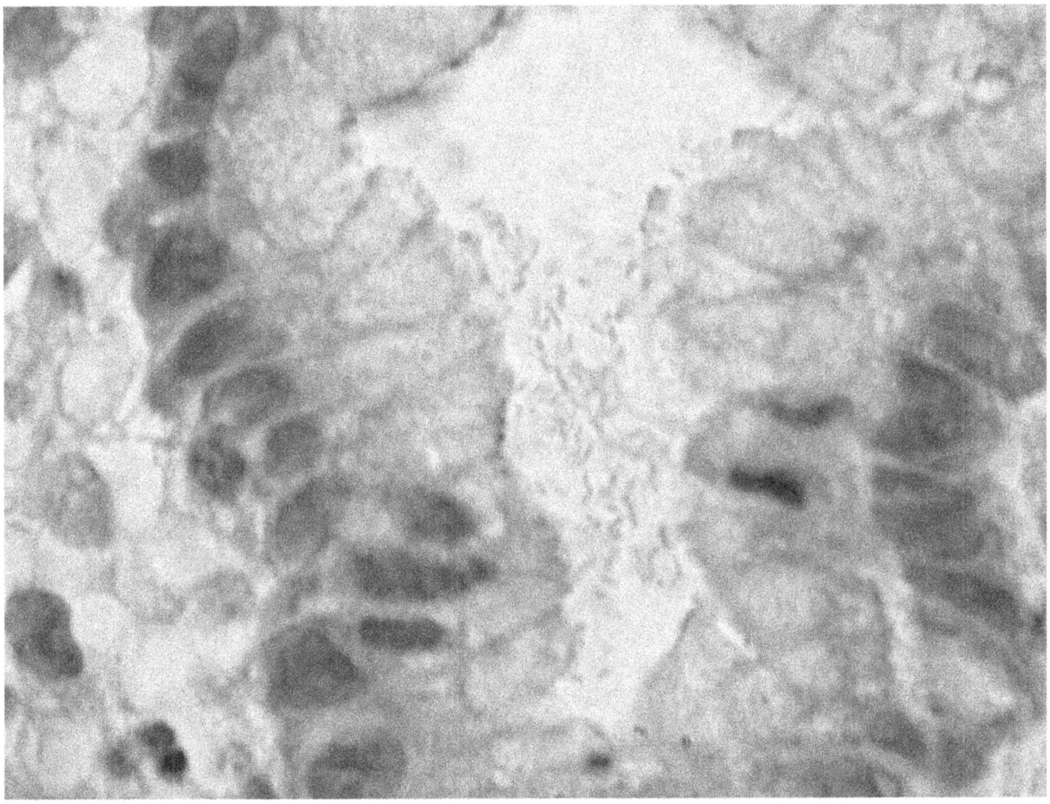

Figure 18.4A: Helicobacter pylori gastritis (H&E). Curved/seagull-shaped bacilli lying within surface mucus of gastric foveolar epithelium; underlying chronic active inflammation. (Source: Ed Uthman, Flickr/Wikimedia Commons, CC BY 2.0.)

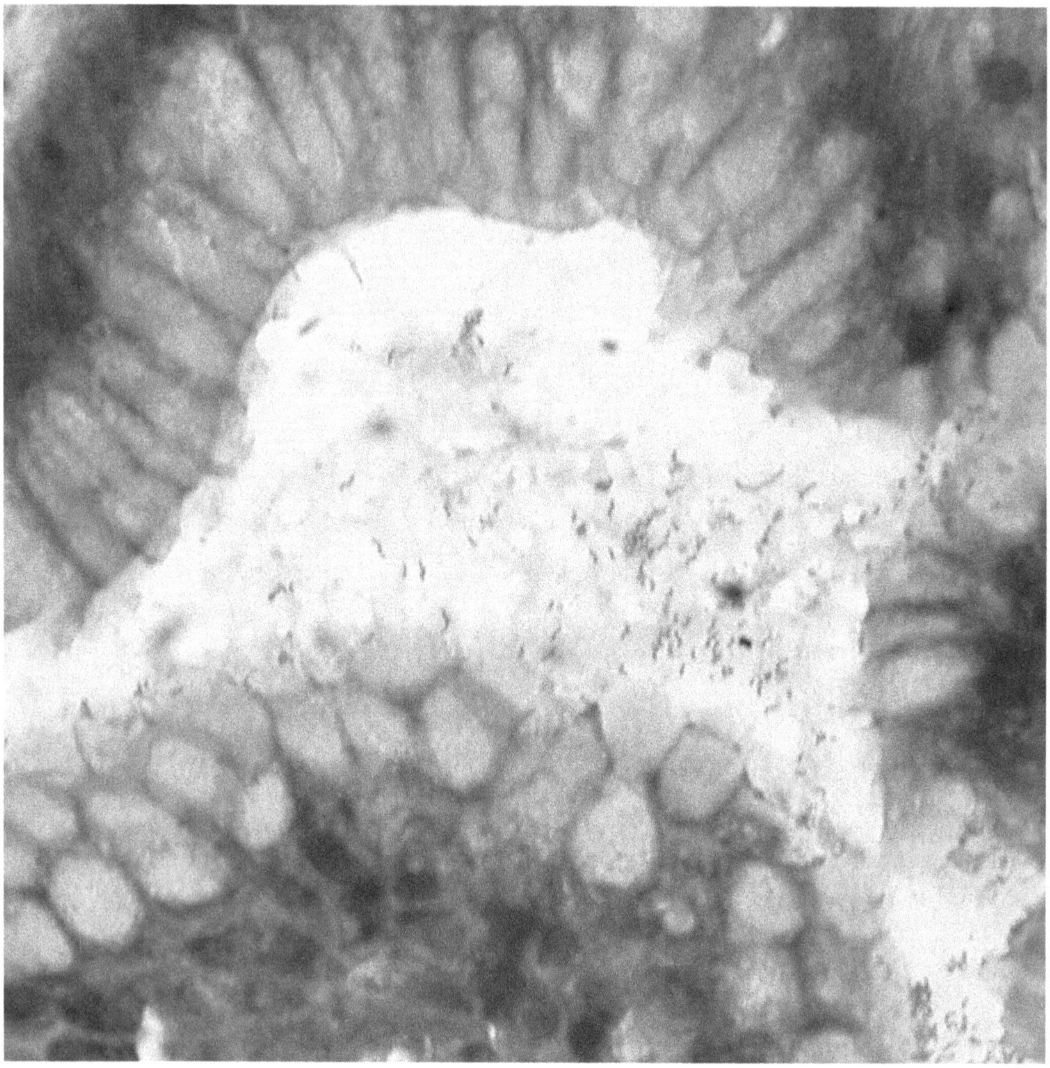

Figure 18.4B: H. pylori — Giemsa stain (same organism highlighted). Bacilli appear dark blue along foveolar epithelial surface, confirming organisms readily missed on routine H&E. (Source: Ed Uthman, Flickr/Wikimedia Commons, CC BY 2.0.)

A viva hook to consider: Why does H. pylori cause both duodenal ulcer AND gastric carcinoma, apparently contradictory outcomes? The answer lies in the topography of gastritis. Antral-predominant gastritis increases acid output (by destroying D cells that produce somatostatin, releasing G cells from inhibition), leading to duodenal ulceration. Pangastritis or corpus-predominant gastritis destroys parietal cells, reduces acid output, promotes atrophy and intestinal metaplasia, and follows the Correa cascade toward carcinoma.

Autoimmune (metaplastic atrophic) gastritis is an organ-specific autoimmune disease characterised by autoantibodies against parietal cells and intrinsic factor. It targets the oxyntic (body/fundic) mucosa, causing progressive destruction of parietal and chief cells with resulting hypochlorhydria, intrinsic factor deficiency (leading to vitamin B12 malabsorption and pernicious anaemia), and compensatory gastrin hypersecretion from antral G cells. Histologically, the body mucosa shows deep chronic inflammation, oxyntic gland atrophy, intestinal metaplasia, and pyloric metaplasia (replacement of oxyntic glands by mucous glands resembling pyloric-type). **Enterochromaffin-like (ECL) cell hyperplasia** is a characteristic consequence of hypergastrinaemia and is the precursor to type I gastric neuroendocrine tumours.

The distinction from H. pylori gastritis rests on the topography: autoimmune gastritis is body-predominant with antral sparing, while H. pylori gastritis is antral-predominant or pangastric. Gastrin immunostain on antral biopsies is positive (confirming antral origin), while body biopsies show loss of parietal cells and ECL hyperplasia (highlighted by chromogranin IHC).

Other forms of gastritis include **reactive (chemical) gastropathy** caused by bile reflux, NSAIDs, or alcohol, showing foveolar hyperplasia ('corkscrew glands'), mucinous depletion, smooth muscle extension between glands, and minimal inflammation. **Lymphocytic gastritis** (more than 25 intraepithelial lymphocytes per 100 epithelial cells) is associated with H. pylori infection and celiac disease.

Feature	H. pylori Gastritis	Autoimmune Gastritis
Topography	Antral-predominant	Body/fundic-predominant
Antibodies	None	Anti-parietal cell, anti-intrinsic factor
Acid output	Increased (antral) or decreased (pangastric)	Markedly decreased (achlorhydria)
Serum gastrin	Normal or slightly increased	Markedly increased (G-cell hyperplasia)
Key histology	Active inflammation, lymphoid follicles, organisms visible	Oxyntic atrophy, pyloric/intestinal metaplasia, ECL hyperplasia
B12 status	Normal	Deficient (pernicious anaemia)
Neoplasia risk	Adenocarcinoma, MALT lymphoma	Type I NET, adenocarcinoma (less common)

Quick Recall: Gastritis

H. pylori gastritis: Antral; active chronic inflammation; lymphoid follicles; Correa cascade to carcinoma.

Autoimmune gastritis: Body; anti-parietal cell Ab; pernicious anaemia; ECL hyperplasia; Type I NET risk.

Reactive gastropathy: Corkscrew foveolar hyperplasia; bile/NSAIDs; minimal inflammation.

Updated Sydney System: Grade: inflammation, activity, atrophy, IM, H. pylori; antrum + corpus biopsies.

CagA: Virulence factor injected via type IV secretion system; higher carcinoma risk.

Peptic Ulcer Disease

Peptic ulcers result from an imbalance between mucosal defence mechanisms (mucus-bicarbonate barrier, prostaglandins, mucosal blood flow) and aggressive factors (acid, pepsin, H. pylori, NSAIDs). **Duodenal ulcers** are more common than gastric ulcers and are almost always associated with H. pylori or NSAID use. **Gastric ulcers** may be benign (H. pylori, NSAIDs) or malignant (ulcerated carcinoma), and any gastric ulcer requires biopsy to exclude malignancy.

Histologically, a chronic peptic ulcer shows four distinct zones from the lumen to the base: (1) a fibrinopurulent exudate (necrotic debris), (2) a zone of fibrinoid necrosis, (3) granulation tissue with active angiogenesis and inflammation, and (4) a fibrotic scar base. The muscularis propria is typically destroyed at the ulcer site and replaced by fibrosis. Complications include haemorrhage (erosion into a vessel), perforation (penetration through the serosa), and pyloric stenosis (fibrotic narrowing). Stress ulcers (Curling ulcers in burns, Cushing ulcers in CNS injury) are acute, superficial erosions occurring in critically ill patients (see Chapter 4).

Diagnostic Tests for H. pylori

Detection of H. pylori uses both invasive (biopsy-based) and non-invasive methods. Invasive tests include histology (H&E, Giemsa, or immunohistochemistry on gastric biopsy; IHC is the most sensitive), rapid urease test (CLO test, based on the organism's potent urease activity), and culture (gold standard for antibiotic susceptibility testing but technically demanding). Non-invasive tests include the urea breath test (UBT, using ^{13}C or ^{14}C-labelled urea; excellent sensitivity and specificity for active infection), stool antigen test, and serology (detects prior exposure but cannot distinguish active from past infection). PPI use can cause false-negative results on UBT, stool antigen test, and histology; PPIs should be stopped for at least 2 weeks before testing. On biopsy, *the key diagnostic clue for H. pylori is the combination of active chronic gastritis (neutrophils plus lymphoplasmacytic infiltrate) with prominent lymphoid follicles in antral mucosa. Always request immunohistochemistry if organisms are not visible on routine stains, particularly after eradication therapy.*

Test	Type	Sensitivity	Specificity	Notes
Histology (IHC)	Invasive	95%	>95%	Gold standard on biopsy; also allows assessment of gastritis
Rapid urease test	Invasive	85-95%	>95%	Quick (minutes to hours); false negative with PPI/antibiotics
Urea breath test	Non-invasive	>95%	>95%	Best non-invasive test for active infection; stop PPI 2 weeks before
Stool antigen	Non-	>90%	>90%	Useful for post-eradication confirmation

	invasive			
Serology (IgG)	Non-invasive	>90%	80-90%	Cannot distinguish active from past infection; not for follow-up

Table 18.1: Diagnostic tests for H. pylori infection.

The Pathologist's Eye: Approach to Gastric Endoscopic Biopsies

The Updated Sydney System recommends a minimum of five biopsies: two from the antrum (lesser and greater curvature), one from the incisura, and two from the corpus (lesser and greater curvature). Report each parameter (inflammation, activity, atrophy, IM, H. pylori) separately for antrum and corpus. Atrophy is best assessed in well-oriented biopsies; tangential cutting can falsely suggest gland loss. Intestinal metaplasia can be highlighted by Alcian blue-PAS stain (goblet cells stain blue). If clinical suspicion for H. pylori is high but organisms are not seen on H&E, request Giemsa or IHC before reporting as negative.

Gastric Polyps and Dysplasia

Gastric polyps are common incidental findings. **Fundic gland polyps** are the most common, associated with PPI use (which causes parietal cell hypertrophy via gastrin feedback). They show dilated oxyntic glands and are almost always non-dysplastic; however, multiple or dysplastic fundic gland polyps should raise suspicion for familial adenomatous polyposis (FAP). **Hyperplastic polyps** arise in the setting of chronic gastritis (H. pylori or autoimmune), show foveolar hyperplasia ('corkscrew glands') and oedematous inflamed stroma, and carry a very low risk of dysplasia (less than 2%). **Gastric adenomas** (intestinal type and foveolar type) are true neoplastic polyps with dysplastic epithelium and carry a significant malignant potential (up to 30% harbour carcinoma).

Gastric dysplasia is classified as low-grade or high-grade, using morphological criteria analogous to dysplasia elsewhere in the GI tract. Low-grade dysplasia shows pencillate, hyperchromatic, pseudostratified nuclei confined to the lower half of the cell with preserved architecture. High-grade dysplasia shows marked atypia, loss of polarity, and complex/cribriform architecture. When faced with a gastric biopsy showing dysplasia, the first question to ask is whether it is arising in a background of intestinal metaplasia (suggesting the Correa pathway) or in non-metaplastic mucosa (suggesting a foveolar pathway, which may progress more rapidly) (Figures 18.4A–B, 18.5).

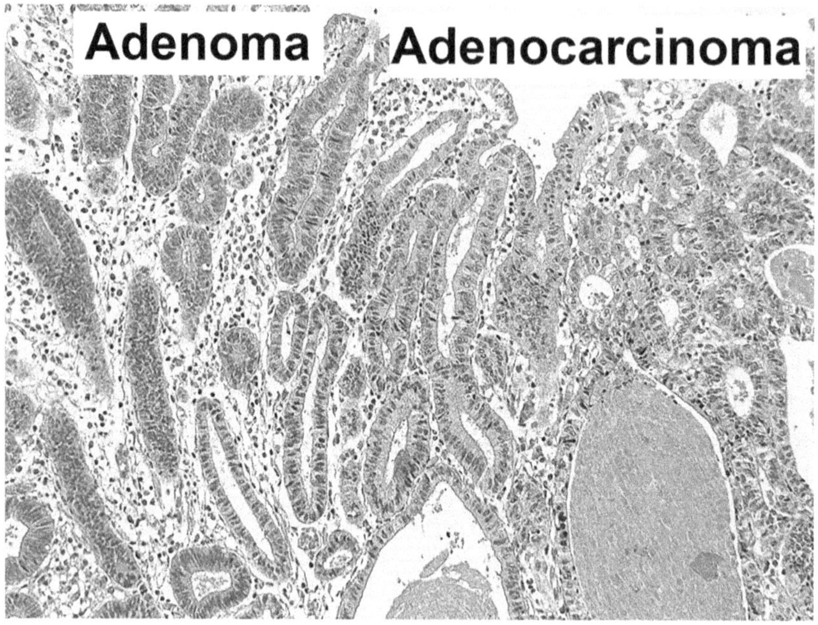

Figure 18.5: Gastric adenoma-to-adenocarcinoma transition (H&E). Adenomatous dysplasia (left) with adjacent invasive adenocarcinoma (right); yellow dashed line marks the boundary. (Source: Green et al., Wikimedia Commons, CC BY 4.0.)

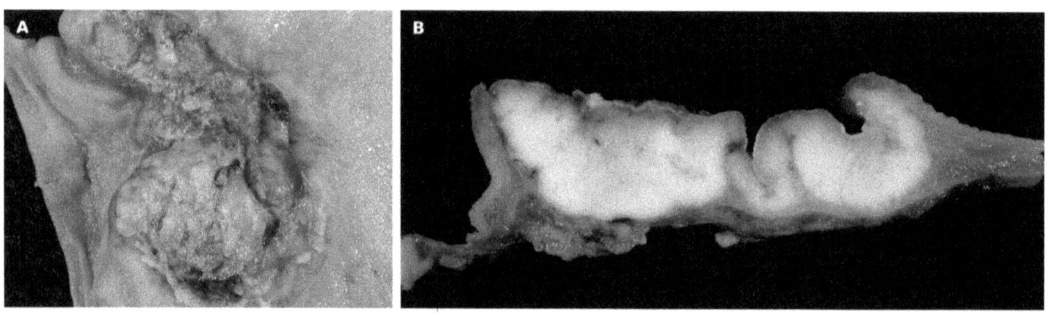

Figure 18.6: Gastric adenocarcinoma. (A) Gross specimen: ulcerated, fungating mass with raised, irregular borders and central necrosis. (Source: Ed Uthman, Wikimedia Commons, CC BY 2.0.) (B) Cut surface: firm, white, scirrhous tumour infiltrating the gastric wall. (Source: Ed Uthman, Flickr/Wikimedia Commons, CC BY 2.0.)

GASTRIC ADENOCARCINOMA

Definition: Malignant epithelial neoplasm of the gastric mucosa. Fifth most common cancer worldwide. In South Asia: male predominance, younger age of onset, predilection for non-cardia subsites.

Etiology: H. pylori chronic infection (intestinal type); CDH1 germline mutations (hereditary diffuse type); EBV (~10%); dietary factors (smoked/salted foods, nitrosamines); chronic atrophic gastritis with intestinal metaplasia.

Pathogenesis (intestinal type): H. pylori infection → Chronic active gastritis → Mucosal atrophy → Intestinal metaplasia → Dysplasia (low → high grade) → Invasive adenocarcinoma (Correa cascade)

Laurén classification: Intestinal type (well-formed glands, cohesive growth, H. pylori/IM pathway, older males, better prognosis) vs Diffuse type (**signet ring cells, discohesive single-cell infiltration, linitis plastica**, younger patients, CDH1/E-cadherin loss, worse prognosis). Indeterminate/mixed types exist.

Gross: Borrmann classification: Type I (polypoid), Type II (fungating, ulcerated with raised margins), Type III (ulcero-infiltrative), Type IV (diffuse/linitis plastica — leather bottle stomach with rigid, thickened wall).

Microscopy: Intestinal type: tubular/papillary glands with nuclear pleomorphism. Diffuse type: **signet ring cells** (eccentric nucleus displaced by intracytoplasmic mucin vacuole), discohesive infiltration, desmoplastic stroma. Early gastric cancer = confined to mucosa/submucosa regardless of nodal status.

IHC/Molecular: HER2 testing mandatory (IHC ± FISH); MMR/MSI testing; PD-L1 CPS; EBV (EBER ISH). TCGA molecular subtypes: CIN (~50%, HER2), EBV (~10%, PD-L1 high), GS (~20%, CDH1), MSI (~20%, immunotherapy responsive).

Hereditary: HDGC (CDH1 mutations) — prophylactic total gastrectomy recommended. Lynch syndrome — gastric cancer screening.

Exam yield: ★★★ HIGH — Laurén classification, Correa cascade, signet ring cell morphology, linitis plastica, HER2/MSI testing, and TCGA subtypes are all heavily tested.

The Cancer Genome Atlas (TCGA) molecular classification divides gastric carcinoma into four subtypes with distinct therapeutic implications:

Subtype	Frequency	Key Features	Morphology	Therapeutic Relevance
Chromosomally unstable (CIN)	~50%	TP53 mutations, HER2 amplification	Intestinal type	HER2-targeted therapy
Genomically stable (GS)	~20%	CDH1, RHOA mutations	Diffuse/signet ring	Limited targets
Microsatellite unstable (MSI)	~22%	MLH1 methylation/MMR loss	Variable; lymphoid stroma	Immunotherapy (PD-1/PD-L1)
EBV-positive	~8%	PIK3CA, ARID1A; PD-L1 amplified	Lymphoid stroma	Immunotherapy

Current standard practice for newly diagnosed gastric adenocarcinoma includes HER2 testing (IHC and/or FISH), mismatch repair/MSI testing (IHC for MLH1, MSH2, MSH6, PMS2), EBV ISH (EBER), and PD-L1 (CPS scoring). *The HER2 scoring system for gastroesophageal carcinoma differs from breast cancer: heterogeneous, incomplete membranous staining is acceptable for a 2+ or 3+ score because of the intrinsic heterogeneity of HER2 expression in gastric tumours.*

T Stage	Definition

Tis	Carcinoma in situ (high-grade dysplasia)
T1a	Tumour invades lamina propria or muscularis mucosae
T1b	Tumour invades submucosa
T2	Tumour invades muscularis propria
T3	Tumour penetrates subserosal connective tissue without serosal invasion
T4a	Tumour perforates serosa (visceral peritoneum)
T4b	Tumour invades adjacent structures

Table 18.2: T staging of gastric adenocarcinoma (AJCC 8th Edition). Note: tumours with epicentre within 2 cm of the GEJ are staged as oesophageal carcinomas.

Linitis plastica ('leather bottle stomach') is a distinctive macroscopic presentation of diffuse gastric carcinoma in which extensive submucosal infiltration by poorly cohesive carcinoma cells with desmoplastic reaction produces a thickened, rigid, non-distensible stomach wall. The mucosa may appear deceptively normal on endoscopy; deep biopsies are required for diagnosis. *When faced with thickened gastric folds on endoscopy and superficial biopsies that appear negative, the first question to ask is whether the biopsies are deep enough, as diffuse carcinoma often infiltrates the submucosa and muscularis while sparing the mucosal surface.*

The Pathologist's Eye: Signet Ring Cells in Gastric Biopsy

Not all signet ring cells are malignant. Mucin-laden histiocytes (pseudosignet ring cells) can mimic signet ring cell carcinoma on H&E. The distinction is made by IHC: true signet ring carcinoma cells are CK positive and CD68 negative, while histiocytes are CK negative and CD68 positive. In subtle cases of diffuse gastric carcinoma where tumour cells are sparse and interspersed with normal tissue, a cytokeratin stain (AE1/AE3 or CAM5.2) can highlight the neoplastic infiltrate. Always check deeper levels if initial biopsies from a clinically suspicious area appear unremarkable.

Quick Recall: Gastric Carcinoma

Lauren classification: Intestinal (glands, cohesive, older, H. pylori) vs Diffuse (signet ring, infiltrative, younger).

TCGA molecular: CIN (~50%, HER2), GS (~20%, CDH1), MSI (~22%, immunotherapy), EBV (~8%, PD-L1).

HDGC: Germline CDH1 mutation; E-cadherin loss; prophylactic gastrectomy.

Biomarker workup: HER2 IHC/FISH, MMR IHC, EBER ISH, PD-L1 CPS on all new cases.

HER2 scoring: Differs from breast; heterogeneous membranous staining acceptable for 2+/3+.

GASTROINTESTINAL STROMAL TUMOUR (GIST)

Definition: Most common mesenchymal neoplasm of the GI tract, derived from interstitial cells of Cajal (GI pacemaker cells). Stomach (60%) > small intestine (30%) > others.

Pathogenesis: Gain-of-function KIT/PDGFRA mutation → Constitutive receptor tyrosine kinase activation → Uncontrolled proliferation of interstitial cells of Cajal → GIST

Molecular: KIT mutation (~80%, exon 11 most common) → imatinib sensitive. PDGFRA (~10%, D842V most common) → imatinib resistant, avapritinib sensitive. SDH-deficient (~5%, paediatric/Carney triad) → wild-type GIST.

Microscopy: Three patterns: spindle cell (70%, intersecting fascicles), epithelioid (20%), or mixed. **CD117 (KIT) positivity on IHC is the diagnostic hallmark**. Also DOG1+ (95%), CD34+ (70%). Desmin−, S100− (distinguishes from leiomyoma and schwannoma).

Risk stratification: Based on tumour size, mitotic rate (/5 mm^2), and anatomical location. Gastric GISTs have more favourable prognosis than small bowel GISTs at equivalent size/mitotic rate. GISTs do not metastasise to lymph nodes (unlike carcinomas); spread is peritoneal and hepatic.

Exam yield: ★★★ HIGH — KIT/PDGFRA mutations, imatinib therapy, CD117/DOG1 IHC, and risk stratification are core exam topics.

Quick Recall: GIST

Origin: Interstitial cells of Cajal; most common GI mesenchymal tumour.

Molecular: KIT mutation (80%, exon 11 most common); PDGFRA (10%); mutually exclusive.

IHC: DOG1 (most sensitive, 97%), CD117/c-KIT (95%), CD34 (70%).

Risk stratification: Size + mitotic rate + location; gastric > small bowel prognosis.

SDH-deficient: Paediatric/young; epithelioid; loss of SDHB on IHC; Carney-Stratakis; imatinib-resistant.

Therapy: Imatinib (KIT/PDGFRA-mutant); avapritinib (PDGFRA D842V).

Gastric Neuroendocrine Tumours

Well-differentiated gastric neuroendocrine tumours (NETs, formerly 'carcinoids') arise from ECL cells and are classified into three types based on their clinical-pathological context:

Feature	Type I	Type II	Type III
Background	Autoimmune gastritis	MEN1/ZES (gastrinoma)	Sporadic
Gastrin level	High (parietal cell loss)	High (gastrinoma)	Normal
Tumour	Multiple, small (<1 cm)	Multiple, small	Solitary, often >2 cm

number			
Fundic mucosa	Atrophic, ECL hyperplasia	ECL hyperplasia	Normal
Behaviour	Indolent, rarely metastasise	Low-grade; occasional mets	Aggressive; frequent mets
Management	Surveillance ± endoscopic resection	Treat gastrinoma	Surgery ± chemotherapy

Gastric MALT Lymphoma

Extranodal marginal zone lymphoma of mucosa-associated lymphoid tissue (MALT lymphoma) of the stomach is strongly associated with H. pylori infection. The lymphoma arises from the acquired MALT tissue that develops in response to chronic H. pylori stimulation. Histologically, it shows a diffuse to perifollicular infiltrate of small centrocyte-like (monocytoid) lymphocytes with characteristic lymphoepithelial lesions (lymphocytes infiltrating and destroying glandular epithelium). IHC: CD20 positive, CD43 positive (often), CD5/CD10/CD23/cyclin D1 negative. Most localised gastric MALT lymphomas respond to H. pylori eradication therapy alone. Those that are t(11;18)(API2::MALT1)-positive are resistant to antibiotic eradication and require radiation or chemotherapy.

The distinction between florid H. pylori-associated gastritis with prominent lymphoid follicles and early MALT lymphoma can be challenging. Features favouring lymphoma include: destruction of glands by lymphoepithelial lesions (highlighted by CK immunostain), a monotonous lymphoid infiltrate extending beyond the muscularis mucosae, and Dutcher bodies (intranuclear PAS-positive inclusions). Light chain restriction on IHC or flow cytometry and clonal immunoglobulin gene rearrangement on PCR confirm the diagnosis.

Disease	Mechanism	Frequency
Chronic active gastritis	Direct mucosal inflammation	All infected individuals
Duodenal ulcer	Antral gastritis → increased acid → duodenal injury	15-20% of infected
Gastric ulcer	Pangastritis with mucosal damage	Less common than DU
Gastric adenocarcinoma	Correa cascade; CagA+ strains, higher risk	1-3% of infected
MALT lymphoma	Acquired MALT → chronic antigenic stimulation	<0.1% of infected
Iron deficiency	Hypochlorhydria; impaired iron absorption	Variable

anaemia		
Immune thrombocytopenia	Molecular mimicry; anti-platelet antibodies	Rare; variable response to eradication

Table 18.3: Diseases associated with H. pylori infection.

Other Gastric Lesions

Gastric antral vascular ectasia (GAVE), endoscopically known as 'watermelon stomach,' shows dilated mucosal capillaries with fibrin thrombi in a background of reactive gastropathy (foveolar hyperplasia, muscular hyperplasia, and minimal inflammation). The fibrin thrombi within lamina propria capillaries are the key distinguishing histological feature. GAVE is associated with cirrhosis, autoimmune conditions (especially systemic sclerosis), and chronic renal failure. It must be distinguished from **portal hypertensive gastropathy**, which shows dilated submucosal and mucosal vessels without fibrin thrombi, in a background of congestion. Endoscopically, portal hypertensive gastropathy has a 'snake skin' or mosaic pattern, while GAVE has characteristic longitudinal antral folds converging on the pylorus.

Ménétrier disease (hypertrophic gastropathy) is a rare condition characterised by massive foveolar hyperplasia producing giant cerebriform gastric rugal folds, predominantly in the body and fundus. Histologically, there is marked foveolar hyperplasia with cystically dilated glands, reduced parietal cells, and expansion of the mucous cell compartment. The pathogenesis involves excessive TGF-alpha signalling through the EGFR pathway. Clinically, patients present with protein-losing gastropathy (hypoalbuminaemia), hypochlorhydria, and abdominal pain. There is an increased risk of gastric adenocarcinoma. Treatment includes cetuximab (anti-EGFR) and, in refractory cases, gastrectomy.

Ectopic pancreatic tissue (pancreatic heterotopia) is an incidental finding, most commonly in the stomach (antrum), duodenum, and jejunum, presenting as a submucosal nodule. It contains ductular and acinar pancreatic tissue without connection to the native pancreas. It is usually asymptomatic and must be distinguished clinically from GIST and other submucosal tumours.

Quick Recall: Other Gastric Lesions

GAVE: Watermelon stomach; fibrin thrombi in mucosal capillaries; cirrhosis, systemic sclerosis.

Portal hypertensive gastropathy: Snake skin pattern; dilated vessels without fibrin thrombi; no capillary thrombosis.

Ménétrier disease: Giant rugal folds; massive foveolar hyperplasia; TGF-alpha/EGFR; protein-losing gastropathy.

MALT lymphoma: H. pylori-driven; LELs; CD20+, CD43+; t(11;18) = eradication-resistant.

Recent Advances

WHO 5th edition classification of tumours of the digestive system. The 2019 fifth-edition WHO Classification of Tumours of the Digestive System introduced a hierarchical site–category–family–type framework that integrates morphology, immunohistochemistry, and molecular criteria across the oesophagus, stomach, small intestine, appendix, colorectum, anal canal, liver, biliary tract, and pancreas (Nagtegaal et al. Histopathology 2020; 76: 182–188; PMID 31433515). For each entity the volume specifies essential and desirable diagnostic criteria, and replaces the prior dichotomy of low-grade versus high-grade dysplasia in tubular GI lesions with the harmonised two-tier intraepithelial neoplasia terminology endorsed by the Vienna group. The classification incorporates molecular categorisation of gastric and colorectal carcinomas — including microsatellite instability, EBV-associated, chromosomally unstable, and genomically stable subtypes — as well as the neuroendocrine neoplasm framework that distinguishes well-differentiated neuroendocrine tumours (NET G1–G3) from poorly differentiated neuroendocrine carcinomas. Mixed neuroendocrine–non-neuroendocrine neoplasms (MiNENs) are redefined to require at least 30% of each component. Reporting implication: GI biopsy and resection reports should map findings to the WHO 5 entity, include the relevant essential diagnostic criteria, and incorporate molecular and grading data where indicated to support targeted therapy selection.

Artificial intelligence in Barrett surveillance. Deep learning algorithms have been developed for automated detection and grading of Barrett oesophagus dysplasia on digitised H&E slides, with performance approaching expert pathologist concordance. These tools are being integrated into clinical workflows to reduce interobserver variability, which is the Achilles heel of Barrett dysplasia grading. AI-assisted triage could improve detection of low-prevalence dysplasia in high-volume surveillance programmes.

Molecular residual disease in gastric cancer. Circulating tumour DNA (ctDNA) analysis post-gastrectomy is emerging as a powerful tool for detecting molecular residual disease and predicting recurrence. Studies have shown that postoperative ctDNA positivity identifies patients at high risk of relapse who may benefit from adjuvant chemotherapy, while ctDNA-negative patients may be spared unnecessary treatment. Integration of ctDNA with TCGA molecular subtypes is being explored to guide personalised adjuvant strategies.

Claudin 18.2 as a therapeutic target. Claudin 18.2 (CLDN18.2), a tight junction protein highly expressed in gastric carcinoma (particularly diffuse type), has emerged as a novel therapeutic target. Zolbetuximab, an anti-CLDN18.2 monoclonal antibody, demonstrated significant survival benefit in CLDN18.2-positive, HER2-negative advanced gastric cancer in the SPOTLIGHT and GLOW trials. CLDN18.2 IHC testing is becoming a new standard biomarker alongside HER2, MMR, EBV, and PD-L1 in the workup of gastric adenocarcinoma.

Approach to the Histopathology Slide

Step 1: Identify the tissue. Recognise squamous mucosa (oesophagus), oxyntic mucosa (body/fundus: pink parietal cells, purple chief cells), antral mucosa (mucous glands, G cells), or villous mucosa (duodenum). This immediately orientates you to the correct differential diagnosis.

Step 2: For oesophageal biopsies, determine whether the epithelium is squamous or columnar. If columnar with goblet cells = Barrett oesophagus; then assess for dysplasia using the four-line approach. If squamous, assess for oesophagitis pattern: eosinophilic (count per HPF), reflux (basal hyperplasia, papillary elongation), or infectious (look for viral inclusions, fungal organisms).

Step 3: For gastric biopsies, first determine the mucosal type (oxyntic vs antral). Then assess: (a) Is there gastritis? Grade inflammation, activity, atrophy, and IM per the Sydney System. (b) Look for H. pylori organisms at high power. (c) Is there dysplasia? Grade as low or high. (d) For submucosal spindle cell lesions, consider GIST (CD117, DOG1) versus schwannoma (S100) versus leiomyoma (desmin, SMA).

Step 4: For duodenal biopsies, assess villous architecture (villous:crypt ratio, normally 3:1 or greater), count IELs per 100 enterocytes (normally fewer than 25), and look for crypt hyperplasia. Describe findings using the Marsh classification and recommend serological correlation.

Step 5: For neoplastic lesions, determine epithelial (adenocarcinoma, SCC, NET) versus mesenchymal (GIST, schwannoma, leiomyoma) versus lymphoid (MALT lymphoma, DLBCL). Apply the appropriate IHC panel and request molecular testing (HER2, MMR, EBER for gastric carcinoma; KIT/PDGFRA for GIST).

International Frameworks

Vienna Classification of GI Epithelial Neoplasia (2000). Conceived to reconcile the long-standing divergence between Western and Japanese pathologists in diagnosing oesophageal, gastric, and colorectal lesions, the Vienna classification establishes a five-category framework adopted globally for biopsy and resection reporting: (1) negative for neoplasia/dysplasia, (2) indefinite for neoplasia/dysplasia, (3) non-invasive low-grade neoplasia (low-grade adenoma/dysplasia), (4) non-invasive high-grade neoplasia (high-grade adenoma/dysplasia, non-invasive carcinoma, suspicion of invasive carcinoma), and (5) invasive neoplasia (intramucosal, submucosal, or beyond). Application of this scheme increased interobserver agreement substantially (κ 0.31–0.55 across organs versus 0.01–0.27 with conventional terminology). Reporting implication: GI biopsy reports should map findings to a Vienna category in addition to descriptive terminology, particularly when interfacing with international tumour boards or comparing across centres with different historical reporting cultures. Citation: Schlemper RJ, et al. Gut 2000;47(2):251–255. PMID 10896917.

Ultra High-Yield Chapter Summary

Topic	Must Remember
GERD histology	Basal hyperplasia, papillary elongation, scattered eosinophils (<15/HPF), spongiosis
EoE	>15 eosinophils/HPF; eosinophilic microabscesses; atopic triad; rings and furrows
HSV vs CMV oesophagitis	HSV: squamous cells, ulcer edge, 3Ms; CMV: mesenchymal cells, ulcer base, owl's eye
Barrett definition	Columnar epithelium with goblet cells ≥1 cm above gastric folds; ~0.5%/yr cancer risk
Barrett dysplasia	Four-line approach; LGD = pencillate nuclei, basal; HGD = loss of polarity, complex architecture
p53 in Barrett	Aberrant (overexpression or null) = TP53 mutation = supports dysplasia
Oesophageal SCC across the Asian oesophageal cancer belt	Predominant type (>80%); Asian oesophageal-cancer belt highest risk; tobacco, hot beverages
H. pylori pathogenesis	CagA (type IV secretion, oncogenic); VacA (vacuolation, apoptosis); WHO class I carcinogen

Correa cascade	H. pylori → chronic gastritis → atrophy → IM → dysplasia → carcinoma
Autoimmune gastritis	Body-predominant; anti-parietal cell Ab; pernicious anaemia; ECL hyperplasia; Type I NET
Updated Sydney System	Grade 5 parameters (inflammation, activity, atrophy, IM, H. pylori) in antrum + corpus
Gastric carcinoma Lauren	Intestinal (glands, older, H. pylori) vs Diffuse (signet ring, younger, CDH1)
TCGA molecular subtypes	CIN (HER2), GS (CDH1), MSI (immunotherapy), EBV (PD-L1)
HER2 in gastric	Heterogeneous membranous staining acceptable; differs from breast scoring
GIST	Cajal cells; KIT (80%)/PDGFRA (10%); DOG1 most sensitive; risk = size + mitoses + site
SDH-deficient GIST	Young; epithelioid; SDHB loss on IHC; imatinib-resistant; Carney-Stratakis/triad
Gastric NET types	I (autoimmune, indolent); II (MEN1/ZES); III (sporadic, aggressive)
Celiac disease	HLA-DQ2/DQ8; tTG deamidates gliadin; Marsh 3c = total villous atrophy
MALT lymphoma	H. pylori-driven; lymphoepithelial lesions; t(11;18) = resistant to eradication
Claudin 18.2	Novel target in gastric carcinoma (diffuse type); zolbetuximab; emerging biomarker

Diagnostic thinking: intestinal metaplasia + goblet cells + oesophageal biopsy → Barrett oesophagus (risk for adenocarcinoma)

Diagnostic thinking: signet ring cells + diffuse infiltration + linitis plastica → diffuse-type gastric carcinoma (Lauren classification)

Diagnostic thinking: spindle cells + DOG1+/CD117+ + GI mass → GIST

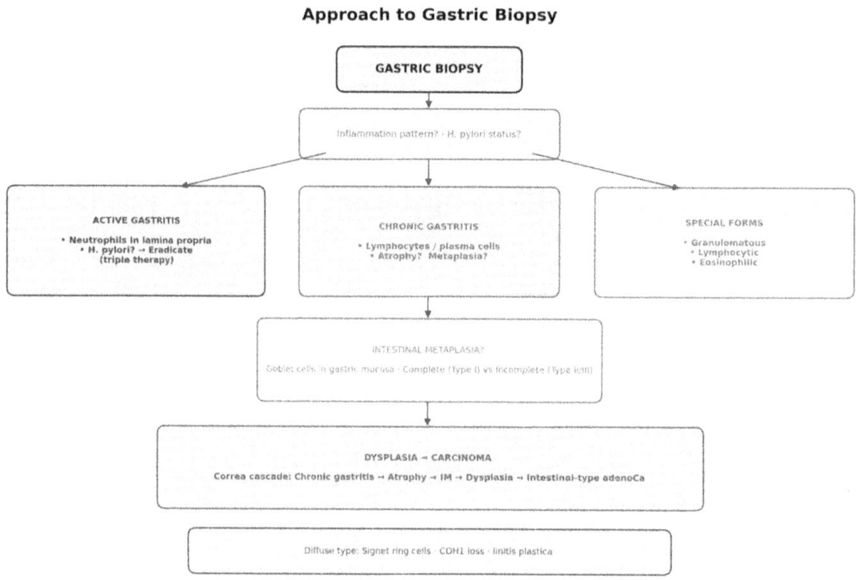

Figure 18.7: Approach to Gastric Biopsy. (Source: Author's original.)

Chapter 19: Gastrointestinal Pathology Part 2: Lower GI

THE BIG PICTURE

The lower gastrointestinal tract, from the jejunum to the rectum and including the appendix, is the site of some of the most commonly examined diseases in pathology: inflammatory bowel disease, colorectal adenomas, colorectal carcinoma, and celiac disease. TB-endemic regions add a unique diagnostic challenge in the form of intestinal tuberculosis, which mimics Crohn disease both clinically and histologically. The differential diagnosis of ulcerative lesions of the intestines, encompassing TB, Crohn disease, ulcerative colitis, typhoid, amoebic colitis, and ischaemic disease, is one of the highest-frequency exam topics. Colorectal carcinoma is the third most common cancer worldwide, and its molecular pathogenesis through the adenoma-carcinoma sequence is one of the best-understood multistep carcinogenesis models. Universal mismatch repair testing on all new colorectal carcinomas is now standard practice, both for prognostic stratification and for identifying Lynch syndrome families.

High-yield topics in this chapter: Ulcerative lesions of the intestines (differential diagnosis); colorectal adenomas (conventional and serrated pathways); adenoma-carcinoma sequence (CIN, MSI, serrated); familial polyposis syndromes (FAP, Lynch); inflammatory bowel disease (Crohn vs UC); intestinal TB vs Crohn disease; IBD-associated dysplasia; celiac disease; colorectal carcinoma (morphology, grading, staging, molecular); MMR/MSI testing; appendiceal tumours; GI neuroendocrine tumours; Hirschsprung disease.

WHO Classification: Lower GI Tumours (5th Ed, 2019) -- Selected

Colorectal epithelial: Conventional adenoma (tubular, tubulovillous, villous); sessile serrated lesion (SSL, replaces SSA/P); traditional serrated adenoma; adenocarcinoma (NOS, mucinous, signet ring, medullary, micropapillary, serrated).

Key change: SSL replaces sessile serrated adenoma/polyp (SSA/P). Two-tier dysplasia grading replaces three-tier in SSL.

Appendiceal: Low-grade appendiceal mucinous neoplasm (LAMN); high-grade (HAMN); goblet cell adenocarcinoma (replaces goblet cell carcinoid); conventional adenocarcinoma.

NE tumours: NET G1/G2/G3 (well-differentiated); NEC large cell and small cell (poorly differentiated). Appendiceal NET (formerly carcinoid) is the most common appendiceal tumour.

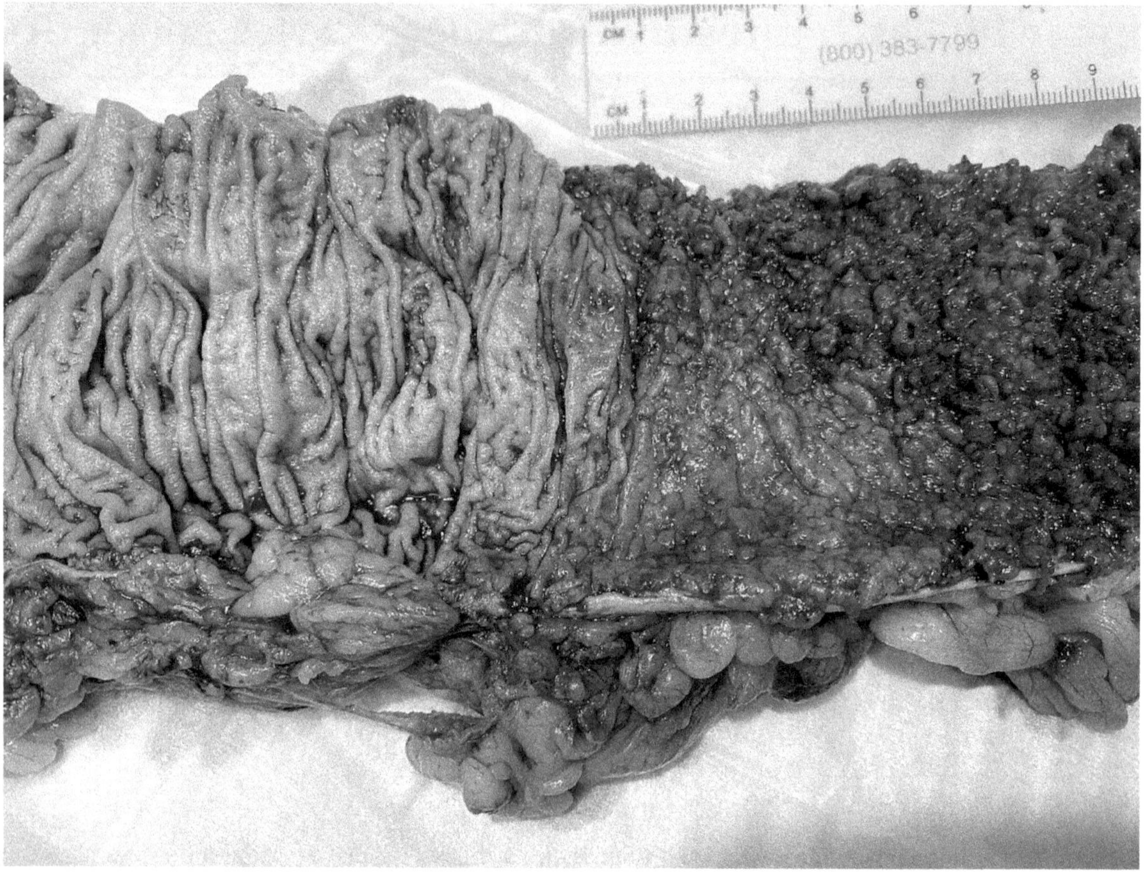

Figure 19.1: Ulcerative colitis, gross appearance. Resected colon showing continuous mucosal involvement extending from the rectum proximally (right-to-left), with granular, friable, hemorrhagic mucosa and loss of haustral folds; adjacent uninvolved mucosa at left shows preserved folds. (Source: Wikimedia Commons, CC BY-SA 4.0.)

The colon processes over a litre of ileal effluent daily, reabsorbing water and electrolytes while harbouring the densest microbial ecosystem in the human body. This constant interplay between luminal contents, commensal flora, and mucosal immunity creates an environment where perturbations in any component, whether genetic (APC mutation), immunological (dysregulated T cell responses in IBD), or infectious (Mycobacterium tuberculosis in the ileum), can initiate a cascade of pathological events. For the pathologist, the lower GI tract demands expertise in polyp classification, dysplasia grading, IBD interpretation, ulcer characterisation, and molecular testing, often on small biopsy material.

Colorectal Polyps and the Adenoma-Carcinoma Sequence

Conventional Adenomas

Conventional colorectal adenomas are neoplastic polyps characterised by dysplastic epithelium with 'picket fence' nuclei: elongated, pencillate, pseudostratified, hyperchromatic nuclei that generally retain basal orientation. They are classified by architecture into **tubular adenoma (TA)** (more than 75%

tubular, most common), **villous adenoma (VA)** (more than 75% villous, larger, higher dysplasia risk), and **tubulovillous adenoma (TVA)** (25 to 75% villous component). The risk of harbouring high-grade dysplasia or malignancy correlates with size (more than 1 cm), villous architecture, and degree of dysplasia.

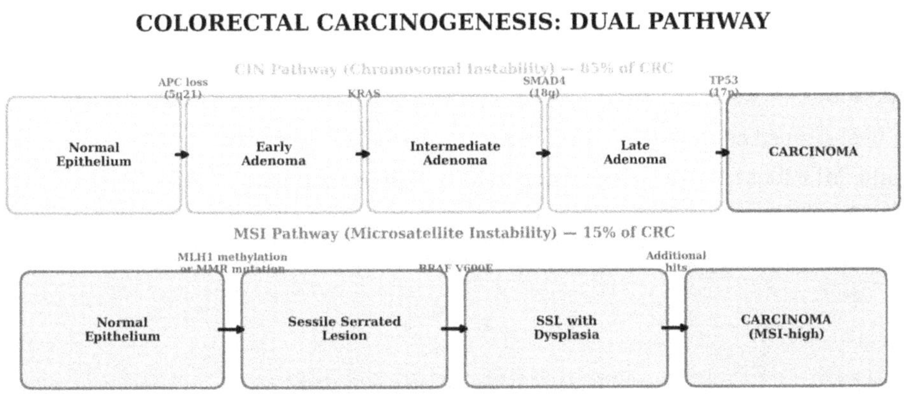

Figure 19.2: Colorectal Carcinogenesis: CIN vs MSI Pathway. (Source: Author's original.)

High-grade dysplasia (HGD) shows significant cytologic pleomorphism with rounded, heaped-up cells, high nuclear-to-cytoplasmic ratio, vesicular 'open' chromatin with prominent nucleoli, loss of basal nuclear orientation, and architectural complexity (cribriform glands, solid nests, intraluminal necrosis). **Intramucosal carcinoma** shows neoplastic cells through the basement membrane into the lamina propria but not through the muscularis mucosae. In the colorectum, intramucosal carcinoma has negligible metastatic risk because the colonic mucosa has sparse lymphatic channels, and it is managed as high-grade dysplasia. True invasive adenocarcinoma requires penetration into the submucosa (pT1), where lymphovascular channels are present.

Normal epithelium → APC mutation → Adenoma → KRAS mutation → Advanced adenoma → TP53 loss → Carcinoma (CIN pathway)

Serrated Polyps

The serrated pathway accounts for approximately 20 to 30% of colorectal carcinomas and proceeds through a distinct set of precursor lesions. **Hyperplastic polyps (HP)** are the most common serrated polyps, typically small (less than 5 mm) and left-sided, showing superficial luminal serrations with proliferation confined to the crypt base. They have no significant malignant potential. **Sessile serrated lesions (SSL, formerly sessile serrated adenoma/polyp)** are typically larger (1 cm or more), right-sided lesions characterised by architectural distortion at the crypt bases: serrations extending to the base, dilated crypt bases with lateral growth producing boot-shaped or 'duck foot' profiles, and asymmetric growth. Only one unequivocal distorted crypt is required for diagnosis.

SSL with dysplasia shows superimposed cytological atypia (often sharply demarcated) and frequently shows loss of MLH1 expression on IHC, indicating progression along the serrated-MSI pathway. **Traditional serrated adenoma (TSA)** is uncommon, shows prominent filiform serrations with eosinophilic, mucin-depleted columnar cells, central pencillate nuclei, and characteristic ectopic crypt foci (slit-like serrations). TSAs harbour either BRAF (from MVHPs) or KRAS (from GCHPs) mutations and progress to microsatellite-stable carcinoma.

Normal → BRAF V600E → MVHP → DNA methylation → SSL → MLH1 promoter methylation → MSI → Dysplasia → Carcinoma (Serrated/MSI pathway)

Quick Recall: Colorectal Polyps

Conventional adenoma: Picket fence nuclei; TA/TVA/VA; CIN pathway (APC→KRAS→TP53).

SSL: Right-sided; boot-shaped crypt bases; BRAF V600E; serrated-MSI pathway.

SSL with dysplasia: MLH1 loss on IHC; progression to MSI-high carcinoma.

Intramucosal carcinoma: Into lamina propria only; negligible metastatic risk in colon; manage as HGD.

TSA: Eosinophilic cells, ectopic crypt foci; BRAF or KRAS; microsatellite-stable carcinoma.

Vienna Classification of Gastrointestinal Epithelial Neoplasia

The Vienna classification (2000, updated 2002) was introduced to reconcile the persistent divergence between Western and Japanese pathologists in reporting gastrointestinal mucosal neoplasia — particularly the classic disagreement over what one tradition calls "high-grade dysplasia" and the other calls "non-invasive carcinoma." It defines six categories applicable across oesophageal, gastric, and colorectal biopsies, and explicitly links each category to a recommended clinical action. The categories are not disease entities but reporting tiers, and Vienna has become the reference framework for biopsy terminology in WHO 5th Edition digestive system tumour classifications.

Table 19.1: Revised Vienna Classification of Gastrointestinal Epithelial Neoplasia (2002)

Category	Terminology	Clinical action
1	Negative for neoplasia or dysplasia	Routine follow-up as clinically indicated.
2	Indefinite for neoplasia or dysplasia	Repeat biopsy after inflammation or reactive changes settle; short-interval follow-up.
3	Mucosal low-grade neoplasia — low-grade adenoma or low-grade dysplasia	Endoscopic resection or follow-up; risk of progression low but non-negligible.
4	Mucosal high-grade neoplasia — subdivided into 4.1 high-grade adenoma/dysplasia, 4.2 non-invasive carcinoma (carcinoma in situ), 4.3 suspicious for invasive carcinoma, 4.4 intramucosal carcinoma	Endoscopic resection in most cases; surgery if en-bloc resection is not feasible or if invasion is suspected.
5	Submucosal invasion by carcinoma	Surgical resection; assess lymph-vascular invasion and depth for oncological

Category	Terminology	Clinical action
		management.
6	Advanced carcinoma (beyond submucosa)	Oncological staging and multidisciplinary management.

Exam point: The Vienna category 4.4 (intramucosal carcinoma) is a useful pivot to emphasise — in the colon, lack of mucosal lymphatics means intramucosal carcinoma confers essentially no metastatic risk, and endoscopic resection alone is curative; in the oesophagus and stomach, mucosal lymphatics are present and intramucosal carcinoma carries a measurable (5-10 percent) nodal-metastasis risk. This organ-specific distinction is a frequent MCQ trap.

Hereditary Polyposis Syndromes

Familial adenomatous polyposis (FAP) results from germline APC mutations (autosomal dominant) with hundreds to thousands of adenomas and virtually 100% CRC risk without prophylactic colectomy. Attenuated FAP: 10–100 polyps, later onset, right-sided. Extracolonic: fundic gland polyps, desmoids, duodenal adenomas, osteomas, CHRPE, cribriform-morular PTC. Gardner = FAP + osteomas/soft tissue tumours. Turcot = polyposis + CNS tumours (medulloblastoma/APC; GBM/MMR).

Lynch syndrome (hereditary non-polyposis colorectal cancer, HNPCC) is caused by germline mutations in mismatch repair (MMR) genes (MLH1, MSH2, MSH6, PMS2) and accounts for 3 to 5% of all colorectal carcinomas. Unlike FAP, patients develop relatively few adenomas, but these progress rapidly to carcinoma (accelerated adenoma-carcinoma sequence). Colorectal carcinomas are characteristically right-sided, mucinous or medullary, with prominent tumour-infiltrating lymphocytes. Lynch syndrome also confers increased risk of endometrial, ovarian, gastric, urinary tract, and other cancers (see Chapter 25). Diagnosis: universal MMR IHC screening on all new CRC specimens. Loss of MLH1/PMS2 triggers BRAF V600E testing and MLH1 promoter methylation analysis to distinguish sporadic (BRAF-positive or methylated) from Lynch (BRAF-negative, unmethylated, requiring germline testing).

Other polyposis syndromes include **Peutz-Jeghers syndrome** (germline STK11/LKB1 mutation; hamartomatous polyps with arborising smooth muscle bands; mucocutaneous melanin pigmentation; increased cancer risk), **juvenile polyposis syndrome** (SMAD4 or BMPR1A mutations; juvenile polyps with oedematous lamina propria and cystically dilated glands), **MUTYH-associated polyposis (MAP)** (autosomal recessive; biallelic MUTYH mutations; phenotype mimics attenuated FAP with 10 to 100 adenomas; also associated with serrated polyps and fundic gland polyps; CRC risk approximately 80% by age 60), and **serrated polyposis syndrome** (more than 5 serrated polyps proximal to rectum, at least 2 being 10 mm or more; OR more than 20 serrated polyps of any size; approximately 25% CRC risk).

Syndrome	Gene / Inheritance	Polyp Type	CRC Risk	Key Extracolonic Features
FAP	APC / AD	Adenomas (>100)	~100%	Desmoids, osteomas, duodenal

				adenomas, CHRPE
Attenuated FAP	APC / AD	Adenomas (10-100)	~70%	Similar to FAP but milder
MUTYH (MAP)	MUTYH / AR	Adenomas + serrated	~80%	Duodenal adenomas; fundic gland polyps
Lynch	MMR genes / AD	Adenomas (few)	40-80%	Endometrial, ovarian, urinary, gastric cancers
Peutz-Jeghers	STK11 / AD	Hamartomatous	~40%	Mucocutaneous melanin; breast, pancreas, GI cancers
Juvenile polyposis	SMAD4, BMPR1A / AD	Juvenile (hamartomatous)	40-50%	HHT if SMAD4 (epistaxis, AVM)
Serrated polyposis	Unknown / sporadic	Serrated (SSL, HP, TSA)	~25%	None

Table 19.2: Hereditary polyposis syndromes (Figure 19.3).

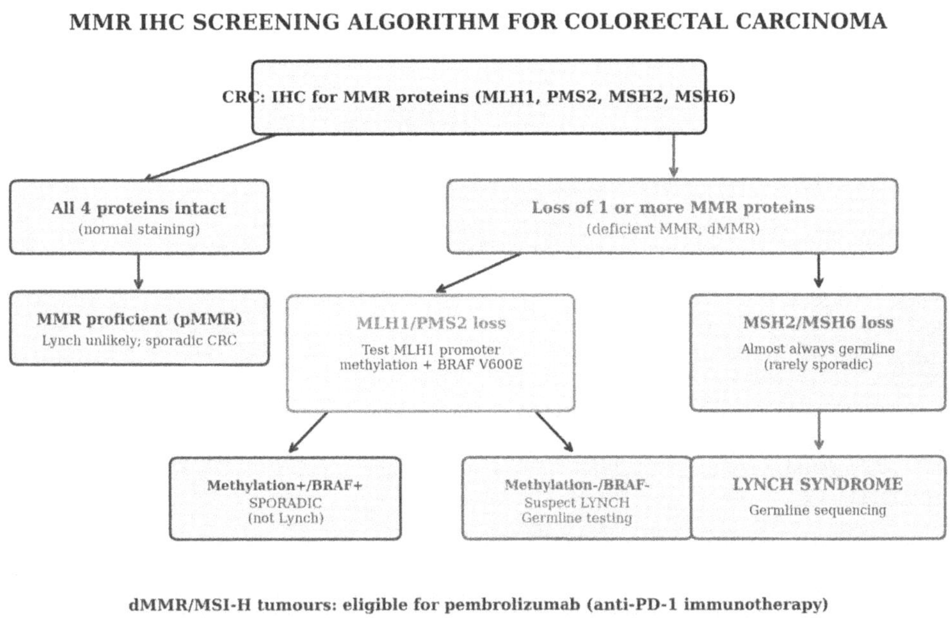

Figure 19.3: MMR immunohistochemistry screening algorithm for colorectal carcinoma. MMR intact indicates sporadic. MSH2/MSH6 or isolated PMS2 loss directs to probable Lynch syndrome and germline testing. MLH1/PMS2 loss requires BRAF V600E/methylation testing: positive indicates sporadic; negative indicates Lynch syndrome. (Source: Author's original.)

Exam Pitfall: Three Molecular Pathways of Colorectal Carcinogenesis

1. Chromosomal instability (CIN) pathway (~85%): APC → KRAS → TP53; conventional adenoma → carcinoma; microsatellite-stable; RAS mutations confer resistance to anti-EGFR therapy (cetuximab).

2. Microsatellite instability (MSI) pathway (~15%): Either sporadic (BRAF V600E → MLH1 methylation, from SSL) or Lynch (germline MMR mutation, from adenoma). MSI-high tumours have better prognosis and respond to checkpoint inhibitors (anti-PD-1).

3. POLE ultramutated pathway (~3%): POLE proofreading domain mutation; ultramutated; excellent prognosis; responsive to immunotherapy.

Quick Recall: Polyposis Syndromes and Molecular Pathways

FAP: APC germline mutation; >100 adenomas; 100% CRC risk; Gardner = osteomas + desmoids.

Lynch: MMR germline mutation; few adenomas, rapid progression; right-sided, mucinous, TILs.

Universal MMR IHC: All new CRC; MLH1/PMS2 loss → BRAF/methylation to distinguish sporadic vs Lynch.

CIN pathway: ~85%; APC→KRAS→TP53; microsatellite-stable; anti-EGFR resistance if RAS-mutant.

Serrated/MSI pathway: BRAF→SSL→MLH1 methylation→MSI-high; checkpoint inhibitor responsive.

Colorectal Carcinoma (Figure 19.4)

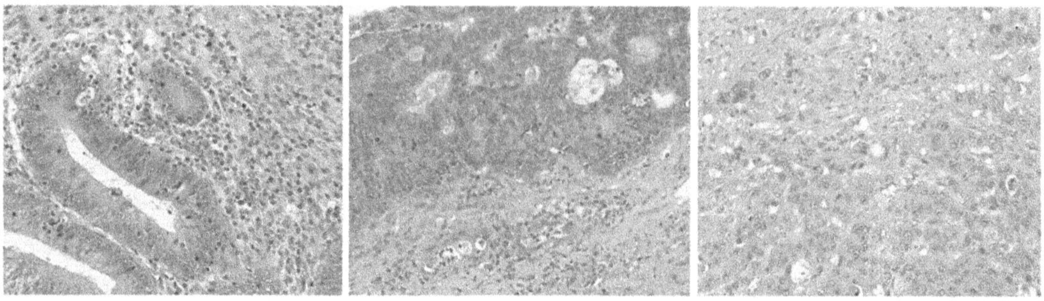

Figure 19.4: Colorectal adenocarcinoma grading (H&E). Left: well-differentiated (>95% gland formation). Centre: moderately differentiated (50\u201395% glands). Right: poorly differentiated (<50% glands, predominantly solid sheets). (Source: Mikael Häggström, Wikimedia Commons.)

Colorectal carcinoma (CRC) is the third most common cancer worldwide. In South Asia, CRC incidence is rising, particularly in urban populations, and patients tend to present at a younger age and more advanced stage than in Western countries. Urban registries report age-adjusted incidence rates of 4 to 6 per 100,000, with a notable increase in individuals under 40 years. Risk factors include processed meat, obesity, low-fibre diet, alcohol, smoking, and chronic IBD. Protective factors include aspirin/NSAIDs, physical activity, and dietary fibre.

Most CRCs are adenocarcinoma NOS with cribriform glands, dirty luminal necrosis, and desmoplastic stroma. Key subtypes: mucinous (>50% mucin; MSI-high enriched), signet ring cell (>50% signet ring cells; worst prognosis; Lynch-associated), medullary (BRAF-mutant, MSI-high; better prognosis despite undifferentiated appearance), and micropapillary (aggressive, early nodal metastasis).

Grading uses gland formation in the least differentiated component: low-grade (well to moderately differentiated, more than 50% gland formation) versus high-grade (poorly differentiated, less than 50% gland formation). Staging follows the AJCC 8th Edition TNM system. Key histological parameters beyond T stage include **tumour budding** (single cells or clusters of fewer than 5 cells at the invasive front; high budding is a significant adverse prognostic factor, representing epithelial-mesenchymal transition), **poorly differentiated clusters** (clusters of 5 or more cells without gland formation), and **extramural venous invasion** (tumour in veins beyond the muscularis propria; risk factor for hepatic metastasis; elastin stain (EVG) may help identify).

The key diagnostic clue when assessing a 'malignant polyp' (adenoma with invasive carcinoma into submucosa) is to evaluate the high-risk features: high-grade histology, positive/close margin (less than 1 mm), lymphovascular invasion, high tumour budding, and deep submucosal invasion (more than 2 mm). If any are present, colectomy with lymph node dissection is recommended rather than endoscopic management alone.

Biomarker	Method	Clinical Utility

MMR/MSI	IHC (MLH1, MSH2, MSH6, PMS2); PCR	Prognosis (MSI-H = better); Lynch screening; immunotherapy eligibility
RAS (KRAS, NRAS)	NGS or PCR	RAS-mutant = anti-EGFR resistance (cetuximab/panitumumab)
BRAF V600E	IHC or molecular	Poor prognosis if MSS; distinguish sporadic from Lynch if MLH1 lost
HER2	IHC/FISH	HER2-amplified = targeted therapy (trastuzumab) in RAS-WT metastatic CRC
NTRK fusions	IHC (pan-TRK)/FISH/NGS	Tumour-agnostic: larotrectinib/entrectinib

Table 19.3: Molecular biomarkers in colorectal carcinoma.

T Stage	Definition
pTis	Carcinoma in situ (HGD) or intramucosal carcinoma (lamina propria only)
pT1	Tumour invades submucosa (through muscularis mucosae)
pT2	Tumour invades muscularis propria
pT3	Tumour invades through muscularis propria into pericolorectal tissues
pT4a	Tumour perforates visceral peritoneum (including through inflammation)
pT4b	Tumour directly invades or adheres to adjacent organs/structures

Table 19.4: T staging of colorectal adenocarcinoma (AJCC 8th Edition). Note: pTis in the colon includes intramucosal carcinoma because the colonic mucosa has negligible metastatic risk.

Pseudo-invasion (misplaced epithelium) is an important mimic of submucosal invasion in colonic polyps, particularly pedunculated left-sided adenomas. It results from mechanical herniation of adenomatous epithelium into the submucosa through the stalk. Features favouring pseudo-invasion include: rounded, well-circumscribed nests without cytological atypia, surrounded by lamina propria (not desmoplastic stroma), haemosiderin-laden macrophages, and an inflamed/fibrotic background. True invasion shows desmoplastic stromal reaction, infiltrative/irregular glands, and cytological atypia without accompanying lamina propria.

The Pathologist's Eye: Assessing the Peritoneal Surface in CRC Resections

Determining pT4a (tumour penetrating the visceral peritoneum) versus pT3 (tumour in pericolorectal fat but not reaching the serosa) is one of the most prognostically important assessments in CRC pathology. Even if tumour does not directly touch the serosal surface, if it is continuous with the surface through a band of inflammation, it qualifies as pT4a. If tumour is close to but not reaching the surface (less than 1 mm), additional levels and sections should be examined, as understaging at this threshold affects adjuvant therapy decisions. Peritoneal elastic stain can help identify the peritoneal surface in difficult cases.

A viva hook to consider: Why is the distinction between pT3 and pT4a so critical in CRC? Because pT4a (peritoneal breach) shifts the stage from potentially curable stage II to stage IIC with a 5-year survival approximately 20% lower, and is an absolute indication for adjuvant chemotherapy, whereas some pT3 patients (stage IIA/B) with favourable features (MSI-H, no LVI, no high budding) may safely avoid chemotherapy.

Quick Recall: Colorectal Carcinoma

Essential/Desirable: Diagnostic Criteria -- Colorectal Adenocarcinoma

Essential: Invasive glandular neoplasm through muscularis mucosae into submucosa (intramucosal carcinoma in the colorectum is managed as high-grade dysplasia, not carcinoma).

Desirable: CK20+/CK7-; CDX2+; MMR IHC on all new CRCs (universal testing); KRAS/NRAS/BRAF status; tumour budding and lymphovascular invasion reported.

Essential/Desirable: Diagnostic Criteria -- Sessile Serrated Lesion (SSL)

Essential: Architectural distortion of ≥1 crypt: dilated crypt base, horizontal extension along muscularis mucosae, boot-shaped or L-shaped or inverted T-shaped crypts, serration extending to crypt base.

Desirable: BRAF V600E mutation; MLH1 promoter methylation (in SSL with dysplasia); right-sided predominance; absence of cytological dysplasia in uncomplicated SSL.

Grading: Low-grade (>50% glands) vs high-grade (<50% glands); based on worst area.

Tumour budding: Single cells/<5 cell clusters at invasive front; high budding = poor prognosis.

MMR testing: Universal on all new CRC; MSI-H = better prognosis + immunotherapy eligible.

RAS testing: KRAS/NRAS mutant = anti-EGFR resistant; test all metastatic CRC.

Mucinous CRC: >50% extracellular mucin; enriched for MSI-high; not inherently worse prognosis.

Ulcerative Lesions of the Intestines

The differential diagnosis of ulcerative lesions of the intestines is among the most frequently examined topics in postgraduate pathology examinations. The pathologist confronted with intestinal ulcers on biopsy or resection must integrate the clinical history, endoscopic findings, distribution, ulcer morphology, and histological features to arrive at a specific diagnosis. In TB-endemic and tropical settings, this differential is particularly complex because tuberculosis, amoebic colitis, and typhoid fever are common and frequently mimic inflammatory bowel disease.

When faced with intestinal ulceration on biopsy, the first question to ask is: What is the distribution (ileocaecal, segmental, diffuse, rectal), what is the ulcer morphology (superficial vs deep fissuring vs transverse vs circumferential), and is there granulomatous inflammation?

Condition	Site	Ulcer Pattern	Key Histology	Granulomas	Distinguishing Feature
Crohn disease	Ileocaecal, any GI; skip lesions	Deep fissuring, 'knife-cut'; aphthous	Focal chronic active inflammation; transmural	Non-caseating (30-60%)	Skip lesions; fistulae; focally enhanced gastritis
Ulcerative colitis	Rectum → continuous proximal	Superficial, broad-based; pseudopolyps	Diffuse mucosal inflammation; crypt distortion	Absent (crypt-rupture only)	Continuous from rectum; basal plasmacytosis
Intestinal TB	Ileocaecal; circumferential	Transverse (perpendicular to long axis)	Submucosal granulomas; caseation	Large, confluent, caseating	Caseation; >5 per section; AFB/GeneXpert
Typhoid	Ileal Peyer patches; longitudinal	Oval, along long axis; 'punched out'	Typhoid nodules (macrophage aggregates)	Absent	Longitudinal ulcers over Peyer patches; erythrophagocytosis
Amoebic colitis	Caecum, ascending colon	Flask-shaped; undermined edges	Trophozoites with ingested RBCs; minimal inflammation	Absent	PAS-positive trophozoites; minimal neutrophils
NSAID enteropathy	Small bowel; 'diaphragm disease'	Circumferential; thin web-like strictures	Submucosal fibrosis; minimal inflammation	Absent	Diaphragm-like strictures; medication history
Ischaemic colitis	Watershed areas (splenic flexure)	Longitudinal; mucosal	'Ghost crypts'; coagulative necrosis; haemosiderin	Absent	Elderly; cardiovascular disease; watershed distribution
Behcet	Ileocaecal	Deep, round,	Vasculitis;	Absent	Oral/genital ulcers;

disease		'punched out'	deep ulceration without granulomas		pathergy; vasculitis
CMV colitis	Any; often right colon	Deep, irregular	Owl-eye nuclear inclusions; granular cytoplasmic inclusions	Absent	Immunosuppressed; CMV IHC confirms
Lymphoma	Ileum (B-cell); jejunum (T-cell)	Large, irregular; may be annular	Atypical lymphoid infiltrate; destructive pattern	Absent	IHC for lineage; EATL if celiac-associated

Table 19.5: Differential diagnosis of ulcerative lesions of the intestines.

Typhoid ulcers deserve specific mention because of their distinctive longitudinal orientation, aligned along the long axis of the bowel over the Peyer patches of the terminal ileum. The ulcers progress through a predictable sequence: (1) first week, lymphoid hyperplasia of Peyer patches; (2) second week, necrosis and ulceration; (3) third week, ulcer base deepens (risk of perforation and haemorrhage); (4) fourth week, healing with scarring. Histologically, the lamina propria and submucosa show aggregates of 'typhoid cells' (activated macrophages with erythrophagocytosis) forming typhoid nodules. Granulomas are absent. Blood culture is positive in the first week; Widal test has limited specificity and should not be used as the sole diagnostic criterion in endemic areas (see Chapter 9).

Amoebic colitis is caused by Entamoeba histolytica and is common in tropical regions. The classic histological finding is flask-shaped ulcers with undermined edges, where the ulcer is narrow at the mucosal surface but widens in the submucosa. The base shows necrotic debris with surprisingly scant inflammatory infiltrate (amoebiasis characteristically elicits minimal neutrophilic response). The diagnostic finding is identification of trophozoites with ingested erythrocytes (erythrophagocytosis), which are PAS-positive. Trophozoites are found at the advancing edge of the ulcer, at the junction of viable and necrotic tissue. The differential from Crohn disease is important: amoebic colitis shows flask-shaped ulcers without granulomas or transmural inflammation, and the clinical presentation is acute dysentery rather than chronic relapsing course. Complications include hepatic abscess (see Chapter 20) and toxic megacolon.

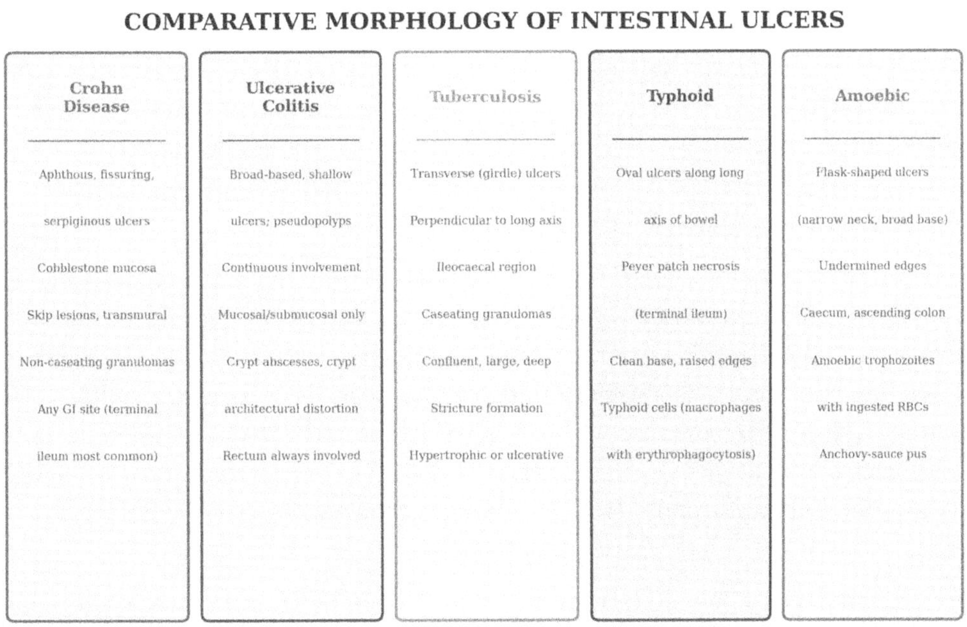

Figure 19.5: Comparative morphology of intestinal ulcers. (A) Crohn disease: deep fissuring longitudinal ulcer; (B) Ulcerative colitis: superficial broad-based ulcer; (C) Tuberculosis: transverse circumferential ulcer; (D) Typhoid: longitudinal ulcer over Peyer patch; (E) Amoebiasis: flask-shaped undermined ulcer. (Source: Author's original.)

Exam Pitfall: Ulcer Orientation as a Diagnostic Clue

Crohn disease: Longitudinal fissuring ulcers (along the long axis), producing 'cobblestone' mucosa.

Tuberculosis: Transverse ulcers (perpendicular to the long axis), circumferential, following lymphatic drainage.

Typhoid: Longitudinal ulcers (along the long axis), but aligned specifically over Peyer patches.

The orientation of the ulcer is a key gross finding that narrows the differential before microscopy. Never confuse TB transverse ulcers with Crohn longitudinal ulcers.

Quick Recall: Ulcerative Lesions

Crohn: Skip lesions, deep fissuring ulcers, non-caseating granulomas, fistulae.

UC: Continuous from rectum, superficial broad ulcers, crypt distortion, no granulomas.

TB: Transverse circumferential ulcers, large caseating granulomas, AFB/GeneXpert.

Typhoid: Longitudinal over Peyer patches, typhoid nodules, erythrophagocytosis.

Amoebic: Flask-shaped undermined ulcers, trophozoites with ingested RBCs, minimal inflammation.

Ischaemic: Watershed areas, ghost crypts, haemosiderin, coagulative necrosis.

Inflammatory Bowel Disease

Pathogenesis of IBD

Inflammatory bowel disease (IBD) encompasses two major chronic, relapsing conditions: **Crohn disease (CD)** and **ulcerative colitis (UC)**. Both result from a dysregulated immune response to intestinal microbiota in genetically susceptible individuals, modulated by environmental triggers. The pathogenesis involves four interconnected elements: genetic susceptibility, epithelial barrier dysfunction, dysbiotic microbiome, and aberrant immune activation.

Genome-wide association studies have identified over 200 susceptibility loci. The strongest genetic risk factor for Crohn disease is **NOD2/CARD15** (chromosome 16q12), an intracellular innate immunity receptor that senses muramyl dipeptide from bacterial peptidoglycan. Loss-of-function NOD2 mutations impair the mucosal innate immune response to commensal bacteria, paradoxically leading to excessive adaptive immune activation. Other key susceptibility genes include **ATG16L1** and **IRGM** (autophagy pathway; defective bacterial clearance in Paneth cells), **IL-23R** (Th17 differentiation), and **HLA-DRB1** (antigen presentation). UC shows stronger HLA associations, reflecting a greater contribution of adaptive immunity.

Genetic susceptibility (NOD2, ATG16L1, IL-23R) → Barrier dysfunction → Dysbiotic microbiome → Aberrant Th1/Th17 (CD) or Th2 (UC) response → Chronic mucosal inflammation

The **epithelial barrier** is compromised in IBD: tight junction proteins (claudins, occludin) are downregulated, mucus layer thickness is reduced (particularly in UC), and Paneth cell defensin production is impaired (particularly in ileal CD). This allows translocation of luminal bacteria into the lamina propria, triggering innate immune activation through pattern recognition receptors (TLRs, NOD-like receptors). In Crohn disease, the immune response is predominantly Th1/Th17-driven (IL-12, IFN-gamma, IL-17, IL-23), while in UC it is Th2-driven (IL-4, IL-5, IL-13). These cytokine profiles explain differential therapeutic responses: anti-TNF (infliximab) works in both; anti-IL-12/23 (ustekinumab) and anti-IL-23 (risankizumab) are particularly effective in CD; JAK inhibitors (tofacitinib) are approved for UC.

Integration: The pathogenesis of IBD involves innate immunity receptors (NOD2), connecting to Chapter 2 (Inflammation), and adaptive immune dysregulation (Th1/Th17 vs Th2), connecting to Chapter 5 (Diseases of the Immune System). The autophagy defects (ATG16L1) link to Chapter 1 (Cell Injury). Extraintestinal manifestations (primary sclerosing cholangitis, erythema nodosum, pyoderma gangrenosum) connect to Chapters 20 (Hepatobiliary) and 28 (Dermatopathology).

Feature	Crohn Disease	Ulcerative Colitis
Distribution	Any GI tract (mouth to anus); skip lesions	Rectum → continuous proximal extension; colon only
Depth	Transmural inflammation	Mucosal and submucosal only

Granulomas	Non-caseating granulomas (30-60%)	Absent (crypt rupture granulomas excluded)
Ulcers	Deep, fissuring, 'knife-cut'; aphthous ulcers	Superficial, broad-based; pseudopolyps
Fistulae	Common (perianal, enteroenteric, enterovesical)	Rare
Terminal ileum	Commonly involved	Usually spared (backwash ileitis only)
Crypt architecture	Focal distortion	Diffuse distortion, branching, shortening
Goblet cell depletion	Focal or absent	Diffuse
Paneth cell metaplasia	Rare	Common (in left colon)
Submucosal fibrosis	Prominent	Minimal
Key molecular pathway	Th1/Th17; NOD2; ATG16L1	Th2; HLA-DRB1; IL-13
Key complication	Strictures, fistulae, malabsorption	Toxic megacolon, haemorrhage
Cancer risk	Increased (small bowel and colon)	Increased (colon; proportional to extent and duration)

Table 19.6: Crohn disease versus ulcerative colitis: comprehensive comparison.

Crohn Disease: Histological Features in Detail

On mucosal biopsy, Crohn disease shows a characteristic pattern of **focal (patchy) chronic active inflammation** with intervening normal mucosa, in contrast to the diffuse continuous involvement of UC. The earliest lesion is the **aphthous ulcer**, a small superficial ulcer overlying a lymphoid follicle. Non-caseating epithelioid granulomas (found in 30 to 60% of biopsies) are the histological hallmark but are not required for diagnosis. Granulomas may be found in the mucosa, submucosa, or even lymph nodes. Other features include focal architectural distortion, pyloric gland metaplasia in the ileum, focal enhanced gastritis in upper GI biopsies (a useful supportive finding), and neural hypertrophy with transmural lymphoid aggregates on resection specimens.

Ulcerative Colitis: Histological Features and Activity Scoring

In UC, the hallmark is diffuse, continuous mucosal and submucosal inflammation beginning at the rectum and extending proximally without skip lesions. The key chronic changes include diffuse crypt architectural distortion (branching, shortening, dropout), **basal plasmacytosis** (plasma cells between the crypt bases and the muscularis mucosae, one of the earliest and most reliable features), goblet cell depletion, and Paneth cell metaplasia in the left colon (an indicator of chronic mucosal injury and regeneration). Active disease shows neutrophilic cryptitis (neutrophils infiltrating crypt epithelium), crypt abscesses (neutrophils filling and distending crypt lumens), and surface erosion or ulceration.

The **Geboes score** grades histological activity on a 0 to 5 scale: grade 0 (structural changes only), grade 1 (chronic inflammation), grade 2 (lamina propria neutrophils), grade 3 (neutrophils in epithelium/cryptitis), grade 4 (crypt destruction/crypt abscess), grade 5 (erosion/ulceration). The **Nancy index** is a validated 5-grade system (0 to 4) focused on three features: ulceration, acute inflammatory infiltrate, and chronic inflammatory infiltrate. Histological remission (Geboes <2, Nancy 0) is now recognised as a treatment target beyond endoscopic remission, as persistent histological activity predicts relapse.

Interpretation of Ileal Biopsies

Terminal ileal biopsies are routinely taken during colonoscopy and their interpretation is frequently examined. The normal terminal ileum shows villi with Peyer patches (organised lymphoid aggregates). A systematic approach to abnormal ileal biopsies includes assessment of villous architecture (blunting suggests chronic injury: Crohn, NSAID enteropathy, celiac disease), inflammation pattern (active ileitis with neutrophils in Crohn, infections such as Yersinia, Salmonella, Campylobacter, TB, CMV, and NSAID injury), granulomas (non-caseating favouring Crohn or Yersinia; large caseating favouring TB), and special features (lymphoid hyperplasia, eosinophilic infiltration, viral inclusions).

When faced with ileal biopsies showing granulomatous inflammation in a patient from a TB-endemic region, the three most important differential diagnoses are, in order: (1) intestinal TB, (2) Crohn disease, and (3) Yersinia infection. The granuloma characteristics (size, caseation, number, location) combined with AFB stain and GeneXpert on biopsy tissue are the cornerstones of distinction.

Dysplasia Surveillance in IBD

Long-standing colitis (more than 8 years, extensive disease) carries a significantly increased risk of colorectal carcinoma: approximately 2% at 10 years, 8% at 20 years, and 18% at 30 years for UC. The risk is proportional to disease extent (pancolitis > left-sided > proctitis), duration, severity of inflammation, presence of primary sclerosing cholangitis (strongest independent risk factor), and family history of CRC.

Dysplasia in IBD is classified as **low-grade dysplasia (LGD)** or **high-grade dysplasia (HGD)**. Indefinite for dysplasia is used when reactive/regenerative changes in an inflamed background cannot be confidently distinguished from true dysplasia. Current guidelines recommend chromoendoscopy-guided targeted biopsies, which have largely replaced the older protocol of random four-quadrant biopsies every 10 cm.

p53 immunohistochemistry is a valuable adjunct in equivocal biopsies. Three abnormal p53 patterns support dysplasia: (1) **overexpression** (strong, diffuse nuclear staining in >50% of crypt epithelium, indicating TP53 missense mutation), (2) **null pattern** (complete absence of staining, indicating TP53 deletion/nonsense mutation), and (3) **cytoplasmic pattern** (rare, aberrant). Normal/wild-type p53 shows scattered weak-to-moderate nuclear staining in the proliferative zone. An abnormal p53 pattern in a morphologically equivocal biopsy supports upgrading to at least low-grade dysplasia. Colitis-associated carcinoma tends to be multifocal, mucinous, and signet ring cell type more frequently than sporadic CRC.

Extraintestinal Manifestations and Complications of IBD

Both Crohn disease and ulcerative colitis are associated with extraintestinal manifestations affecting the joints (seronegative arthritis, ankylosing spondylitis), skin (erythema nodosum in Crohn; pyoderma gangrenosum in UC), eyes (uveitis, episcleritis), liver (primary sclerosing cholangitis, strongly associated with UC), and the biliary tract. PSC-IBD patients carry a particularly high risk of cholangiocarcinoma and colorectal carcinoma, requiring annual surveillance colonoscopy from the time of PSC diagnosis regardless of colitis duration.

Complications specific to Crohn disease include strictures (fibrostenotic disease causing bowel obstruction), fistulae (perianal, enteroenteric, enterovesical, enterocutaneous), intra-abdominal abscess formation, and malabsorption (especially B12 and bile salts when the terminal ileum is affected). Complications specific to ulcerative colitis include toxic megacolon (acute dilatation with impending perforation; mucosal denudation and transmural necrosis on histology; requires emergent colectomy) and massive haemorrhage.

Complication	Crohn Disease	Ulcerative Colitis
Stricture	Common (fibrosis + inflammation)	Rare; if present, exclude carcinoma
Fistula	Common (perianal, enteric, cutaneous)	Rare
Toxic megacolon	Uncommon	Classic complication; mucosal denudation
Cancer risk	Small bowel + colon	Colon (proportional to extent and duration)
PSC association	Uncommon	Strong (up to 5%); increases CRC risk further
Malabsorption	Common (ileal B12, bile salts)	Rare

Table 19.7: Complications of Crohn disease versus ulcerative colitis.

Quick Recall: IBD

Crohn: Transmural; skip lesions; non-caseating granulomas; fissuring ulcers; fistulae; NOD2/CARD15.

UC: Mucosal; continuous from rectum; crypt distortion; basal plasmacytosis; goblet cell depletion; Paneth cell metaplasia.

IBD dysplasia: >8 years extensive colitis; p53 IHC (overexpression or null pattern) helpful; chromoendoscopy surveillance.

TB vs Crohn in TB-endemic regions: Large caseating granulomas = TB; small non-caseating = Crohn; AFB/GeneXpert essential.

Never start immunosuppression for presumed Crohn in TB-endemic regions without excluding TB (ATT trial if doubt).

Histological remission: Geboes <2 or Nancy 0; treatment target beyond endoscopic remission.

Celiac Disease

Celiac disease (gluten-sensitive enteropathy) is an immune-mediated disorder triggered by dietary gluten (wheat, barley, rye) in genetically susceptible individuals carrying HLA-DQ2 (90%) or HLA-DQ8 (10%). It affects approximately 0.5 to 1% of the population globally. In wheat-belt regions of South Asia, prevalence approaches Western figures, reflecting the wheat-based diet, while it is comparatively underdiagnosed in rice-belt regions.

The pathogenesis involves both adaptive and innate immune mechanisms. Tissue transglutaminase (tTG) deamidates gliadin peptides, creating negatively charged epitopes that bind HLA-DQ2/DQ8 on antigen-presenting cells, triggering a CD4+ T-cell Th1 response with production of IFN-gamma. Simultaneously, gliadin peptides activate the innate immune system through IL-15, driving intraepithelial lymphocyte (IEL) expansion and epithelial cytotoxicity. The combined effect is villous atrophy with crypt hyperplasia.

The **Modified Marsh-Oberhuber classification** grades the histological severity: Type 0 (normal, pre-infiltrative), Type 1 (increased IELs, >25 per 100 enterocytes, with normal villous architecture), Type 2 (increased IELs plus crypt hyperplasia), Type 3a (partial villous atrophy), Type 3b (subtotal villous atrophy), Type 3c (total villous atrophy). The biopsy should be taken from the second part of the duodenum (D2, at least 4 biopsies) and the duodenal bulb (1-2 biopsies). *The distinction between celiac disease and other causes of villous atrophy (tropical sprue, autoimmune enteropathy, common variable immunodeficiency, NSAID enteropathy, Whipple disease) rests on the combination of serology (anti-tTG IgA, anti-endomysial antibodies), HLA typing, clinical response to gluten-free diet, and biopsy features.*

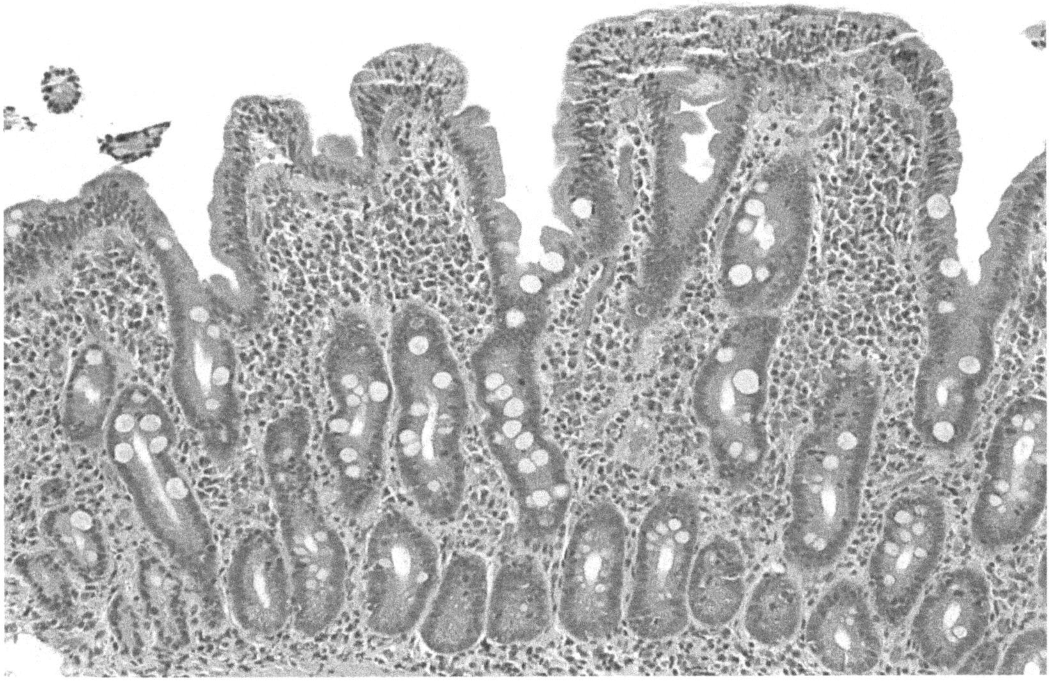

Figure 19.6: Coeliac disease (Marsh 3). Villous atrophy with crypt hyperplasia and markedly increased intraepithelial lymphocytes (>25/100 enterocytes) within a flattened mucosa (H&E, high mag). (Source: Nephron, Wikimedia Commons, CC BY-SA 3.0.)

Complications of celiac disease include refractory celiac disease (type I: polyclonal IELs; type II: monoclonal aberrant IELs, pre-lymphoma), **enteropathy-associated T-cell lymphoma (EATL)** (see GI lymphomas below), and an increased risk of small bowel adenocarcinoma. Dermatitis herpetiformis is the cutaneous manifestation (see Chapter 28).

> **Quick Recall: Celiac Disease**
>
> **Genetics:** HLA-DQ2 (90%) or HLA-DQ8 (10%).
>
> **Key enzyme:** Tissue transglutaminase (tTG) deamidates gliadin → T-cell activation.
>
> **Serology:** Anti-tTG IgA (screening); anti-endomysial IgA (confirmatory); check total IgA (IgA deficiency = false negative).
>
> **Marsh 3c:** Total villous atrophy + crypt hyperplasia + >25 IELs/100 enterocytes.
>
> **Complications:** Refractory CD (type II = pre-lymphoma); EATL; small bowel adenocarcinoma.

Other Colonic Inflammatory Conditions

Ischaemic Colitis

Definition: Colonic ischaemia due to reduced blood flow, most commonly affecting watershed areas (splenic flexure, rectosigmoid junction). Most common form of intestinal ischaemia.

Etiology: Elderly patients with cardiovascular disease, hypotension, mesenteric atherosclerosis, post-surgical low-flow states.

Pathogenesis: Reduced mesenteric blood flow → Mucosal ischaemia (watershed areas) → Coagulative necrosis of surface epithelium → **'Ghost crypts'** (necrotic crypt outlines) → Haemosiderin deposition → Chronic: fibrosis and stricture

Microscopy:

- Acute: Mucosal haemorrhage, oedema, superficial coagulative necrosis with **'ghost' outlines of necrotic crypts** and hyalinised lamina propria.

- Chronic: Fibrosis with stricture formation; haemosiderin-laden macrophages.

- Transmural infarction (gangrenous bowel): full-thickness necrosis requiring emergent surgical resection.

Key DDx vs IBD: Distribution (watershed areas, not rectum), acute onset, presence of ghost crypts and haemosiderin, absence of chronic architectural distortion.

Exam yield: ★★ MODERATE — appears in ulcerative lesions DDx tables.

Microscopic Colitis

Two subtypes with normal endoscopic appearance but chronic watery diarrhoea. Associated with autoimmune conditions and medications (NSAIDs, PPIs, SSRIs). Treatment: budesonide.

COLLAGENOUS COLITIS

Definition: Thickened subepithelial collagen band (>10 μm) with surface epithelial damage and chronic inflammation.

Microscopy: Subepithelial collagen band >10 μm (normal <5 μm), highlighted by **Masson trichrome stain**. Surface epithelial flattening, detachment, and damage. Chronic inflammatory infiltrate in lamina propria.

LYMPHOCYTIC COLITIS

Definition: Increased intraepithelial lymphocytes (>20 per 100 surface epithelial cells) with surface epithelial damage but normal collagen band.

Microscopy: Increased surface IELs (>20/100 epithelial cells), surface epithelial damage, normal collagen thickness. Chronic lamina propria inflammation.

Key DDx: Celiac disease can also show increased IELs; check serology and duodenal biopsies.

Pseudomembranous Colitis

Definition: Antibiotic-associated colitis caused by Clostridioides difficile toxins A and B. Most common cause of nosocomial diarrhoea.

Pathogenesis: Antibiotic therapy → Disruption of colonic microbiome → C. difficile overgrowth → Toxin A (enterotoxin) + Toxin B (cytotoxin) production → Mucosal damage → Pseudomembrane formation

Microscopy: Hallmark finding: **volcano-like pseudomembrane ('summit lesion')** — mushroom-shaped eruption of fibrin, mucus, neutrophils, and cellular debris emerging from a damaged crypt. Intervening mucosa may be relatively preserved.

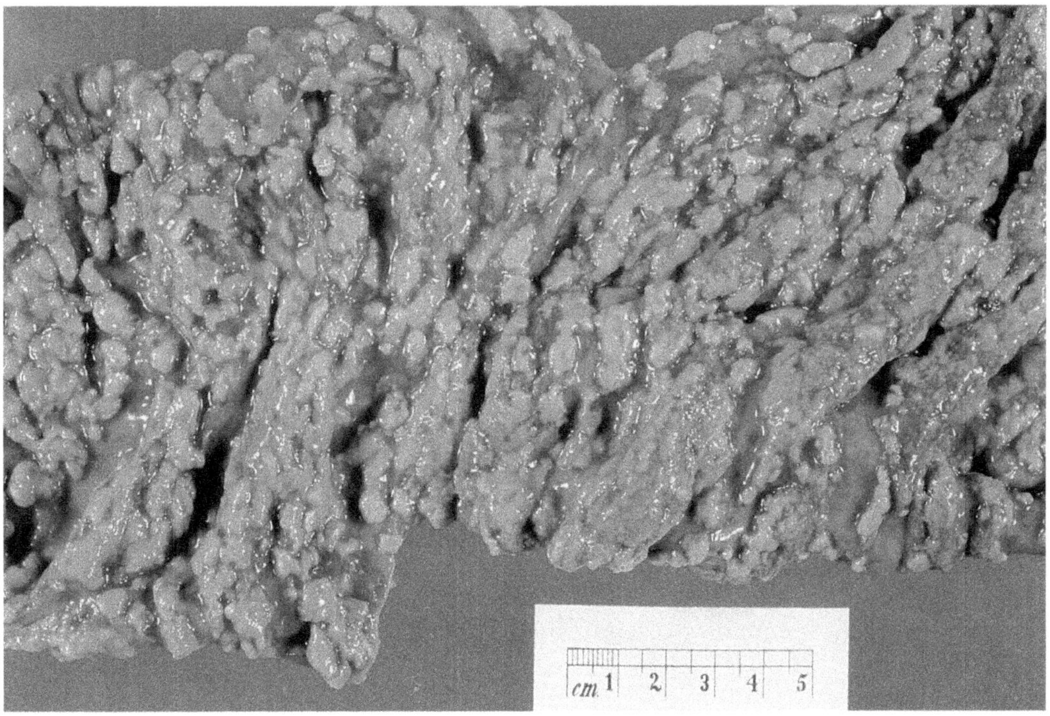

Figure 19.7A: Pseudomembranous colitis (Clostridioides difficile) — gross. Colonic mucosa studded with adherent yellow-tan pseudomembranous plaques of fibrin, mucin, and neutrophilic exudate. (Source: Narraburra, Wikimedia Commons, CC0.)

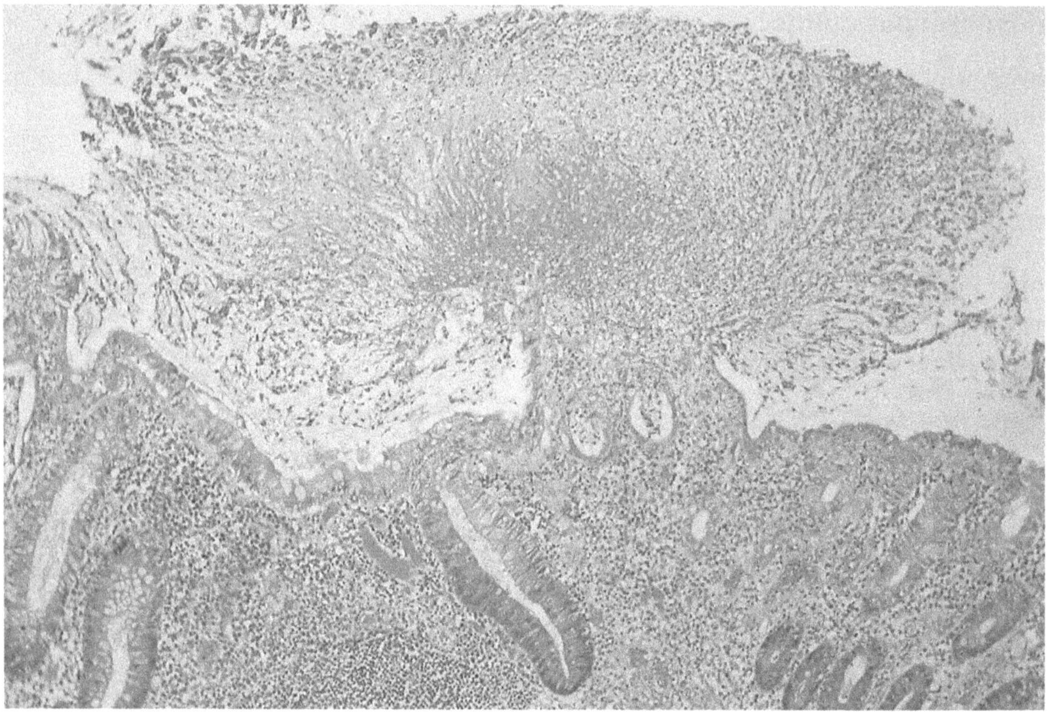

Figure 19.7B: Pseudomembranous colitis (H&E). Characteristic "volcano" summit lesion — mushroom-shaped exudate of fibrin, mucin, and neutrophils erupting from a damaged crypt onto the luminal surface. (Source: Ed Uthman, Flickr/Wikimedia Commons, CC BY 2.0.)

Diagnosis: Stool PCR for C. difficile toxin genes; GDH screening assay followed by toxin EIA confirmation.

Complications: Severe cases progress to toxic megacolon.

Exam yield: ★★★ HIGH — summit/volcano lesion is a classic viva and MCQ image.

Diverticular Disease

Definition: Acquired pseudodiverticula — herniations of mucosa and submucosa through the muscularis propria at points where vasa recta penetrate the bowel wall.

Epidemiology: Extremely common in Western populations (>50% of individuals over 60 years). Sigmoid colon predominance in Western populations; **right-sided predominance in Asian populations**.

Microscopy: Mucosal and submucosal herniation through muscularis propria defect. Muscularis propria adjacent to diverticula shows thickening (**myochosis**). No muscularis propria in the wall of the diverticulum (pseudodiverticulum).

Complications: Diverticulitis, haemorrhage, stricture, fistula formation, perforation with peritonitis.

Exam yield: ★★ MODERATE — definition of true vs pseudo-diverticulum is a classic viva question.

Quick Recall: Other Colonic Inflammatory Conditions

Ischaemic colitis: Watershed areas; ghost crypts; haemosiderin; elderly; cardiovascular disease.

Collagenous colitis: Collagen band >10 µm; normal endoscopy; watery diarrhoea; budesonide treatment.

Lymphocytic colitis: IELs >20/100 epithelial cells; normal endoscopy; NSAID/PPI associated.

C. difficile colitis: Pseudomembrane (volcano/summit lesion); antibiotic-associated; toxin A and B.

Diverticular disease: Pseudodiverticula; sigmoid (West), right-sided (Asia/India); myochosis.

Small Bowel Pathology

Small bowel adenocarcinoma is rare (duodenum > jejunum); risk factors include celiac disease, Crohn, FAP, and Lynch. Meckel diverticulum (rule of 2s): complications include haemorrhage from ectopic gastric mucosa, intussusception, and diverticulitis. Radiation enteritis: acute (crypt apoptosis) and chronic (obliterative vasculopathy, submucosal fibrosis, strictures).**Small bowel adenocarcinoma** is rare, arising most commonly in the duodenum (particularly periampullary) and jejunum. Risk factors include celiac disease, Crohn disease (ileal adenocarcinoma), FAP (duodenal adenomas), Lynch syndrome, and Peutz-Jeghers syndrome. **Meckel diverticulum** is a true diverticulum, the remnant of the vitelline duct, governed by the 'rule of 2s': 2% of population, 2 feet from ileocaecal valve, 2 inches long, 2 types of ectopic mucosa (gastric most common, pancreatic). Complications include haemorrhage from ectopic gastric acid secretion, intussusception, and Meckel diverticulitis mimicking appendicitis. The small bowel is also affected by **radiation enteritis** (acute: mucosal injury with crypt apoptosis; chronic: obliterative vasculopathy with submucosal fibrosis and telangiectasia, producing strictures and malabsorption).

Primary Gastrointestinal Lymphomas

The GI tract is the most common site of extranodal lymphoma, accounting for 30 to 40% of all extranodal non-Hodgkin lymphomas. Primary GI lymphomas are defined as lymphomas presenting with predominant GI involvement, and are staged by the Lugano system. The stomach is the most common GI site overall, but the small bowel and ileocaecal region are the most common sites for primary intestinal lymphoma (see Chapter 18 for gastric MALT lymphoma).

Diffuse large B-cell lymphoma (DLBCL) is the most common GI lymphoma subtype, presenting as large masses or ulcerated lesions. It can arise de novo or through transformation from a low-grade MALT lymphoma. Histology shows sheets of large atypical lymphoid cells with vesicular nuclei, prominent nucleoli, and frequent mitoses. IHC: CD20+, CD10/BCL6/MUM1 for cell-of-origin classification. **Extranodal marginal zone lymphoma (MALT lymphoma)** of the intestine resembles gastric MALT lymphoma but is less clearly linked to a specific infectious agent. Immunoproliferative small intestinal disease (IPSID, 'alpha heavy chain disease'), endemic in the Middle East and Mediterranean, is a variant of intestinal MALT lymphoma producing truncated alpha heavy chains.

Enteropathy-associated T-cell lymphoma (EATL) is a high-grade T-cell lymphoma of the jejunum, strongly associated with refractory celiac disease (type II). The tumour shows large pleomorphic lymphoid cells with necrosis and ulceration. IHC: CD3+, CD7+, CD103+, CD30+ (variable), CD4−, CD8−

(often double-negative). EATL type II (now termed monomorphic epitheliotropic intestinal T-cell lymphoma, MEITL) shows monomorphic medium-sized cells, is CD8+/CD56+, and is not associated with celiac disease. **Mantle cell lymphoma** can present as multiple lymphomatous polyposis of the GI tract, mimicking FAP endoscopically. Diagnosis relies on CD5+/CD20+/Cyclin D1+ immunophenotype and t(11;14) confirmation. **Burkitt lymphoma** presents in the ileocaecal region, especially in endemic (African) and immunodeficiency-associated forms. The classic 'starry sky' pattern with high Ki-67 (approaching 100%) and MYC translocation t(8;14) are diagnostic.

The key diagnostic clue when a lymphoma is suspected on GI biopsy is a destructive, monomorphic lymphoid infiltrate that effaces the mucosal architecture. Always request a broad IHC panel (CD20, CD3, CD5, CD10, CD30, cyclin D1, Ki-67) and consider flow cytometry on fresh tissue for lineage determination.

Gastrointestinal Neuroendocrine Tumours

Well-differentiated neuroendocrine tumours (NETs) of the GI tract arise from enteroendocrine cells distributed throughout the gut. They are classified by site and graded by the WHO system based on mitotic count and Ki-67 proliferation index: **G1** (mitoses <2/10 HPF, Ki-67 <3%), **G2** (mitoses 2-20/10 HPF, Ki-67 3-20%), and **G3** (mitoses >20/10 HPF, Ki-67 >20%). Poorly differentiated neuroendocrine carcinomas (NECs, small cell and large cell types) are high-grade by definition and biologically distinct from G3 NETs.

Histologically, well-differentiated NETs show nests, trabeculae, ribbons, or acini of uniform cells with 'salt-and-pepper' chromatin, inconspicuous nucleoli, and moderate eosinophilic cytoplasm. IHC: synaptophysin positive, chromogranin A positive, INSM1 positive. Cytokeratin shows characteristic perinuclear 'dot-like' staining. Site-specific considerations: small bowel (ileal) NETs are the most common site, frequently multifocal, and associated with carcinoid syndrome (serotonin secretion causing flushing, diarrhoea, wheezing, and right-sided valvular heart disease) when hepatic metastases bypass first-pass metabolism.

Integration: Gastric NETs (types I-III, see Chapter 18), carcinoid syndrome (right-sided heart disease connects to Chapter 14), and MEN1 syndrome (connects to Chapter 27, Endocrine Pathology). GI NET grading system applies across all GI sites.

Grade	Mitotic Rate (/10 HPF)	Ki-67 Index	Terminology
G1	<2	<3%	Well-differentiated NET, low-grade
G2	2-20	3-20%	Well-differentiated NET, intermediate-grade
G3	>20	>20%	Well-differentiated NET, high-grade
NEC	>20	>20%	Poorly differentiated NEC (small cell or

			large cell)

Table 19.8: WHO grading system for GI neuroendocrine neoplasms. Note the critical distinction between G3 NET (well-differentiated, retains organoid architecture) and NEC (poorly differentiated, sheet-like growth, TP53/RB1 mutations).

Appendiceal Pathology

ACUTE APPENDICITIS

Definition: Most common abdominal surgical emergency. Histological diagnosis requires **neutrophilic infiltration of the muscularis propria** (not just the mucosa, which can be reactive). Periappendicitis (serosal inflammation without mural involvement) suggests extra-appendiceal source (salpingitis, Meckel diverticulitis). Granulomatous appendicitis: Crohn, sarcoidosis, Yersinia, mycobacteria, foreign body.

Always examine the appendix tip for incidental tumours.

APPENDICEAL NEUROENDOCRINE TUMOUR

Definition: Most common appendiceal neoplasm (~1% of appendectomies). Typically at the tip; younger age than NETs elsewhere.

Management: <1 cm confined to appendix = excellent prognosis (>95% survival), appendectomy alone sufficient. 1–2 cm: assess LVI, mesoappendiceal invasion >3 mm, grade → right hemicolectomy if high-risk features.

LOW-GRADE APPENDICEAL MUCINOUS NEOPLASM (LAMN)

Definition: Mucinous neoplasm with pushing invasive front and loss of normal lamina propria/muscularis mucosae (replaced by fibrosis).

Microscopy: Villous or flat mucinous epithelium with low-grade cytological atypia. Abundant luminal mucin that may dissect through the wall. **Pushing invasion, no desmoplasia, loss of lamina propria** — these features distinguish LAMN from appendiceal adenocarcinoma (infiltrative invasion with desmoplastic stroma).

Complication: When mucin (± epithelial cells) escapes to peritoneum → **pseudomyxoma peritonei (PMP)** — progressive gelatinous ascites. PMP graded: low-grade (acellular/paucicellular, from LAMN) vs high-grade (cellular with signet ring cells, from adenocarcinoma). Treatment: cytoreductive surgery + HIPEC.

Exam yield: ★★★ HIGH — LAMN vs adenocarcinoma distinction and PMP are favourite viva topics.

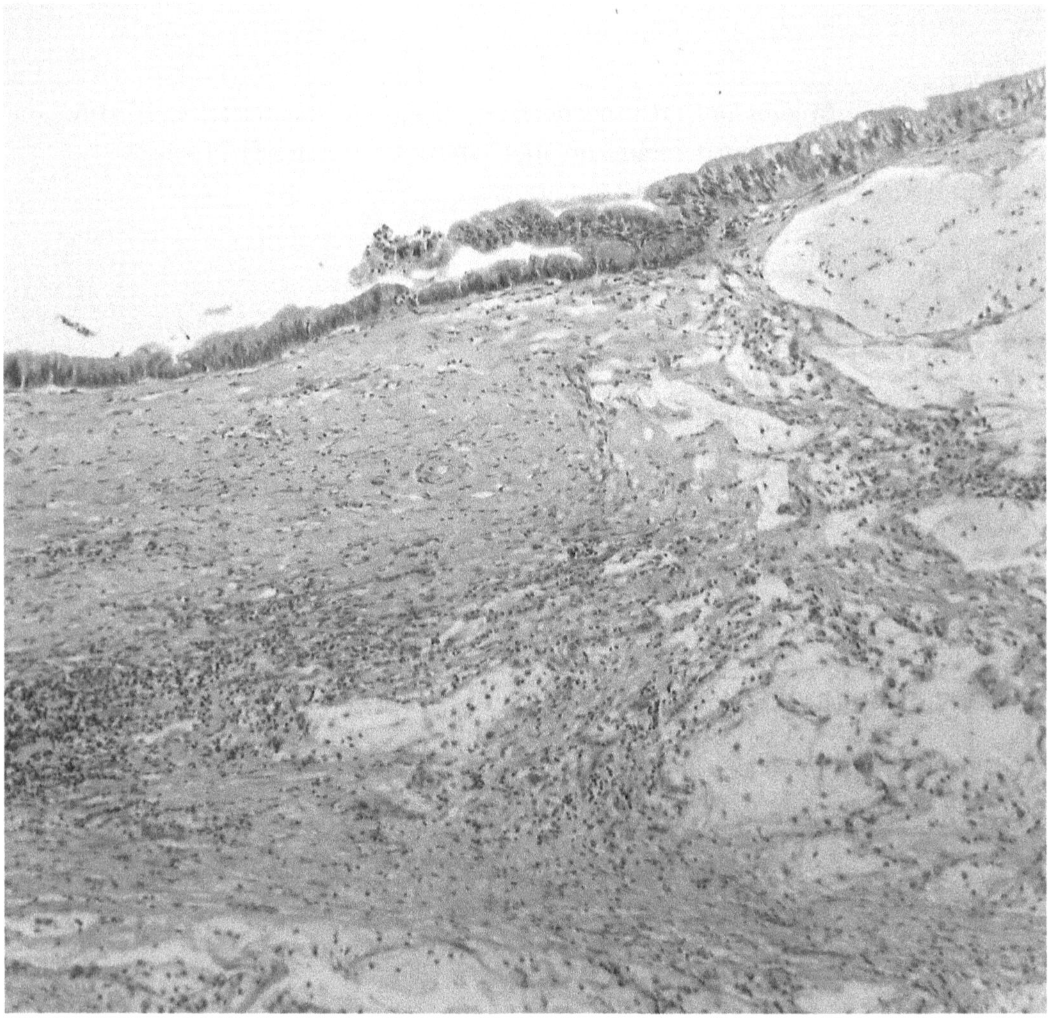

Figure 19.8: Low-grade appendiceal mucinous neoplasm (LAMN). Villous/undulating mucinous epithelium with low-grade cytology, abundant luminal mucin, and loss of lamina propria with fibrotic wall replacement ("pushing" pattern of invasion) (H&E). (Source: Sarahkayb, Wikimedia Commons, CC BY-SA 4.0.)

Rectal Cancer: Special Considerations

Rectal cancers are treated differently from colon cancers: most locally advanced rectal cancers (cT3 or node-positive) receive neoadjuvant chemoradiation before surgery. The pathologist's role in the post-neoadjuvant resection specimen is critical. **Tumour regression grading (TRG)** assesses the degree of treatment response. The Modified Ryan/AJCC system scores: TRG 0 (complete response, no viable tumour cells), TRG 1 (moderate response, single cells or small groups), TRG 2 (minimal response, residual cancer with fibrosis), TRG 3 (poor response, minimal or no tumour kill). The quality of the total mesorectal excision (TME) is graded as complete, nearly complete, or incomplete. The **circumferential**

resection margin (CRM) is positive if tumour is within 1 mm of the inked non-peritonealised margin, and is the strongest predictor of local recurrence.

Peritoneal Pathology

Primary peritoneal tumours include well-differentiated papillary mesothelioma (indolent) and malignant mesothelioma (aggressive, linked to asbestos, see Chapter 16), and **desmoplastic small round cell tumour** (EWSR1::WT1 fusion, affects young males, peritoneal masses). Secondary peritoneal disease is far more common, with peritoneal carcinomatosis from gastric, ovarian, colorectal, and appendiceal carcinomas. Peritoneal involvement is staged as M1c in CRC. The Peritoneal Cancer Index (PCI) quantifies disease distribution and guides selection for cytoreductive surgery with HIPEC.

Quick Recall: Appendix and Peritoneum

Appendiceal NET: Most common appendiceal tumour; tip; <1 cm + no LVI = appendectomy alone sufficient.
LAMN: Pushing invasion; loss of lamina propria; low-grade mucinous epithelium; risk of PMP.
PMP: Gelatinous ascites from ruptured LAMN or appendiceal adenocarcinoma; HIPEC treatment.
Rectal TRG: 0 = complete response; 3 = poor response; assess on post-neoadjuvant specimens.
CRM: Positive if tumour <1 mm from non-peritonealised margin; strongest predictor of local recurrence.

Hirschsprung Disease

Definition: Congenital disorder characterised by absence of ganglion cells in the myenteric (Auerbach) and submucosal (Meissner) plexuses of the distal bowel, resulting from failure of neural crest cell migration during embryogenesis.

Pathogenesis: Failed neural crest cell migration (craniocaudal) → Aganglionic distal segment (rectosigmoid in 80%) → Tonic contraction → Functional obstruction with proximal dilatation

Genetics: RET proto-oncogene mutations are the most common genetic association (see Chapter 8).

Diagnosis (rectal suction biopsy):

1. **Absence of ganglion cells** in myenteric and submucosal plexuses.

2. Nerve trunk hypertrophy (S100 IHC).

3. **Calretinin IHC negative** in the lamina propria and muscularis mucosae of the aganglionic segment.

4. AChE histochemistry (frozen section): increased thickened nerve fibres in lamina propria.

Exam yield: ★★★ HIGH — calretinin IHC negativity is a classic MCQ and viva image.

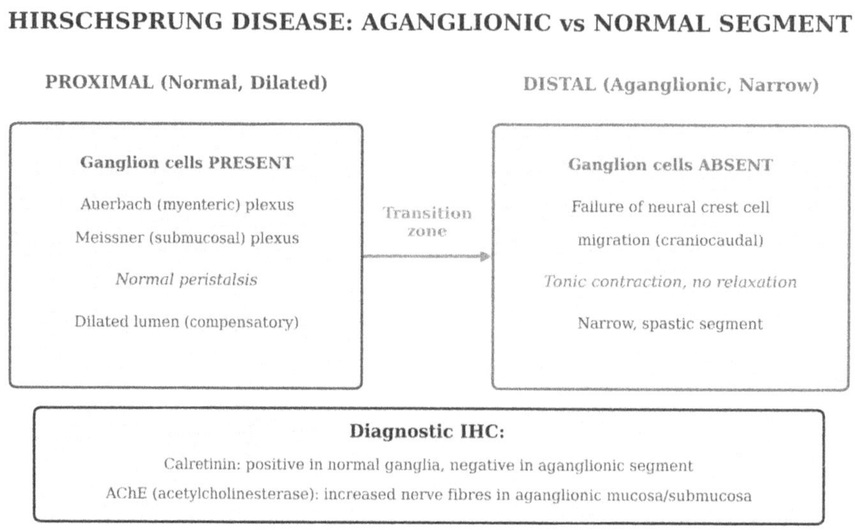

Figure 19.9: Hirschsprung disease: comparison of aganglionic segment (distal, contracted) versus normal segment (proximal, dilated), with rectal suction biopsy showing absent ganglion cells and calretinin immunohistochemistry negativity in the lamina propria. (Source: Author's original.)

Other Lower GI Conditions

Whipple disease (Tropheryma whipplei): rare systemic infection with malabsorption and arthralgias. Duodenal biopsy: foamy PAS-positive (diastase-resistant) macrophages in lamina propria with villous blunting. Differential: MAI in immunocompromised (also PAS-positive but AFB-positive).

Melanosis coli: benign brown-black colonic pigmentation from chronic anthraquinone laxative use (lipofuscin in lamina propria macrophages; Fontana-Masson negative, PAS positive). Highlights adenomas as pale unpigmented areas.

Solitary rectal ulcer syndrome (SRUS): rectal bleeding with fibromuscular obliteration of the lamina propria (smooth muscle extending between crypts), surface erosion, and thickened muscularis mucosae. Pitfall: regenerative changes may mimic dysplasia or adenocarcinoma.*The key diagnostic pitfall is misinterpreting the regenerative epithelial changes and distorted crypts as dysplasia or even adenocarcinoma; awareness of the clinical setting and the fibromuscular obliteration pattern prevents this error.*

The Pathologist's Eye: IBD vs Infectious Colitis on Mucosal Biopsy

> The distinction between inflammatory bowel disease (IBD) and infectious colitis on mucosal biopsy is a frequent diagnostic challenge. Features favouring IBD include: basal plasmacytosis (plasma cells between crypt bases and muscularis mucosae, the earliest and most reliable histological sign of chronicity), crypt architectural distortion (branching, shortening, irregular spacing), Paneth cell metaplasia in the left colon, and basal lymphoid aggregates. Infectious colitis, by contrast, typically shows preserved crypt architecture with a neutrophilic infiltrate concentrated in the superficial lamina propria and crypt epithelium (cryptitis and crypt abscesses without structural distortion). The practical rule: if crypt architecture is preserved and the infiltrate is predominantly neutrophilic without basal plasmacytosis, consider infection first. However, early IBD (first presentation, pre-treatment) may lack architectural distortion, and some infections (particularly Clostridioides difficile, CMV, and intestinal TB) can mimic chronic colitis. Always correlate with clinical history, stool cultures, and endoscopic findings. GMS and PAS stains for fungi, Ziehl-Neelsen for AFB, and CMV immunostain should be performed when the clinical context warrants.

Recent Advances

Consensus molecular subtypes of colorectal cancer. An international consortium reconciled six independent gene-expression classification systems for colorectal cancer into a single robust framework of four consensus molecular subtypes (Guinney et al. Nature Medicine 2015; 21: 1350–1356; PMID 26457759). CMS1 (microsatellite-instability immune; 14% of cases) is hypermutated, microsatellite-unstable, and characterised by strong immune activation; CMS2 (canonical; 37%) is epithelial with marked WNT and MYC signalling; CMS3 (metabolic; 13%) is epithelial with overt metabolic dysregulation and a high frequency of KRAS mutation; CMS4 (mesenchymal; 23%) shows transforming-growth-factor-beta activation, stromal infiltration, and angiogenesis. Approximately 13% of tumours show mixed features, interpreted as transitional phenotypes or intratumoural heterogeneity. The CMS framework underpins immunotherapy selection in CMS1 (deficient mismatch repair / high microsatellite instability now treated with first-line pembrolizumab per KEYNOTE-177), informs prognostication (CMS4 carries the worst overall survival), and is increasingly used to stratify clinical trials. For the surgical pathologist, CMS-aligned reporting begins with comprehensive MMR-IHC and adds molecular profiling (KRAS, NRAS, BRAF, microsatellite status) on every primary colorectal carcinoma to permit subtype assignment by integrated histological–molecular criteria.

Circulating tumour DNA for minimal residual disease in CRC. Post-surgical ctDNA detects MRD in stage II/III CRC. The DYNAMIC trial showed ctDNA-guided adjuvant chemotherapy reduced unnecessary treatment by 50% without compromising outcomes. CIRCULATE-Japan extends this to stage III.

Immunotherapy in MSI-high CRC. Pembrolizumab is first-line for MSI-high/dMMR metastatic CRC (KEYNOTE-177). The NICHE-2 trial showed 67% pathological complete response with neoadjuvant ipilimumab plus nivolumab in dMMR colon cancer.

Approach to the Histopathology Slide

Step 1: Identify the specimen. Is this a biopsy (mucosal), polypectomy (with stalk/base), or resection? For resections, orient and identify the mucosal surface, muscularis propria, serosa, and mesentery.

Step 2: For polyps, classify immediately: conventional adenoma (tubular/villous with picket fence nuclei) vs serrated polyp (HP: superficial serrations only; SSL: boot-shaped bases; TSA: eosinophilic, ectopic crypts). Assess for dysplasia grade. For 'malignant polyps,' evaluate all high-risk features (margin, LVI, budding, depth, grade).

Step 3: For IBD biopsies, assess architecture (focal vs diffuse distortion), inflammatory pattern (activity, chronicity, basal plasmacytosis), granulomas, and distribution across sites. Always compare biopsies from multiple levels (terminal ileum to rectum). Report whether features favour Crohn, UC, or are indeterminate. In TB-endemic regions, always comment on the need to exclude TB.

Step 4: For carcinoma resections, report: histological type and grade, depth of invasion (T stage), lymph node status (N stage), tumour budding, venous invasion (large vessel; consider EVG stain), circumferential resection margin (for rectal cancers), and MMR IHC status. Request RAS/BRAF testing for metastatic CRC.

Step 5: For appendix, always section the tip; report any incidental tumour (NET, LAMN, SSL). For mucinous lesions, distinguish LAMN (pushing invasion, loss of lamina propria) from adenocarcinoma (infiltrative invasion with desmoplasia) and from ruptured diverticulum (benign epithelium with lamina propria intact).

International Frameworks

Universal MMR/MSI screening for colorectal cancer (ASCO/ESMO 2015). The American Society of Clinical Oncology endorsed the ESMO Familial Risk-Colorectal Cancer guideline, which recommends that the possibility of a hereditary cancer syndrome be assessed at the time of every colorectal cancer diagnosis through review of personal and family history together with reflex tumour testing for DNA mismatch-repair deficiency (MMR-IHC for MLH1, MSH2, MSH6, PMS2) and/or microsatellite instability. Approximately 5–6% of colorectal cancers arise from inherited germline mutations, and screening based on Bethesda or Amsterdam criteria alone misses roughly one in four Lynch syndrome cases. Reporting requirement: pathologists should report MMR-IHC results on every primary colorectal cancer resection (or biopsy if resection is not planned), distinguishing concordant loss patterns (MLH1/PMS2, MSH2/MSH6, isolated PMS2, isolated MSH6) and reflex-testing MLH1/PMS2-deficient cases for BRAF V600E and MLH1 promoter hypermethylation to discriminate sporadic from Lynch-associated tumours. Citation: Stoffel EM, et al. J Clin Oncol 2015;33(2):209–217. PMID 25452455.

Ultra High-Yield Chapter Summary

Topic	Must Remember

Conventional adenoma	Picket fence nuclei; TA/TVA/VA; CIN pathway (APC→KRAS→TP53)
SSL	Right-sided; boot-shaped crypt bases; BRAF V600E; ≥1 distorted crypt for Dx
CIN pathway	~85% CRC; APC→KRAS→TP53; microsatellite-stable; RAS-mut = anti-EGFR resistant
Serrated/MSI pathway	BRAF→SSL→MLH1 methylation→MSI-H; better prognosis; immunotherapy
FAP	APC germline; >100 adenomas; 100% CRC risk; Gardner = osteomas + desmoids
Lynch syndrome	MMR germline (MLH1/MSH2/MSH6/PMS2); universal MMR IHC on all CRC
MMR IHC algorithm	MLH1/PMS2 loss → BRAF/methylation → sporadic vs Lynch; MSH2/MSH6 loss → Lynch
CRC grading	Low-grade (>50% glands) vs high-grade (<50% glands); worst area
Tumour budding	<5 cell clusters at invasive front; high budding = adverse prognostic factor
Ulcerative lesions DD	TB (transverse, caseating); Crohn (fissuring, non-caseating); typhoid (longitudinal over Peyer patches); amoebic (flask-shaped)
Crohn disease	Transmural; skip lesions; non-caseating granulomas; fistulae; NOD2/CARD15
Ulcerative colitis	Mucosal; continuous from rectum; crypt distortion; basal plasmacytosis; Paneth cell metaplasia
TB vs Crohn (TB-endemic regions)	Large confluent caseating granulomas = TB; small discrete non-caseating = Crohn; never immunosuppress without excluding TB
IBD dysplasia	>8 yr extensive colitis; p53 IHC (overexpression/null); chromoendoscopy; Geboes/Nancy scoring
Celiac disease	HLA-DQ2/DQ8; anti-tTG IgA; Marsh 3c = total villous atrophy; EATL

	risk
Hirschsprung	Absent ganglion cells; calretinin IHC negative in lamina propria; RET mutations
Appendiceal NET	Most common appendiceal tumour; tip; <1 cm = excellent prognosis
LAMN	Pushing invasion; loss of lamina propria; mucin can cause pseudomyxoma peritonei
GI lymphomas	DLBCL most common; EATL in refractory celiac; MCL = lymphomatous polyposis; Burkitt = ileocaecal, starry sky
ctDNA in CRC	MRD detection post-surgery; DYNAMIC trial; guides adjuvant chemotherapy decisions
Immunotherapy CRC	Pembrolizumab first-line for MSI-H metastatic CRC; KEYNOTE-177; NICHE-2

Diagnostic thinking: skip lesions + transmural inflammation + non-caseating granulomas + fissuring ulcers → Crohn disease

Diagnostic thinking: continuous mucosal inflammation + crypt abscesses + pseudopolyps + limited to colon → ulcerative colitis

Diagnostic thinking: serrated architecture + basal dilation + mucin cap + absence of dysplasia → sessile serrated lesion

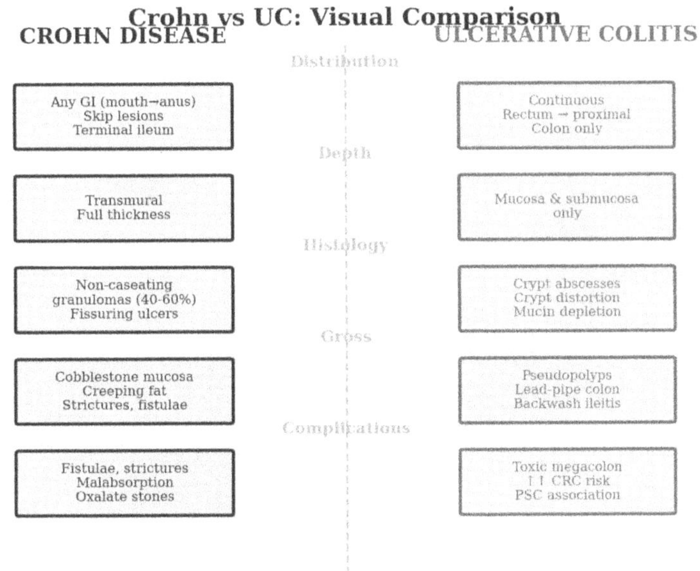

Figure 19.10: Crohn vs UC: Visual Comparison. (Source: Author's original.)

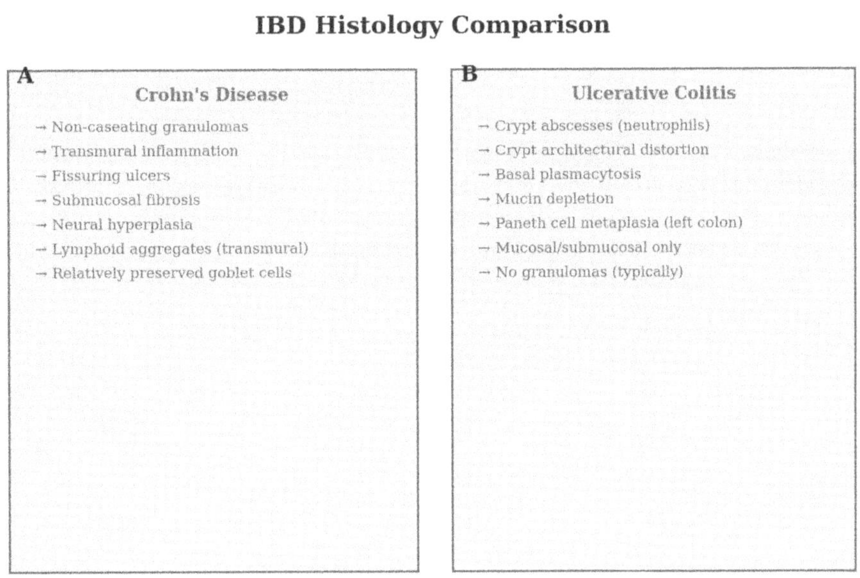

Figure 19.11A: Crohn disease — gross specimen of jejunum showing the classic cobblestone mucosal pattern. Linear longitudinal and transverse ulcers separated by islands of preserved oedematous mucosa create the characteristic cobblestoning. The bowel wall is thickened and the disease is segmental and sharply demarcated — features that distinguish Crohn disease from the diffuse, continuous mucosal involvement of ulcerative colitis. (Source: Jaroslav Cehovsky, Wikimedia Commons, Public Domain.)

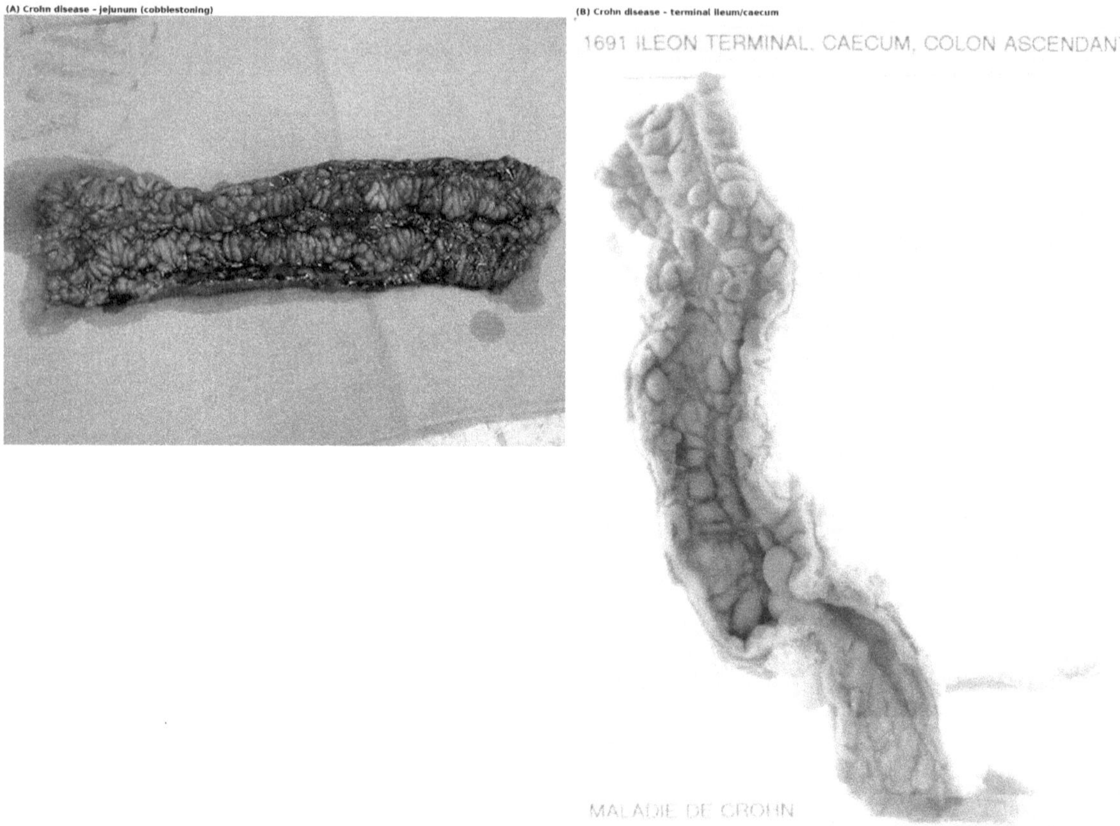

Figure 19.11B: Crohn disease — gross specimen of terminal ileum, caecum, and ascending colon. The mucosa shows pseudopolypoid nodules of preserved mucosa surrounded by deep linear ulceration (cobblestoning). Skip lesions and segmental disease are evident, with abrupt transition between affected and uninvolved bowel — a hallmark distinguishing Crohn disease from the diffuse continuous involvement of ulcerative colitis. (Source: Laval University, Wikimedia Commons, CC BY-SA 4.0.)

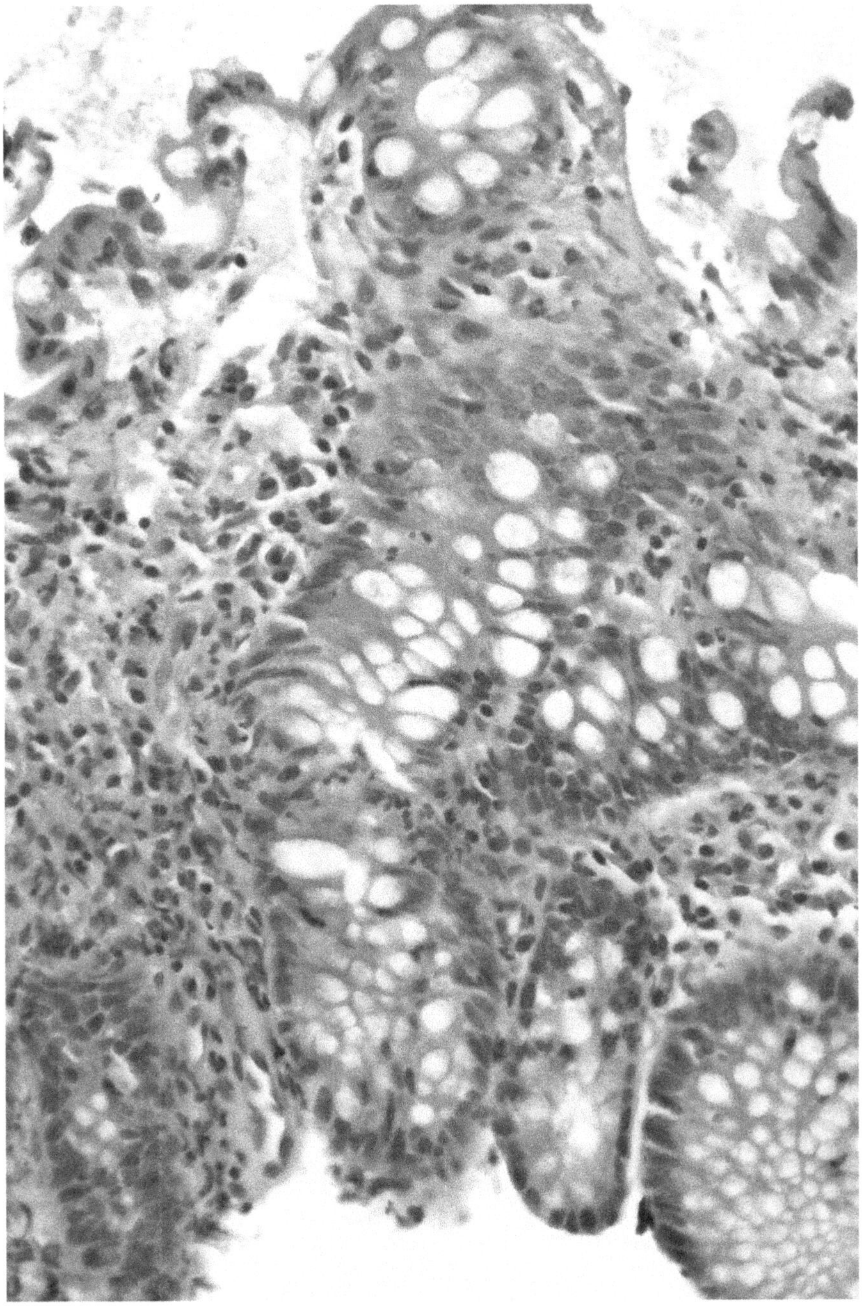

Figure 19.11C: Ulcerative colitis: Active cryptitis with numerous neutrophils (H&E, high mag). (Source: Nephron, Wikimedia Commons, CC BY-SA 3.0.)

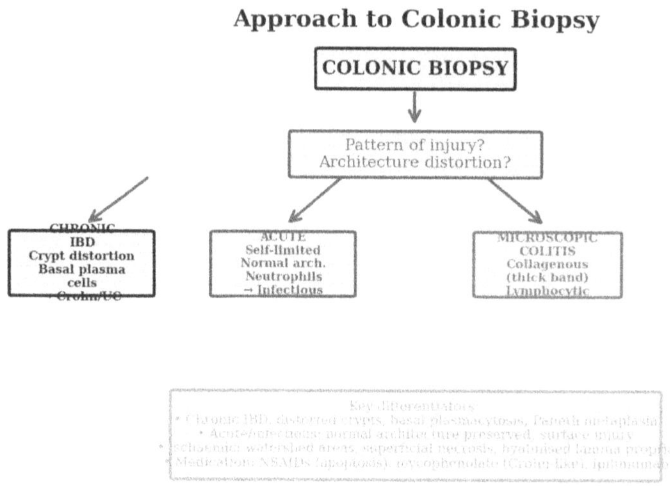

Figure 19.12: Approach to Colonic Biopsy. (Source: Author's original.)

Chapter 20: Hepatobiliary Pathology

THE BIG PICTURE

The liver occupies a unique position in pathology: it is simultaneously a metabolic organ, an immunological filter, and a frequent target of systemic disease. Hepatobiliary pathology encompasses a vast spectrum from viral hepatitis and metabolic steatohepatitis to cirrhosis, primary hepatocellular and cholangiocarcinoma, and biliary disorders. The pathologist's role is pivotal in interpreting liver biopsies, grading chronic hepatitis, staging fibrosis, distinguishing benign hepatocellular nodules from well-differentiated hepatocellular carcinoma, and evaluating transplant pathology. Mastery of hepatobiliary pathology requires integrating clinical biochemistry, serological markers, histomorphology, immunohistochemistry, and increasingly, molecular diagnostics.

High-yield topics in this chapter: Chronic viral hepatitis (HBV, HCV) and grading/staging systems; NAFLD/NASH (MASLD/MASH) and the NASH-CRN scoring system; cirrhosis, portal hypertension, and ascites; hepatocellular carcinoma and precursor lesions (dysplastic nodules, small-cell and large-cell change); autoimmune hepatitis; metabolic liver disease (Wilson, hemochromatosis, alpha-1 antitrypsin deficiency); cholestatic liver disease (PBC, PSC); biliary atresia; fibrolamellar HCC; liver biopsy interpretation; jaundice and bilirubin metabolism; hepatic complications of organ transplantation.

The liver processes nearly 1.5 litres of blood every minute, filtering toxins, synthesising proteins, and regulating metabolism with a regenerative capacity unmatched by any other solid organ. Yet this remarkable resilience also means that liver disease often remains clinically silent until fibrosis or cirrhosis is well established. For the pathologist, a liver biopsy is rarely a simple diagnosis; it is an exercise in pattern recognition, where the distribution of inflammation, the type of hepatocyte injury, the presence or absence of fibrosis, and the status of bile ducts must all be integrated with clinical, serological, and radiological data to reach a meaningful conclusion.

WHO Classification: Hepatobiliary Tumours (5th Ed, 2019) -- Selected

HCC subtypes: Conventional; steatohepatitic; macrotrabecular-massive; scirrhous; chromophobe; fibrolamellar (distinct entity, young patients, CK7+, no cirrhosis, DNAJB1::PRKACA fusion); clear cell; neutrophil-rich; lymphocyte-rich.

Combined HCC-CCA: Both hepatocellular and cholangiocellular differentiation confirmed by IHC; not a collision tumour.

Intrahepatic CCA: Small duct type (peripheral, CK7+/CK19+, IDH1/2 mutations, FGFR2 fusions); large duct type (perihilar, mucin+, KRAS/TP53 mutations).

Hepatocellular adenoma: Four subtypes: HNF1A-inactivated (steatotic, no malignant risk); inflammatory (SAA/CRP+, telangiectatic); beta-catenin-activated (highest HCC risk); unclassified.

Applied Anatomy and Histology

The liver is divided into a right and left lobe by the falciform ligament, with the caudate and quadrate lobes defined by hepatic vein and portal structures. The functional unit is the hepatic lobule, a hexagonal arrangement of hepatocytes radiating from a central vein, with portal triads (hepatic artery branch, portal vein branch, and bile ductule) at the periphery. The acinar model of Rappaport divides the parenchyma into three metabolic zones: zone 1 (periportal, richest in oxygen), zone 2 (intermediate), and zone 3 (pericentral, most susceptible to ischaemic and toxic injury).

Stellate cells store vitamin A; their activation into collagen-producing myofibroblasts drives hepatic fibrosis (see Chapter 3, Section 3.4 for TGF-β signalling in fibrosis) (Figure 20.1).

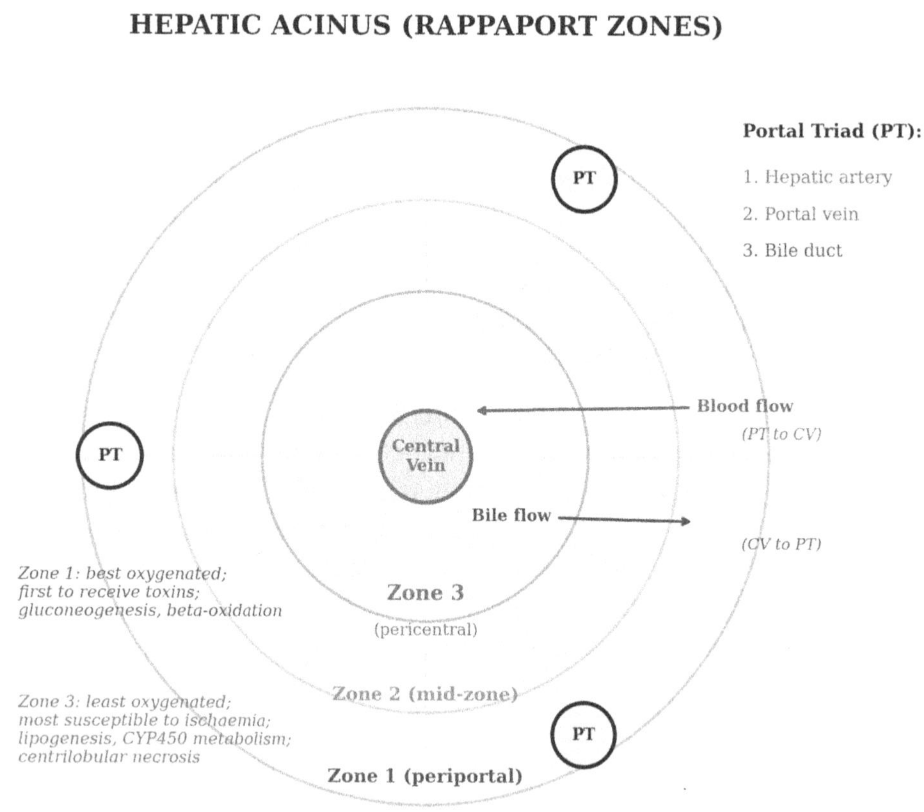

Figure 20.1: Hepatic acinus (Rappaport model) showing zones 1–3 relative to the portal triad and central vein, sinusoidal architecture, space of Disse, Kupffer cells, and hepatic stellate cells. (Source: Author's original.)

Jaundice and Bilirubin Metabolism

Jaundice, the clinical manifestation of hyperbilirubinaemia (serum bilirubin > 2 mg/dL), is a frequent examination topic and a cornerstone of hepatobiliary diagnostics. Bilirubin is produced from haem degradation in the reticuloendothelial system, transported to the liver bound to albumin (unconjugated, indirect), conjugated with glucuronic acid by UDP-glucuronosyltransferase (UGT1A1), and excreted into bile.

Haem → biliverdin → unconjugated bilirubin (albumin-bound) → hepatocyte uptake → conjugation (UGT1A1) → bile canaliculus → gut → urobilinogen

Type	Mechanism	Key Causes	Urine Bilirubin	Urine Urobilinogen
Pre-hepatic (unconjugated)	Excess bilirubin production	Haemolysis, ineffective erythropoiesis, Gilbert syndrome, Crigler-Najjar	Absent	Increased
Hepatic (mixed)	Hepatocyte dysfunction	Viral hepatitis, alcoholic hepatitis, cirrhosis, drug injury	Present	Variable
Post-hepatic (conjugated)	Bile duct obstruction	Gallstones, pancreatic head carcinoma, cholangiocarcinoma, biliary stricture	Present (dark urine)	Absent (pale stools)

The key diagnostic clue in evaluating jaundice is the proportion of conjugated versus unconjugated bilirubin: a predominantly unconjugated hyperbilirubinaemia points to haemolysis or inherited conjugation defects, whereas a predominantly conjugated fraction indicates hepatocellular or obstructive pathology.

Inherited disorders of bilirubin metabolism deserve brief mention. Gilbert syndrome (reduced UGT1A1 activity, 5–10% prevalence) causes mild unconjugated hyperbilirubinaemia precipitated by fasting or stress. Crigler-Najjar type I (absent UGT1A1) presents with severe neonatal jaundice requiring phototherapy and liver transplantation, while type II (reduced activity) responds to phenobarbitone. Dubin-Johnson syndrome and Rotor syndrome are inherited conjugated hyperbilirubinaemias with benign prognosis; Dubin-Johnson livers show characteristic black pigmentation due to lysosomal lipofuscin-like material.

Quick Recall: Jaundice and Bilirubin

Gilbert syndrome: Reduced UGT1A1, unconjugated, benign, 5–10% prevalence.

Crigler-Najjar type I: Absent UGT1A1, severe neonatal jaundice, requires transplant.

Dubin-Johnson: Conjugated, black liver, defective canalicular excretion (MRP2 mutation).
Rotor: Conjugated, no liver pigmentation, defective hepatic storage.
Obstructive jaundice triad: Dark urine, pale stools, pruritus.

Viral Hepatitis

Viral hepatitis remains the most important cause of chronic liver disease worldwide and is among the most frequently examined topics in postgraduate pathology. Five major hepatotropic viruses are recognised: HAV and HEV (faecal-oral, typically acute and self-limited), and HBV, HCV, and HDV (parenteral, with significant chronicity risk).

Acute Viral Hepatitis

Acute viral hepatitis presents with lobular disarray, diffuse lobular inflammation (lymphocytes and scattered neutrophils), hepatocyte ballooning and swelling, acidophil bodies (apoptotic hepatocytes), and hepatocyte regeneration. Portal and periportal inflammation is mild. Crucially, there is no fibrosis in pure acute hepatitis; its presence suggests chronic or acute-on-chronic disease. Hepatitis A (HAV) and hepatitis E (HEV) are transmitted by the faecal-oral route and produce only acute infection. HEV is a leading cause of acute viral hepatitis across South Asia: it carries a mortality rate of 15–25% in pregnant women, particularly in the third trimester, due to fulminant hepatic failure.

Fulminant hepatitis (acute liver failure) is defined as the onset of hepatic encephalopathy within 8 weeks of the first symptoms of liver disease in a patient without pre-existing chronic liver disease. Histologically, it shows massive or submassive hepatic necrosis with collapse of the reticulin framework. The major causes are acute viral hepatitis (HAV, HBV, HEV), drug reactions (acetaminophen toxicity is the leading cause in Western countries), Wilson disease, and autoimmune hepatitis.

Hepatitis B Virus (HBV)

Definition: Partially double-stranded DNA virus (Hepadnaviridae). India: intermediate endemicity (HBsAg prevalence 3–4%). Chronicity: 5% immunocompetent adults, 90% neonates (perinatal). Cirrhosis risk 15–25%; leading cause of HCC globally.

Pathogenesis: HBV infection → Immune-mediated hepatocyte injury (CD8+ T cells target HBsAg/HBcAg on hepatocyte surface) → Chronic necroinflammation → Stellate cell activation → Fibrosis → Cirrhosis → HCC (insertional mutagenesis also contributes)

Microscopy: Portal lymphocytic infiltrates with variable interface hepatitis. Key findings: **ground-glass hepatocytes** (cytoplasm packed with HBsAg-laden smooth ER, highlighted by orcein or Victoria blue stain) and **sanded nuclei** (HBcAg accumulation).

IHC: HBsAg (cytoplasmic/membranous) and HBcAg (nuclear in replicative phase, cytoplasmic in integrative phase).

Special pattern — fibrosing cholestatic hepatitis: Severe cholestasis, ductular reaction, rapid progression to liver failure in immunosuppressed patients (post-transplant). Represents aggressive viral replication unchecked by immune control.

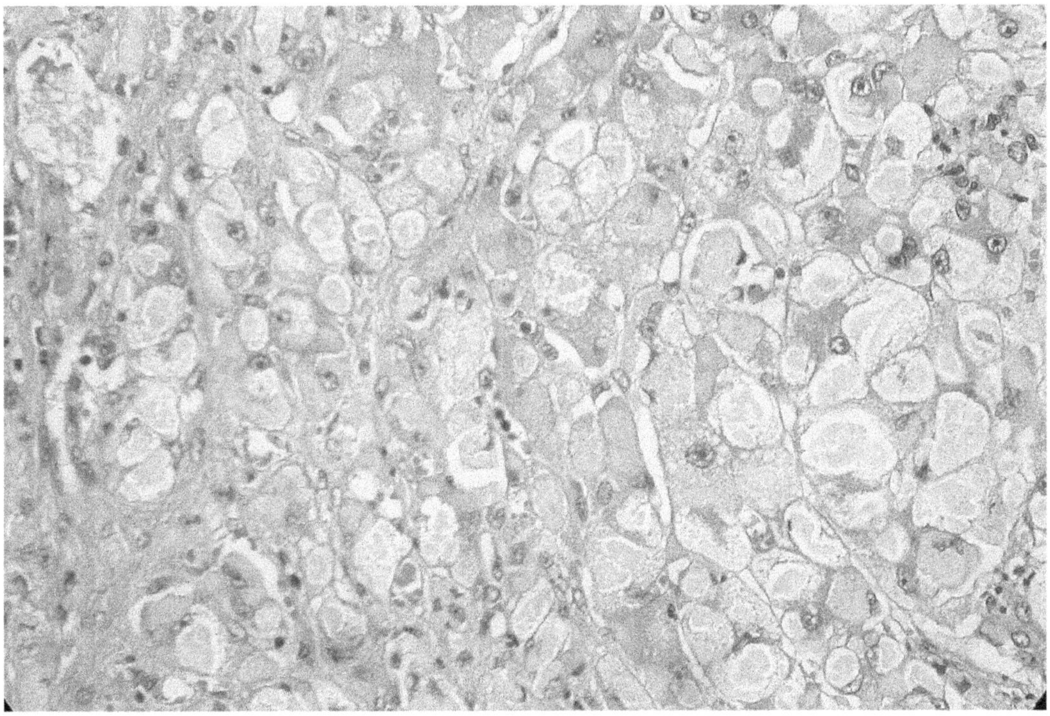

Figure 20.2: Chronic hepatitis B — ground-glass hepatocytes. Hepatocytes with finely granular, eosinophilic "ground-glass" cytoplasm representing accumulated HBsAg in dilated smooth endoplasmic reticulum (H&E, high mag). (Source: Ed Uthman, Flickr/Wikimedia Commons, CC BY 2.0.)

Hepatitis C Virus (HCV)

Definition: RNA virus (Flaviviridae). ~80% develop chronic infection; 20–30% progress to cirrhosis over 2–3 decades.

Microscopy: Portal **lymphoid aggregates** (sometimes with germinal centres), interface hepatitis, scattered acidophil bodies, mild bile duct damage, steatosis (especially genotype 3).

Treatment: Direct-acting antivirals (DAAs, e.g., sofosbuvir/ledipasvir): SVR rates >95%. Transformed HCV management.

Grading and Staging of Chronic Hepatitis

Grading (necroinflammatory activity) and staging (fibrosis) are central to liver biopsy reporting. Multiple systems exist; the METAVIR system is the most widely used for HCV, while Ishak scoring provides greater granularity.

System	Activity Grade	Fibrosis Stage
METAVIR	A0 (none) to A3 (severe)	F0 (none) to F4 (cirrhosis)
Ishak (modified HAI)	0–18 (necroinflammatory score)	0–6 (fibrosis stage)
Batts-Ludwig	Grade 0–4 (portal/interface/lobular)	Stage 0–4

This finding, when seen alongside portal lymphoid aggregates and mild bile duct injury in a patient with risk factors, points strongly towards chronic HCV infection.

Table 20.1 compares the key features of the five hepatotropic viruses.

Feature	HAV	HBV	HCV	HDV	HEV
Genome	RNA	DNA	RNA	RNA (defective)	RNA
Transmission	Faecal-oral	Parenteral, sexual, vertical	Parenteral	Parenteral (requires HBV)	Faecal-oral, waterborne
Chronicity	Never	5% adults, 90% neonates	80%	5% co-infection, 80% super-infection	Rare (immunosuppressed)
Cirrhosis risk	No	15–25%	20–30%	Accelerated with HBV	No (except chronic)
HCC risk	No	Yes (major)	Yes	Yes (with HBV)	No
Vaccine	Yes	Yes	No	HBV vaccine protects	Yes (in some countries)
Diagnostic hallmark on biopsy	Lobular hepatitis, no chronicity	Ground-glass cells, sanded nuclei	Lymphoid aggregates, steatosis	Severe interface hepatitis	Cholestatic hepatitis

Quick Recall: Viral Hepatitis

Faecal-oral: HAV, HEV. Both acute; HEV dangerous in pregnancy (20% mortality).

Parenteral: HBV, HCV, HDV. HDV requires HBV co-infection.

HBV hallmarks: Ground-glass hepatocytes (HBsAg), sanded nuclei (HBcAg).

HCV hallmarks: Portal lymphoid aggregates, steatosis (genotype 3), interface hepatitis.
METAVIR: A0–A3 activity, F0–F4 fibrosis. F4 = cirrhosis.
Fibroscan: Non-invasive fibrosis assessment replacing biopsy in many centres.

Autoimmune Hepatitis

Definition: Chronic progressive hepatitis with circulating autoantibodies, hypergammaglobulinaemia (elevated IgG), and characteristic histology. Strong female predominance (F:M 3.6:1); peaks in adolescence and 4th–6th decades.

Types: Type 1 (ANA and/or SMA positive, more common). Type 2 (anti-LKM-1 positive, predominantly children/young adults).

Microscopy — hallmark triad:

1. Dense portal **lymphoplasmacytic interface hepatitis** extending into the lobule.

2. **Hepatocyte rosette formation** (regenerating hepatocytes in rosettes).

3. **Emperipolesis** (lymphocytes within hepatocyte cytoplasm).

Plasma cells are characteristic but NOT required; their absence does not exclude AIH.

Diagnosis: Simplified IAIHG score: autoantibodies + IgG + histology + absence of viral markers. Score ≥6 = probable; ≥7 = definite.

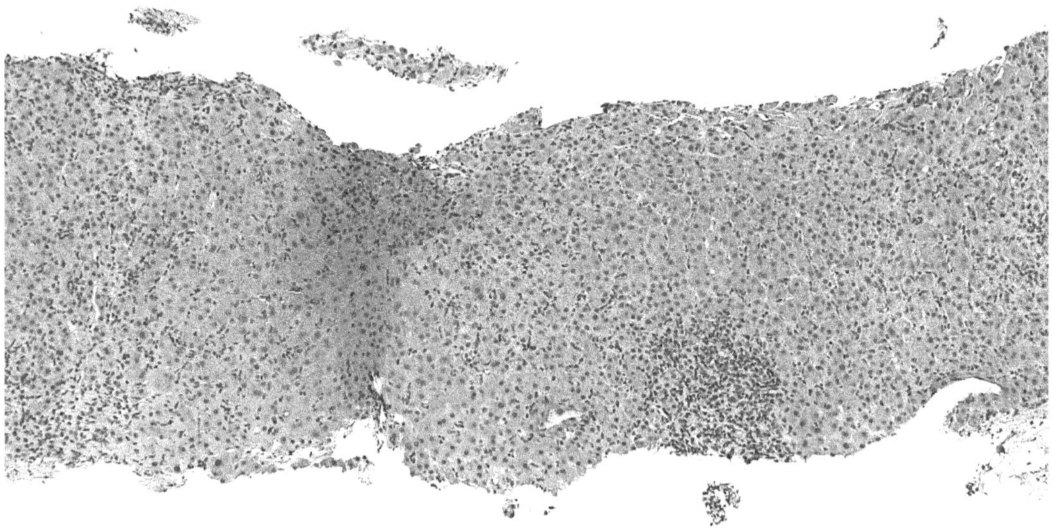

Figure 20.3: Autoimmune hepatitis. Interface hepatitis with portal lymphoplasmacytic infiltrate, hepatocyte rosetting, and emperipolesis. (Source: Nephron, Wikimedia Commons, CC BY-SA 3.0.)

Integration: Autoimmune hepatitis shares pathogenic mechanisms with other autoimmune diseases (see Chapter 5). AIH-PBC and AIH-PSC overlap syndromes occur and require combined assessment.

> **Exam Pitfall**
>
> Plasma cells are characteristic of AIH but not pathognomonic. Drug-induced liver injury, viral hepatitis (especially HCV), and even rejection can show plasma cell-rich infiltrates. Always correlate with serology, IgG levels, and the Simplified IAIHG score before diagnosing AIH on biopsy.

Non-Alcoholic Fatty Liver Disease (NAFLD/MASLD)

Definition: Most common chronic liver disease globally. Spectrum: simple steatosis (NAFL) → steatohepatitis (NASH/MASH) → fibrosis → cirrhosis → HCC. Renamed **MASLD** (metabolic dysfunction-associated steatotic liver disease) in 2023; requires cardiometabolic risk factor. South Asian prevalence: 9–32%.

Pathogenesis: Insulin resistance → Hepatic steatosis → Lipotoxicity + Oxidative stress + ER stress → Hepatocyte injury → Inflammation (NASH/MASH) → Stellate cell activation → Pericellular fibrosis (zone 3) → Cirrhosis. PNPLA3 I148M polymorphism is a major genetic risk factor (with high allele frequency in South Asian populations).

Microscopy — NASH triad (all three required):

1. **Macrovesicular steatosis** (>5% of hepatocytes).

2. **Lobular inflammation** (lymphocytes and neutrophils).

3. **Hepatocyte ballooning** (swollen, pale hepatocytes with loss of cytoplasmic detail).

Supportive features: Mallory-Denk bodies (ubiquitinated CK aggregates) and **pericellular ('chicken-wire') fibrosis in zone 3**.

NAS score (NASH-CRN): Steatosis (0–3) + Lobular inflammation (0–3) + Ballooning (0–2) = 0–8. Used for clinical trials.

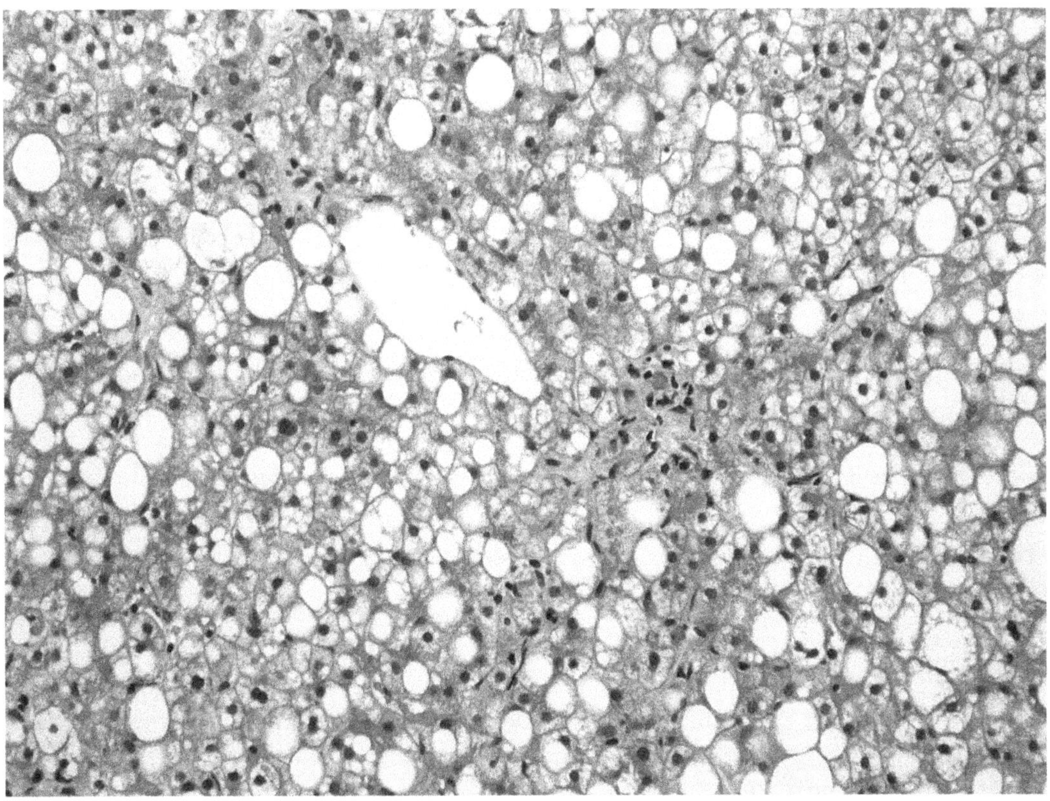

Figure 20.4: Non-alcoholic steatohepatitis (NASH/MASH). Macrovesicular steatosis with delicate pericellular ("chicken-wire") perisinusoidal fibrosis on Masson trichrome; hepatocyte ballooning and Mallory-Denk bodies may be seen in more active lesions. (Source: Nephron, Wikimedia Commons, CC BY-SA 3.0.)

Component	Score 0	Score 1	Score 2	Score 3
Steatosis	<5%	5–33%	34–66%	>66%
Lobular	None	<2	2–4	>4

inflammation (foci per 20× field)				
Hepatocyte ballooning	None	Few	Many/prominent	—

Quick Recall: NAFLD/NASH

NASH triad: Steatosis + lobular inflammation + hepatocyte ballooning.

NAS score: Steatosis (0–3) + inflammation (0–3) + ballooning (0–2) = 0–8.

Zone 3 pericellular fibrosis: Earliest and most characteristic fibrosis pattern in NASH.

MASLD: New nomenclature (2023) replacing NAFLD; requires cardiometabolic risk factor.

Mallory-Denk bodies: Also seen in alcoholic hepatitis, Wilson disease, HCC.

Alcoholic Liver Disease

Definition: Spectrum: steatosis (reversible) → alcoholic hepatitis → cirrhosis.

Pathogenesis: Ethanol → Alcohol dehydrogenase + CYP2E1 → Acetaldehyde (directly hepatotoxic) → Oxidative stress + Lipid peroxidation + Immune activation → Hepatocyte injury → Fibrosis

Microscopy (alcoholic hepatitis): Hepatocyte ballooning, **Mallory-Denk bodies** (ropey cytoplasmic inclusions of ubiquitinated CK8/18), **neutrophilic 'satellitosis'** (neutrophils surrounding injured hepatocytes), macrovesicular steatosis.

Fibrosis pattern: Zone 3 pericellular and perisinusoidal → Bridging fibrosis → Micronodular cirrhosis.

Clinical clue: AST:ALT ratio >2 (pyridoxal phosphate/B6 depletion impairs ALT production).

Drug-Induced Liver Injury (DILI)

Drug-induced liver injury is a major diagnostic consideration in any unexplained liver abnormality. Two principal mechanisms operate: intrinsic (predictable, dose-dependent, as in acetaminophen toxicity) and idiosyncratic (unpredictable, not dose-dependent, often immune-mediated). DILI can mimic virtually any pattern of liver disease: acute hepatitis, cholestatic hepatitis, bland cholestasis, steatohepatitis, granulomatous hepatitis, sinusoidal obstruction syndrome, and even autoimmune hepatitis.

Acetaminophen (paracetamol) toxicity, the most common cause of acute liver failure in Western countries, produces characteristic zone 3 (centrilobular) coagulative necrosis with relatively little inflammation. The toxic metabolite NAPQI, normally detoxified by glutathione conjugation, overwhelms hepatic glutathione stores at supratherapeutic doses. N-acetylcysteine is the specific antidote. Herbal and dietary supplements are an increasingly recognised and often overlooked cause of hepatotoxicity, particularly relevant where Ayurvedic, traditional, or herbal preparations are widely used.

Histological clues to DILI include: prominent eosinophils in the infiltrate, sharply demarcated zone 3 necrosis (intrinsic toxicity), cholestasis out of proportion to hepatocyte injury, and granulomas without an obvious infectious aetiology. The Roussel Uclaf Causality Assessment Method (RUCAM) score is the standard tool for establishing causality in suspected DILI cases.

> **Exam Pitfall**
>
> Drug-induced liver injury is the great mimicker of hepatobiliary pathology. Any histological pattern can be drug-related. When a liver biopsy shows features that do not fit neatly into a recognised category, always obtain a detailed medication and supplement history.

Metabolic and Storage Liver Diseases

Hereditary Hemochromatosis

Definition: AR disorder, most commonly HFE C282Y mutation. Excessive intestinal iron absorption → progressive iron deposition in parenchymal organs.

Microscopy: Iron accumulates initially in **periportal (zone 1) hepatocytes**, then extends to zone 3, bile duct epithelium, and Kupffer cells. **Perl's Prussian blue stain**: coarse blue granules in periportal-predominant distribution.

Quantification: Hepatic iron concentration (HIC); hepatic iron index (HIC/age) >1.9 supports HH.

Clinical triad: Cirrhosis + diabetes mellitus ('bronze diabetes') + skin pigmentation. HCC risk increased 200-fold in HH-related cirrhosis.

Key DDx: Periportal hepatocyte-predominant iron = HH; Kupffer cell-predominant = secondary hemosiderosis (transfusional, haemolytic).

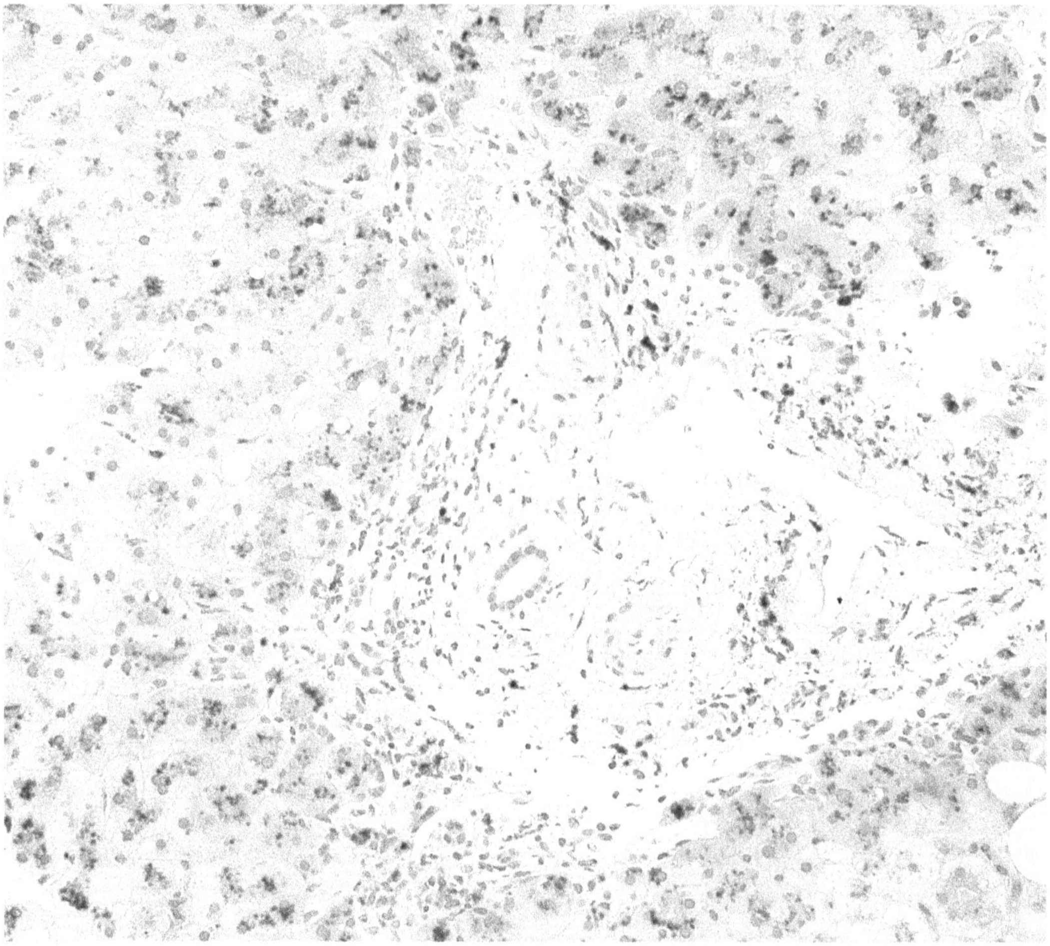

Figure 20.5: Hereditary haemochromatosis — Perls Prussian blue stain. Coarse blue granular iron deposition predominantly in periportal hepatocytes with involvement of Kupffer cells; grade 3–4 iron load with periportal (zone 1) gradient. (Source: Nephron, Wikimedia Commons, CC BY-SA 3.0.)

Wilson Disease

Definition: AR disorder caused by ATP7B mutations. Impaired biliary copper excretion → copper accumulation in liver, brain, cornea (Kayser-Fleischer rings).

Microscopy: Variable and non-specific: steatohepatitis with glycogenated nuclei (early), chronic hepatitis, or fulminant hepatic failure. **Rhodanine or rubeanic acid stains** demonstrate hepatocyte copper (negative stain does not exclude diagnosis).

Gold standard: Hepatic copper quantification >250 µg/g dry weight on fresh tissue.

Laboratory clues: Low serum ceruloplasmin, elevated 24-hour urine copper, AST:ALT >2.2, disproportionately low ALP:total bilirubin ratio (<4) in acute presentations.

Alpha-1 Antitrypsin Deficiency

Definition: SERPINA1 gene mutations; PiZZ phenotype causes clinically significant liver disease.

Pathogenesis: Misfolded A1AT protein → Accumulation in hepatocyte ER → ER stress → Hepatocyte injury → Chronic hepatitis and cirrhosis

Microscopy: Characteristic **eosinophilic, PAS-diastase-resistant globules** in periportal hepatocytes.

Presentation: Neonates: neonatal cholestasis. Adults: chronic hepatitis and cirrhosis.

Diagnosis: Serum A1AT levels, protein phenotyping, or genotyping.

> **Quick Recall: Metabolic Liver Disease**
> **Hemochromatosis:** HFE C282Y, periportal iron (zone 1), Perl's stain, HIC/age >1.9.
> **Wilson disease:** ATP7B, copper, Kayser-Fleischer rings, low ceruloplasmin, rhodanine stain.
> **A1AT deficiency:** PiZZ, PAS-D resistant globules (periportal), SERPINA1 gene.
> **Distinguishing iron pattern:** HH = hepatocyte-first (zone 1); secondary = Kupffer cell-first.

Cirrhosis and Its Complications

Cirrhosis is defined as diffuse hepatic fibrosis with formation of regenerative nodules, representing the end-stage of chronic liver disease regardless of aetiology. It is both a morphological and a clinical diagnosis. The two essential histological criteria are: (1) fibrous septa bridging portal tracts and central veins, and (2) regenerative nodules of hepatocytes bounded by fibrous tissue.

Classification by nodule size (micronodular, less than 3 mm, and macronodular, greater than 3 mm) has limited aetiological specificity but provides a morphological framework. Micronodular cirrhosis is typical of alcohol and metabolic disease; macronodular of viral hepatitis and autoimmune hepatitis. In South Asia, major causes include chronic HBV infection, alcohol, NAFLD/NASH, and chronic HCV.

Chronic injury → stellate cell activation → collagen deposition → sinusoidal capillarisation → portal hypertension → regenerative nodule formation → cirrhosis

Complications of cirrhosis include portal hypertension (causing oesophageal varices, splenomegaly, ascites, caput medusae), hepatorenal syndrome, hepatopulmonary syndrome, spontaneous bacterial peritonitis, hepatic encephalopathy, and increased risk of hepatocellular carcinoma. The pathogenesis of ascites involves a combination of sinusoidal portal hypertension, splanchnic vasodilatation, reduced effective arterial blood volume, activation of the renin-angiotensin-aldosterone system and sympathetic nervous system, and hypoalbuminaemia.

Why does liver biopsy matter even after cirrhosis is diagnosed clinically? Because biopsy can identify the underlying aetiology (viral markers, iron, copper, PAS-D globules, autoimmune features), detect superimposed hepatocellular carcinoma or dysplastic nodules, and assess the degree of ongoing inflammation, which guides treatment decisions.

Quick Recall: Cirrhosis

Definition: Diffuse hepatic fibrosis + regenerative nodules.
Micro/macronodular: <3 mm (alcohol, metabolic) vs >3 mm (viral, autoimmune).
Ascites pathogenesis: Portal HTN + splanchnic vasodilatation + RAAS activation + hypoalbuminaemia.
Child-Pugh score: Albumin, bilirubin, INR, ascites, encephalopathy. Classes A/B/C.
MELD score: Bilirubin, INR, creatinine. Used for transplant allocation.

Cholestatic and Biliary Diseases

Primary Biliary Cholangitis (PBC)

Definition: Autoimmune disease targeting intrahepatic bile ducts. Middle-aged women predominantly. Hallmark serology: **anti-mitochondrial antibody (AMA), M2 subtype** (>90% of cases).

Microscopy: Diagnostic lesion: **'florid duct lesion'** — granulomatous destruction of interlobular bile ducts with lymphocytic cholangitis and non-caseating granulomas. Progressive bile duct loss (ductopenia) → Cholestasis → Periportal copper accumulation → Biliary cirrhosis with 'jigsaw' fibrosis pattern.

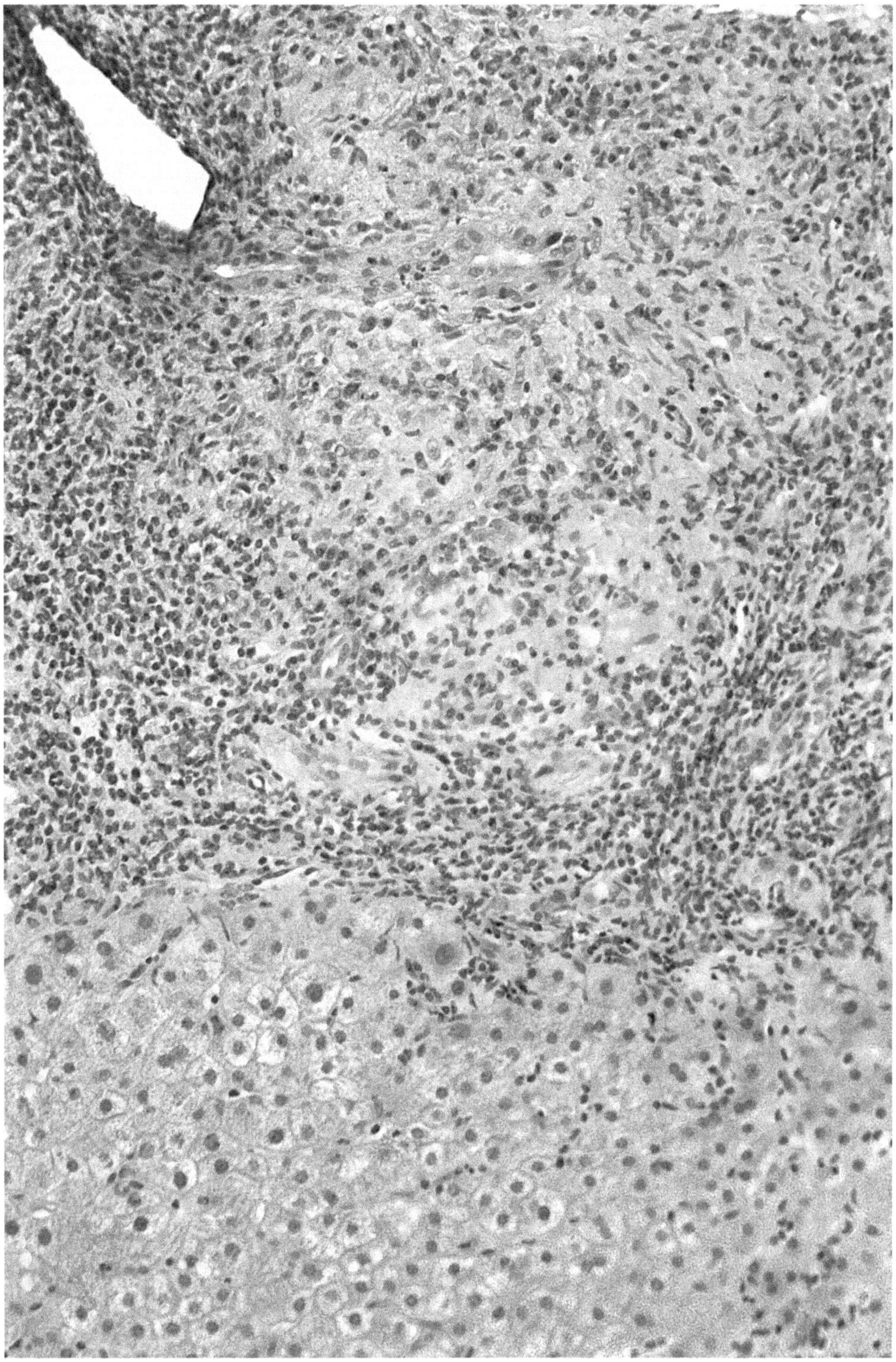

Figure 20.6: Primary biliary cholangitis — florid duct lesion. Granulomatous destruction of an interlobular bile duct with dense periductal lymphoplasmacytic infiltrate and epithelioid histiocytes damaging the duct epithelium (H&E, intermediate mag). (Source: Nephron, Wikimedia Commons, CC BY-SA 3.0.)

Primary Sclerosing Cholangitis (PSC)

Definition: Progressive fibrosis and stricturing of intrahepatic and extrahepatic bile ducts. Strong association with UC (60–80% of PSC patients have IBD). Young to middle-aged men.

Diagnosis: Cholangiography: 'beaded' pattern of multifocal strictures and dilatations.

Microscopy: Classic finding: **concentric periductal fibrosis ('onion-skin' pattern)** — though infrequently seen on needle biopsy.

Complications: Cholangiocarcinoma (lifetime risk 10–15%). Annual surveillance colonoscopy for CRC from PSC diagnosis.

Biliary Atresia

Definition: Fibroinflammatory destruction of extrahepatic bile ducts. Most common indication for liver transplantation in infants.

Presentation: Neonatal conjugated hyperbilirubinaemia, acholic stools, hepatomegaly.

Microscopy: Features of large duct obstruction: portal oedema, **bile ductular proliferation (ductular reaction)**, canalicular and ductular cholestasis, portal neutrophilic infiltration.

Treatment: Kasai portoenterostomy as bridge to transplantation.

Integration: PSC is closely linked to IBD, particularly ulcerative colitis (see Chapter 19). The cholestatic liver diseases share pathogenic overlap with autoimmune disorders (see Chapter 5).

Hepatocellular Tumours

Focal Nodular Hyperplasia (FNH)

FNH is the second most common benign liver lesion (after haemangioma). It is a regenerative hyperplastic response to a local vascular abnormality, not a true neoplasm. Typically found in young women, FNH presents as a well-circumscribed nodule with a central stellate scar containing dystrophic blood vessels, fibrous septae, and bile ductular proliferation. Hepatic plates are normal in thickness (1–2 cells). Glutamine synthetase IHC shows a characteristic "map-like" staining pattern, distinguishing FNH from hepatocellular adenoma and well-differentiated HCC.

Hepatocellular Adenoma (HCA)

Hepatocellular adenoma is a benign neoplasm associated with oral contraceptive use, anabolic steroids, and metabolic syndrome. The current WHO classification recognises four molecular subtypes with distinct morphological, immunohistochemical, and prognostic features.

Subtype	Frequency	Molecular Alteration	IHC Signature	Malignant Risk

HNF1α-inactivated	~30%	Biallelic HNF1A inactivation	Loss of LFABP	Low
Inflammatory	~40%	IL6/JAK/STAT activation	SAA and CRP positive	Low
β-catenin-activated	~20%	CTNNB1 activating mutations	Diffuse GS, nuclear β-catenin	Highest
Unclassified	~10%	None of the above	No specific pattern	Variable

Dysplastic Nodules and Precursor Lesions

In cirrhotic livers, the progression from regenerative nodule to dysplastic nodule to hepatocellular carcinoma follows a well-recognised morphological spectrum. Dysplastic nodules are divided into low-grade and high-grade based on the degree of cytological and architectural atypia. Small-cell change (increased nuclear-to-cytoplasmic ratio, cytoplasmic basophilia, decreased cell volume) is more strongly associated with progression to HCC than large-cell change (nuclear enlargement, pleomorphism). Reticulin stain is the critical ancillary tool: preserved reticulin framework supports a dysplastic nodule, while reticulin loss (plates >2 cells thick) indicates HCC.

Hepatocellular Carcinoma (HCC)

Definition: Most common primary malignant liver tumour; third leading cause of cancer death globally. In South Asia: HBV is the leading cause, followed by HCV, alcohol, and NAFLD/NASH. Most arise in cirrhotic livers. AFP elevated in ~60–70%.

Microscopy: Widened hepatic plates (**>2 cells thick, demonstrated by reticulin loss**), trabecular/pseudoacinar/solid growth, unpaired arteries (without accompanying bile ducts), endothelial wrapping. **Bile production by tumour cells is virtually diagnostic.** Diffuse sinusoidal CD34 staining ('capillarisation') supports HCC.

IHC panel: HepPar-1+, arginase-1+ (more sensitive for poorly differentiated), glypican-3+ (positive in HCC, negative in benign lesions — key malignancy marker).

Grading: Four-tier: G1 (well-differentiated) to G4 (undifferentiated).

Key subtypes: Fibrolamellar HCC (young, non-cirrhotic, DNAJB1-PRKACA fusion, lamellar fibrosis, CK7+/CD68+, normal AFP); Steatohepatitic HCC (NASH-associated); Macrotrabecular-massive HCC (trabeculae >10 cells, aggressive, TP53).

T Stage	Definition

T1a	Solitary tumour ≤2 cm
T1b	Solitary tumour >2 cm without vascular invasion
T2	Solitary with vascular invasion, or multiple tumours ≤5 cm
T3	Multiple tumours, at least one >5 cm
T4	Tumour involving a major branch of portal or hepatic vein, or direct invasion of adjacent organs (other than gallbladder), or perforation of visceral peritoneum

Hepatoblastoma

Hepatoblastoma is the most common malignant liver tumour in children (peak incidence 1–2 years). Serum AFP is markedly elevated. Histologically, it shows a spectrum of epithelial and mesenchymal differentiation recapitulating hepatic ontogenesis. Epithelial patterns include fetal (thin trabeculae of hepatocyte-like cells with clear to eosinophilic cytoplasm, the best prognosis), embryonal (solid nests with basophilic cytoplasm, pseudorosettes, more mitoses), and small cell undifferentiated (SCUD, worst prognosis, may show INI1 loss). Mesenchymal elements include osteoid, cartilage, and fibrous tissue. Frequent WNT/β-catenin pathway mutations are present. Association with Beckwith-Wiedemann syndrome and familial adenomatous polyposis (FAP) should be considered.

The Pathologist's Eye

Distinguishing well-differentiated HCC from hepatocellular adenoma and high-grade dysplastic nodules on core biopsy is among the most challenging diagnoses in liver pathology. The reticulin stain is your most reliable tool: loss of the reticulin framework with plates greater than 2 cells thick is the single most important criterion for HCC. Complement this with glypican-3 (positive in HCC, negative in benign lesions), diffuse CD34 (sinusoidal capillarisation), and Ki-67 (significantly elevated above background). When the findings are equivocal, reporting as "well-differentiated hepatocellular neoplasm" with a comment explaining the limitations is preferable to an incorrect definitive diagnosis.

Quick Recall: Hepatocellular Lesions

Essential/Desirable: Diagnostic Criteria -- Hepatocellular Carcinoma

Essential: Hepatocellular differentiation (widened trabeculae >2 cells, bile production, or IHC: HepPar1+/arginase-1+). Reticulin loss with CD34 sinusoidal capillarisation.

Desirable: Glypican-3+ (distinguishes from adenoma/FNH); cirrhotic background; unpaired arteries; radiological correlation (LIRADS-5 on CT/MRI); AFP elevation.

FNH: Central scar, map-like GS, not a neoplasm, no malignant potential.

HCA subtypes: HNF1α (LFABP loss), inflammatory (SAA/CRP), β-catenin (highest HCC risk).

Dysplastic nodule: Preserved reticulin; small-cell change more worrisome than large-cell.
HCC diagnosis: Reticulin loss + glypican-3 + diffuse CD34 + elevated Ki-67.
Fibrolamellar HCC: Young, non-cirrhotic, DNAJB1-PRKACA, CK7+, CD68+, normal AFP.

Staging and Prognostication of Hepatocellular Carcinoma: Milan Criteria and BCLC

Hepatocellular carcinoma is one of the few solid tumours for which staging is determined not only by tumour size and nodal or metastatic spread, but also by the degree of underlying hepatic dysfunction. The Milan criteria (Mazzaferro, 1996) remain the single most widely cited selection tool for liver transplantation, while the Barcelona Clinic Liver Cancer (BCLC) staging system integrates tumour burden, liver function (Child-Pugh), and performance status to recommend a treatment stage. Both are exam staples, especially in the context of HBV-related and NAFLD-related HCC prevalent across South Asia.

Table 20.2: Milan Criteria for Liver Transplantation in HCC (Mazzaferro, 1996)

Criterion	Threshold for transplant eligibility
Single tumour	Diameter not exceeding 5 cm.
Multiple tumours	Up to three lesions, none exceeding 3 cm in diameter.
Vascular invasion	Absent on imaging (macrovascular invasion excludes).
Extrahepatic spread	Absent.
Outcome if met	5-year survival 70 percent, recurrence less than 15 percent.

Table 20.3: BCLC Staging System for HCC (2022 update)

Stage	Tumour burden	Liver function / PS	Recommended treatment
0 (very early)	Single tumour ≤2 cm, carcinoma in situ.	Preserved (Child-Pugh A), PS 0.	Ablation or resection; transplant if portal hypertension.
A (early)	Single tumour or up to 3 nodules each ≤3 cm.	Preserved (Child-Pugh A or B), PS 0.	Resection, ablation, or transplant (Milan).
B (intermediate)	Multinodular, beyond Milan, no vascular invasion or spread.	Preserved (Child-Pugh A or B), PS 0.	Trans-arterial chemoembolisation (TACE); transplant in selected down-staging candidates.
C (advanced)	Macrovascular (portal vein) invasion or extrahepatic spread.	Preserved (Child-Pugh A or B), PS 1-2.	Systemic therapy: atezolizumab + bevacizumab (first-line); sorafenib,

Stage	Tumour burden	Liver function / PS	Recommended treatment
			lenvatinib alternatives.
D (terminal)	Any tumour burden.	End-stage (Child-Pugh C) or PS 3-4.	Best supportive care.

Table 20.4: NASH Clinical Research Network (NASH CRN) Fibrosis Staging in NAFLD/MASLD

Stage	Histological pattern	Clinical correlate
F0	No fibrosis.	Simple steatosis; favourable prognosis.
F1a / F1b / F1c	Mild (1a) or moderate (1b) perisinusoidal fibrosis in zone 3; (1c) portal or periportal fibrosis only.	Steatohepatitis without bridging fibrosis.
F2	Perisinusoidal and portal or periportal fibrosis.	Intermediate risk of progression.
F3	Bridging fibrosis (portal-portal, portal-central).	Advanced fibrosis; candidate for intensified monitoring and trial entry.
F4	Cirrhosis.	Risk of hepatic decompensation and HCC (1-2 percent annual incidence).

Note: South Asian adult NAFLD prevalence is estimated at 25-30 percent (composite estimates), and NASH-related cirrhosis and HCC are rising rapidly in parallel with diabetes and metabolic syndrome. The F3 versus F4 distinction in NASH CRN staging is the cutoff that selects patients for hepatology referral and HCC surveillance. BCLC stage C HCC is managed with systemic therapy (atezolizumab + bevacizumab as the current first-line) rather than locoregional therapy, a shift from the sorafenib era.

Cholangiocarcinoma and Biliary Neoplasms

INTRAHEPATIC CHOLANGIOCARCINOMA (iCCA)

Definition: Second most common primary hepatic malignancy.

Two pathways: Large duct type (perihilar, associated with PSC and liver flukes, progresses through BilIN, KRAS/TP53 mutations). Small duct type (peripheral, associated with cirrhosis/hepatitis, IDH1/2 mutations, FGFR2 fusions).

Microscopy: Tubular or glandular architecture with desmoplastic stroma. IHC: CK7+, CK19+, MOC31+; albumin ISH supports intrahepatic origin. HepPar-1 and arginase-1 negative (distinguishes from HCC).

Combined HCC-CCA: Biphenotypic tumour with separate areas of hepatocytic and cholangiocytic differentiation on H&E; not a collision tumour.

Gallbladder Pathology

CHOLELITHIASIS AND CHOLECYSTITIS

Cholelithiasis affects 10–15% of adults. Types: cholesterol stones (80% Western, associated with obesity/oestrogen), black pigment stones (haemolytic diseases), brown pigment stones (biliary infections). Chronic cholecystitis: mucosal atrophy, **Rokitansky-Aschoff sinuses** (mucosal herniations into the muscular wall), mural fibrosis, chronic inflammation.

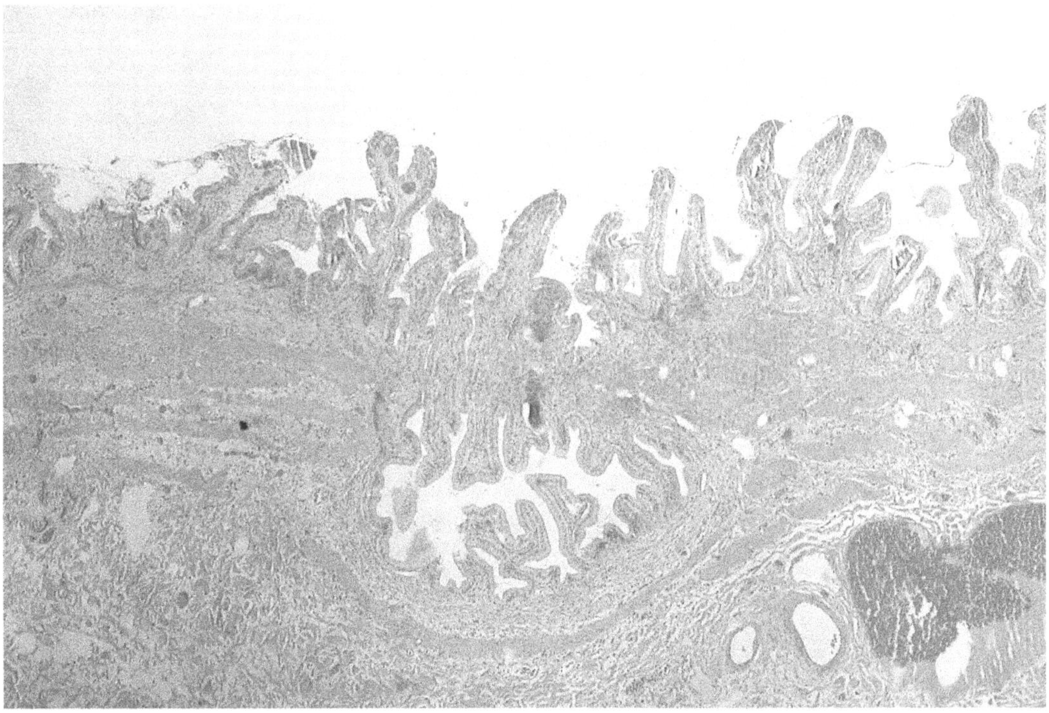

Figure 20.7: Chronic cholecystitis. Mucosal glands with Rokitansky–Aschoff sinuses (herniations into the thickened muscular wall), chronic inflammatory infiltrate, and mural fibrosis. H&E. (Source: Ed Uthman, Flickr/Wikimedia Commons, CC BY 2.0.)

GALLBLADDER CARCINOMA

Definition: Most common biliary tract malignancy. Marked female predominance (F:M 3:1). Most are adenocarcinomas.

Risk factors: Porcelain gallbladder (mural calcification), large gallstones (>3 cm), anomalous pancreaticobiliary junction, chronic Salmonella typhi carriage.

Prognosis: Incidental T1a (lamina propria only) = excellent prognosis after cholecystectomy. T2 and beyond = radical re-resection required.

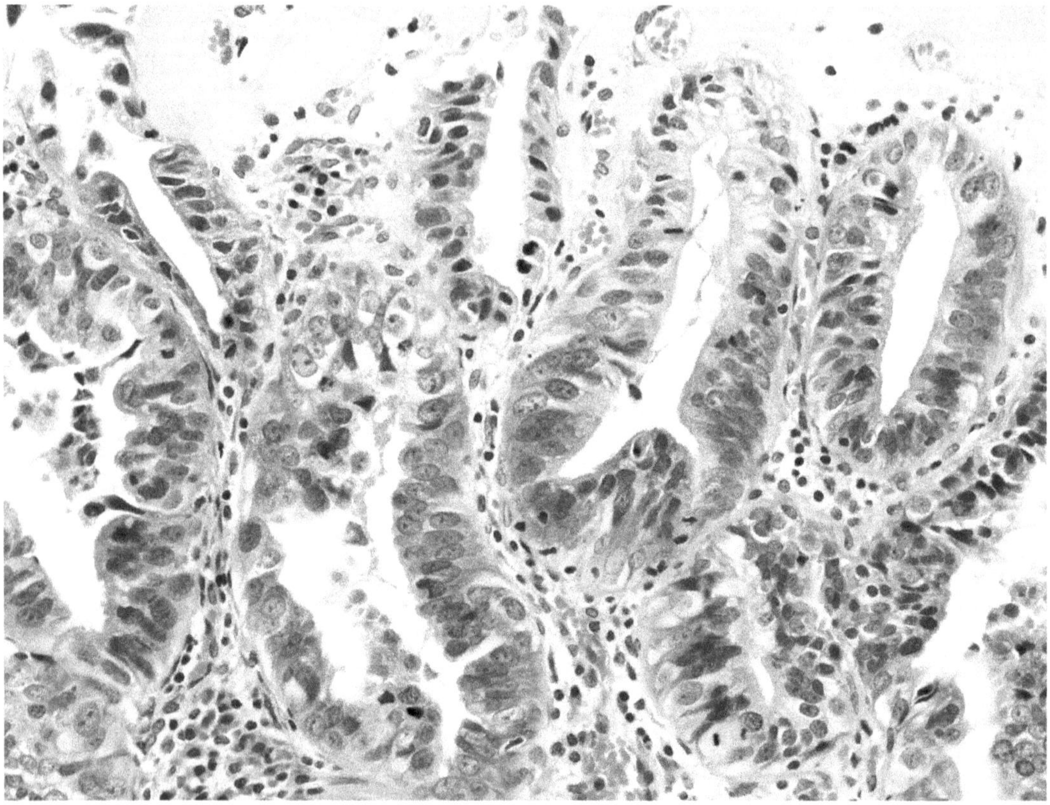

Figure 20.8: Gallbladder adenocarcinoma. Malignant glandular epithelium with nuclear pleomorphism, pseudostratification, and stromal invasion. H&E, high magnification. (Source: KGH, Wikimedia Commons, CC BY-SA 3.0.)

Transplant Hepatology

Liver biopsy is essential in the post-transplant setting for diagnosing rejection, recurrent disease, drug toxicity, and opportunistic infection. T cell-mediated (acute cellular) rejection, the most common form, is characterised by a triad of (1) mixed portal inflammation with activated lymphocytes and eosinophils, (2) bile duct damage (lymphocytic cholangitis with epithelial apoptosis), and (3) venous endothelialitis (subendothelial lymphocytic infiltration). The Banff global assessment grades rejection as indeterminate, mild, moderate, or severe.

Chronic rejection manifests as progressive bile duct loss (ductopenia, bile ducts present in <50% of portal tracts), foam cell arteriopathy, and eventual ductopenic rejection. Antibody-mediated rejection is diagnosed when compatible histology (portal vascular dilation, endothelial hypertrophy, microvasculitis), diffuse C4d staining (>50% of portal venous/sinusoidal endothelium), positive donor-specific antibodies, and exclusion of other causes are all present.

IHC Panel: Liver Tumour Differential Diagnosis

Marker	Interpretation
HepPar1	Hepatocellular differentiation; sensitivity ~80% for HCC; may be focal in

	poorly differentiated HCC
Arginase-1	Hepatocellular; more sensitive than HepPar1 for poorly differentiated HCC
Glypican-3	Positive in HCC (70-80%), hepatoblastoma; negative in benign hepatocellular lesions (FNH, adenoma) -- key malignancy marker
CK7	Cholangiocytes, cholangiocarcinoma; positive in some HCC (poor prognosis); hepatic progenitor cell marker
CK19	Cholangiocarcinoma; HCC with CK19+ has worse prognosis; positive in ductular reaction
CK20/CDX2	Colorectal origin if both positive; helps identify metastatic CRC to liver
TTF-1	Lung/thyroid origin; positive metastatic lung adenocarcinoma to liver

DDx: Hepatic Tumours

Entity	**Key Features**
HCC	Widened plates (>2 cells), reticulin loss, CD34 diffuse sinusoidal, unpaired arteries, bile production; HepPar1+, arginase-1+, glypican-3+
Cholangiocarcinoma	Glandular, desmoplastic stroma, mucin+; CK7+, CK19+; small duct: IDH1/2, FGFR2; large duct: KRAS, TP53
Metastatic carcinoma	CK7/CK20 profile + organ-specific markers (TTF-1 lung, CDX2 colon, PAX8 kidney/GYN); multiple nodules; no cirrhosis
Hepatoblastoma	Paediatric; epithelial (fetal/embryonal) +/- mesenchymal; AFP markedly elevated; beta-catenin nuclear+
FNH	Central scar with thick-walled vessels, ductular reaction at interface; map-like glutamine synthetase pattern; no reticulin loss
Hepatocellular adenoma	Subtype-specific IHC: LFABP loss (HNF1A); SAA/CRP+ (inflammatory); beta-catenin nuclear+ (activated); no glutamine synthetase map pattern

Pattern-Based Approach to Liver Biopsy

Liver Function Tests and Clinicopathological Correlation

Liver function tests (LFTs) are essential for correlating biopsy findings with clinical context. They assess two broad categories: hepatocyte integrity (transaminases) and synthetic/excretory function (albumin, bilirubin, INR, alkaline phosphatase).

Test	Reflects	Elevated In	Clinical Significance
AST (SGOT)	Hepatocyte injury (also muscle, heart)	Hepatitis, cirrhosis, MI, haemolysis	AST:ALT >2 suggests alcoholic or advanced liver disease
ALT (SGPT)	Hepatocyte injury (more liver-specific)	Viral hepatitis, NAFLD, drug injury	ALT > AST in most chronic hepatitis
Alkaline phosphatase (ALP)	Biliary epithelial damage, cholestasis	Obstructive jaundice, PBC, PSC, infiltrative disease	Confirm hepatic origin with GGT
GGT	Biliary damage, enzyme induction	Cholestasis, alcohol, drugs	Elevated with ALP confirms hepatic source
Serum albumin	Hepatic synthetic function	Decreased in cirrhosis, chronic liver disease	Half-life 20 days; reflects chronic dysfunction
INR/PT	Coagulation factor synthesis	Prolonged in acute or chronic liver failure	Best marker of acute synthetic failure (short half-life factors)
Serum bilirubin	Bilirubin metabolism and excretion	Jaundice, hepatitis, obstruction, haemolysis	Fractionation distinguishes conjugated from unconjugated

In acute hepatitis, transaminases are markedly elevated (often >10× normal), whereas in cholestatic disease, ALP and GGT predominate. In cirrhosis with synthetic failure, albumin is low, INR is prolonged, and transaminases may be only mildly elevated. The pattern of LFT abnormality guides the pre-biopsy differential and determines which ancillary investigations (viral serology, autoantibodies, iron studies, ceruloplasmin) to request.

Pattern Recognition on Biopsy

A systematic pattern-based approach is the most efficient method for liver biopsy interpretation. The pathologist should sequentially evaluate: (1) portal tracts (inflammation type, interface activity, bile duct status, fibrosis), (2) lobular parenchyma (hepatocyte injury pattern, steatosis, cholestasis, iron/copper), (3) central veins (congestion, endothelialitis), and (4) overall architecture (fibrosis stage, nodularity).

Primary Pattern	Key Features	Main Differential Diagnosis
Portal chronic inflammation	Interface hepatitis, lymphoplasmacytic infiltrate	Chronic viral hepatitis, AIH, drug reaction, overlap syndromes
Lobular injury/disarray	Acidophil bodies, lobulitis, ballooning	Acute viral hepatitis, drug reaction, autoimmune flare
Steatohepatitis	Steatosis + ballooning + lobular inflammation	NASH, alcoholic hepatitis, drug-induced, Wilson
Cholestatic	Bile ductular reaction, oedema, neutrophils	Large duct obstruction, PBC, PSC, drug reaction, sepsis
Granulomatous	Portal or lobular granulomas	PBC, sarcoidosis, infections (TB, fungal), drugs
Vascular	Sinusoidal dilatation, congestion, necrosis	Congestive hepatopathy, Budd-Chiari, SOS, shock liver

In South Asia, the most likely causes of chronic hepatitis are HBV infection and increasingly NAFLD/NASH. Always request hepatitis B and C serology, autoimmune markers, and metabolic workup alongside every chronic hepatitis liver biopsy.

Recent Advances

EASL Clinical Practice Guidelines on the management of hepatocellular carcinoma. The 2018 European Association for the Study of the Liver Clinical Practice Guidelines provide the international consensus framework for surveillance, diagnosis, staging, and treatment of hepatocellular carcinoma (European Association for the Study of the Liver. Journal of Hepatology 2018; 69: 182–236; PMID 29628281). Surveillance is recommended every six months in patients with cirrhosis or chronic hepatitis B with abdominal ultrasound; alpha-fetoprotein has limited additional value. Diagnosis in cirrhotic livers is established radiologically by characteristic arterial-phase hyperenhancement with portal-venous-phase washout on contrast-enhanced CT or MRI for nodules over one centimetre, and biopsy is reserved for indeterminate lesions. Histopathological grading follows a four-tier scheme, with reticulin loss and immunohistochemistry (glypican-3, glutamine synthetase, heat-shock protein 70) used to distinguish well-differentiated HCC from high-grade dysplastic nodules. Treatment is allocated by the Barcelona Clinic

Liver Cancer (BCLC) algorithm — resection, ablation, transplantation, transarterial chemoembolisation, or systemic therapy — with first-line systemic therapy for advanced disease evolving from sorafenib (the original EASL recommendation) toward combination atezolizumab plus bevacizumab on the basis of subsequent IMbrave150 evidence already noted in this chapter.

The nomenclature revision from NAFLD to MASLD (metabolic dysfunction-associated steatotic liver disease) in 2023 reflects a paradigm shift towards positive diagnostic criteria based on cardiometabolic risk factors, replacing the diagnosis-of-exclusion approach. MASH (metabolic dysfunction-associated steatohepatitis) replaces NASH. This reclassification is expected to improve patient identification and reduce stigma.

Resmetirom, a thyroid hormone receptor-beta (THR-β) agonist, became the first FDA-approved drug for MASH with liver fibrosis (stages F2–F3) in March 2024. The MAESTRO-NASH trial demonstrated significant resolution of MASH without worsening fibrosis, marking a milestone in MASH therapeutics. Other agents in advanced trials include obeticholic acid (FXR agonist), semaglutide (GLP-1 agonist), and lanifibranor (pan-PPAR agonist).

In hepatocellular carcinoma, the combination of atezolizumab (anti-PD-L1) and bevacizumab (anti-VEGF) has become the first-line systemic therapy for unresectable HCC, based on the IMbrave150 trial. Liquid biopsy approaches, including circulating tumour DNA (ctDNA) and methylation markers, are emerging for HCC surveillance and early detection, with potential to supplement or even replace AFP in high-risk populations (see Chapter 41). Additionally, spatial transcriptomics and single-cell RNA sequencing studies are refining our understanding of the tumour microenvironment in HCC and cholangiocarcinoma, revealing distinct immunological niches that may guide immunotherapy selection.

International Frameworks

WHO Classification of Tumours, 5th edition — hepatobiliary tumours and AJCC 8 staging integration. The 5th edition WHO Classification of Tumours of the Digestive System (2019) restructured hepatobiliary nomenclature around morphological subtypes with distinct molecular signatures and clinical behaviour. Hepatocellular carcinoma is now formally subclassified into eight recognised variants — steatohepatitic HCC (associated with metabolic dysfunction-associated steatotic liver disease and IL6/JAK/STAT activation), clear-cell HCC, macrotrabecular-massive HCC (associated with TP53 mutation, FGF19 amplification, and aggressive behaviour), scirrhous HCC (with TGF-β signature and aberrant CK7 and CK19 expression), chromophobe HCC, fibrolamellar carcinoma (the DNAJB1–PRKACA fusion in young adults without cirrhosis), neutrophil-rich HCC, and lymphocyte-rich HCC. Combined hepatocellular-cholangiocarcinoma is retained as a discrete entity for tumours with unequivocal dual differentiation; the previously separate intermediate cell carcinoma category is now classified within the cholangiocarcinoma family. Cholangiocarcinoma is split anatomically into intrahepatic, perihilar (Klatskin), and distal subtypes. Intrahepatic cholangiocarcinoma is further divided morphologically and molecularly into a small-duct subtype (arising on chronic liver disease, sharing IDH1/IDH2 mutations and FGFR2 fusions with HCC, and amenable to targeted therapy with ivosidenib and pemigatinib) and a large-duct subtype (arising on primary sclerosing cholangitis or hepatobiliary fluke infection, with KRAS and TP53 mutations and a desmoplastic mucin-producing morphology). Hepatoblastoma is subclassified into epithelial (foetal, embryonal, small-cell undifferentiated, cholangioblastic, macrotrabecular) and mixed epithelial-mesenchymal subtypes, with prognostic stratification by the Children's Hepatic Tumours International Collaboration (CHIC) risk system. Gallbladder adenocarcinoma is classified histologically into biliary, intestinal, mucinous, and signet-ring variants, and AJCC 8 staging now distinguishes T2a (peritoneal-side perimuscular invasion) from T2b (hepatic-side perimuscular invasion) — a clinically important refinement, because hepatic-side invasion confers significantly worse outcome. AJCC 8 staging for HCC integrates tumour size, multifocality, and vascular invasion, with microvascular invasion driving stage migration; tumours of any size with major vascular invasion or multiple tumours larger than five centimetres are stage T3 or T4. The diagnostic IHC algorithm for hepatocellular versus metastatic adenocarcinoma pivots on HepPar1 (granular cytoplasmic), arginase-1 (the most specific hepatocellular marker, both cytoplasmic and nuclear), and glypican-3 (more sensitive in poorly differentiated HCC); CK7 and CK19 co-expression in HCC predicts a cholangiocellular phenotype with worse prognosis. Citation: Calderaro J, Couchy G, Imbeaud S, et al. Histological subtypes of hepatocellular carcinoma are related to gene mutations and molecular tumour classification. J Hepatol 2017; 67: 727–738. PMID 28532995.

Approach to the Histopathology Slide

When presented with a liver biopsy slide in the practical examination, adopt a systematic approach.

Step 1: Low power. Assess overall architecture. Is the normal lobular architecture preserved, or is there nodularity with fibrous septa (cirrhosis)? Note the distribution of any abnormality: portal-predominant, lobular-predominant, or both.

Step 2: Portal tracts. Evaluate portal inflammation (lymphocytic, lymphoplasmacytic, mixed, granulomatous), interface hepatitis, bile duct status (intact, damaged, absent), and fibrosis (trichrome).

Step 3: Lobular parenchyma. Look for steatosis (type and zone), hepatocyte injury (ballooning, acidophil bodies, Mallory-Denk bodies), cholestasis, iron or copper deposition, and infiltrative lesions.

Step 4: Central veins. Assess for congestion, endothelialitis, or sinusoidal dilatation.

Step 5: Special features. Ground-glass hepatocytes (HBV), PAS-D resistant globules (A1AT), Perl's positive iron (hemochromatosis), "fried egg" cells (clear cell HCC), lamellar fibrosis (fibrolamellar HCC).

Synthesise findings into a pattern-based diagnosis and correlate with available clinical and serological data (Figure 20.9).

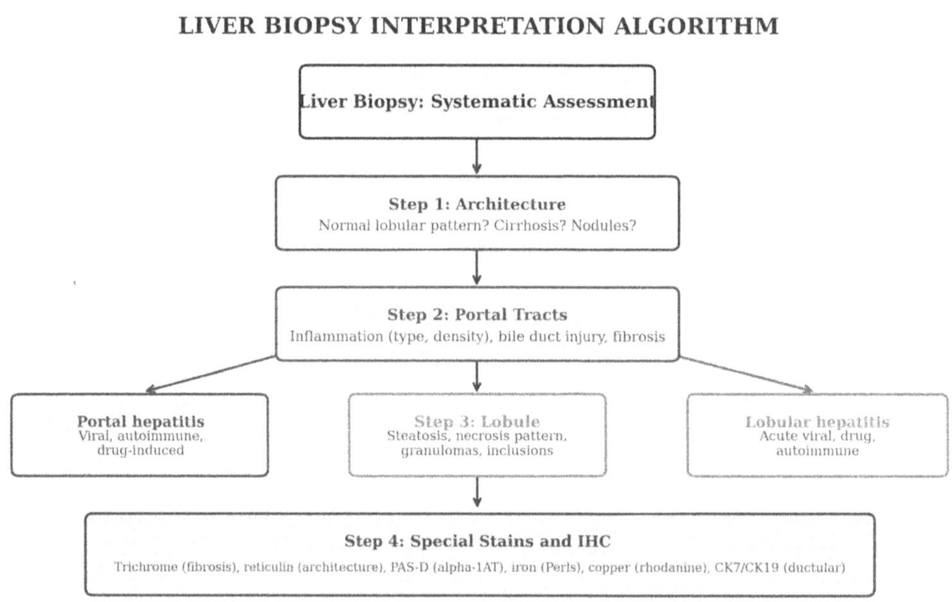

Figure 20.9: Algorithmic approach to liver biopsy interpretation. Flowchart progressing from architectural assessment through portal tract evaluation, lobular assessment, and vascular evaluation to pattern-based differential diagnosis. (Source: Author's original.)

Ultra High-Yield Chapter Summary

Topic	Must Remember
Jaundice classification	Pre-hepatic (unconjugated), hepatic (mixed), post-hepatic (conjugated); urine bilirubin and urobilinogen distinguish them
Gilbert syndrome	UGT1A1 deficiency, 5–10% prevalence, benign unconjugated hyperbilirubinaemia
HBV hallmarks	Ground-glass hepatocytes (HBsAg), sanded nuclei (HBcAg); orcein/Victoria blue stain
HCV hallmarks	Portal lymphoid aggregates, steatosis (genotype 3), interface hepatitis; >80% chronicity

METAVIR system	Activity A0–A3, Fibrosis F0–F4; F4 = cirrhosis
Autoimmune hepatitis	Lymphoplasmacytic interface hepatitis, rosettes, emperipolesis; ANA/SMA/LKM-1; Simplified score ≥7 definite
NASH triad	Steatosis + lobular inflammation + hepatocyte ballooning; NAS score 0–8; zone 3 pericellular fibrosis
MASLD (2023)	New nomenclature for NAFLD; requires cardiometabolic risk factor
Hemochromatosis	HFE C282Y; periportal hepatocyte iron (zone 1); Perl's stain; HIC/age >1.9
Wilson disease	ATP7B; low ceruloplasmin; AST:ALT >2.2; hepatic Cu >250 µg/g dry weight
A1AT deficiency	PiZZ; PAS-D resistant globules, periportal; SERPINA1 gene
Cirrhosis	Diffuse fibrosis + regenerative nodules; micronodular (<3 mm) vs macronodular (>3 mm)
PBC	AMA (M2), florid duct lesion, granulomatous bile duct destruction, ductopenia
PSC	Onion-skin fibrosis, cholangiographic beading, UC association, cholangiocarcinoma risk 10–15%
Biliary atresia	Most common indication for infant liver transplant; ductular reaction, portal oedema, cholestasis
FNH vs HCA	FNH: central scar, map-like GS, no malignant risk.
HCC diagnosis	Reticulin loss (plates >2 cells), glypican-3+, diffuse CD34+, Hepar-1+, arginase-1+
Fibrolamellar HCC	Young, non-cirrhotic, DNAJB1-PRKACA fusion, CK7+, CD68+, normal AFP
iCCA	CK7+/CK19+, albumin ISH+, desmoplastic stroma; large duct (PSC, flukes) vs small duct (cirrhosis)
Transplant rejection	T cell-mediated: portal inflammation + bile duct damage + endothelialitis; Banff grading

Diagnostic thinking: widened hepatic plates + reticulin loss + HepPar1+/glypican-3+ → hepatocellular carcinoma

Diagnostic thinking: bridging fibrosis + regenerative nodules + ductular reaction → cirrhosis (identify aetiology by pattern)

Diagnostic thinking: CK7+/CK19+ + desmoplastic stroma + bile duct morphology → cholangiocarcinoma (Figure 20.11)

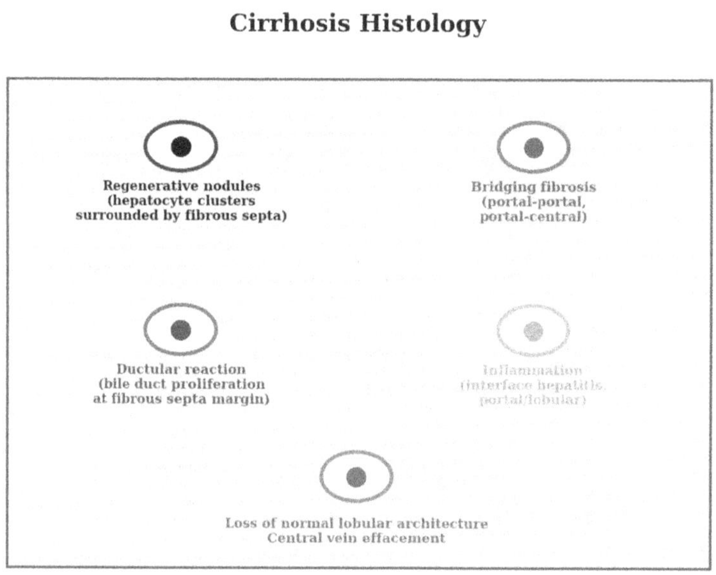

Figure 20.10A: Cirrhosis Histology. (Source: Author's original.)

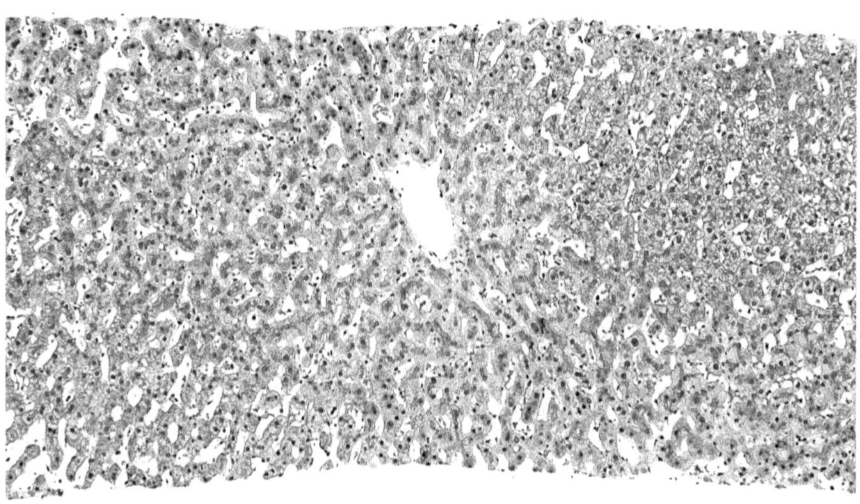

Figure 20.10B: Liver cirrhosis: Fibrous expansion with Trichrome stain delineating collagen (blue) bridges (Masson Trichrome, intermed mag). (Source: Nephron, Wikimedia Commons, CC BY-SA 3.0.)

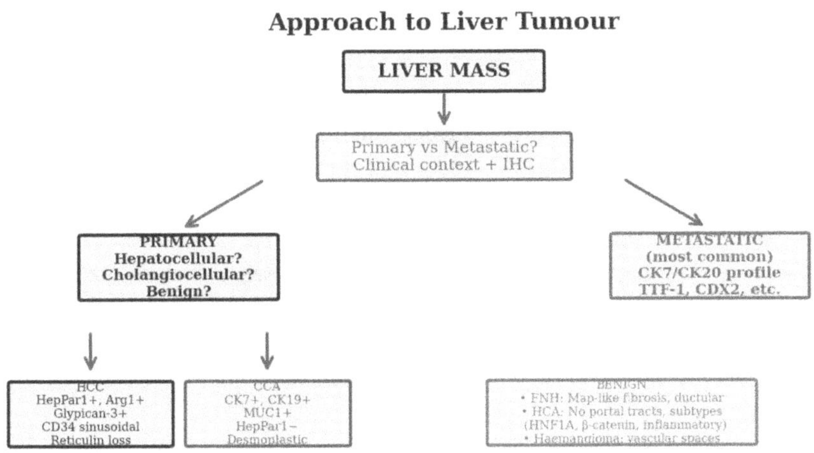

Figure 20.11: Approach to Liver Tumour. (Source: Author's original.)

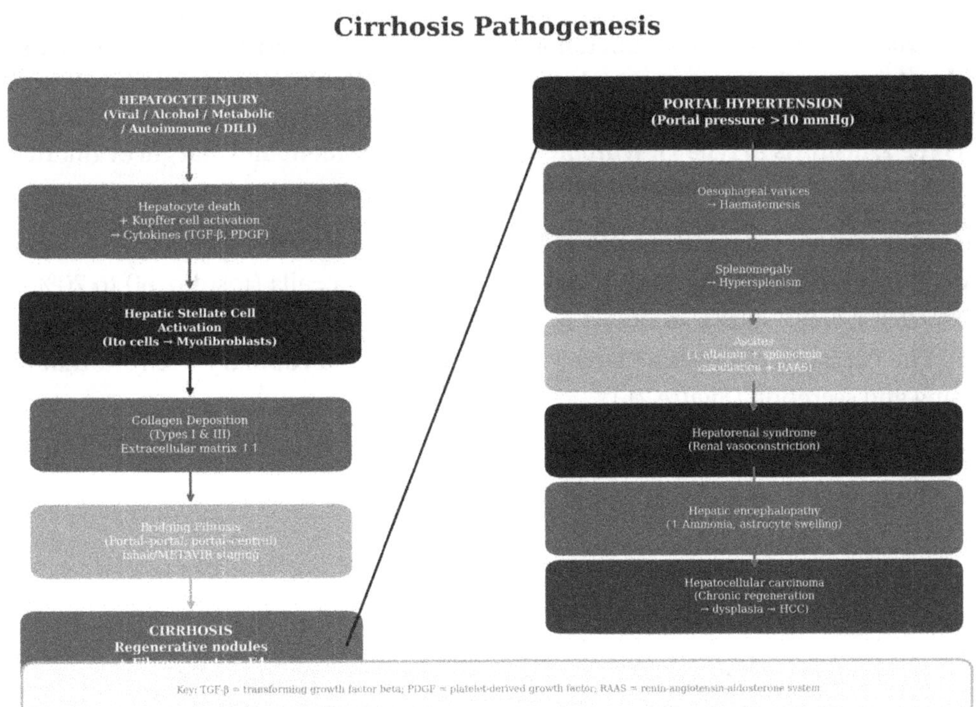

Figure 20.12: Cirrhosis Pathogenesis. (Source: Author's original.)

Chapter 21: Pancreas Pathology

THE BIG PICTURE

The pancreas is a dual-function gland whose exocrine and endocrine compartments generate distinct disease spectra. Exocrine pathology spans acute and chronic pancreatitis — including autoimmune pancreatitis with its characteristic IgG4 signature — and a well-defined family of precursor lesions and neoplasms: pancreatic intraepithelial neoplasia (PanIN), cystic neoplasms (IPMN, MCN, SCN, SPN), and pancreatic ductal adenocarcinoma (PDAC), the lethal archetype of stromal-rich cancer. The endocrine pancreas contributes a separate population of neuroendocrine tumours whose behaviour is dictated by grade and functional status, as well as the systemic morphological footprint of diabetes mellitus in the islet compartment. This chapter organises these entities around their histological architecture, molecular alterations, and diagnostic IHC profiles, emphasising the patterns most frequently tested in postgraduate pathology examinations.

High-yield topics in this chapter: Normal pancreatic anatomy, ductal system, and islet architecture; Acute pancreatitis (pathogenesis of enzyme activation, gross and microscopic features, complications); Chronic pancreatitis (aetiology, calcifying and obstructive forms, differential with PDAC); Autoimmune pancreatitis type 1 (IgG4-related) and type 2 (idiopathic duct-centric); Pancreatic ductal adenocarcinoma (morphology, histological subtypes, IHC panel, molecular alterations including KRAS, TP53, SMAD4, CDKN2A); Precursor lesions — PanIN 1, 2, 3 and their molecular progression; Cystic pancreatic neoplasms (IPMN main-duct and branch-duct, MCN with ovarian-type stroma, SCN with central scar, SPN with nuclear beta-catenin); Pancreatic neuroendocrine tumours (functional vs non-functional, WHO 2019 grading with Ki-67, insulinoma/gastrinoma/glucagonoma syndromes); Rare exocrine tumours (acinar cell carcinoma, pancreatoblastoma); Pathology of the endocrine pancreas in diabetes mellitus (amyloid in type 2, insulitis in type 1); Whipple specimen assessment and margin evaluation; Approach to the pancreatic mass on biopsy and resection.

The endocrine pancreas consists of the islets of Langerhans (approximately 1 to 2% of pancreatic mass, numbering about one million in the adult gland), containing beta cells (insulin, 60 to 70%), alpha cells (glucagon, 20 to 25%), delta cells (somatostatin, 5 to 10%), PP cells (pancreatic polypeptide), and epsilon cells (ghrelin). The islets are richly vascularised with a fenestrated capillary network that allows direct hormone sensing and secretion (Figure 21.1).

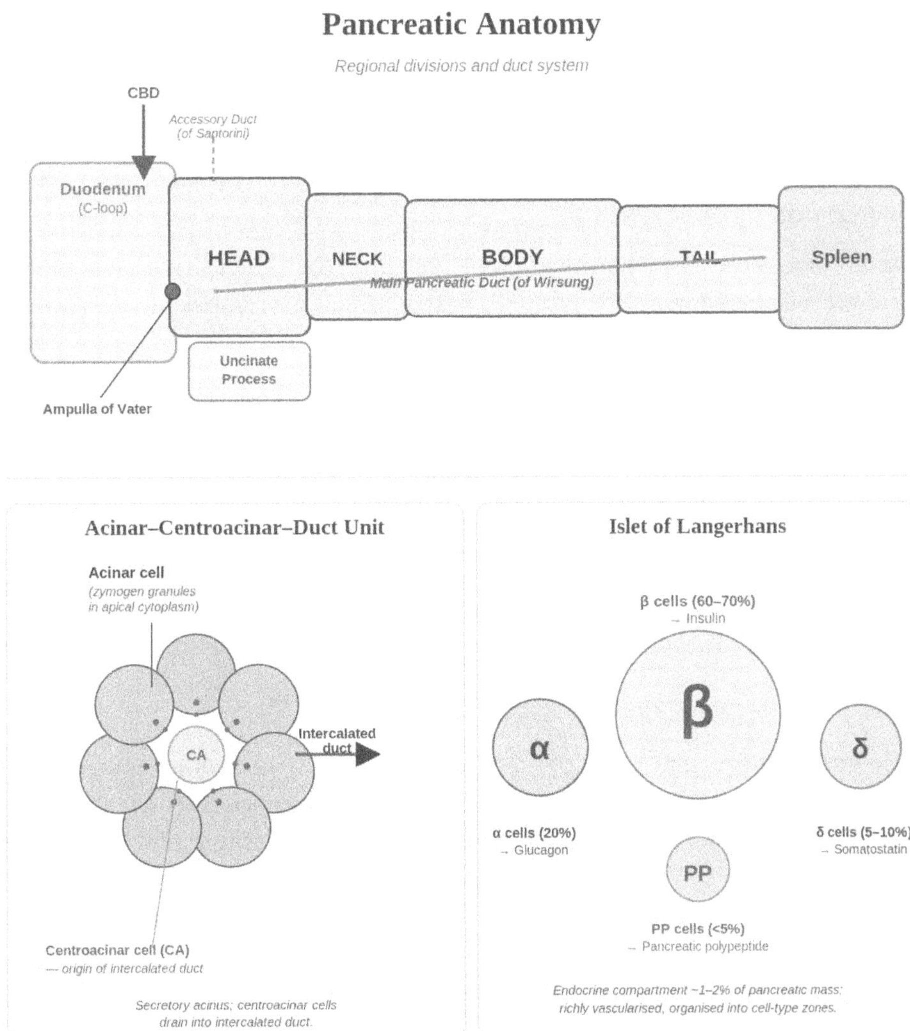

Figure 21.1: Pancreatic anatomy: regional divisions, duct system (Wirsung and Santorini), acinar-centroacinar-duct unit, and islet of Langerhans architecture. (Source: Author's original.)

21.2 Pancreatitis

21.2.1 Acute Pancreatitis

Definition: Acute inflammatory condition from inappropriate activation of pancreatic enzymes within the gland. Ranges from mild interstitial oedematous pancreatitis (80–90%) to severe necrotising pancreatitis (10–20%, mortality 20–30%).

Etiology/Associations: Gallstones (40%) and alcohol (30%) = ~70%. Others: hypertriglyceridaemia (>1000 mg/dL), hypercalcaemia, drugs (azathioprine, valproic acid, thiazides), ERCP, trauma, infections (mumps, coxsackievirus), pancreas divisum, genetic (PRSS1, SPINK1, CFTR). Idiopathic 10–20%.

Pathogenesis: Three converging mechanisms: (1) duct obstruction → increased intraductal pressure; (2) direct acinar injury → co-localisation of zymogens and lysosomes; (3) defective intracellular transport. All exceed SPINK1/mesotrypsin protective capacity.

Duct obstruction/acinar injury → Premature trypsinogen activation → Trypsin cascade (elastase, phospholipase A2, lipase) → Autodigestion → Fat necrosis + proteolysis + haemorrhage → Oedematous or necrotising pancreatitis

Gross: Chalky white fat necrosis (saponification — calcium soap deposition), haemorrhagic necrosis (dark red-black from elastase-mediated vascular destruction), peritoneal fat necrosis extending into omentum/mesentery.

Microscopy: Oedematous type: marked oedema, mild neutrophils, preserved acinar architecture. Necrotising type: coagulative necrosis, **basophilic calcium deposits in fat necrosis (saponification)**, extensive neutrophils, vascular thrombosis, haemorrhage.

Complications/Prognosis: Pseudocyst (6–12 weeks), infected necrosis, abscess, ARDS, DIC, splenic vein thrombosis. Revised Atlanta: mild (no organ failure), moderate (transient <48 h), severe (persistent >48 h).

Exam yield: ★★★ HIGH — Pathogenesis arrow chain and saponification are exam staples.

21.2.2 Laboratory Diagnosis and Serum Enzymes in Pancreatic Disease

Serum pancreatic enzymes are central to the diagnosis of acute pancreatitis and are among the most frequently tested laboratory topics in examinations. Serum amylase rises within 6 to 12 hours of symptom onset, peaks at 24 to 48 hours, and normalises within 3 to 5 days due to rapid renal clearance. Serum lipase rises within 4 to 8 hours, peaks at 24 hours, and remains elevated for 8 to 14 days, making it the preferred diagnostic marker when presentation is delayed. A threefold or greater elevation of either enzyme, combined with characteristic abdominal pain and/or imaging findings, meets the Revised Atlanta criteria for diagnosing acute pancreatitis (two of three criteria required).

The key diagnostic clue in serum enzyme interpretation is that lipase is more specific for pancreatic disease than amylase. Amylase has multiple non-pancreatic sources: salivary glands (salivary-type amylase, S-type), fallopian tubes (ectopic pregnancy), and the intestine. Conditions causing hyperamylasaemia without pancreatitis include parotitis, macroamylasaemia (amylase-immunoglobulin complexes too large for renal filtration), intestinal obstruction or perforation, renal failure (decreased clearance), and ruptured ectopic pregnancy. In contrast, lipase is produced almost exclusively by pancreatic acinar cells, and elevated lipase with normal amylase may indicate pancreatitis with delayed presentation or chronic pancreatitis with sufficient acinar reserve for lipase but not amylase release.

Table 21.1: Serum Pancreatic Enzymes in Clinical Practice

Feature	Amylase	Lipase
Source	Pancreas, salivary glands, fallopian tubes, intestine	Pancreas (predominant), gastric lipase (minor)

Rise after onset	6–12 hours	4–8 hours
Peak	24–48 hours	24 hours
Duration of elevation	3–5 days	8–14 days
Specificity for pancreatitis	Lower (many non-pancreatic sources)	Higher (pancreas is dominant source)
Preferred marker	Not preferred alone	Yes; preferred single marker for acute pancreatitis
False elevation	Parotitis, macroamylasaemia, renal failure, bowel obstruction, ectopic pregnancy	Renal failure, bowel obstruction (rare)
Isoenzymes	P-type (pancreatic) and S-type (salivary); P-type isoamylase improves specificity	Not clinically subtyped
Chronic pancreatitis	May be normal (burned-out gland)	May be normal or mildly elevated

Other useful laboratory investigations in pancreatic disease include serum calcium (hypocalcaemia from saponification is a marker of severity), C-reactive protein (>150 mg/L at 48 hours predicts severe disease), serum triglycerides (both a cause and consequence), liver function tests (elevated bilirubin and ALP suggest gallstone aetiology), and urinary trypsinogen-2 (a rapid bedside test with high sensitivity). The Revised Atlanta Classification (2012) categorises severity as mild (no organ failure, no local complications), moderately severe (transient organ failure <48 hours or local complications), and severe (persistent organ failure >48 hours). CT severity scoring (Balthazar) and the APACHE II system complement laboratory assessment for prognosis.

Pseudocysts, encapsulated collections of enzyme-rich fluid lacking an epithelial lining, develop in approximately 10% of acute pancreatitis cases, typically 4 to 6 weeks after the acute episode. They are lined by granulation tissue and fibrous capsule, not epithelium, which distinguishes them from true cystic neoplasms. Walled-off necrosis (WON) is an encapsulated collection of pancreatic and/or peripancreatic necrosis that has developed a well-defined inflammatory wall; unlike pseudocysts, WON contains solid necrotic debris.

When faced with a peripancreatic cystic lesion, the first question to ask is whether it arises in the setting of recent pancreatitis (pseudocyst or WON) or represents a de novo cystic neoplasm. Cyst fluid analysis is invaluable: pseudocyst fluid shows high amylase (>250 U/L) and low CEA (<5 ng/mL), while mucinous neoplasms show elevated CEA (>192 ng/mL, 75% sensitivity) and variable amylase depending on duct communication.

Table 21.2: Pancreatic Cyst Fluid Analysis

Parameter	Pseudocyst	Serous Cystadenoma	Mucinous (IPMN/MCN)	Interpretation
CEA	<5 ng/mL	<5 ng/mL	>192 ng/mL	CEA >192: 75% sensitive, 84% specific for mucinous
Amylase	Very high (>250 U/L)	Low	Variable (high if IPMN communicates with duct)	High amylase = duct communication or pancreatitis
Cytology	Macrophages, debris	Cuboidal glycogen-rich cells	Columnar mucinous cells, mucin	Cytology specificity high but sensitivity low
Molecular markers	Not applicable	VHL mutation	KRAS, GNAS mutations	KRAS mutation 96% specific for mucinous cyst
Viscosity	Low (watery)	Low	High (string sign positive)	Mucinous fluid is characteristically viscous

Quick Recall: Acute Pancreatitis and Serum Enzymes

Aetiology: Gallstones (40%) + alcohol (30%) = 70%; GET SMASHED mnemonic.

Lipase > amylase: Lipase is more specific and stays elevated longer (8–14 days vs 3–5 days).

Amylase pitfalls: Elevated in parotitis, macroamylasaemia, renal failure, ectopic pregnancy; P-type isoamylase improves specificity.

Atlanta criteria: 2 of 3: characteristic pain + enzymes ≥3× ULN + imaging. Severity: mild/moderately severe/severe.

CRP >150 at 48h: Predicts severe disease. Hypocalcaemia = saponification (poor prognostic sign).

Pseudocyst: NO epithelial lining; enzyme-rich; cyst fluid: high amylase, low CEA.

21.2.3 Chronic Pancreatitis

Definition: Progressive, irreversible destruction of pancreatic parenchyma with fibrosis, leading to exocrine and eventually endocrine insufficiency.

Etiology/Associations: Alcohol (60–70%). TIGAR-O: Toxic-metabolic, Idiopathic, Genetic (PRSS1, SPINK1, CFTR), Autoimmune, Recurrent acute, Obstructive.

Repeated injury → Necrosis-fibrosis sequence → Acinar atrophy + duct dilation/calcification → Exocrine insufficiency → Endocrine failure (late)

Microscopy: Acinar atrophy with **dense fibrosis and chronic inflammatory infiltrates (lymphocytes, plasma cells)**. Dilated ducts with proteinaceous plugs and calcifications. Residual islets in fibrous tissue. Perineural inflammation (not invasion). Faecal elastase-1: <200 = insufficiency; <100 = severe.

Key DDx: Chronic pancreatitis vs well-differentiated PDAC — most challenging distinction. SMAD4 loss supports carcinoma (never lost in chronic pancreatitis). Perineural invasion (not inflammation) favours carcinoma.

Exam yield: ★★★ HIGH — DDx with PDAC is a classic viva question. TIGAR-O classification frequently asked.

Exam Pitfall: Chronic Pancreatitis versus Well-Differentiated PDAC

This is one of the most challenging distinctions in surgical pathology. Both show glandular structures in a fibrotic stroma.

Favouring chronic pancreatitis: preserved lobular architecture, complete rounded glandular lumina with minimal atypia, no perineural invasion (perineural inflammation is acceptable), calcifications, uniform nuclear size.

Favouring PDAC: haphazard gland distribution disrupting lobular architecture, incomplete lumina, perineural invasion (tumour cells wrapping around ≥one-third of nerve circumference), vascular invasion, marked nuclear size variation (>4:1 ratio), single infiltrating cells or small clusters, glands adjacent to muscular vessels.

IHC: SMAD4 (DPC4) loss supports carcinoma (lost in ~55% of PDAC, always retained in chronic pancreatitis). p53 overexpression (missense mutation pattern) also supports carcinoma.

21.2.4 Autoimmune Pancreatitis

Definition: Two distinct subtypes. Type 1 = pancreatic manifestation of IgG4-related disease. Type 2 = idiopathic duct-centric pancreatitis.

Etiology/Associations: Type 1: IgG4-RD; older men (median 60). Type 2: IBD association (UC in 20–30%); younger (median 40).

Microscopy: Type 1: Dense lymphoplasmacytic infiltrates with **IgG4+ plasma cells (>10/HPF), storiform fibrosis, obliterative phlebitis**. Serum IgG4 >135 mg/dL. HISORt criteria. Type 2: **Granulocytic epithelial lesions (GELs)** — neutrophils in duct epithelium. No IgG4 elevation. Groove pancreatitis (paraduodenal): dense fibrosis in groove, myoid Brunner gland proliferation, duodenal wall cysts, neural hyperplasia; mimics carcinoma.

Key DDx: Both types mimic PDAC on imaging. Type 1: sausage-shaped pancreas. Both respond to corticosteroids. Type 1 has higher relapse rate.

Exam yield: ★★★ HIGH — Type 1 vs Type 2, GELs, storiform fibrosis, and groove pancreatitis as carcinoma mimic are all exam favourites.

Quick Recall: Pancreatitis

Acute: Gallstones (40%) + alcohol (30%); fat necrosis = saponification; Revised Atlanta severity.

Chronic: Irreversible; acinar atrophy, fibrosis, calcifications, duct dilation; TIGAR-O classification.

AIP type 1: IgG4-RD; storiform fibrosis, obliterative phlebitis, >10 IgG4+ plasma cells/HPF; steroid-responsive.

AIP type 2: GELs (neutrophils in ducts), no IgG4 elevation, IBD association, younger patients.

Groove pancreatitis: Paraduodenal, mimics carcinoma, alcohol-related, Brunner gland hyperplasia, duodenal wall cysts.

Faecal elastase-1: <200 µg/g = exocrine insufficiency; <100 = severe.

21.3 Pancreatic Ductal Adenocarcinoma

Definition: Most common pancreatic malignancy (~90%). Fourth leading cause of cancer death worldwide.

Etiology/Associations: Age 60–70s, M:F 1.3:1. Smoking (2-fold). Chronic pancreatitis (4% at 20 years). Hereditary: Peutz-Jeghers (132-fold), BRCA2 (3.5–10-fold), Lynch (8.6-fold), FAMMM/CDKN2A, PRSS1 (50-fold). 60–70% in head (Courvoisier sign).

Normal epithelium → PanIN-1 (KRAS, telomere shortening) → PanIN-2 (+ CDKN2A/p16 loss) → PanIN-3 (+ TP53, SMAD4 loss) → Invasive PDAC

Gross: Firm, grey-white scirrhous mass with infiltrative borders. Desmoplastic stroma 50–80% of tumour (chemoresistance via hypovascular microenvironment).

Microscopy: Infiltrating duct-like glands in dense desmoplasia. Mucin production, haphazard distribution, incomplete lumina, nuclear pleomorphism. **Perineural invasion in >80%** (diagnostic clue + spread route). Lymphovascular invasion common.

Molecular/Genetics: Tetrad: KRAS (>90%, G12D), CDKN2A/p16 (>90%), TP53 (60–70%), SMAD4/DPC4 (55% — IHC loss distinguishes from chronic pancreatitis). ~5–7% HRD (BRCA1/2, PALB2 → PARP inhibitor eligible). ~1% MMR-deficient.

Complications/Prognosis: 5-year survival ~10%. Whipple: SMA/uncinate margin most critical. NCCN: germline testing for all new PDAC.

Exam yield: ★★★ HIGH — Molecular tetrad, perineural invasion, Whipple margins, SMAD4 IHC are all exam staples.

21.3.1 Histological Subtypes

Definition: Histological variants of PDAC with prognostic significance.

Microscopy: **Adenosquamous**: ≥30% squamous; worse prognosis. **Colloid (mucinous non-cystic)**: >80% extracellular mucin pools; better prognosis; from intestinal-type IPMN; CDX2+. **Medullary**: syncytial growth + TILs; often MMR-deficient; checkpoint inhibitor responsive. **Undifferentiated with osteoclast-like giant cells**: CD68+ giant cells + mononuclear tumour cells.

Exam yield: ★★ MODERATE — Colloid (CDX2+, better prognosis) and medullary (MMR-deficient) are exam favourites.

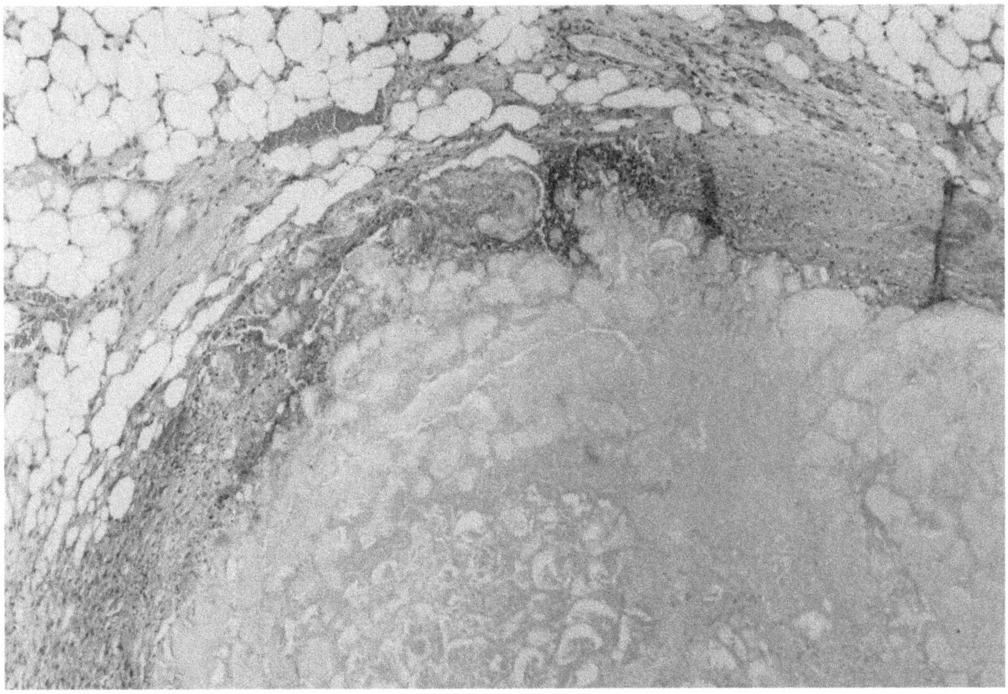

Figure 21.2: Acute pancreatitis with fat necrosis and saponification (H&E). Areas of coagulative necrosis of adipocytes with basophilic calcium soap deposits are characteristic. (Source: Patho, Wikimedia Commons, CC BY-SA 3.0.)

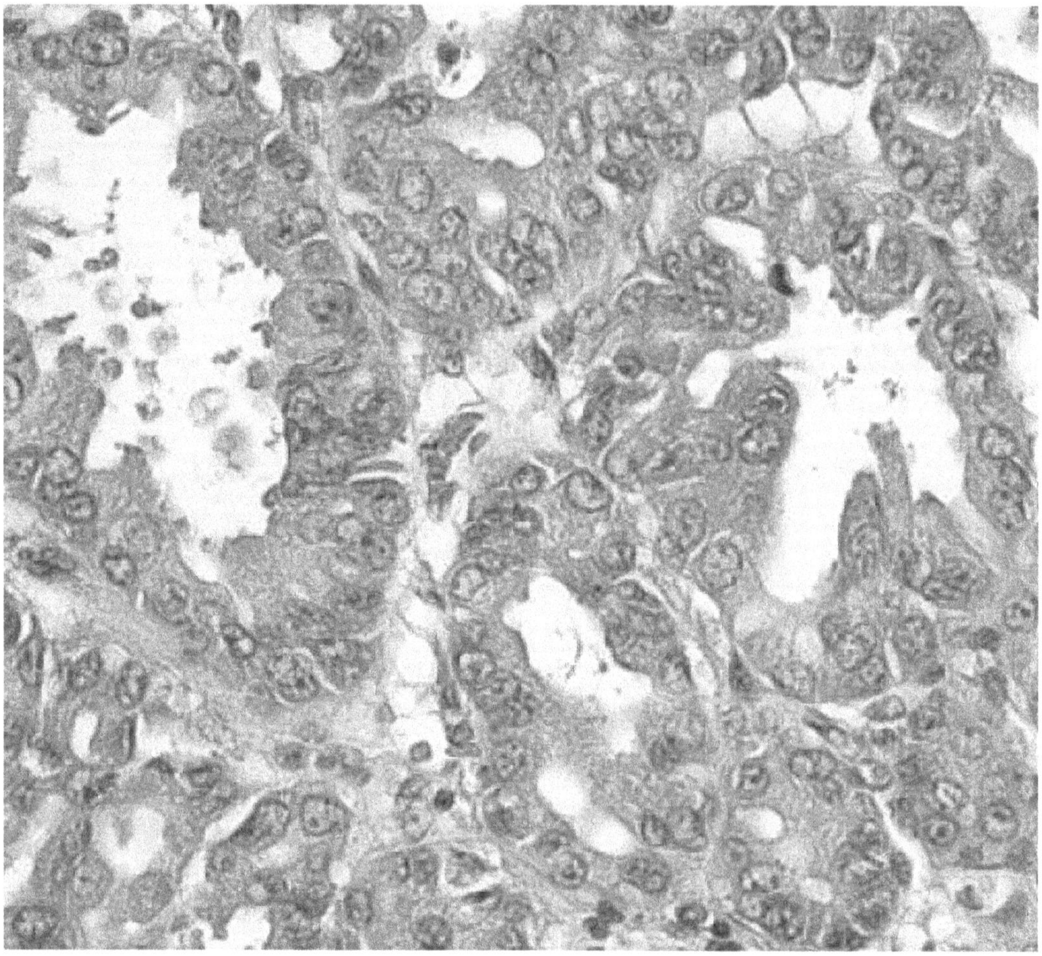

Figure 21.3: Intraductal papillary mucinous neoplasm (IPMN), pancreatobiliary subtype. Complex papillary proliferation of mucinous epithelium within a dilated pancreatic duct. H&E. (Source: Shibata et al., Wikimedia Commons, CC BY 4.0.)

21.3.2 Staging and Whipple Specimen Assessment

PDAC is staged using the AJCC/UICC TNM 8th edition. Key T stage landmarks: T1 (tumour limited to pancreas, ≤2 cm; T1a ≤0.5 cm, T1b 0.5–1 cm, T1c 1–2 cm), T2 (>2 cm but ≤4 cm, limited to pancreas), T3 (>4 cm, limited to pancreas), and T4 (tumour involving the coeliac axis or superior mesenteric artery; unresectable). Note that the 8th edition no longer considers extrapancreatic extension as a staging criterion; size alone drives T stage. N staging is also size-based: N1 (1–3 positive nodes), N2 (≥4 positive nodes).

The Whipple pancreaticoduodenectomy specimen includes the head and uncinate process of the pancreas, duodenum, distal common bile duct, and gallbladder. The systematic gross examination must identify and ink all margins. Critical margins include: the superior mesenteric artery (SMA/retroperitoneal/uncinate) margin (the most commonly positive margin and strongest predictor of local recurrence, inked separately), the pancreatic neck (transection) margin, the bile duct margin, and the anterior and posterior surfaces. R0 denotes microscopically clear margins; R1 denotes microscopic tumour at the margin. The

Royal College of Pathologists (UK) defines R1 as tumour within 1 mm of the margin, while the College of American Pathologists (US) defines R1 as tumour at the inked margin.

Pathological assessment should document tumour size, histological type and grade (well, moderate, poor), margin status (R0 vs R1 with distances), lymph node status (with total count), perineural invasion, lymphovascular invasion, and tumour regression grade if neoadjuvant therapy was administered. The CAP four-tier tumour regression grading system ranges from grade 0 (complete response, no viable tumour) to grade 3 (poor response, extensive residual cancer with minimal tumour kill).

Quick Recall: PDAC

Frequency: 90% of pancreatic neoplasms; 60–70% in head; Courvoisier sign (painless jaundice + palpable GB).

Molecular tetrad: KRAS (>90%), TP53 (60–70%), CDKN2A (>90%), SMAD4 (55%).

SMAD4 IHC: Loss supports carcinoma (never lost in chronic pancreatitis). Correlates with metastatic phenotype.

Perineural invasion: Present in >80%; key diagnostic feature and route of retroperitoneal spread.

Whipple margins: SMA/uncinate margin most critical; R1 definition differs between RCPath (≤1 mm) and CAP (at ink).

Neoadjuvant: CAP 4-tier regression grading: 0 = complete response, 3 = poor response.

21.4 Precursor Lesions: PanIN

Definition: Most common precursor of PDAC. Microscopic (<5 mm) intraductal lesions.

Microscopy: PanIN-1: flat/papillary mucinous epithelium, minimal atypia. PanIN-2: nuclear enlargement, pseudostratification. **PanIN-3 (carcinoma in situ)**: severe atypia, cribriform growth, luminal necrosis, atypical mitoses.

Molecular/Genetics: PanIN-1 (KRAS, telomere shortening) → PanIN-2 (CDKN2A/p16) → PanIN-3 (TP53, SMAD4, BRCA2). KRAS present even in low-grade — cyst fluid KRAS cannot distinguish grade alone.

Exam yield: ★★★ HIGH — PanIN progression model with molecular events is a classic exam diagram.

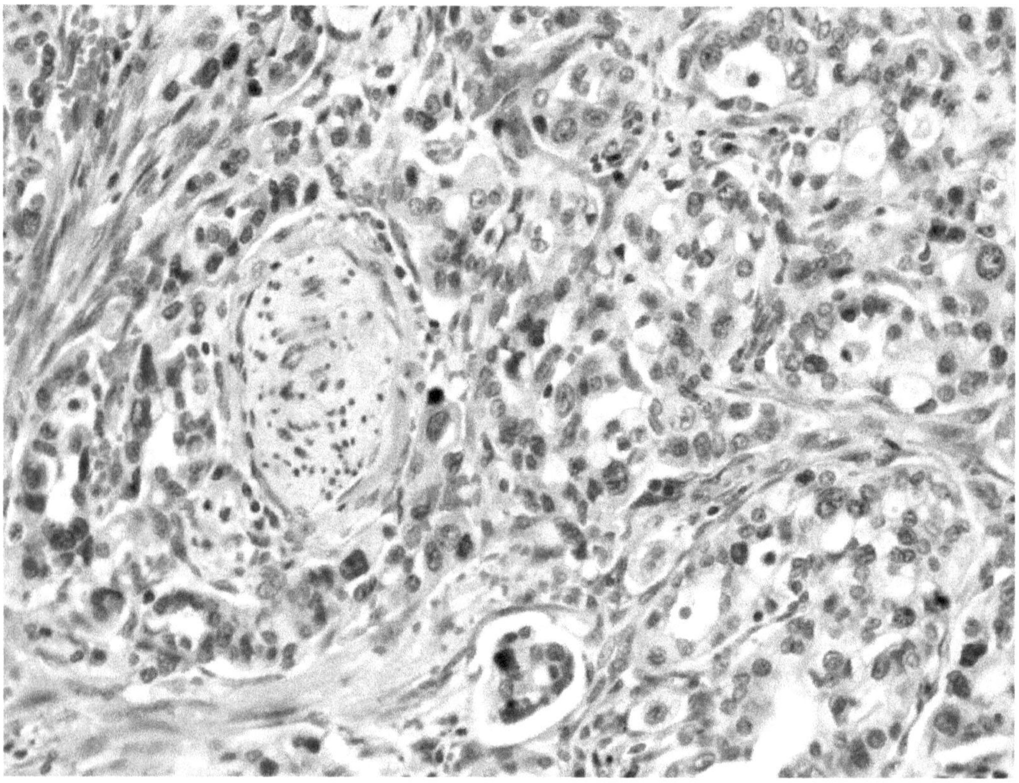

Figure 21.4: Pancreatic ductal adenocarcinoma — infiltrating glands in desmoplastic stroma with perineural invasion (H&E). (Source: KGH, Wikimedia Commons, CC BY-SA 3.0.)

The pathogenesis explains the morphology: because KRAS activation is the earliest event, even low-grade PanIN-1 lesions harbour KRAS mutations. This has important implications: KRAS mutations in cyst fluid or pancreatic juice cannot distinguish low-grade from high-grade dysplasia. Additional molecular events (TP53, SMAD4 loss) are needed to identify high-risk lesions (Figure 21.5).

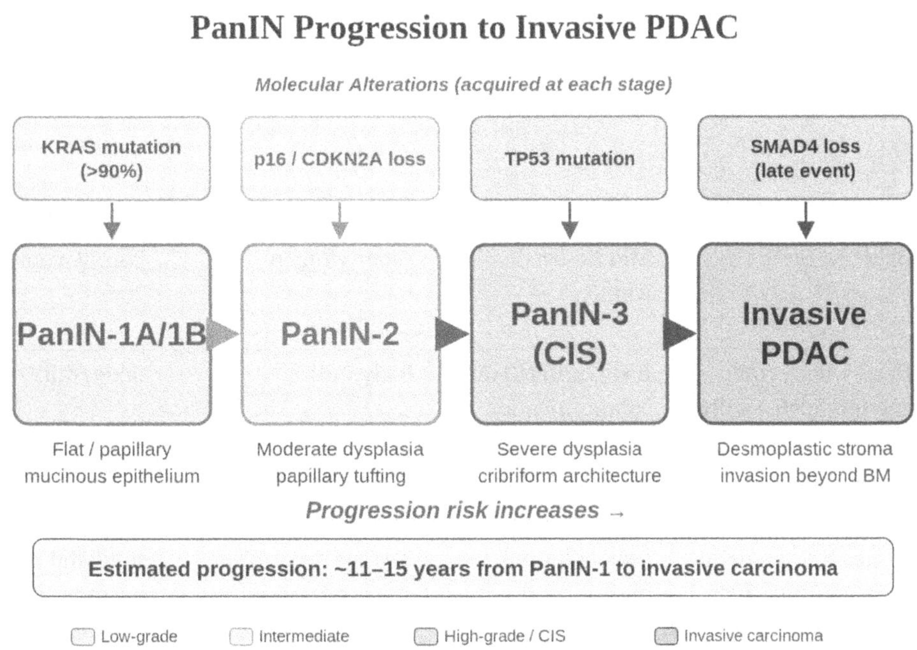

Figure 21.5: PanIN progression model: stepwise molecular and histological changes from PanIN-1 to invasive pancreatic ductal adenocarcinoma. (Source: Author's original.)

21.5 Cystic Pancreatic Neoplasms

Cystic pancreatic neoplasms are a diverse group with vastly different malignant potential. The increasing use of cross-sectional imaging has made incidental pancreatic cysts a common clinical problem; approximately 2 to 3% of CT scans and 20% of MRI scans detect pancreatic cysts. Accurate classification is essential because management ranges from observation to surgical resection.

WHO 5th Edition Classification: Epithelial Tumours of the Exocrine Pancreas (selected)

Benign: Serous cystadenoma; acinar cell cystadenoma

Precursor lesions: PanIN (low-grade and high-grade); IPMN with low-grade or high-grade dysplasia; MCN with low-grade or high-grade dysplasia

Malignant (common): Ductal adenocarcinoma (and variants); IPMN with associated invasive carcinoma; MCN with associated invasive carcinoma

Malignant (uncommon): Acinar cell carcinoma; pancreatoblastoma; solid pseudopapillary neoplasm

Neuroendocrine: Well-differentiated NET G1/G2/G3; poorly differentiated NEC (small cell, large cell)

Note: WHO 5th Edition (2019) uses a two-tier system for dysplasia (low-grade and high-grade) replacing the former three-tier system in both IPMN and MCN.

Table 21.3: Cystic Pancreatic Neoplasms: Comparison

Feature	IPMN	MCN	Serous Cystadenoma	SPN
Age/Sex	Older, M=F	Middle-aged women	Older women	Young women (20–30s)
Location	Head > body/tail; communicates with duct	Body/tail; NO duct communication	Body/tail	Body/tail
Gross	Papillary growths in dilated duct; mucin from ampulla (fish-mouth papilla)	Thick-walled, unilocular or multilocular	Microcystic (sponge-like) with central stellate scar	Large, encapsulated, solid and cystic with haemorrhage
Epithelium	Tall columnar mucinous with papillae; gastric, intestinal, pancreatobiliary, oncocytic subtypes	Tall columnar mucinous, no papillae	Cuboidal, glycogen-rich, clear cytoplasm (PAS+, PAS-D−)	Solid sheets, pseudopapillae around hyalinised fibrovascular cores
Stroma	No ovarian stroma	Ovarian-type stroma (ER/PR+, inhibin+)	No ovarian stroma	Hyalinised fibrovascular stalks
Key IHC	CK7+, MUC variable by subtype	CK7+, ER/PR+ (stroma), inhibin+ (stroma)	Inhibin+, CAIX+, GLUT1+, MUC6+	β-catenin nuclear+, CD10+, CD56+, E-cadherin lost
Malignant potential	Yes; main-duct > branch-duct	Yes; increases with size	Almost none	Low (~15%)
Key molecular	GNAS (60%), KRAS	KRAS, RNF43	VHL mutations	CTNNB1 (β-catenin) mutations

Definition: Intraductal papillary mucinous neoplasm. Communicates with duct system (vs MCN).

Etiology/Associations: Older adults, M=F. Head > body/tail. Main-duct vs branch-duct drives management.

Gross: Papillary growths in dilated duct; mucin from ampulla (fish-mouth papilla). Main-duct ≥10 mm = 40–60% invasive carcinoma.

Microscopy: Subtypes: **gastric (most common, foveolar, MUC5AC+, lowest risk)**, intestinal (CDX2+, MUC2+, → colloid Ca), pancreatobiliary (MUC1+, highest risk), oncocytic (IOPN per WHO 2019). Cyst fluid: CEA >192, KRAS/GNAS mutations.

Complications/Prognosis: Fukuoka high-risk stigmata (jaundice + head cyst, mural nodule ≥5 mm, duct ≥10 mm) → resect. Worrisome features → EUS.

Exam yield: ★★★ HIGH — IPMN subtypes and Fukuoka algorithm are frequently examined.

> **Exam Pitfall: MCN vs IPMN**
>
> MCN is defined by the presence of ovarian-type stroma (confirmed by inhibin, ER, PR immunohistochemistry). Without ovarian-type stroma, a mucinous cystic lesion communicating with the ductal system is an IPMN, not an MCN. This distinction has direct management implications: MCNs are always resected (any size), while branch-duct IPMNs <3 cm without worrisome features can be surveilled.
> **Key rule:** MCN never communicates with the pancreatic duct; IPMN always does. MCN occurs almost exclusively in the body/tail of women; IPMN has no sex predilection.

21.6 Pancreatic Neuroendocrine Tumours

Definition: Islet cell neoplasms, 2–5% of pancreatic neoplasms. Functional (hormone syndromes) or non-functional (60–90%).

Etiology/Associations: Sporadic or syndromic: MEN1 (menin, multiple tumours), VHL (clear cell morphology), tuberous sclerosis, NF1.

Microscopy: Organoid architecture: nests, trabeculae, ribbons. **Finely stippled salt-and-pepper chromatin**, moderate eosinophilic cytoplasm, inconspicuous nucleoli.

Special stains/IHC: Synaptophysin (most sensitive), chromogranin A (most specific), INSM1 (nuclear). Ki-67 hot-spot (≥500 cells) mandatory for grading.

Molecular/Genetics: NET: MEN1, DAXX/ATRX, mTOR. NEC: TP53, RB1 (no MEN1/DAXX/ATRX). NET G3 vs NEC: same Ki-67 >20% but different biology, treatment, prognosis.

Exam yield: ★★★ HIGH — WHO grading Ki-67 cut-offs, NET G3 vs NEC, and functional tumour syndromes are high-yield.

Table 21.4: WHO 2022 Grading of Pancreatic Neuroendocrine Neoplasms

Category	Differentiation	Grade	Mitoses (/10 HPF)	Ki-67 Index	Key Molecular
NET G1	Well differentiated	Low	<2	<3%	MEN1, DAXX/ATRX, mTOR pathway

NET G2	Well differentiated	Intermediate	2–20	3–20%	MEN1, DAXX/ATRX, mTOR pathway
NET G3	Well differentiated	High	>20	>20%	MEN1, DAXX/ATRX; TP53/RB1 intact
NEC, small cell	Poorly differentiated	High	>20 (often >>20)	>20% (often >55%)	TP53, RB1 mutations; no MEN1/DAXX/ATRX
NEC, large cell	Poorly differentiated	High	>20 (often >>20)	>20% (often >55%)	TP53, RB1 mutations; no MEN1/DAXX/ATRX

The critical distinction between well-differentiated NET G3 and poorly differentiated NEC matters greatly for prognosis and treatment. Despite sharing a high Ki-67 (>20%), NET G3 retains organised architecture, shows typical salt-and-pepper chromatin, and harbours MEN1/DAXX/ATRX alterations (ATRX or DAXX loss by IHC). NECs show sheet-like growth, geographic necrosis, crush artefact, moulding (small cell type), and TP53/RB1 mutations with retained ATRX/DAXX. NET G3 is treated with temozolomide-based regimens; NEC responds to platinum-etoposide, analogous to small cell lung carcinoma (see Chapter 16).

Table 21.5: Functional Pancreatic Neuroendocrine Tumours

Tumour	Hormone	Syndrome	Location	% Malignant	Key Features
Insulinoma	Insulin	Hypoglycaemia (Whipple triad)	Pancreas (even distribution)	~10%	Most common functional PanNET; 90% benign, solitary, <2 cm; rule of 10s does NOT apply
Gastrinoma	Gastrin	Zollinger-Ellison (peptic ulcers, diarrhoea)	Duodenum (70%) > pancreas	60–90%	Gastrinoma triangle; 25% associated with MEN1
Glucagonoma	Glucagon	4D syndrome: Dermatitis (NME), Diabetes, DVT, Depression	Body/tail	60–80%	Necrolytic migratory erythema pathognomonic

VIPoma	VIP	WDHA (watery diarrhoea, hypokalaemia, achlorhydria)	Body/tail	40–70%	Verner-Morrison syndrome; pancreatic cholera
Somatostatinoma	Somatostatin	Diabetes, gallstones, steatorrhoea	Head/duodenum	70%	Inhibits all other hormones; psammoma bodies (duodenal)

In a viva, the examiner may ask: How do you distinguish an incidental small pancreatic NET from an insulinoma? The answer lies in clinical correlation rather than morphology: insulinomas produce Whipple's triad (symptoms of hypoglycaemia, documented low blood glucose <55 mg/dL, and symptom relief with glucose administration). Proinsulin and C-peptide levels are elevated (excluding exogenous insulin). On IHC, insulin staining is positive but is unreliable for diagnosis because even non-functional NETs may show focal insulin expression.

Quick Recall: Pancreatic Neuroendocrine Tumours

Grading: Ki-67: G1 (<3%), G2 (3–20%), G3 (>20%); NEC is poorly differentiated with TP53/RB1.

IHC: Synaptophysin (most sensitive), chromogranin A (most specific), INSM1. Ki-67 on hot-spot (≥500 cells).

NET G3 vs NEC: G3: organised architecture + MEN1/DAXX/ATRX; NEC: sheet-like + TP53/RB1. Treatment differs.

Insulinoma: Most common functional; Whipple triad; 90% benign, solitary, <2 cm.

MEN1: 10% of PanNETs; AD; pituitary + parathyroid + pancreas (3 Ps).

Gastrinoma: 70% in duodenum; 25% MEN1; gastrinoma triangle (CBD, 2nd/3rd duodenum, neck/body junction).

Integration: PanNETs share grading principles with GI NETs (see Chapter 19) and connect to endocrine tumour syndromes (MEN1, VHL; see Chapter 27). Gastrinoma relates to peptic ulcer disease (see Chapter 18). Cystic pancreatic changes in VHL (serous cystadenomas, PanNETs) overlap with renal pathology (see Chapter 23).

21.7 Other Pancreatic Tumours

21.7.1 Acinar Cell Carcinoma

Definition: Rare (1–2% of pancreatic neoplasms) with acinar differentiation.

Microscopy: Solid sheets/acinar structures. **Granular eosinophilic cytoplasm (zymogen granules) + prominent single nucleoli**. No dense desmoplasia (unlike PDAC).

Special stains/IHC: Trypsin, chymotrypsin positive. BCL10 (nuclear/cytoplasmic) useful surrogate. Mixed acinar-NE carcinoma: each component ≥30%.

Complications/Prognosis: Lipase hypersecretion syndrome (10–15%): subcutaneous fat necrosis, polyarthralgia, eosinophilia.

Exam yield: ★★ MODERATE — BCL10 and lipase hypersecretion syndrome are the exam points.

21.7.2 Solid Pseudopapillary Neoplasm (SPN)

Definition: Low-grade malignant tumour; almost exclusively young women (mean 25–30, F:M >9:1).

Gross: Large, well-encapsulated, solid and cystic with extensive haemorrhagic degeneration.

Microscopy: Monotonous cells around hyalinised fibrovascular stalks; degeneration creates **pseudopapillary pattern**. Eosinophilic globules, foamy histiocytes, cholesterol clefts, nuclear grooves.

Special stains/IHC: Nuclear β-catenin (CTNNB1 mutations virtually 100%), CD10+, CD56+, vimentin+. **E-cadherin lost** (diagnostic). Synaptophysin focal dot-like; chromogranin NEGATIVE (vs PanNET).

Complications/Prognosis: Resection curative in >95%. Even metastatic disease is indolent.

Exam yield: ★★★ HIGH — Young woman + nuclear β-catenin + E-cadherin loss + chromogranin negative = SPN.

21.7.3 Pancreatoblastoma

Definition: Most common pancreatic neoplasm in children (peak 1–8 years).

Microscopy: Mixed acinar, endocrine, ductal differentiation with **squamoid corpuscles (morules with optically clear nuclei)**. AFP may be elevated.

Molecular/Genetics: WNT/β-catenin pathway mutations. Loss of 11p (imprinting). Better prognosis in children than rare adult form.

Exam yield: ★★ MODERATE — Squamoid corpuscles = pancreatoblastoma.

Table 21.6: IHC Panel for Pancreatic Tumour Differential Diagnosis

Marker	PDAC	PanNET	Acinar Cell CA	SPN	Pancreatoblastoma
CK7	+	−/+	+/−	−	+
CK19	+	−/+	−	−	+
Synaptophysin	−	+	−/+ (focal)	−/+ (focal, dot-like)	+/−
Chromogranin	−	+	−/+ (focal)	−	+/−

Trypsin/Chymotrypsin	–	–	++	–	++
BCL10	–	–	+	–	+
β-catenin (nuclear)	–	–	–	+ (diagnostic)	–/+ (in morules)
CD10	–	–	–	+	–
E-cadherin (membranous)	+	+	+	Lost (diagnostic)	+
SMAD4 (DPC4)	Lost in ~55%	Retained	Retained	Retained	Retained
INSM1	–	+	–/+	–	+/–

21.8 Pathology of the Endocrine Pancreas in Diabetes Mellitus

Definition: Islet pathology underlying type 1 and type 2 diabetes mellitus.

Pathogenesis: T1DM: autoimmune CD8+ T cell beta cell destruction in HLA-DR3/DR4/DQ8 individuals. T2DM: peripheral insulin resistance + progressive beta cell failure (obesity, glucotoxicity, lipotoxicity).

Microscopy: T1DM: **Insulitis (lymphocytic infiltration, CD8+ T cells)** → progressive beta cell loss → atrophic fibrotic islets. Serological: anti-GAD65 (most sensitive). T2DM: **Islet amyloid (IAPP/amylin)** — eosinophilic amorphous on H&E, apple-green birefringence on Congo red. Beta cell mass reduced 40–60%.

Key DDx: Insulitis (T1DM, pathognomonic) vs islet amyloid (T2DM). Amyloid may occur in small amounts in aged non-diabetics.

Exam yield: ★★★ HIGH — Insulitis vs amyloid and Congo red birefringence are classic exam questions.

Quick Recall: Endocrine Pancreas and Diabetes

T1DM islets: Insulitis (CD8+ T cells), progressive beta cell loss, eventual atrophy. Serological: anti-GAD65 most sensitive.

T2DM islets: Islet amyloid (IAPP/amylin), 40–60% beta cell mass reduction, hyalinised vessels. NO insulitis.

FCPD: Young, lean, tropical patient; large calculi; ketosis-resistant; SPINK1/CFTR variants; PDAC risk.

Congo red: Islet amyloid shows apple-green birefringence under polarised light.

The Pathologist's Eye: Pancreatic Cyst Lining Recognition: Mucinous vs Serous vs IPMN

The pathologist must distinguish three main pancreatic cystic neoplasms by their lining epithelium.

Serous cystadenoma shows a single layer of cuboidal cells with clear, glycogen-rich cytoplasm (PAS-positive, diastase-sensitive) and small, round, centrally placed nuclei without atypia; the cysts are typically small (microcystic or honeycomb pattern) and filled with serous fluid. Mucinous cystic neoplasm (MCN) shows tall columnar mucinous epithelium (resembling gastric foveolar or endocervical epithelium) with underlying ovarian-type stroma (ER/PR positive); this stroma is the defining diagnostic criterion. Intraductal papillary mucinous neoplasm (IPMN) shows papillary proliferation of mucinous epithelium within a dilated pancreatic duct, classified by subtype: gastric (most common, foveolar-type), intestinal (villous, MUC2/CDX2 positive), pancreatobiliary (complex papillae, MUC1 positive, worst prognosis), and oncocytic (abundant eosinophilic granular cytoplasm). On cyst fluid analysis, CEA greater than 192 ng/mL and amylase elevation favour mucinous over serous cysts. KRAS and GNAS mutations in cyst fluid support mucinous neoplasm (IPMN).

DDx: Pancreatic Cystic Neoplasms

Entity	Key Features
Serous cystadenoma (SCN)	Microcystic/honeycomb; cuboidal clear cells (glycogen-rich, PAS+/diastase-sensitive); central scar; VHL association; benign, no malignant potential
Mucinous cystic neoplasm (MCN)	Unilocular/oligocystic; tall columnar mucinous epithelium; ovarian-type stroma (ER/PR+, mandatory for diagnosis); body/tail; exclusively women; no duct communication
IPMN	Papillary mucinous epithelium within dilated pancreatic duct; communicates with duct system; subtypes: gastric, intestinal (MUC2/CDX2+), pancreatobiliary (MUC1+), oncocytic; cyst fluid: CEA >192, KRAS/GNAS mutations
Solid pseudopapillary neoplasm (SPN)	Young women; solid-cystic; pseudopapillae around hyalinised vessels; nuclear beta-catenin+, CD10+, PR+; CTNNB1 mutation; low malignant potential

21.9 Recent Advances

ISGPS 2016 update — postoperative pancreatic fistula redefined. The International Study Group in Pancreatic Surgery revised the 2005 definition of postoperative pancreatic fistula after eleven years of clinical experience (Bassi et al. Surgery 2017; 161: 584–591; PMID 28040257). A clinically relevant postoperative pancreatic fistula is now defined as drain output of any measurable volume on or after postoperative day 3 with a fluid amylase activity exceeding three times the upper limit of institutional normal serum amylase, accompanied by a clinically relevant condition directly attributable to the leak. The former grade A category, which lacked clinical consequence, has been renamed a biochemical leak and is no longer considered a true fistula. Grade B requires a change in postoperative management — prolonged drainage beyond three weeks, repositioning of drains, percutaneous or endoscopic intervention, antibiotics, or somatostatin analogues. Grade C requires reoperation, leads to single or multiple organ failure, or causes mortality directly attributable to the fistula. For the pathologist, the implication is that synoptic reporting on pancreaticoduodenectomy and distal pancreatectomy specimens should record the pancreatic-stump margin status, duct diameter, and parenchymal texture (soft, intermediate, hard) — all established preoperative and intraoperative predictors of postoperative fistula severity in the updated ISGPS framework.

Molecular profiling of PDAC has identified actionable targets beyond the four core drivers. Approximately 5 to 7% of PDAC harbour homologous recombination deficiency (HRD) from germline BRCA1/2 or PALB2 mutations, rendering tumours sensitive to platinum-based chemotherapy and PARP inhibitors. The POLO trial demonstrated olaparib maintenance significantly improved progression-free survival in germline BRCA-mutated metastatic PDAC. Current NCCN guidelines recommend germline testing for all newly diagnosed PDAC patients for BRCA1/2, PALB2, ATM, and other DNA damage repair genes, as results may influence both treatment and family screening. Approximately 1% of PDACs are MMR-deficient/microsatellite unstable and eligible for pembrolizumab (tumour-agnostic approval). KRAS G12C inhibitors (sotorasib, adagrasib) are under investigation for the subset of KRAS G12C-mutant PDAC (approximately 1 to 2%).

AI-powered algorithms for pancreatic cyst fluid analysis and EUS-FNA cytology are demonstrating improved accuracy for distinguishing mucinous from non-mucinous cysts and detecting high-grade dysplasia. Machine learning models integrating clinical features, imaging characteristics, and molecular markers (KRAS, GNAS, TP53, SMAD4 in cyst fluid) are being validated to refine the Fukuoka guidelines for IPMN surveillance. Neoadjuvant chemotherapy regimens (FOLFIRINOX, gemcitabine plus nab-paclitaxel) are increasingly used for borderline resectable and locally advanced PDAC, and standardised pathological tumour regression grading (CAP system) is becoming essential in Whipple specimen reporting.

In the neuroendocrine tumour space, peptide receptor radionuclide therapy (PRRT) using 177-Lu-DOTATATE (lutetium-177) has established itself as a standard treatment for somatostatin receptor-positive advanced PanNETs (NETTER-1 trial). Belzutifan, a HIF-2α inhibitor, has been approved for VHL-associated PanNETs. For NET G3, temozolomide-capecitabine (CAPTEM) remains the preferred regimen, and genomic profiling to confirm MEN1/DAXX/ATRX status helps solidify the distinction from NEC.

Essential/Desirable: Diagnostic Criteria -- PanNET vs NEC Distinction

Essential: Ki-67 proliferation index is the cornerstone: NET G1 (<3%), G2 (3-20%), G3 (>20% but well-differentiated morphology). NEC: >20% Ki-67 with poorly differentiated morphology (small cell or large cell type).

Desirable: G3 NET: ATRX/DAXX loss by IHC, p53/Rb intact, alternative lengthening of telomeres (ALT). NEC: p53 aberrant (overexpression or null), Rb loss, ATRX/DAXX intact. This distinction is critical as PanNET G3 and NEC have different biology and treatment.

Essential/Desirable: Diagnostic Criteria -- Pancreatic Ductal Adenocarcinoma

Essential: Invasive glandular neoplasm with marked desmoplastic stroma and perineural invasion; cytological atypia exceeding reactive changes.

Desirable: KRAS mutation (>90%); SMAD4 loss by IHC (60%, correlates with widespread metastases); associated PanIN precursor lesions; p53 aberrant expression.

21.10 Approach to the Histopathology Slide

Pancreatic specimens in examinations may include Whipple resections, distal pancreatectomies, biopsies, and EUS-FNA cytology slides. The following systematic approach applies.

Step 1: Specimen type. Whipple (pancreaticoduodenectomy) or distal pancreatectomy. Identify duodenum, CBD, pancreatic duct, ampulla. On cytology, identify the cell block.

Step 2: Solid or cystic? Solid masses: PDAC, PanNET, acinar cell carcinoma, SPN, metastasis. Cystic lesions: IPMN, MCN, serous cystadenoma, pseudocyst, SPN (cystic component).

Step 3: Epithelial pattern. Ductal/glandular with desmoplasia (PDAC); solid nests/trabeculae with salt-and-pepper chromatin (PanNET); acinar with granular cytoplasm (acinar cell CA); pseudopapillary with hyalinised cores (SPN); mucinous papillary (IPMN).

Step 4: Stroma. Dense desmoplasia (PDAC, chronic pancreatitis); ovarian-type stroma (MCN); minimal delicate stroma (PanNET); hyalinised fibrovascular stalks (SPN).

Step 5: Special features. Perineural invasion (PDAC); mucin production (PDAC, IPMN, MCN); squamoid corpuscles (pancreatoblastoma); nuclear β-catenin (SPN); salt-and-pepper chromatin (PanNET); saponification (fat necrosis in pancreatitis).

Step 6: IHC strategy. For solid tumours: CK7, synaptophysin, chromogranin, β-catenin, trypsin, SMAD4. For NET grading: Ki-67 (hot-spot method). For PDAC confirmation: SMAD4 loss, p53 aberrant pattern.

The Pathologist's Eye: Three Traps in Pancreatic Pathology

1. PDAC vs chronic pancreatitis on biopsy: Look for haphazard glands adjacent to muscular vessels, incomplete lumina, and perineural invasion. SMAD4 loss by IHC clinches the diagnosis of carcinoma. Isolated gland atypia in a fibrotic background is not sufficient for a malignant diagnosis.

2. Contaminant epithelium on EUS-FNA: Duodenal and gastric epithelial fragments may be picked up during transgastric/transduodenal EUS-FNA. These show orderly honeycomb sheets without haphazard architecture. Do not overcall as adenocarcinoma.

3. PanNET G3 vs NEC: Both have Ki-67 >20%, but treatment differs dramatically. NET G3 retains organoid architecture and salt-and-pepper chromatin; NEC shows sheet-like growth, geographic necrosis, and moulding. IHC for ATRX/DAXX (lost in NET G3) and p53/Rb (aberrant in NEC) resolves most cases (Figure 21.6).

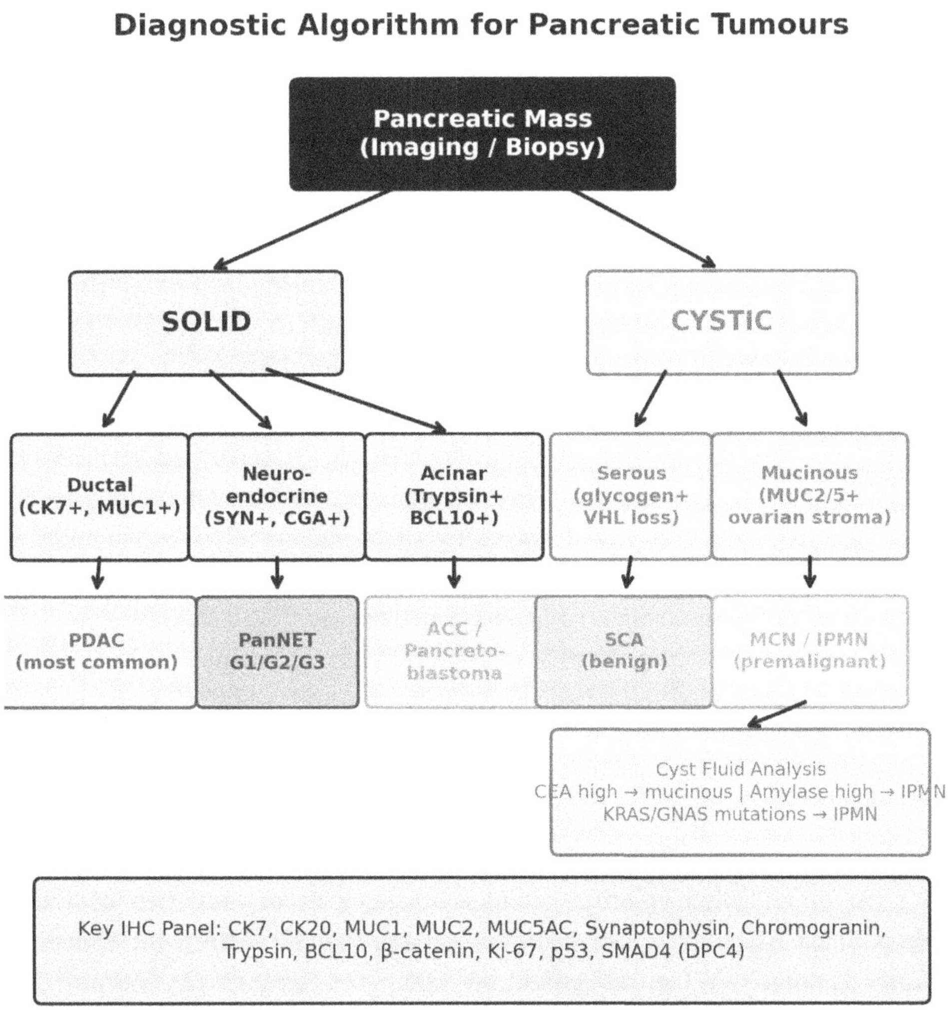

Figure 21.6: Diagnostic algorithm for pancreatic tumours: solid versus cystic, epithelial pattern, IHC panel, and cyst fluid analysis pathway. (Source: Author's original.)

International Frameworks

International frameworks for pancreatic pathology — WHO 5th edition tumour classification and the Atlanta 2012 revised classification of acute pancreatitis. Pancreatic pathology operates within two complementary international frameworks that the FRCPath candidate must apply to every specimen. The 5th edition WHO Classification of Tumours of the Digestive System (2019) recognises pancreatic ductal adenocarcinoma (PDAC) as the dominant malignancy with named morphological variants — adenosquamous, colloid, hepatoid, medullary, signet-ring cell, undifferentiated (anaplastic), and undifferentiated with osteoclast-like giant cells — and codifies precursor lesions as a graded continuum: pancreatic intraepithelial neoplasia (PanIN, low-grade and high-grade per the 2015 Baltimore consensus), intraductal papillary mucinous neoplasm (IPMN, with subtypes gastric, intestinal, pancreatobiliary, and oncocytic; graded as low-grade dysplasia, high-grade dysplasia, or with associated invasive carcinoma), intraductal oncocytic papillary neoplasm (IOPN, separated from IPMN as a distinct entity in the 5th edition with characteristic PRKACA fusions), intraductal tubulopapillary neoplasm (ITPN), and mucinous cystic neoplasm (MCN, occurring almost exclusively in women and characterised by ovarian-type stroma). Pancreatic neuroendocrine neoplasms are stratified by the WHO/ENETS scheme into well-differentiated PanNET (graded G1: Ki-67 less than 3 per cent; G2: 3 to 20 per cent; G3: greater than 20 per cent) and poorly differentiated pancreatic neuroendocrine carcinoma (PanNEC, small cell or large cell), with PanNET-G3 distinguished from PanNEC by retention of DAXX/ATRX and well-differentiated morphology. Solid pseudopapillary neoplasm, acinar cell carcinoma, and pancreatoblastoma complete the morphological spectrum. AJCC 8 staging for PDAC anchors T1, T2, and T3 to tumour size (less than or equal to 2 cm, 2 to 4 cm, and greater than 4 cm respectively, regardless of organ confinement), with T4 reserved for involvement of the coeliac axis, superior mesenteric artery, or common hepatic artery. The Atlanta 2012 revised classification of acute pancreatitis establishes diagnosis on any two of three criteria — characteristic abdominal pain, serum lipase or amylase greater than three times the upper limit of normal, and characteristic findings on contrast-enhanced computed tomography. Acute pancreatitis is morphologically dichotomised into interstitial oedematous pancreatitis (the dominant phenotype, with a homogeneously enhancing gland) and necrotising pancreatitis (further subdivided into parenchymal, peripancreatic, or both). Severity is stratified into mild (no organ failure, no local or systemic complications), moderately severe (transient organ failure resolving within 48 hours, or local complications), and severe (persistent organ failure beyond 48 hours, with hospital mortality of approximately 30 per cent). Local complications evolve along a defined timeline: acute peripancreatic fluid collection in the first four weeks of interstitial oedematous pancreatitis, organising into pancreatic pseudocyst beyond four weeks; acute necrotic collection in the first four weeks of necrotising pancreatitis, organising into walled-off necrosis with a mature wall beyond four weeks. Citation: Banks PA, Bollen TL, Dervenis C, et al; Acute Pancreatitis Classification Working Group. Classification of acute pancreatitis—2012: revision of the Atlanta classification and definitions by international consensus. Gut 2013; 62: 102–111. PMID 23100216.

Ultra High-Yield Chapter Summary

Topic	Must Remember
Acute pancreatitis	Gallstones + alcohol = 70%; lipase > amylase (more specific, longer elevation); fat necrosis = saponification; Revised Atlanta Classification (mild/mod severe/severe)
Serum amylase vs lipase	Amylase: rises 6–12h, normalises 3–5d, many non-pancreatic sources.
Pseudocyst vs WON	Pseudocyst: NO epithelial lining, enzyme-rich fluid, high amylase, low CEA.
Cyst fluid analysis	CEA >192 ng/mL = mucinous (75% sensitive); KRAS mutation 96% specific; high amylase = duct communication or pancreatitis
Chronic pancreatitis	Irreversible fibrosis, acinar atrophy, calcifications; alcohol most common; TIGAR-O classification; mimics PDAC
AIP type 1 vs type 2	Type 1: IgG4-RD, storiform fibrosis, obliterative phlebitis, older men.
Groove pancreatitis	Paraduodenal, mimics carcinoma, Brunner gland hyperplasia, duodenal wall cysts, alcohol-related
PDAC molecular tetrad	KRAS (>90%), TP53, CDKN2A, SMAD4; SMAD4 loss by IHC relatively specific to PDAC
PanIN sequence	PanIN-1 (KRAS) → PanIN-2 (p16 loss) → PanIN-3 (TP53, SMAD4) → invasive PDAC
PDAC variants	Adenosquamous (worse); colloid (better, CDX2+); medullary (MSI, TILs); undifferentiated with OGCs
Whipple margins	SMA/uncinate margin most critical; R1 varies: RCPath ≤1 mm, CAP at ink; CAP 4-tier regression grading
IPMN	Intraductal, communicates with duct; GNAS + KRAS; gastric subtype most common; main-duct risk > branch-duct
MCN	Ovarian-type stroma (ER/PR/inhibin+), body/tail, women, NO duct communication; always resect

Serous cystadenoma	Microcystic, glycogen-rich clear cells (PAS+, PAS-D−), VHL mutations, central stellate scar, benign
SPN	Young women, nuclear β-catenin, CD10+, loss of E-cadherin, >95% cured by resection
PanNET grading	G1 Ki-67 <3%, G2 3–20%, G3 >20%; NEC is poorly differentiated with TP53/RB1
NET G3 vs NEC	G3: organoid + DAXX/ATRX loss; NEC: sheet-like + p53/Rb aberrant.
Insulinoma	Most common functional PanNET; 90% benign, solitary, <2 cm; Whipple triad
Gastrinoma	ZE syndrome; 70% duodenal; 25% MEN1; gastrinoma triangle
T1DM vs T2DM islets	T1: insulitis (CD8+ T cells), beta cell loss.
FCPD	Tropical chronic pancreatitis; young, lean; large calculi; SPINK1/CFTR; ketosis-resistant; PDAC risk
Faecal elastase-1	<200 μg/g = exocrine insufficiency; <100 = severe; non-invasive test for chronic pancreatitis
PDAC germline testing	All PDAC: test BRCA1/2, PALB2, ATM; PARP inhibitors (olaparib) for BRCA-mutant; 1% MSI (pembrolizumab eligible)
PRRT	177-Lu-DOTATATE for SSTR+ advanced PanNETs (NETTER-1 trial); belzutifan for VHL-associated NETs
CP vs PDAC on biopsy	PDAC: haphazard glands, PNI, incomplete lumina, SMAD4 loss, p53 aberrant.

Diagnostic thinking: infiltrating glands in desmoplastic stroma + perineural invasion + KRAS/TP53/SMAD4 mutated → pancreatic ductal adenocarcinoma

Diagnostic thinking: well-circumscribed + salt-and-pepper chromatin + CgA+/Syn+ + Ki-67 stratifies grade → pancreatic neuroendocrine tumour

Diagnostic thinking: solid-pseudopapillary pattern + young woman + nuclear beta-catenin+ → solid pseudopapillary neoplasm (Figure 21.7)

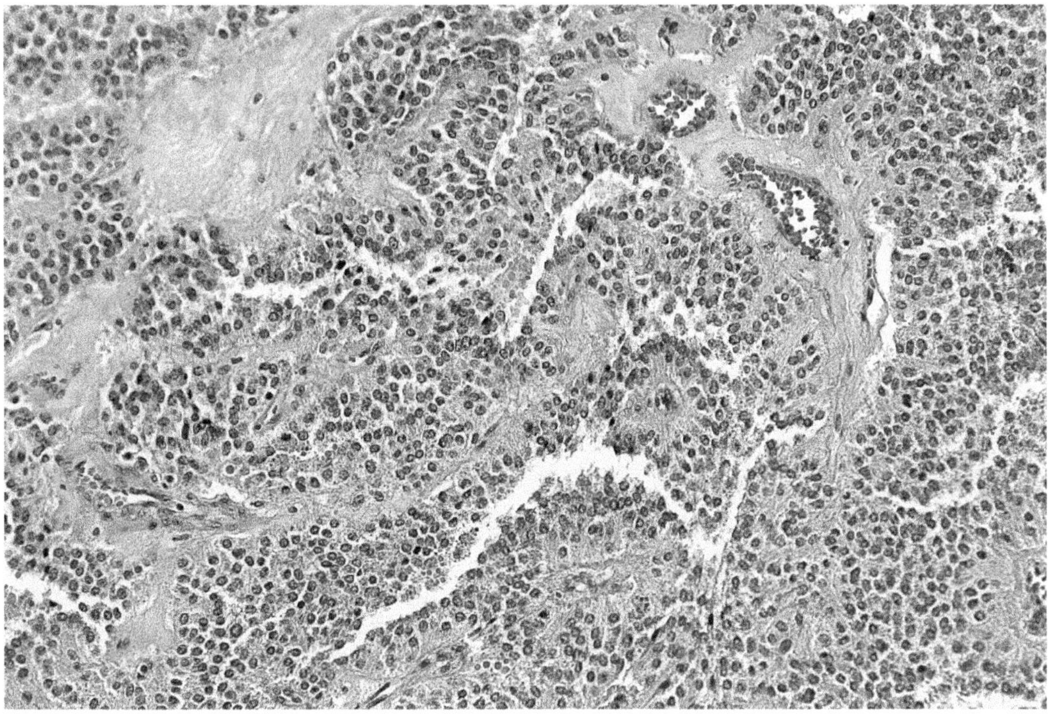

Figure 21.7: Solid pseudopapillary neoplasm of the pancreas. Monotonous neoplastic cells arranged around hyalinised fibrovascular stalks producing the characteristic pseudopapillary pattern, with cholesterol clefts and foamy macrophages in degenerative areas. H&E, high magnification. (Source: Nephron, Wikimedia Commons, CC BY-SA 3.0.)

Chapter 22: Renal Pathology Part 1: Glomerular

THE BIG PICTURE

The glomerulus is a uniquely structured capillary tuft designed for plasma ultrafiltration, and its diseases produce some of the most distinctive clinicopathological syndromes in medicine. Glomerulonephritis (GN) remains a leading cause of chronic kidney disease and end-stage renal disease worldwide, and South Asia carries a disproportionate burden of post-infectious, IgA, and lupus nephritis. Diagnosis rests on the triad of light microscopy, immunofluorescence, and electron microscopy; no single modality suffices. The WHO and ISN/RPS classification systems provide a standardised framework for reporting, and the understanding of podocyte biology, complement pathways, and anti-PLA2R antibodies has transformed both classification and targeted therapy.

High-yield topics in this chapter: Clinical syndromes of glomerular disease (nephrotic vs nephritic); Mechanisms of glomerular injury (immune complex, anti-GBM, complement); Minimal change disease; Focal segmental glomerulosclerosis; Membranous nephropathy and PLA2R; IgA nephropathy; Post-infectious GN; Rapidly progressive (crescentic) GN; Lupus nephritis (ISN/RPS classification); Diabetic nephropathy; Role of immunofluorescence and electron microscopy; Hereditary glomerulopathies (Alport syndrome).

The glomerulus filters approximately 180 litres of plasma every day through a barrier only 300 nanometres thick. When this barrier is breached, the consequences are immediate and measurable: protein spills into the urine, red cells escape into Bowman's space, and the filtration rate falls. Glomerular diseases are the most intellectually demanding area of renal pathology because their diagnosis requires the integration of three microscopy modalities, clinical syndromic classification, serological data, and an understanding of the molecular events at the slit diaphragm and basement membrane. For the postgraduate examination, this chapter is indispensable: approach to glomerular disease, crescentic GN, and the role of IF/EM appear repeatedly.

22.1 Normal Glomerular Structure and the Filtration Barrier

Each kidney contains approximately one million glomeruli. The glomerulus is a tuft of fenestrated capillaries invaginated into Bowman's capsule. The filtration barrier consists of three layers: the fenestrated capillary endothelium, the glomerular basement membrane (GBM), and the visceral epithelial cells (podocytes) with their interdigitating foot processes bridged by the slit diaphragm. Each layer contributes to selective permeability; disruption at any level produces proteinuria.

The GBM is a trilaminar structure (lamina rara interna, lamina densa, lamina rara externa) composed primarily of type IV collagen (alpha-3, alpha-4, alpha-5 chains), laminin, nidogen, and heparan sulphate proteoglycans. The negative charge of heparan sulphate provides the charge barrier that repels albumin (pI 4.7). The slit diaphragm is a specialised cell junction between adjacent podocyte foot processes; its key molecular components include nephrin (NPHS1 gene), podocin (NPHS2), CD2AP, and TRPC6. Mutations in these genes cause hereditary nephrotic syndrome in children.

The mesangium provides structural support and contains mesangial cells embedded in mesangial matrix. Mesangial cells are modified smooth muscle cells with contractile, phagocytic, and secretory functions. They regulate glomerular blood flow and clear immune complexes deposited in the mesangium. Parietal epithelial cells line Bowman's capsule and can proliferate to form crescents in rapidly progressive GN (Figure 22.1).

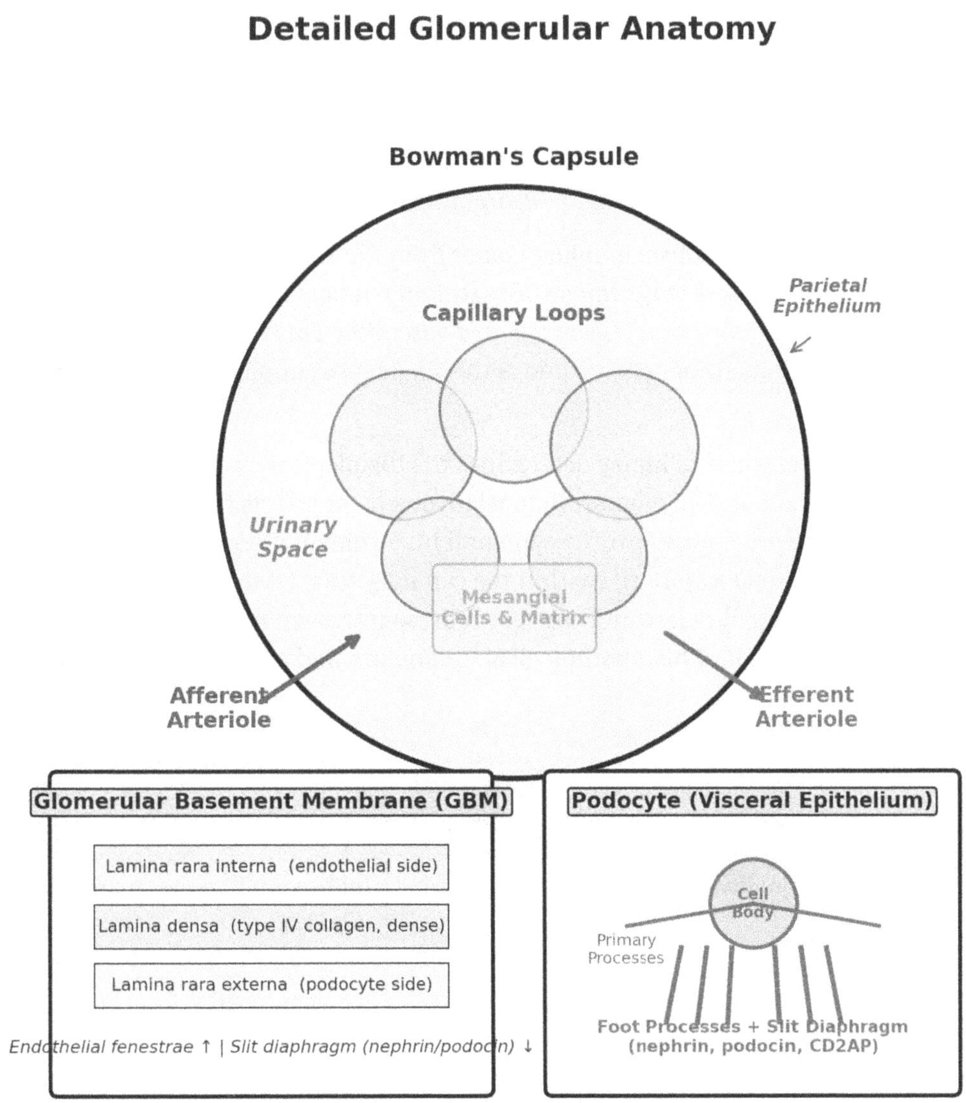

Figure 22.1: Detailed glomerular anatomy: capillary loop, GBM layers, podocyte foot processes with slit diaphragm, mesangial cells, and Bowman\'s capsule. (Source: Author's original.)

22.2 Mechanisms of Glomerular Injury

Glomerular injury is overwhelmingly immune-mediated (complement pathways are detailed in Chapter 5, Section 5.3). The principal mechanisms are: (1) deposition of circulating immune complexes (e.g. post-streptococcal GN, lupus nephritis), (2) in-situ immune complex formation (e.g. anti-PLA2R in membranous nephropathy, anti-GBM disease), (3) complement activation via the alternative pathway (C3 glomerulopathy), (4) antibody-mediated endothelial injury (ANCA in pauci-immune GN), and (5) cell-mediated immunity (T cells in minimal change disease). Non-immune mechanisms include haemodynamic injury, metabolic deposition, and structural defects (Alport syndrome).

Antigen exposure → Immune complex formation (circulating or in-situ) → Complement/Fc receptor activation → Neutrophil/macrophage recruitment → Cytokine/protease release → GBM damage + Podocyte injury → Proteinuria/Haematuria

The key diagnostic clue to the mechanism of injury comes from the immunofluorescence pattern: granular deposits indicate immune complex disease, linear GBM staining indicates anti-GBM disease, and pauci-immune (negative IF) pattern indicates ANCA-associated vasculitis. This triad forms the foundation of the diagnostic approach to glomerulonephritis and is the single most important concept for the postgraduate examination.

The pattern of glomerular response to injury determines the histological classification. Diffuse involvement affects more than 50% of glomeruli; focal involvement affects fewer than 50%. Global involvement affects the entire glomerular tuft; segmental involvement affects only a portion. Proliferative changes may be endocapillary (within the capillary tuft), extracapillary (crescent formation in Bowman's space), or mesangial. Sclerosing changes represent irreversible collagenous replacement. These descriptors form the standard histopathological vocabulary and appear in every examination question on GN.

Histological Pattern	Definition	Classic Example
Diffuse	More than 50% of glomeruli affected	Diffuse proliferative lupus nephritis (Class IV)
Focal	Fewer than 50% of glomeruli affected	IgA nephropathy, focal lupus nephritis (Class III)
Global	Entire glomerular tuft involved	Diffuse membranous nephropathy
Segmental	Part of glomerular tuft involved	FSGS
Proliferative (endocapillary)	Increased cellularity within capillary lumen	Post-infectious GN

Proliferative (extracapillary)	Crescent formation in Bowman's space	RPGN (Types I, II, III)
Membranous	GBM thickening without proliferation	Primary membranous nephropathy
Membranoproliferative	GBM thickening + mesangial proliferation + double contours	C3 glomerulopathy, immune complex MPGN
Sclerosing	Collagenous obliteration of capillary loops	End-stage any GN

22.3 Clinical Syndromes of Glomerular Disease

Glomerular diseases present with a limited number of clinical syndromes. Recognising these syndromes is the first step in the diagnostic algorithm and guides further investigation including renal biopsy.

Syndrome	Key Features	Common Causes
Nephrotic syndrome	Proteinuria >3.5 g/day, hypoalbuminaemia, oedema, hyperlipidaemia, lipiduria	MCD (children), FSGS, Membranous (adults), Diabetic, Amyloid
Nephritic syndrome	Haematuria (RBC casts), mild-moderate proteinuria, hypertension, oliguria, azotaemia	Post-infectious GN, IgA nephropathy, Lupus nephritis, MPGN
Rapidly progressive GN	Nephritic syndrome with rapid decline in GFR over days to weeks; crescents on biopsy	Anti-GBM (Type I), Immune complex (Type II), Pauci-immune/ANCA (Type III)
Chronic GN	Persistent proteinuria/haematuria progressing to CKD	End-stage of any GN
Asymptomatic haematuria/proteinuria	Isolated urinary abnormalities without overt syndrome	IgA nephropathy, thin BM disease, Alport

The distinction between nephrotic and nephritic syndromes is the first question the examiner expects to see in any answer on glomerular disease. Nephrotic syndrome reflects podocyte injury with loss of the charge and size barriers; nephritic syndrome reflects endothelial and mesangial injury with inflammatory breach of the capillary wall. Some diseases (membranoproliferative GN, advanced lupus nephritis, advanced diabetic nephropathy) produce mixed nephrotic-nephritic features.

Quick Recall: Clinical Syndromes

Nephrotic: Podocyte injury → massive proteinuria (>3.5 g/day) → hypoalbuminaemia → oedema + hyperlipidaemia.

Nephritic: Endothelial/mesangial inflammation → haematuria (RBC casts) + hypertension + oliguria.

RPGN: Crescents on biopsy; loss of function in days-weeks; three immunopathological types.

Most common nephrotic in children: Minimal change disease. In adults: Membranous nephropathy (primary) or FSGS.

22.4 Primary Glomerulonephritides

22.4.1 Minimal Change Disease

Definition: Most common cause of nephrotic syndrome in children (70–80%). 10–15% of adult nephrotic syndrome.

Pathogenesis: T-cell dysfunction → Circulating permeability factor → Podocyte injury → Foot process effacement → Massive selective proteinuria.

Microscopy: LM: **Glomeruli entirely normal**. Lipid-laden proximal tubular cells. IF: Negative. EM (diagnostic): **Diffuse podocyte foot process effacement**. Only GN diagnosed primarily by EM.

Key DDx: Normal LM + negative IF + nephrotic = MCD until EM proves it. Early FSGS may mimic.

Complications/Prognosis: Excellent steroid response (>90% children). Frequent relapses. Steroid-resistant: test NPHS2/NPHS1 mutations.

Exam yield: ★★★ HIGH — Normal LM + negative IF + foot process effacement on EM = MCD.

22.4.2 Focal Segmental Glomerulosclerosis

Definition: Pattern of injury (not single disease). Most common nephrotic syndrome cause in some adult populations.

Etiology/Associations: Primary (circulating factor). Secondary/adaptive (obesity, reduced renal mass, sickle cell). Genetic (NPHS2, ACTN4, TRPC6, APOL1). Virus-associated (HIV → collapsing variant).

Podocyte injury → Foot process effacement → Podocyte detachment → Bare GBM → Synechiae → Segmental sclerosis → Global sclerosis

Microscopy: Columbia classification: NOS, perihilar, **tip (best prognosis)**, cellular, **collapsing (worst prognosis, hallmark of HIVAN — capillary tuft collapse + podocyte hypertrophy/hyperplasia)**. IF: Non-specific IgM/C3 trapping. EM: Foot process effacement.

Key DDx: Primary vs secondary: management differs (immunosuppression vs treat cause). South Asian biopsy registries: FSGS is the most common primary glomerulopathy causing nephrotic syndrome in adults.

Exam yield: ★★★ HIGH — Columbia classification (collapsing = HIVAN, tip = best prognosis) and primary vs secondary distinction.

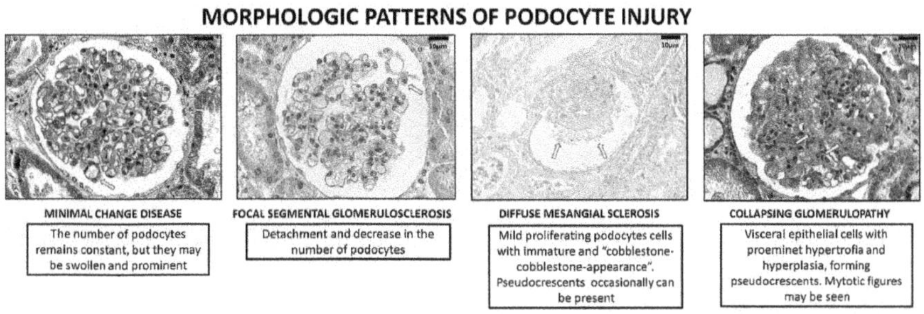

Figure 22.2: Morphologic patterns of podocyte injury. Left to right: minimal change disease (swollen podocytes, normal number), focal segmental glomerulosclerosis (podocyte detachment and loss), diffuse mesangial sclerosis (proliferating immature podocytes with cobblestone appearance), and collapsing glomerulopathy (prominent podocyte hypertrophy and hyperplasia with pseudocrescents). (Source: Mikael Häggström, Wikimedia Commons, CC BY 4.0.)

Podocyte injury (circulating factor / genetic / haemodynamic / viral) → Foot process effacement → Podocyte detachment from GBM → Bare GBM → Synechiae → Segmental sclerosis → Global sclerosis

When faced with FSGS on biopsy, the first question to ask is whether it is primary or secondary, because management differs fundamentally: primary FSGS is treated with immunosuppression, while secondary FSGS requires treatment of the underlying cause. South Asian biopsy registries report FSGS as the most common primary glomerulopathy causing nephrotic syndrome in adults, surpassing MCD.

22.4.3 Membranous Nephropathy

Definition: Most common primary nephrotic syndrome in white adults (30–60 years). 70–80% due to anti-PLA2R IgG4 antibodies.

Etiology/Associations: Primary: anti-PLA2R (70–80%), anti-THSD7A (3–5%). Secondary (20–25%): SLE Class V, HBV, malignancy (screen if >65), NSAIDs.

Anti-PLA2R IgG4 → Podocyte PLA2R binding → In-situ subepithelial immune complex → C5b-9 MAC insertion → Sublytic podocyte injury → Proteinuria

Microscopy: LM: Diffuse capillary wall thickening, no proliferation. **Jones silver: subepithelial spikes (pathognomonic)**. IF: Granular capillary wall IgG (IgG4) + C3. EM: Subepithelial deposits. Ehrenreich-Churg: I–IV staging.

Key DDx: Primary (PLA2R+) vs secondary (PLA2R−). Rule of thirds: ~1/3 remit, ~1/3 persistent, ~1/3 ESRD. Rituximab first-line (MENTOR trial).

Exam yield: ★★★ HIGH — Silver stain spikes, anti-PLA2R, Ehrenreich-Churg staging, rule of thirds are all exam staples.

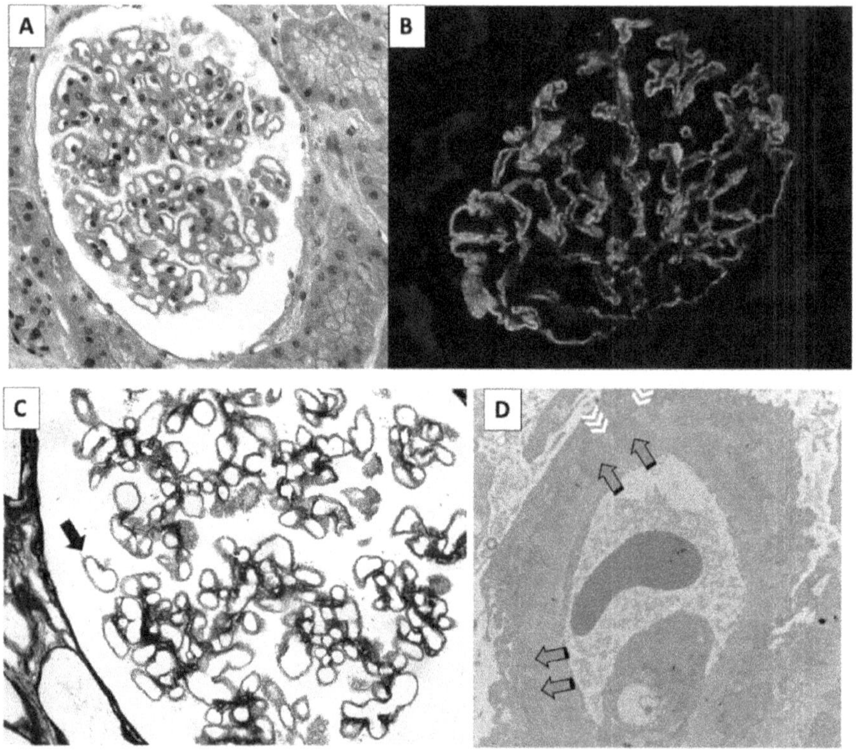

Figure 22.3: Membranous nephropathy — multi-modality composite. (A) Glomerulus with global thickening of the capillary wall (Masson trichrome, ×40). (B) High-intensity granular deposits along glomerular capillary walls (immunofluorescence, ×40). (C) Capillary walls with characteristic spikes at the basement membrane, stage 2 membranous nephropathy (silver methenamine, ×100). (D) Electron microscopy — subepithelial electron-dense deposits (blue arrows) and basement-membrane projections enveloping the deposits (white chevrons). (Source: dos Reis MA et al., Braz J Nephrol 2023; 45(2):e20230046 — PMC10627124, CC BY 4.0.)

Quick Recall: Membranous Nephropathy

Anti-PLA2R: Present in 70-80% of primary MN; IgG4 subclass; serological biomarker for diagnosis and monitoring.

Silver stain spikes: Pathognomonic; represent GBM reaction to subepithelial deposits.

Rule of thirds: Approximately one-third remit spontaneously, one-third have persistent proteinuria, one-third progress to ESRD.

Secondary causes to exclude: SLE, HBV, malignancy (especially in elderly), drugs (NSAIDs, gold, penicillamine).

Treatment: Rituximab is now first-line for primary MN (MENTOR trial); cyclophosphamide-based regimens as alternative.

22.4.4 IgA Nephropathy

Definition: Most common GN worldwide. Most common cause of recurrent gross haematuria in young adults.

Mucosal trigger → Galactose-deficient IgA1 (Gd-IgA1) → Anti-Gd-IgA1 autoantibodies → Immune complex → Mesangial deposition → Complement activation → Mesangial proliferation

Microscopy: LM: **Mesangial proliferation and matrix expansion**. Crescents in severe cases. IF (diagnostic): **Dominant mesangial IgA** (with C3, often IgG/IgM). EM: Mesangial electron-dense deposits.

Key DDx: IgA nephropathy vs HSP nephritis: identical histology; HSP has systemic vasculitis. Oxford MEST-C scoring: M, E, S, T, C. 20–40% progress to ESRD over 20 years.

Exam yield: ★★★ HIGH — Mesangial IgA on IF is the defining feature. Oxford MEST-C and Gd-IgA1 pathogenesis frequently asked.

The Oxford MEST-C classification (2009, updated 2016) provides a standardised histological scoring system: M (mesangial hypercellularity), E (endocapillary hypercellularity), S (segmental glomerulosclerosis), T (tubular atrophy/interstitial fibrosis), C (crescents). Each variable is independently associated with renal outcome and guides treatment decisions. Henoch-Schonlein purpura (IgA vasculitis) is considered the systemic form of IgA nephropathy, with identical renal histology.

> **Exam Pitfall: Post-Infectious GN vs IgA Nephropathy**
>
> Both present with haematuria after infection, but the timing differs critically:
>
> **IgA nephropathy:** Haematuria within 1-2 days of mucosal infection (synpharyngitic); normal complement; mesangial IgA on IF.
>
> **Post-infectious GN:** Haematuria 1-3 weeks after pharyngitis/skin infection; low C3; subepithelial humps on EM; granular "starry sky" IgG/C3 on IF.
>
> Confusing these two in an exam answer is a common and costly error.

22.4.5 Membranoproliferative Glomerulonephritis and C3 Glomerulopathy

Definition: Pattern of injury: mesangial proliferation, capillary wall thickening, GBM duplication. Reclassified: immune complex-mediated MPGN vs complement-mediated C3 glomerulopathy.

Etiology/Associations: IC-MPGN: HCV/cryoglobulinaemia, autoimmune, paraprotein. C3 glomerulopathy: C3GN and DDD — alternative complement dysregulation (C3 nephritic factor, Factor H mutations).

Microscopy: LM: Lobular accentuation, **GBM duplication (tram-track on silver/PAS)**. IF: IC type → Ig + C3; C3 glomerulopathy → isolated C3 (≥2 orders above Ig). EM: C3GN → mesangial/subendothelial. **DDD → electron-dense ribbon-like intramembranous deposits (pathognomonic)**.

Key DDx: Serum complement workup: C3 low, C4 distinguishes classical vs alternative. HCV, cryoglobulins, paraprotein screen.

Exam yield: ★★★ HIGH — Tram-tracking, IC-MPGN vs C3G reclassification, DDD intramembranous deposits are exam staples.

22.4.6 Post-Infectious (Post-Streptococcal) Glomerulonephritis

Definition: Prototype post-infectious immune complex GN. Most common GN in children. 1–4 weeks after streptococcal pharyngitis or 3–6 weeks after skin infection.

Etiology/Associations: Group A β-haemolytic strep (nephritogenic M types 1, 2, 4, 12, 49). Also staph, viral, parasitic.

Strep infection → Antibodies against NAPlr/SpeB → In-situ + circulating immune complexes → Classical complement activation (C3↓, C4 low-normal) → Neutrophil infiltration → Endocapillary proliferative GN

Microscopy: LM: Diffuse endocapillary proliferative GN — hypercellular glomeruli with **neutrophil infiltration (lumpy-bumpy)**. IF: Granular starry-sky IgG + C3. EM: **Subepithelial humps (dome-shaped deposits)** — characteristic but transient.

Key DDx: PSGN vs IgA: timing (1–4 wk latency vs synpharyngitic), complement (C3↓ in PSGN vs normal), IF (IgG-dominant vs IgA-dominant). C3 normalises in 6–8 weeks.

Exam yield: ★★★ HIGH — Subepithelial humps and starry-sky IF are classic exam identifiers.

Quick Recall: Post-Infectious GN

Latent period: 1-3 weeks (pharyngitis) or 3-6 weeks (skin); low C3 (normalises in 6-8 weeks).

LM: Diffuse endocapillary proliferative GN with neutrophils.

IF: Granular "starry sky" IgG + C3 along capillary walls and mesangium.

EM: Subepithelial humps (pathognomonic).

Prognosis: Excellent in children (>95% recovery); guarded in adults.

22.5 Rapidly Progressive (Crescentic) Glomerulonephritis

Definition: Rapid renal function loss (weeks–months). Crescents (≥50% glomeruli) = parietal epithelial cells + macrophages in Bowman space.

Etiology/Associations: Type I (anti-GBM, 10–15%): linear IgG. Type II (immune complex, 25–30%): granular Ig+C3 (lupus, IgA, PSGN). Type III (pauci-immune, 55–60%): negative IF, ANCA-associated (GPA = c-ANCA/PR3; MPA = p-ANCA/MPO).

GBM disruption → Fibrin leakage into Bowman space → Parietal cell proliferation + macrophages → Cellular crescent → Fibrocellular → Fibrous crescent (irreversible)

Microscopy: Crescents filling Bowman space in ≥50% glomeruli. Cellular (reversible) vs fibrous (irreversible). Fibrinoid necrosis in pauci-immune type. IF determines type.

Key DDx: Type I vs II vs III by IF. Anti-GBM + ANCA double-positive in ~5%. Goodpasture = anti-GBM + pulmonary haemorrhage.

Exam yield: ★★★ HIGH — Three-type RPGN classification by IF pattern is among the most asked renal topics.

Type	IF Pattern	Mechanism	Diseases	Serology
Type I (Anti-GBM)	Linear IgG along GBM	Autoantibodies against alpha-3 chain of type IV collagen	Goodpasture syndrome (with pulmonary haemorrhage); Anti-GBM nephritis (kidney only)	Anti-GBM antibodies positive
Type II (Immune complex)	Granular Ig + C3	Immune complex deposition with severe inflammatory response	Post-infectious GN, Lupus nephritis (Class IV), IgA nephropathy (severe), MPGN	Depends on underlying disease (ANA, C3, ASO)
Type III (Pauci-immune)	Negative or scanty IF	ANCA-mediated neutrophil activation and endothelial injury	GPA (Wegener), MPA, EGPA (Churg-Strauss), Renal-limited vasculitis	c-ANCA/PR3 (GPA) or p-ANCA/MPO (MPA)

Type I (Anti-GBM disease) accounts for approximately 10 to 15% of RPGN. Autoantibodies target the NC1 domain of the alpha-3 chain of type IV collagen, which is expressed in glomerular and alveolar basement membranes. When both kidneys and lungs are involved (pulmonary haemorrhage with haemoptysis plus RPGN), the condition is called Goodpasture syndrome. The diagnosis is confirmed by detecting circulating anti-GBM antibodies (ELISA) and the characteristic linear IgG staining along the GBM on IF. Treatment includes plasmapheresis (to remove circulating antibodies), corticosteroids, and cyclophosphamide.

Type II (Immune complex) accounts for approximately 25 to 30% and represents severe immune complex-mediated GN of any aetiology with crescent formation. The IF pattern is granular, and the specific pattern (IgA-dominant, "full house," IgG + C3) identifies the underlying disease. Treatment targets the primary disease.

Type III (Pauci-immune/ANCA-associated) is the most common type of RPGN overall (approximately 55 to 60%). The hallmark is extensive crescent formation with absent or minimal IF staining. Approximately 90% of patients are ANCA-positive. ANCA-associated vasculitides include granulomatosis with polyangiitis (GPA, formerly Wegener's; c-ANCA/PR3), microscopic polyangiitis (MPA; p-ANCA/MPO), eosinophilic granulomatosis with polyangiitis (EGPA; p-ANCA/MPO), and renal-limited vasculitis. The pathogenesis involves ANCA-mediated activation of primed neutrophils, which adhere to endothelium and release reactive oxygen species and proteases, causing necrotising vasculitis and glomerulonephritis. Standard treatment is rituximab or cyclophosphamide with corticosteroids; avacopan (C5a receptor inhibitor) is a recent addition (see Recent Advances).

Why is pauci-immune the term used for Type III RPGN? Because immunofluorescence is negative or shows only scanty staining, yet the injury is antibody-mediated (ANCA). The antibodies activate neutrophils in the circulation rather than depositing in the glomerulus, explaining the discrepancy between severe histological damage and "empty" IF.

Morphologically, crescents evolve through cellular (fibrin, macrophages, parietal epithelial cells), fibrocellular, and fibrous stages. Cellular crescents are potentially reversible with aggressive immunosuppression; fibrous crescents represent irreversible scarring. The proportion of fibrous versus cellular crescents on biopsy is a critical prognostic indicator (Figure 22.4).

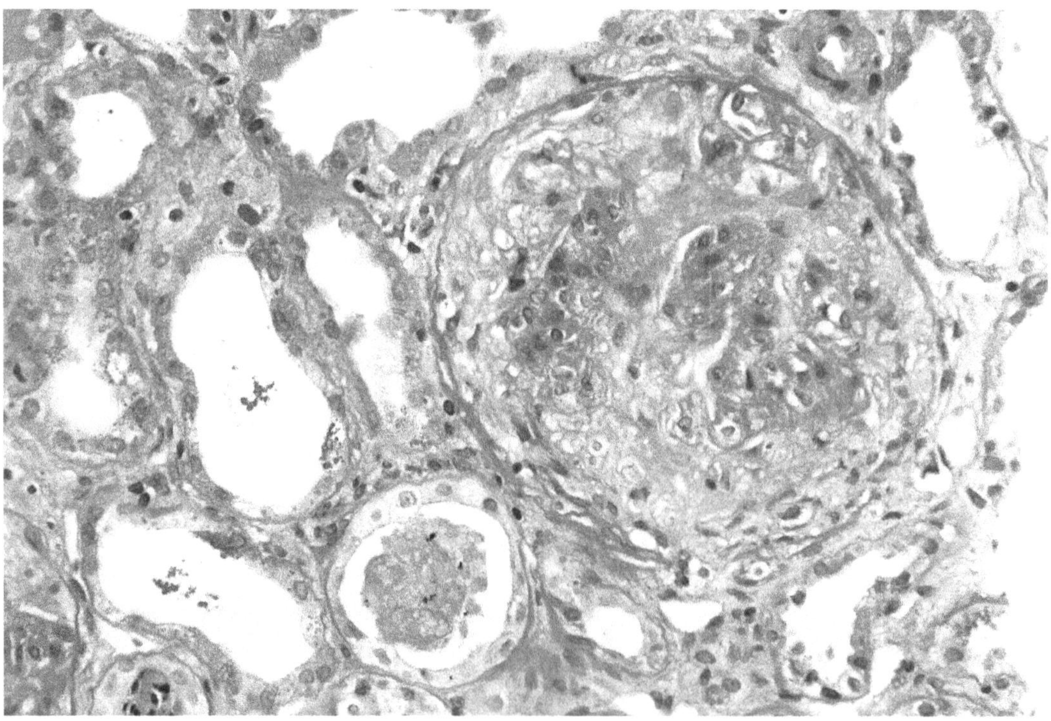

Figure 22.4: Crescentic glomerulonephritis. Left: PAS stain showing a cellular crescent (proliferating parietal epithelial cells and macrophages) compressing the glomerular tuft. Right: Immunofluorescence showing linear IgG staining along the glomerular basement membrane, characteristic of anti-GBM (Type I) disease. (Source: Koya et al., Wikimedia Commons, CC BY 2.0.)

Quick Recall: RPGN/Crescentic GN

Definition: Rapid GFR decline + >50% crescents on biopsy.

Type I (10-15%): Linear IgG on IF; anti-GBM; Goodpasture = kidney + lung.

Type II (25-30%): Granular IF; immune complex (any cause with severe injury).

Type III (55-60%): Pauci-immune (negative IF); ANCA-associated; most common type overall.

Crescent composition: Parietal epithelial cells + macrophages + fibrin.

Crescent evolution: Cellular (reversible) → Fibrocellular → Fibrous (irreversible).

Emergency: Untreated RPGN → ESRD in weeks.

Viva hook: "A 25-year-old presents with rapidly deteriorating renal function and haemoptysis. The renal biopsy shows crescentic GN with linear IgG on IF. What is the diagnosis, and why does the lung bleed?" Answer: Goodpasture syndrome (anti-GBM disease). Anti-GBM antibodies target the alpha-3 chain of type IV collagen, which is present in both glomerular and alveolar basement membranes. Pulmonary haemorrhage occurs because the alveolar basement membrane shares the same antigen. Smoking, infection, or inhaled hydrocarbons increase alveolar capillary permeability, exposing the normally sequestered antigen to circulating antibodies.

Integration: RPGN connects to vasculitis (see Chapter 13 for systemic vasculitis classification, Chapel Hill Consensus), SLE/lupus nephritis (see Section 22.6.1 and Chapter 5), and pulmonary-renal syndromes (see Chapter 15).*

22.6 Secondary Glomerular Diseases

22.6.1 Lupus Nephritis

Definition: Renal manifestation of SLE (~50–70% of patients). ISN/RPS 6-class system. Major determinant of morbidity and mortality.

Anti-dsDNA + nucleosome complexes → Mesangial deposition (I–II) → Subendothelial (III–IV, nephritic) → Subepithelial (V, nephrotic) → Complement activation

Microscopy: Class I: minimal mesangial. II: mesangial proliferative. III: focal (<50%). **Class IV: diffuse (≥50%) — most common/severe; wire-loop deposits (subendothelial)**. V: membranous. VI: advanced sclerotic (>90%). IF: **Full-house (IgG, IgA, IgM, C3, C1q)**. C1q positivity strongly suggestive of lupus.

Key DDx: Full-house IF: lupus first. Wire-loop deposits near-pathognomonic for Class IV. Activity index (reversible) vs chronicity index (irreversible) guide treatment. Class III/IV: aggressive immunosuppression (MMF or cyclophosphamide + steroids).

Exam yield: ★★★ HIGH — ISN/RPS classification, full-house IF, wire-loop deposits, Class IV most common/severe are all exam staples.

ISN/RPS Class	Pattern	LM Features	Clinical Correlation
Class I: Minimal mesangial	Normal LM, mesangial deposits on IF/EM only	Normal glomeruli	Subclinical; mild proteinuria
Class II: Mesangial proliferative	Mesangial hypercellularity	Mesangial expansion and proliferation	Haematuria, mild proteinuria
Class III: Focal lupus nephritis	Focal (<50% glomeruli) endocapillary +/- extracapillary GN	Active: proliferation, necrosis; Chronic: sclerosis	Active nephritic/nephrotic; subclassified as A, A/C, C
Class IV: Diffuse lupus nephritis	Diffuse (>50% glomeruli) endocapillary +/- extracapillary GN	"Wire-loop" deposits, crescents, necrosis	Severe nephritic/nephrotic; worst prognosis; most common class biopsied
Class V: Membranous lupus nephritis	Diffuse membranous pattern	GBM thickening with subepithelial deposits	Nephrotic syndrome; may overlap with III or IV
Class VI: Advanced sclerosing	>90% globally sclerosed glomeruli	End-stage scarring	CKD/ESRD; not amenable to immunosuppression

The hallmark IF pattern in lupus nephritis is "full house": simultaneous positivity for IgG, IgA, IgM, C3, and C1q. This pattern is virtually diagnostic of lupus nephritis and distinguishes it from other immune complex GNs. Class IV is the most common and most severe form; it is characterised by "wire-loop" thickening of capillary walls (massive subendothelial deposits) and extensive crescent formation. EM shows subendothelial (Class III/IV), subepithelial (Class V), and mesangial deposits, often with characteristic tubuloreticular inclusions ("interferon footprints") in endothelial cells.

The ISN/RPS class determines therapy: Classes I and II require conservative management; Classes III and IV require aggressive immunosuppression (mycophenolate mofetil or cyclophosphamide with corticosteroids); Class V is treated with immunosuppression if proteinuria is significant; Class VI is beyond immunosuppressive rescue. (For detailed SLE immunology, see Chapter 5.)

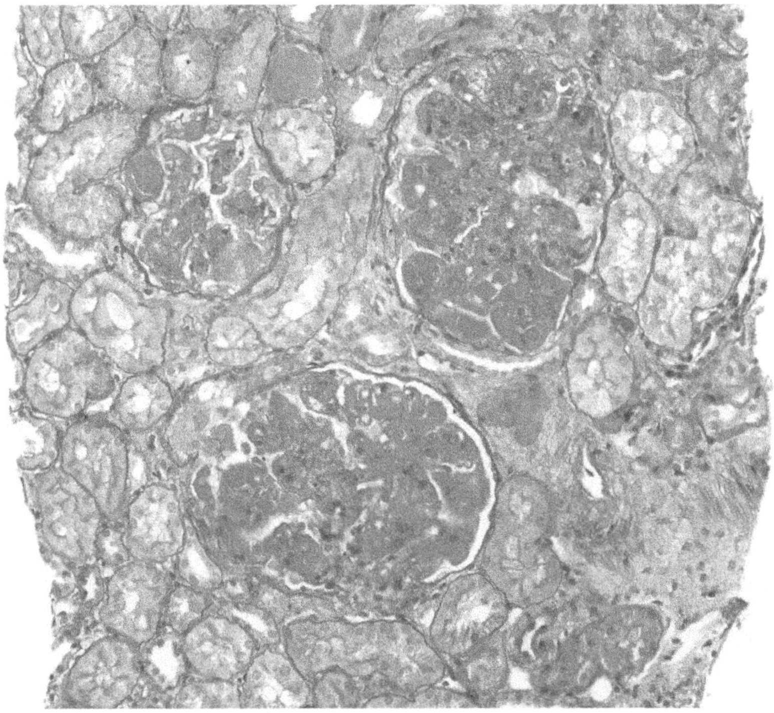

Figure 22.5: Lupus nephritis, Class IV (diffuse proliferative). High-magnification view showing endocapillary hypercellularity with wire-loop deposits (prominent subendothelial immune complex deposits thickening the capillary wall) and infiltrating neutrophils. PAS stain highlights the thickened basement membranes. (Source: Nephron, Wikimedia Commons, CC BY-SA 3.0.)

Quick Recall: Lupus Nephritis

"Full house" IF: IgG, IgA, IgM, C3, C1q = virtually pathognomonic of lupus.

Class IV (Diffuse): Most common biopsied class; worst prognosis; "wire-loop" lesions; crescents.

Wire-loop: Massive subendothelial immune complex deposits thickening the capillary wall.

Tubuloreticular inclusions: EM finding; "interferon footprints"; seen in SLE and HIV.

Activity vs chronicity indices: Guide treatment decisions; active lesions (proliferation, necrosis, crescents) are treatable; chronic lesions (sclerosis, fibrosis) are not.

22.6.2 Diabetic Nephropathy

Definition: Leading cause of ESRD worldwide. Develops in ~30–40% of T1DM and T2DM.

Hyperglycaemia → AGEs + polyol + PKC → GBM thickening + mesangial expansion → Diffuse glomerulosclerosis → Kimmelstiel–Wilson nodules → ESRD

Microscopy: Diffuse glomerulosclerosis (earliest): GBM thickening + mesangial expansion. **Kimmelstiel–Wilson nodules (nodular glomerulosclerosis)**: PAS+ acellular nodules, pathognomonic. Capsular drop, fibrin cap, **afferent AND efferent arteriolar hyalinosis** (unique to diabetes).

Key DDx: Nodular sclerosis DDx: diabetes (most common), amyloidosis (Congo red+), LCDD (kappa/lambda restricted), MPGN, idiopathic.

Exam yield: ★★★ HIGH — KW nodules, afferent + efferent hyalinosis, and nodular sclerosis DDx are high-yield.

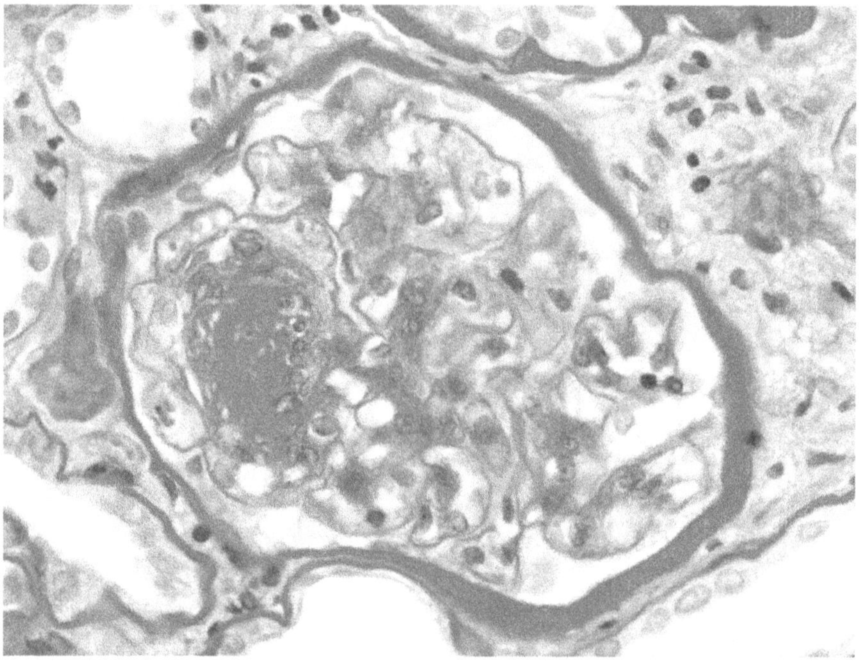

Figure 22.6: Diabetic glomerulosclerosis: Kimmelstiel–Wilson nodules (nodular mesangial sclerosis) with diffuse mesangial matrix expansion and thickened glomerular basement membranes. PAS stain. (Source: KGH, Wikimedia Commons, CC BY-SA 3.0.)

22.6.3 Renal Amyloidosis

Definition: Renal involvement in systemic amyloidosis; kidney is commonly affected.

Etiology/Associations: AL (light chain, plasma cell dyscrasia). AA (reactive: TB, RA, FMF, osteomyelitis). LECT2, fibrinogen, transthyretin (rarer).

Microscopy: Eosinophilic amorphous material in mesangium, capillary walls, arterioles, interstitium. **Congo red: apple-green birefringence under polarised light**. EM: Non-branching fibrils 7–12 nm, randomly arranged.

Special stains/IHC: Typing essential: AL = kappa/lambda restricted. AA = anti-SAA. Mass spectrometry on LCM tissue is gold standard.

Key DDx: Amyloid (Congo red+, fibrils) vs LCDD (granular, kappa-dominant, Congo red−) vs diabetic nodular sclerosis.

Exam yield: ★★★ HIGH — Congo red birefringence and AL vs AA distinction are classic exam questions.

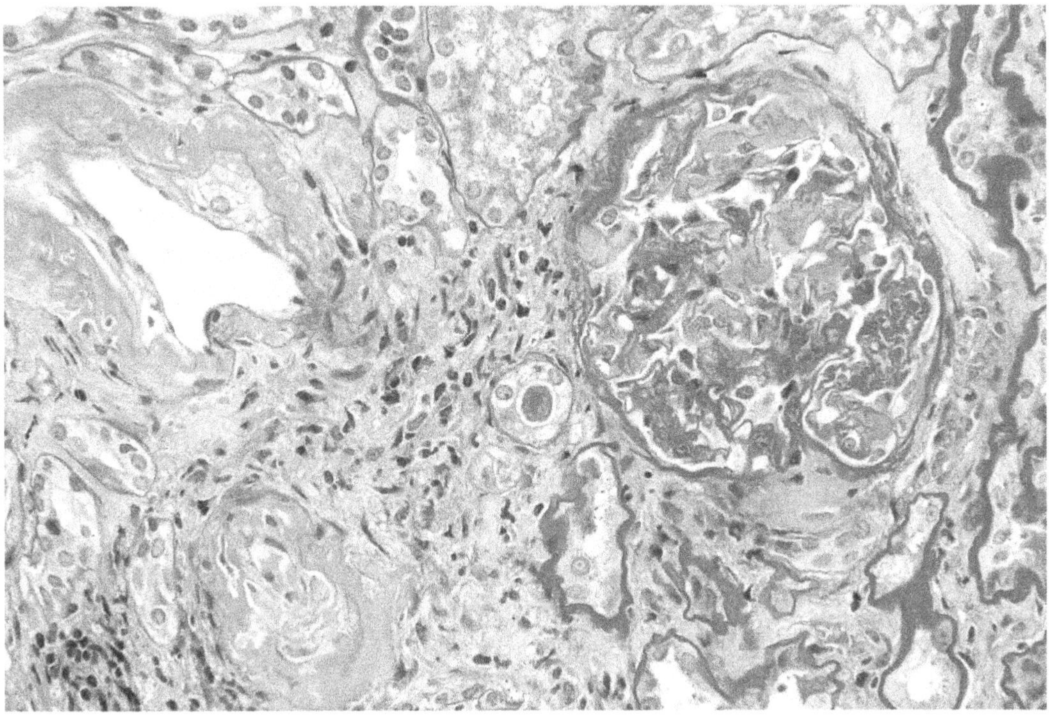

Figure 22.7: Renal amyloidosis. A glomerulus (right) expanded by amorphous pale eosinophilic amyloid deposits within the mesangium and capillary walls, obscuring the capillary tuft architecture and producing the characteristic smudgy acellular appearance. The adjacent tubular basement membranes are also thickened by amyloid deposition. PAS, ×400. (Congo red with apple-green birefringence under polarised light remains the diagnostic gold standard.) (Source: Nephron, Wikimedia Commons, CC BY-SA 3.0.)

22.7 Hereditary Glomerulopathies

22.7.1 Alport Syndrome

Definition: Hereditary nephropathy from COL4A3/A4/A5 mutations affecting GBM, lens, cochlea.

Etiology/Associations: X-linked (COL4A5, 80–85%), autosomal recessive (COL4A3/A4), AD (rare). Males: ESRD by 20–30s.

Microscopy: LM: Non-specific, FSGS pattern late. IF: **Absent α5 chain of type IV collagen** (X-linked males). EM: **Basket-weave pattern — irregular thickening, thinning, splitting, lamellation of GBM** with electron-dense granules.

Key DDx: Alport (basket-weave + deafness) vs TBMD (uniform thinning + benign haematuria).

Complications/Prognosis: Triad: nephropathy (haematuria → ESRD), sensorineural deafness, anterior lenticonus.

Exam yield: ★★★ HIGH — Basket-weave GBM + deafness + lenticonus triad is a classic exam identifier.

22.7.2 Thin Basement Membrane Disease

Definition: Benign familial haematuria from heterozygous COL4A3/A4 mutations.

Microscopy: LM: Normal. IF: Normal. EM: **Uniform GBM thinning (<250 nm)** without splitting or lamellation.

Key DDx: TBMD vs early Alport: basket-weave develops over time in Alport. Genetic testing definitive.

Complications/Prognosis: Excellent prognosis. Persistent microscopic haematuria, minimal proteinuria.

Exam yield: ★★ MODERATE — Uniform GBM thinning vs Alport basket-weave is a commonly tested comparison.

22.7.3 Fabry Disease

Definition: X-linked lysosomal storage disease from α-galactosidase A deficiency. Globotriaosylceramide (Gb3) accumulation.

Microscopy: LM: Enlarged vacuolated podocytes/tubular cells. EM: **Zebra bodies (myeloid/lamellated inclusions)** in podocytes, endothelial, tubular cells.

Key DDx: Other zebra body causes: chloroquine/hydroxychloroquine nephrotoxicity (drug-induced phospholipidosis).

Complications/Prognosis: Proteinuria → ESRD. Cardiomyopathy, angiokeratomas, painful neuropathy, stroke. Enzyme replacement available.

Exam yield: ★★ MODERATE — Zebra bodies + angiokeratomas + α-galactosidase deficiency = Fabry.

> **Quick Recall: Hereditary Glomerulopathies**
>
> **Alport:** COL4A3/A4/A5 mutations; basket-weave GBM on EM; haematuria + deafness + lenticonus; absent alpha-5 collagen on IF.
>
> **Thin BM disease:** Heterozygous COL4A3/A4; uniform GBM thinning <250 nm on EM; benign haematuria; excellent prognosis.
>
> **Fabry:** Alpha-galactosidase A deficiency; zebra bodies on EM; proteinuria to ESRD; enzyme replacement therapy.

22.8 Role of Immunofluorescence and Electron Microscopy in Glomerular Diagnosis

The diagnosis of glomerular disease requires a triad of light microscopy (LM), immunofluorescence (IF), and electron microscopy (EM). No single modality is sufficient. IF reveals the immunopathological mechanism; EM identifies the ultrastructural location of deposits and podocyte/GBM changes. Together, they provide the definitive classification.

IF Pattern	Interpretation	Diseases
Linear IgG along GBM	Anti-GBM antibody binding	Goodpasture/Anti-GBM disease

Granular IgG + C3 (capillary wall)	Immune complex deposition	Membranous nephropathy, Post-infectious GN, MPGN
Granular IgG + C3 (mesangial)	Mesangial immune complex deposition	IgA nephropathy (IgA dominant), Lupus (Class II)
"Full house" (IgG, IgA, IgM, C3, C1q)	Multiple immune complex types	Lupus nephritis (especially Class IV)
Dominant C3 (no/minimal Ig)	Complement pathway dysregulation	C3 glomerulopathy (C3GN, DDD)
Pauci-immune (negative/scanty)	ANCA-mediated (no immune complex deposition)	ANCA-associated vasculitis/RPGN Type III
Negative IF	Non-immune mechanism or podocytopathy	MCD, FSGS, Alport, Thin BM disease, Diabetic nephropathy

EM Finding	Disease
Subepithelial humps	Post-infectious GN
Subepithelial deposits with spikes	Membranous nephropathy
Subendothelial deposits	Lupus nephritis (Class III/IV), Immune complex MPGN
Mesangial deposits	IgA nephropathy, Lupus (Class II), HSP nephritis
Intramembranous dense deposits (ribbon-like)	Dense deposit disease (C3 glomerulopathy)
Diffuse foot process effacement (no deposits)	MCD, primary FSGS
GBM basket-weave lamellation	Alport syndrome
Uniform GBM thinning (<250 nm)	Thin basement membrane disease

Zebra bodies (lamellar inclusions in podocytes)	Fabry disease
Fibrils 8-12 nm (random)	Amyloidosis
Fibrils 10-30 nm (organised)	Fibrillary GN
Microtubules 30-50 nm (hollow core)	Immunotactoid glomerulopathy
Tubuloreticular inclusions in endothelium	SLE, HIV ("interferon footprints")

IHC Panel: RCC Subtyping

Marker	**Clear Cell**	**Papillary**	**Chromophobe**	**Oncocytoma**	**TFE3-rearranged**	**FH-deficient**
PAX8	+	+	+	+	+	+
CA-IX	Diffuse box-like +	-	-	-	Variable	+/-
CK7	-	+ (type 1 diffuse)	Diffuse +	-/focal	Variable	-
CD117	-	-	Diffuse +	Diffuse +	-	-
AMACR	+/-	+ (strong)	-	-	+	+/-
TFE3	-	-	-	-	Nuclear +	-
FH (2SC)	Intact	Intact	Intact	Intact	Intact	FH lost / 2SC+

Essential/Desirable: Clear Cell Renal Cell Carcinoma

Essential: Clear and/or eosinophilic cells in alveolar/nested pattern; sinusoidal vasculature; CA-IX diffuse membranous (box-like) positive; PAX8 positive.

Desirable: VHL mutation or 3p loss by FISH/NGS; ISUP nucleolar grade; sarcomatoid/rhabdoid features; staging.

Fig 22.1 — Glomerular Injury Mechanisms

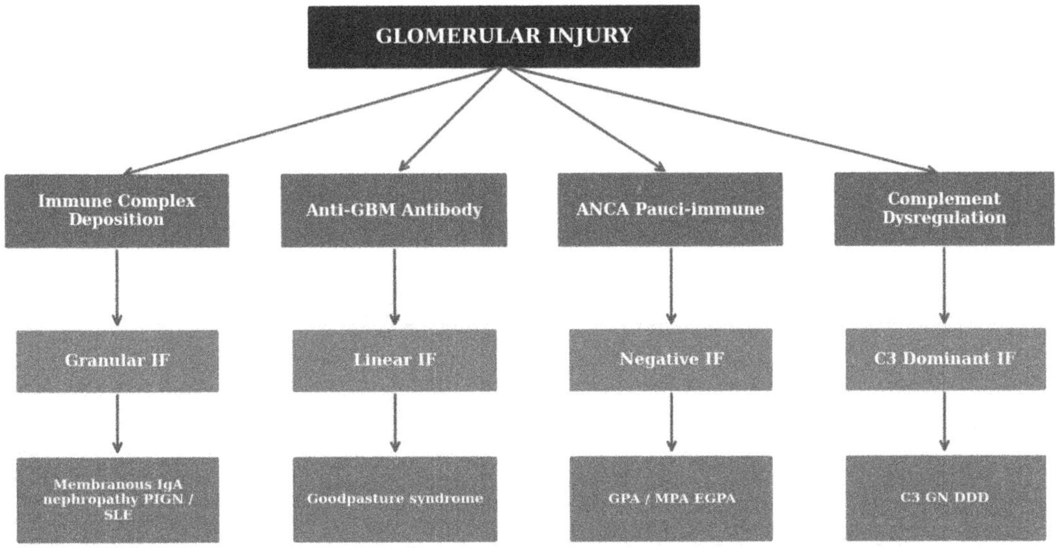

Figure 22.8: IF Pattern: IgA Nephropathy — dominant mesangial IgA. (Source: Author's original.)

Fig 22.2 — IF Pattern Composite Illustrated

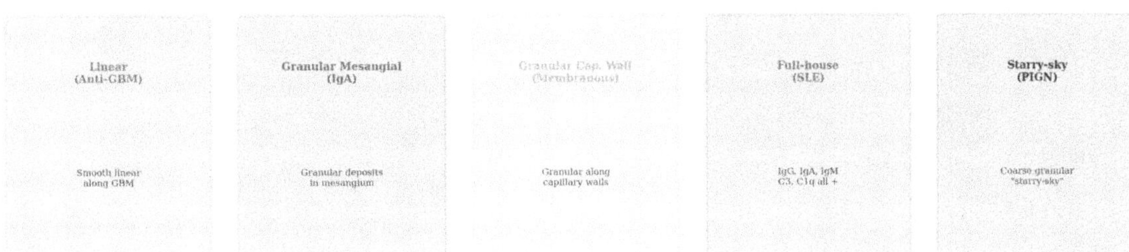

Figure 22.9: IF Pattern: Membranous Nephropathy — granular capillary wall IgG. (Source: Author's original.)

Fig 22.3 — EM Deposit Location Illustrated

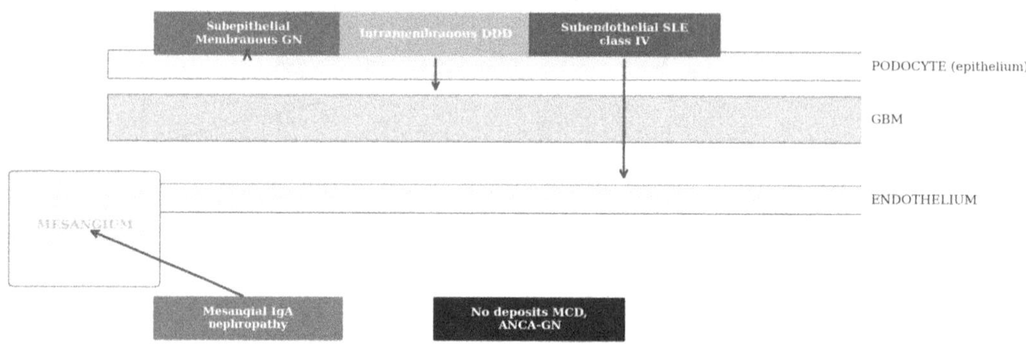

Figure 22.10: IF Pattern: Lupus Nephritis — full-house pattern. (Source: Author's original.)

Fig 22.4 — Nephrotic vs Nephritic Comparison

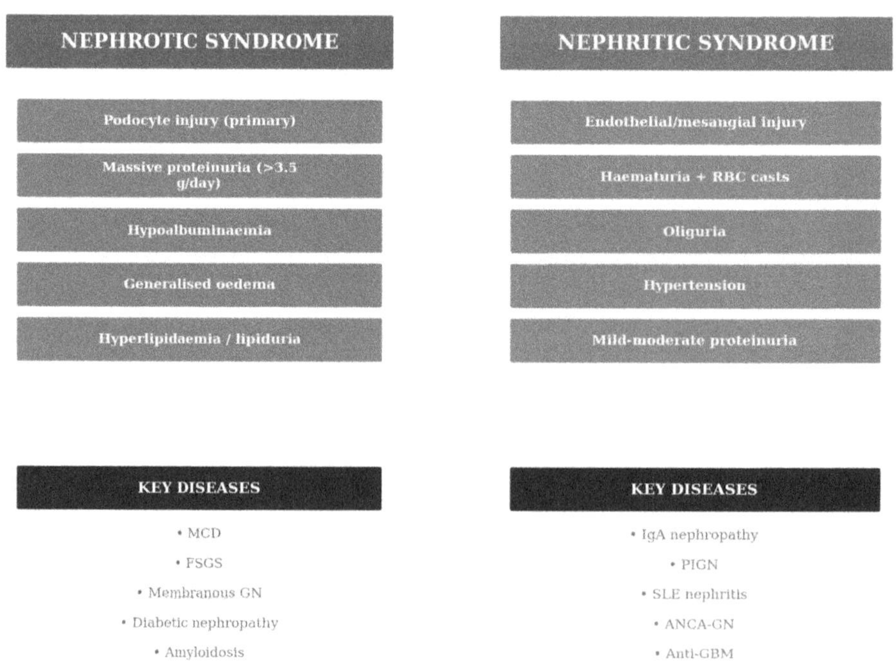

Figure 22.11: EM: Membranous Nephropathy — subepithelial deposits, spike-and-dome. (Source: Author's original.)

Fig 22.5 — Glomerular Patterns Composite

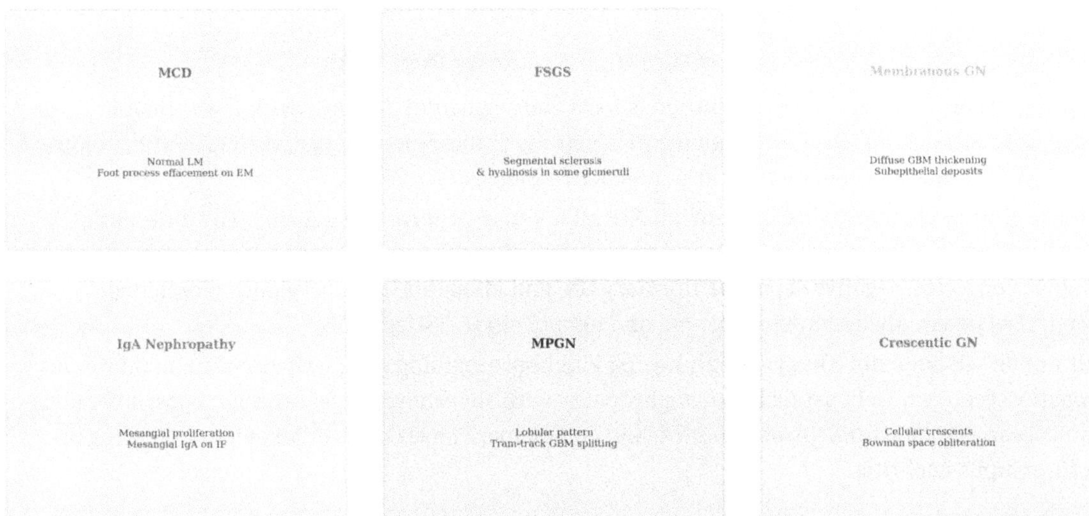

Figure 22.12: EM: IgA Nephropathy — mesangial electron-dense deposits. (Source: Author's original.)

Fig 22.6 — Approach to Renal Biopsy (Glomerular)

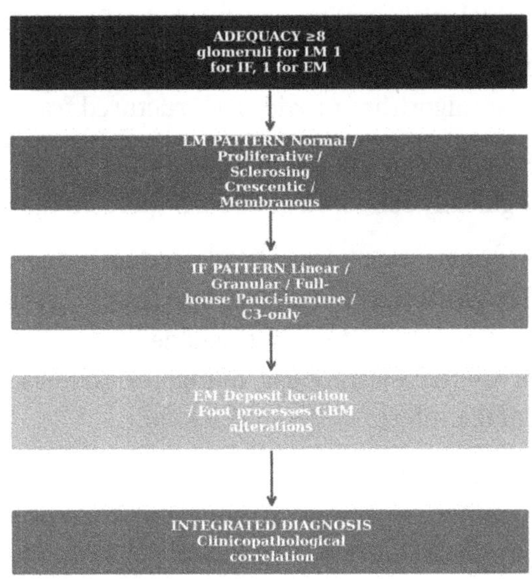

Figure 22.13: EM: MCD/FSGS — podocyte foot process effacement. (Source: Author's original.)

Integration: The techniques of IF and EM connect to Chapter 36 (IHC principles), Chapter 37 (molecular pathology), and Chapter 35 (tissue processing for EM). Lupus nephritis connects to Chapter 5 (SLE immunology). Diabetic nephropathy connects to Chapter 27 (endocrine pathology). Hereditary glomerulopathies connect to Chapter 8 (genetic disorders). TMA and vascular renal disease are covered in Chapter 23.*

The Pathologist's Eye: Three Traps in Glomerular Biopsy Reporting

1. Sampling error in FSGS: FSGS by definition is focal and segmental. A biopsy with fewer than 8 glomeruli risks missing the diagnostic lesion entirely. If the clinical picture suggests FSGS but the biopsy appears normal, request deeper sections and consider re-biopsy.

2. Nodular glomerulosclerosis differential: Not all nodular patterns are diabetic. The differential includes amyloidosis (Congo red positive), light chain deposition disease (kappa or lambda restriction on IF, granular Congo red-negative deposits), fibrillary GN, and idiopathic nodular glomerulosclerosis (smoking-associated). Always order Congo red and light chain IF/ISH.

3. "Full house" IF does not always mean lupus: Full house staining can rarely occur in membranous nephropathy secondary to hepatitis B, IgA nephropathy with superimposed features, and post-infectious GN. Clinical correlation with ANA, anti-dsDNA, and complement levels is essential before rendering a diagnosis of lupus nephritis.

22.9 Approach to the Histopathology Slide: Renal Biopsy (Glomerular)

A systematic approach to the renal biopsy is essential for the postgraduate practical and viva examination. The following six-step algorithm provides a structured framework.

Step 1: Adequacy. Confirm at least 8 glomeruli are present for non-focal diseases; 10 or more for optimal assessment. Note the number of globally sclerosed glomeruli (percentage of obsolescent glomeruli indicates chronicity).

Step 2: Glomerular pattern recognition. Evaluate: (a) Cellularity: Is there mesangial, endocapillary, or extracapillary (crescent) proliferation? (b) GBM: Is it thickened (membranous, diabetic), split (MPGN, Alport), or normal? (c) Deposits: Are there wire-loops, humps, or nodules visible? (d) Distribution: Diffuse vs focal, global vs segmental, uniform vs heterogeneous.

Step 3: Tubulointerstitial compartment. Assess tubular atrophy, interstitial fibrosis, inflammation (tubulitis, interstitial infiltrate), and casts. Tubular atrophy and interstitial fibrosis are the strongest histological predictors of long-term renal outcome regardless of glomerular diagnosis.

Step 4: Vessels. Look for arteriolar hyalinosis (diabetic, hypertensive), fibrinoid necrosis (malignant hypertension, vasculitis), intimal fibrosis, and thrombotic microangiopathy (TMA).

Step 5: Special stains. PAS (GBM, mesangial matrix), Jones silver (GBM spikes, double contours), Masson trichrome (fibrosis, immune deposits), Congo red (amyloid).

Step 6: Correlate with IF and EM. State the IF pattern (linear, granular, full house, pauci-immune, negative) and EM findings (deposit location, foot process effacement, GBM ultrastructure). Synthesise into a final diagnosis using the appropriate classification (ISN/RPS for lupus, Oxford MEST-C for IgA, Columbia for FSGS) (Figure 22.14).

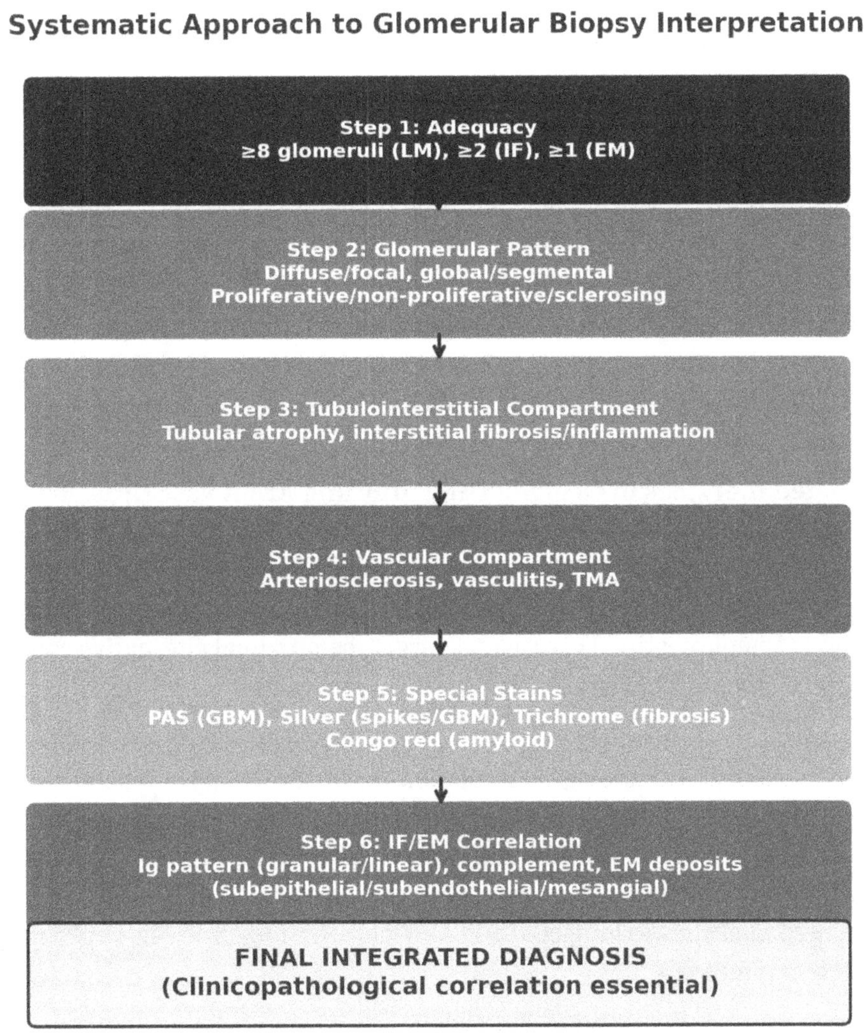

Figure 22.14: Systematic approach to glomerular biopsy interpretation: adequacy, glomerular pattern, tubulointerstitial, vascular, special stains, and IF/EM correlation. (Source: Author's original.)

Viva hook: "You receive a renal biopsy showing a membranoproliferative pattern on LM. What is the single most important next step?" Answer: Examine the immunofluorescence. If IF shows immunoglobulin + complement, it is immune complex-mediated MPGN (screen for infections and autoimmune disease). If IF shows dominant C3 without immunoglobulin, it is C3 glomerulopathy (investigate alternative complement pathway dysregulation). The LM pattern alone does not determine the disease category.

22.10 Recent Advances

Oxford Classification of IgA nephropathy 2016 — MEST-C update. The IgA Nephropathy Classification Working Group updated the 2009 Oxford MEST scoring system to incorporate crescents as an independent predictor of renal outcome (Trimarchi et al. Kidney International 2017; 91: 1014–1021; PMID 28341274). The revised MEST-C system retains the four original lesions — mesangial hypercellularity (M0/M1), endocapillary hypercellularity (E0/E1), segmental sclerosis (S0/S1), and tubular atrophy or interstitial fibrosis (T0/T1/T2) — and adds crescents (C0, no crescents; C1, crescents in less than one-quarter of glomeruli; C2, crescents in at least one-quarter). M, S, and T lesions predict outcome irrespective of immunosuppression, whereas E lesion outcome prediction is restricted to patients without immunosuppressive therapy. A web-based educational tool was developed to address documented interobserver variability in scoring of M and E lesions. Adequate scoring requires a minimum of eight glomeruli on the biopsy. The Working Group demonstrated that MEST-C combined with clinical data at biopsy provides prognostic discrimination equivalent to two years of clinical follow-up. Reporting implication: native renal biopsies showing IgA nephropathy on immunofluorescence should be reported with an explicit MEST-C score in addition to the descriptive histology to permit risk-stratified treatment decisions and entry into international registries.

Complement-targeted therapies in C3 glomerulopathy and ANCA vasculitis. Avacopan, a selective C5a receptor antagonist, was approved for ANCA-associated vasculitis (ADVOCATE trial, 2021), representing the first complement-targeted therapy in GN and allowing significant steroid reduction. Iptacopan (Factor B inhibitor) and danicopan (Factor D inhibitor) are in phase 2/3 trials for C3 glomerulopathy and IgA nephropathy. These agents target the proximal alternative complement pathway, addressing the root mechanism in complement-driven GN.

Anti-PLA2R and precision nephrology. Anti-PLA2R antibody monitoring has become standard of care in membranous nephropathy. Immunological remission (antibody disappearance) precedes clinical remission by months and predicts sustained response. Rituximab has emerged as first-line therapy for primary MN (MENTOR and RI-CYCLO trials), with anti-PLA2R titres guiding retreatment decisions. Novel targets including NELL-1 (neural epidermal growth factor-like 1), SEMA3B, and exostosin 1/2 (EXT1/EXT2) have been identified as antigens in PLA2R-negative membranous nephropathy, expanding the precision medicine framework.

SGLT2 inhibitors and non-steroidal MRAs in diabetic and non-diabetic CKD. The DAPA-CKD and EMPA-KIDNEY trials demonstrated that SGLT2 inhibitors (dapagliflozin, empagliflozin) reduce the risk of kidney disease progression in both diabetic and non-diabetic CKD, including IgA nephropathy. Finerenone, a non-steroidal mineralocorticoid receptor antagonist, reduces cardiovascular and kidney events in diabetic kidney disease (FIDELIO-DKD, FIGARO-DKD trials). Sparsentan, a dual endothelin/angiotensin receptor antagonist, received accelerated approval for IgA nephropathy (PROTECT trial, 2023) based on proteinuria reduction, and has been submitted for FSGS. These agents represent a paradigm shift from purely immunosuppressive therapy to integrated cardio-renal-metabolic protection.

International Frameworks

Revised ISN/RPS classification of lupus nephritis (2018). The 2018 consensus revision by the international nephropathology working group convened in Leiden refined the ISN/RPS classification by clarifying definitions of mesangial hypercellularity, endocapillary hypercellularity (replacing the prior term endocapillary proliferation), and crescent subtypes (cellular, fibrocellular, fibrous). The class IV-S and IV-G subdivisions were eliminated, and the active/chronic designations within class III/IV lesions were replaced by modified NIH activity (range 0–24) and chronicity (range 0–12) indices applied across all classes. Fibrinoid necrosis is now included as a discrete activity-index descriptor. Reporting requirement: lupus nephritis biopsies should be reported with both the lesion class (I–VI) and the modified NIH activity and chronicity scores, since these indices guide induction-versus-maintenance therapy and predict long-term renal outcome. Citation: Bajema IM, et al. Kidney Int 2018;93(4):789–796. PMID 29459092.

Ultra High-Yield Chapter Summary

Topic	Must Remember
Filtration barrier	Three layers: fenestrated endothelium, GBM (type IV collagen), podocytes (nephrin/podocin slit diaphragm)
IF pattern: Linear IgG	Anti-GBM disease (Goodpasture); alpha-3 type IV collagen target
IF pattern: Granular	Immune complex disease (membranous, post-infectious, lupus, IgA, MPGN)
IF pattern: Full house	Lupus nephritis (IgG + IgA + IgM + C3 + C1q)
IF pattern: Dominant C3	C3 glomerulopathy (alternative complement pathway dysregulation)
IF pattern: Pauci-immune	ANCA-associated vasculitis (GPA, MPA); most common RPGN type
MCD	Normal LM/IF; foot process effacement on EM; steroid responsive; most common nephrotic in children
FSGS	Focal segmental sclerosis; Columbia classification (5 variants); collapsing = worst prognosis (HIV)
Membranous nephropathy	Anti-PLA2R (70-80%); subepithelial deposits; spikes on silver; Ehrenreich-Churg stages I-IV
IgA nephropathy	Most common GN worldwide; Gd-IgA1; synpharyngitic haematuria;

	mesangial IgA; Oxford MEST-C
MPGN reclassification	IF-based: immune complex (Ig + C3) vs C3 glomerulopathy (C3 only); tram-track GBM
Post-infectious GN	Low C3; starry sky IF; subepithelial humps on EM; latent period 1-3 weeks
RPGN Type I	Anti-GBM; linear IgG; Goodpasture (+ lung); plasmapheresis
RPGN Type II	Immune complex (any severe GN with crescents); granular IF
RPGN Type III	Pauci-immune; ANCA (c-ANCA/PR3 = GPA; p-ANCA/MPO = MPA); most common RPGN
Crescent evolution	Cellular (reversible) → Fibrocellular → Fibrous (irreversible)
Lupus nephritis	ISN/RPS Classes I-VI; Class IV = worst; wire-loops; full house IF
Diabetic nephropathy	Kimmelstiel-Wilson nodules; diffuse mesangial expansion; afferent + efferent hyalinosis; AGE/RAGE pathway
Alport syndrome	COL4A3/A4/A5; basket-weave GBM on EM; deafness; lenticonus; absent alpha-5 on IF
Thin BM disease	Uniform GBM thinning <250 nm; benign haematuria; normal LM/IF
Amyloid vs diabetic	Both nodular; amyloid = Congo red positive; diabetic = Congo red negative
Renal biopsy adequacy	Minimum 8 glomeruli; IF and EM mandatory for diagnosis
Anti-PLA2R	Serological biomarker for primary membranous; guides treatment (rituximab) and monitoring
Avacopan	C5a receptor inhibitor; approved for ANCA vasculitis; steroid-sparing
SGLT2 inhibitors	Renal protection in diabetic AND non-diabetic CKD (DAPA-CKD, EMPA-KIDNEY)

Table 22.1: Differential Diagnosis of Glomerular Diseases

Disease	LM	IF	EM	Clinical
MCD	Normal (lipid in tubules)	Negative/trace	Foot process effacement (diffuse)	Nephrotic (children); steroid-responsive
FSGS	Segmental sclerosis; hyalinosis	IgM, C3 (trapped)	Foot process effacement (segmental)	Nephrotic; steroid-resistant; progression to CKD
Membranous	Thickened GBM; spikes (silver stain)	Granular IgG, C3 along GBM	Subepithelial deposits	Nephrotic (adults); PLA2R-associated
IgA Nephropathy	Mesangial proliferation	Mesangial IgA (dominant)	Mesangial electron-dense deposits	Recurrent haematuria; commonest GN worldwide
MPGN	Mesangial proliferation; GBM splitting (tram-tracking)	C3 +/- Ig along GBM	Subendothelial (Type I) or intramembranous dense (DDD)	Nephrotic/nephritic; hypocomplementaemia
RPGN	Crescents (>50% glomeruli)	Linear (anti-GBM), granular (immune complex), pauci-immune (ANCA)	Varies by type	Rapidly progressive renal failure

Table 22.2: Immunofluorescence Pattern Master Table

IF Pattern	Ig/Complement	Disease(s)	Diagnostic Significance
Linear GBM	IgG	Anti-GBM (Goodpasture)	Pathognomonic; anti-GBM antibodies
Granular mesangial	IgA (dominant), C3	IgA nephropathy	Mesangial IgA dominance is diagnostic
Granular capillary wall	IgG, C3	Membranous nephropathy	Subepithelial immune complexes
Full-house	IgG, IgA, IgM, C3, C1q	Lupus nephritis	All Ig classes + complement
Pauci-immune	Negative/minimal	ANCA vasculitis (GPA, MPA)	Diagnosis by serology (MPO/PR3-ANCA)
Starry sky (C3 dominant)	C3 only	C3 glomerulopathy (DDD, C3GN)	Alternative pathway dysregulation

Table 22.3: EM Deposit Location and Disease Correlation

Deposit Location	Appearance	Disease	Mnemonic
Subepithelial	Humps (dome-shaped)	PSGN, Membranous (stage II-III)	SubEpithelial = SidE of Epithelium
Subendothelial	Irregular, wire-loop	Lupus (Class III/IV), MPGN Type I	SubENDOthelial = ENDOluminal side
Mesangial	Electron-dense in mesangium	IgA nephropathy, HSP nephritis	Most common deposit site overall
Intramembranous	Ribbon-like dense deposits	Dense deposit disease (C3GN/DDD)	Within GBM itself

Table 22.4: Lupus Nephritis ISN/RPS Classification (2003/2018 Revised)

Class	LM	IF	EM	Clinical
I (Minimal mesangial)	Normal	Mesangial deposits	Mesangial deposits only	Normal/mild proteinuria
II (Mesangial proliferative)	Mesangial hypercellularity	Mesangial Ig/C	Mesangial deposits	Mild haematuria/proteinuria
III (Focal)	<50% glomeruli; segmental endo/extracapillary	Full-house	Subendothelial deposits	Active nephritis; mod proteinuria
IV (Diffuse)	>50% glomeruli; wire-loop deposits	Full-house	Subendothelial (prominent)	Severe nephritis; worst prognosis without Rx
V (Membranous)	Thickened GBM	Granular capillary IgG	Subepithelial deposits	Nephrotic syndrome
VI (Sclerosing)	>90% globally sclerosed	Variable	Variable	Chronic renal failure; irreversible

Table 22.5: Oxford Classification MEST-C Scoring (IgA Nephropathy)

Score	Feature	Definition	Prognostic Impact
M0/M1	Mesangial hypercellularity	M1: >50% glomeruli with >3 cells/mesangial area	Independent predictor of ESRD

E0/E1	Endocapillary hypercellularity	E1: Any glomerulus with endocapillary proliferation	Predicts steroid responsiveness
S0/S1	Segmental sclerosis	S1: Any segmental glomerulosclerosis	Independent predictor of ESRD
T0/T1/T2	Tubular atrophy/interstitial fibrosis	T0: 0-25%; T1: 26-50%; T2: >50%	Strongest predictor of outcome
C0/C1/C2	Crescents	C0: none; C1: <25%; C2: >25% glomeruli	Added 2017; predicts immunosuppression benefit

Table 22.6: IHC Panel for RCC Subtyping

Marker	Clear cell	Papillary	Chromophobe	Oncocytoma	TFE3-rearranged	FH-deficient
PAX8	+	+	+	+	+	+
CA-IX (diffuse)	+++	-/focal	-	-	+/-	+/-
CK7	-/focal	+ (type 1)	+++ (diffuse)	-/focal	-	-
CD117 (c-KIT)	-	-	+++	+++	-	+/-
AMACR	-/+	+++ (type 1)	-	-	+/-	-
TFE3 nuclear	-	-	-	-	+++	-
FH (loss)	Retained	Retained	Retained	Retained	Retained	Lost
2SC	-	-	-	-	-	+++

Essential and Desirable Diagnostic Criteria: Clear Cell RCC (WHO 5th Ed)

ESSENTIAL: Clear to eosinophilic cytoplasm with delicate sinusoidal vasculature; PAX8+; CA-IX diffuse membranous positivity; loss of VHL (3p25) by FISH or sequencing

DESIRABLE: ISUP nucleolar grade (replaces Fuhrman); negative CK7, CD117; exclude FH-deficient and TFE3-rearranged mimics; staging per AJCC 8th edition

PITFALL: Eosinophilic variant of clear cell RCC can mimic chromophobe or oncocytoma. CA-IX remains diffuse membranous even in eosinophilic areas, distinguishing it from mimics.

The diagnostic thinking line in glomerular pathology: every renal biopsy must be read as a triplet (LM + IF + EM). No single modality is sufficient. A crescentic GN on LM with pauci-immune IF points to ANCA vasculitis; the same crescents with linear IgG point to anti-GBM disease. The IF pattern determines the category; the LM pattern determines the activity and chronicity.

Think of nephrotic vs nephritic not as separate diseases but as overlapping clinical syndromes mapping onto specific glomerular compartment injuries: podocyte (nephrotic) vs endothelial/mesangial (nephritic). Membranous starts nephrotic but may acquire nephritic features with superimposed crescents.

When you see full-house IF on a renal biopsy, always think lupus nephritis first. But confirm with clinical correlation: full-house IF can occasionally occur in post-infectious GN and membranoproliferative patterns. The subendothelial wire-loop deposit on EM is the confirmatory finding for Class IV lupus (Figures 22.8–22.10).

[MORPHOLOGY: Fig 22.X -- Glomerular Patterns Composite (6-panel). A: Normal glomerulus. B: Mesangial proliferation (IgA). C: Membranous (spike and dome). D: Crescentic. E: MPGN (tram-tracking). F: FSGS (segmental sclerosis). Source: Author's original.]

Chapter 23: Renal Pathology Part 2: Tubulointerstitial, Vascular, and Neoplastic

THE BIG PICTURE

The renal tubule is not merely a passive conduit for urine. It is a metabolically demanding structure, exquisitely sensitive to ischaemia and toxins, and the site where many systemic diseases leave their earliest morphological footprint. The spectrum of tubulointerstitial, vascular, cystic, and neoplastic diseases of the kidney collectively generates some of the most commonly tested questions, demanding both a mechanistic understanding of pathogenesis and confident pattern recognition at the microscope.

High-yield topics in this chapter: Acute tubular injury (ischaemic vs nephrotoxic; KIM-1/NGAL as early biomarkers); Tubulointerstitial nephritis (drug-induced and analgesic nephropathy); Pyelonephritis including chronic, reflux, and xanthogranulomatous forms; Cystic diseases of the kidney (ADPKD, ARPKD, medullary cystic/nephronophthisis, acquired cystic disease); Renal vascular diseases (benign and malignant nephrosclerosis, thrombotic microangiopathies); Clear cell renal cell carcinoma and its morphological and molecular subtypes; Papillary, chromophobe, and collecting duct carcinomas; WHO 5th Edition (2022) additions: FH-deficient, SDH-deficient, ELOC-mutated, eosinophilic solid and cystic (ESC), and ALK-rearranged renal cell carcinomas; Oncocytoma and angiomyolipoma (PEComa family); Wilms tumour (nephroblastoma); Renal medullary carcinoma and INI1/SMARCB1 loss; Renal transplant pathology including Banff rejection categories and BK virus nephropathy; Staging and prognostic markers for RCC; Emerging targeted therapies (belzutifan for VHL-associated RCC, nivolumab + ipilimumab, TKI-IO combinations).

Tubular and Interstitial Diseases

Acute Tubular Injury

Definition: Irreversible or reversible injury to renal tubular epithelial cells causing AKI. Most common cause of AKI in hospitalised patients. Term “injury” now preferred over “necrosis.”

Etiology: Ischaemic: shock, haemorrhage, sepsis, major surgery (S3 segment, medullary thick ascending limb most vulnerable). Nephrotoxic: aminoglycosides, amphotericin B, cisplatin, radiocontrast, heavy metals, myoglobin, haemoglobin.

Pathogenesis: Ischaemia/Toxin → Proximal tubular injury → Loss of brush border + cell polarity → Cell detachment → Tubular cast formation → Obstruction + Backleak → ↓GFR → AKI

Gross: Swollen, pale kidneys.

Microscopy: Ischaemic: patchy necrosis, skip lesions, multiple segments. Nephrotoxic: uniform, diffuse, proximal tubules. BM typically intact (regeneration possible).

Key finding: Tubular epithelial simplification — flattened cells, loss of brush border, sloughed cells, muddy brown granular casts.

Phases: Initiation → Maintenance (oliguria) → Recovery (polyuria). Reversible if BM intact; 1–2 weeks.

Exam yield: ★★★ HIGH

Fig 23.1 — TIN Diagnostic Algorithm

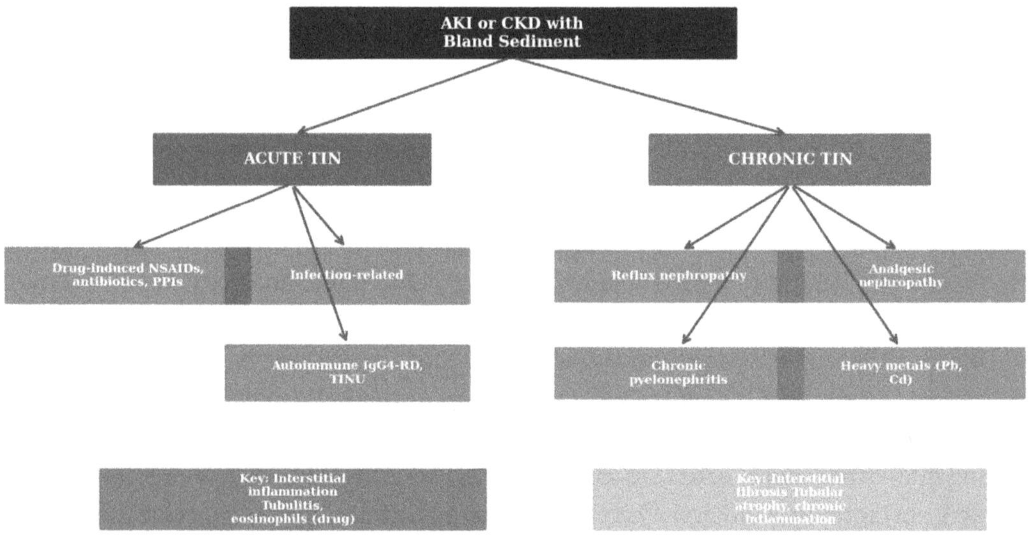

Figure 23.1: Tubulointerstitial nephritis (TIN) diagnostic algorithm. Acute TIN (drug-induced, infection-related, autoimmune) vs Chronic TIN (reflux nephropathy, analgesic, heavy metals). (Source: Author's original.)

Integration: *ATI connects to haemodynamic disorders (shock, DIC, see Chapter 4), drug toxicity and environmental pathology (see Chapter 10), and forms the tubulointerstitial component of many glomerular diseases discussed in Chapter 22.*

Tubulointerstitial Nephritis

Definition: Inflammation primarily of interstitium and tubules, sparing glomeruli/vessels.

Etiology: Acute drug-induced (most common): penicillins, cephalosporins, NSAIDs, PPIs, rifampicin. Other: infections, autoimmune, sarcoidosis, IgG4-RD.

Pathogenesis: Drug hapten → T-cell mediated interstitial inflammation → Tubular injury → ↓GFR

Microscopy: Acute: interstitial oedema, lymphocytes, eosinophils, plasma cells; tubulitis. Granulomas in sarcoidosis/TB/drug reactions. Chronic: fibrosis + tubular atrophy.

Key finding: Interstitial eosinophils + tubulitis with normal glomeruli.

Exam yield: ★★★ HIGH

Definition: Chronic TIN from prolonged analgesic combinations (phenacetin/aspirin/caffeine, chronic NSAIDs).

Pathogenesis: Chronic analgesics → Toxic metabolite concentration in medulla → Oxidative injury → Papillary necrosis → Cortical TIN → CKD

Key finding: Papillary necrosis + chronic TIN. Risk of urothelial carcinoma of renal pelvis.

Exam yield: ★★ MODERATE

> **Quick Recall: Tubulointerstitial Nephritis**
>
> **ATI vs TIN:** ATI shows tubular injury with casts; TIN shows interstitial inflammation with tubulitis.
>
> **Drug-induced TIN triad:** Fever, rash, eosinophilia (not always complete).
>
> **Analgesic nephropathy:** Chronic TIN + papillary necrosis; NSAID combinations; risk of TCC of renal pelvis.
>
> **Granulomatous TIN:** Think sarcoidosis, TB, drug reaction (rifampicin), IgG4-RD (Figure 23.1).

Pyelonephritis

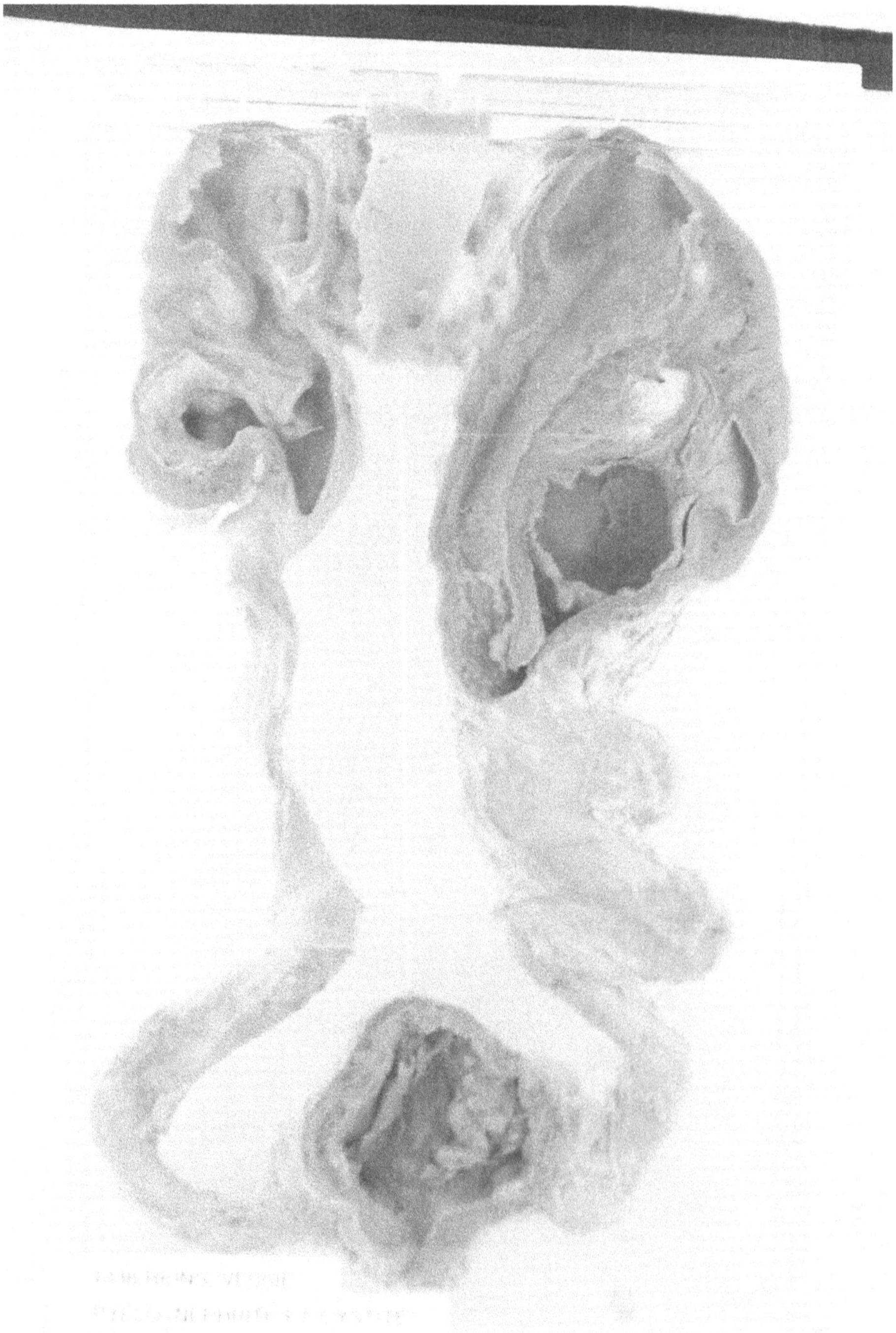

Figure 23.2: Chronic pyelonephritis (gross): irregular cortical scars and blunted, dilated calyces. (Source: Laval University, Wikimedia Commons, CC BY-SA 4.0.)

Pyelonephritis is a bacterial infection of the renal pelvis, calyces, and parenchyma. It is one of the most common renal diseases and a significant cause of morbidity, particularly in women, diabetic patients, and those with urinary obstruction.

Definition: Acute bacterial infection of renal pelvis, calyces, and parenchyma from ascending UTI.

Etiology: E. coli (>80%), Proteus, Klebsiella. Predisposing: VUR, obstruction, catheter, pregnancy, DM.

Pathogenesis: Ascending infection → Neutrophilic infiltration of tubules/interstitium → Microabscess formation

Gross: Enlarged kidney, cortical surface abscesses, yellowish streaks from pelvis to cortex.

Key finding: Neutrophils within tubular lumina + interstitial microabscesses (vs drug-induced TIN: eosinophils).

Exam yield: ★★★ HIGH

Chronic Pyelonephritis — Definition: Chronic TIN from recurrent/persistent infection. Irregular cortical scars overlying blunted calyces.

Etiology: Reflux nephropathy (VUR + infection) or obstructive (calculi, BPH).

Pathogenesis: Recurrent infection → Chronic inflammation → Fibrosis + tubular atrophy → Scarring → CKD

Gross: Asymmetric irregular cortical scars overlying dilated, blunted calyces.

Key finding: Thyroidisation — atrophic dilated tubules with eosinophilic colloid-like casts resembling thyroid follicles.

Variant: Xanthogranulomatous pyelonephritis: foamy macrophages, Proteus, staghorn calculi; mimics RCC.

Exam yield: ★★★ HIGH

Quick Recall: Pyelonephritis

Acute: E. coli; ascending infection; neutrophilic tubulitis and microabscesses.

Chronic: Irregular scars + blunted calyces; thyroidisation; reflux or obstruction.

Xanthogranulomatous: Foamy macrophages; Proteus; staghorn calculi; mimics RCC.

Papillary necrosis: Diabetes, sickle cell, analgesics, pyelonephritis, obstruction (mnemonic: NSAID).

Cystic Diseases of the Kidney

Renal cysts are morphologically diverse and range from trivial incidental findings to life-threatening systemic disorders. A practical classification divides them into genetic (hereditary) and non-genetic (acquired) categories.

Category	Entity	Key Features
Genetic: Autosomal Dominant	ADPKD (PKD1, PKD2)	Bilateral large cystic kidneys; liver cysts; berry aneurysms; adult onset
Genetic: Autosomal Recessive	ARPKD (PKHD1)	Bilateral symmetrical cystic kidneys; congenital hepatic fibrosis; neonatal/infantile
Genetic: Other	Nephronophthisis (NPHP genes)	Medullary cysts; tubular atrophy; childhood/juvenile CKD
Genetic: Other	Medullary cystic kidney disease	Adult onset; medullary cysts; UMOD mutations
Genetic: Syndromic	Von Hippel-Lindau	Cysts + clear cell RCC; VHL gene
Genetic: Syndromic	Tuberous sclerosis	Cysts + angiomyolipomas; TSC1/TSC2
Acquired	Simple renal cysts	Common; cortical; benign; incidental finding
Acquired	Acquired cystic disease	In ESRD/dialysis patients; risk of RCC
Acquired	Medullary sponge kidney	Dilated collecting ducts; medullary calcifications

Autosomal Dominant Polycystic Kidney Disease (ADPKD)

Definition: Most common hereditary cystic kidney disease (~1:400–1:1000). Progressive bilateral cystic enlargement → ESRD by 5th–6th decade.

Genetics: PKD1 (chr 16p, ~85%, ESRD ~54y) and PKD2 (chr 4q, ~15%, ESRD ~74y). AD.

Pathogenesis: PKD1/PKD2 mutation → Defective polycystin → Ciliary dysfunction → ↓Ca^{2+} → ↑cAMP → mTOR/MAPK activation → Proliferation + Fluid secretion → Cyst expansion

Gross: Massively enlarged kidneys, multiple variable-sized cysts in cortex and medulla.

Key finding: Bilateral massive cysts from all nephron segments + family history. Extrarenal: hepatic cysts (~40%), berry aneurysms (SAH risk), MVP.

Treatment: Tolvaptan (V2 receptor antagonist, reduces cAMP, slows cyst growth).

Exam yield: ★★★ HIGH

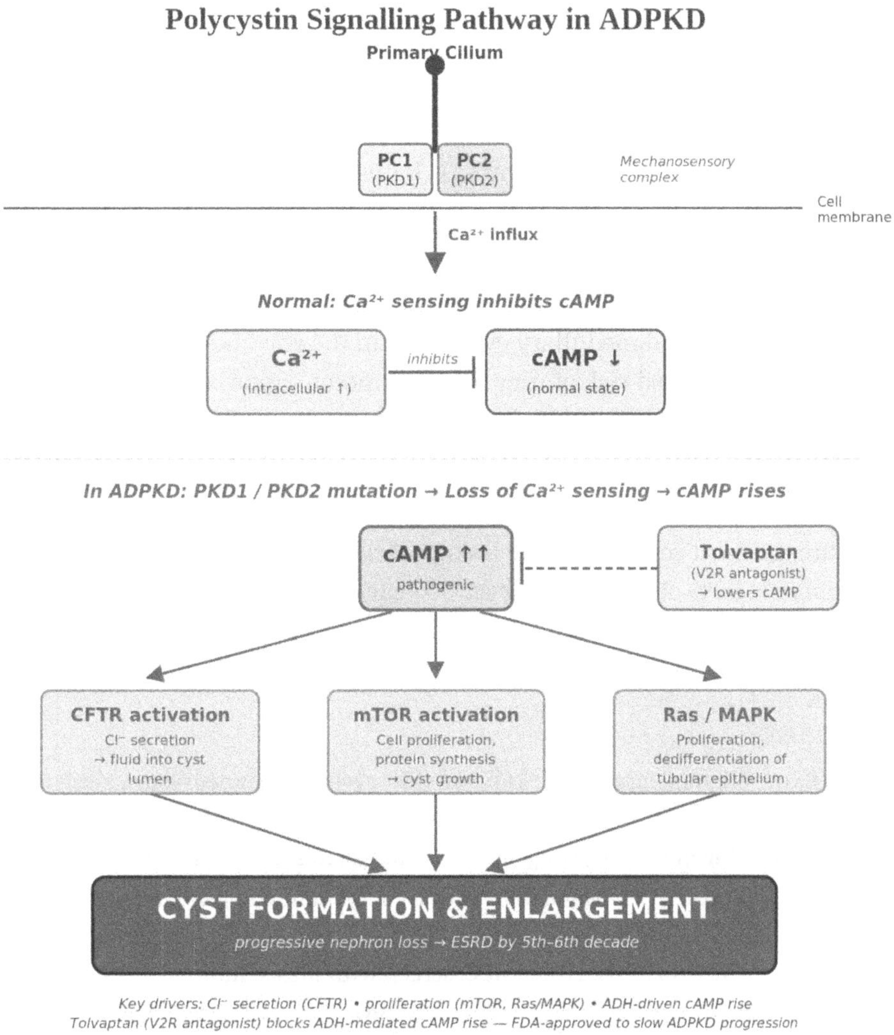

Figure 23.4: Polycystin signalling pathway in ADPKD: primary cilium, PC1/PC2, calcium-cAMP axis, mTOR, CFTR, and tolvaptan mechanism of action. (Source: Author's original.)

Autosomal Recessive Polycystic Kidney Disease (ARPKD)

Definition/Genetics: AR cystic kidney disease. PKHD1 gene (chr 6p21, fibrocystin). Neonatal/infantile presentation.

Pathogenesis: PKHD1 mutation → Defective fibrocystin → Ciliary dysfunction in collecting ducts → Fusiform dilatation → Bilateral renal enlargement

Key finding: Fusiform collecting duct dilatation arranged radially (vs ADPKD: variable cysts, all segments). Congenital hepatic fibrosis always present.

Exam yield: ★★★ HIGH

Definition: Most common genetic cause of childhood ESRD. AR ciliopathy. NPHP genes (>20).

Pathogenesis: NPHP mutation → Ciliary dysfunction → TBM disruption → TI fibrosis + Corticomedullary cysts → ESRD

Key finding: Small kidneys with corticomedullary junction cysts + diffuse TI fibrosis (vs ADPKD/ARPKD: enlarged kidneys).

Associations: Senior-Løken (retinitis pigmentosa), Joubert (cerebellar hypoplasia), MCKD (adult AD counterpart).

Exam yield: ★★ MODERATE

Acquired cystic disease develops in kidneys of patients with end-stage renal disease undergoing long-term dialysis. Multiple cortical and medullary cysts form in the shrunken, fibrotic kidneys. The critical clinical significance is the increased risk of renal cell carcinoma (approximately 7-fold), particularly acquired cystic disease-associated RCC (a WHO 5th Edition recognised entity) characterised by cribriform architecture with oxalate crystals. Screening ultrasonography is recommended in long-term dialysis patients.

Simple renal cysts are the most common cystic lesions of the kidney, increasing in frequency with age (present in approximately 50% of individuals over 50 years). They are cortical, unilocular, lined by flattened epithelium, contain clear fluid, and are clinically insignificant. The Bosniak classification (I through IV) stratifies complex cystic renal lesions by imaging characteristics to guide management.

Quick Recall: Cystic Diseases of the Kidney

ADPKD: AD; PKD1/PKD2; bilateral large cystic kidneys; liver cysts; berry aneurysms; adult onset; tolvaptan.

ARPKD: AR; PKHD1; collecting duct cysts; congenital hepatic fibrosis; neonatal/infantile.

Nephronophthisis: AR; ciliopathy; corticomedullary cysts; most common genetic cause of childhood ESRD.

Acquired cystic disease: ESRD/dialysis; risk of RCC; screen with ultrasound.

Simple cysts: Common, benign, cortical, increase with age; Bosniak classification for complex cysts.

Exam Pitfall: ADPKD vs ARPKD

Do not confuse ADPKD and ARPKD. ADPKD presents in adults with variable-sized cysts from all nephron segments; ARPKD presents in neonates/infants with uniform, radially arranged collecting duct cysts. ARPKD always has congenital hepatic fibrosis (ductal plate malformation); ADPKD has hepatic cysts (simple cysts, not fibrosis).

Renal Vascular Diseases

Nephrosclerosis

Definition: Sclerosis of renal arterioles/small arteries from chronic HTN or ageing.

Pathogenesis: Chronic HTN → Hyaline arteriolosclerosis (plasma protein insudation) → Luminal narrowing → Ischaemia → Glomerulosclerosis + Tubular atrophy + Fibrosis

Gross: Symmetrically contracted, finely granular cortical surface.

Key finding: Hyaline arteriolosclerosis — homogeneous, pink, glassy arteriolar wall thickening (PAS+).

Exam yield: ★★★ HIGH

Definition: Severe acute HTN (diastolic >120 mmHg) with end-organ damage.

Pathogenesis: Severe HTN → Endothelial injury → Fibrinoid necrosis + Hyperplastic arteriolosclerosis ("onion-skinning") → Luminal obliteration → Ischaemia

Gross: "Flea-bitten kidney" — petechial haemorrhages on cortical surface.

Key finding: Onion-skin hyperplastic arteriolosclerosis + fibrinoid necrosis ("necrotising arteriolitis").

Key DDx: Benign nephrosclerosis (hyaline, granular) vs malignant HTN (onion-skin, flea-bitten) vs TMA (capillary thrombi, schistocytes).

Exam yield: ★★★ HIGH

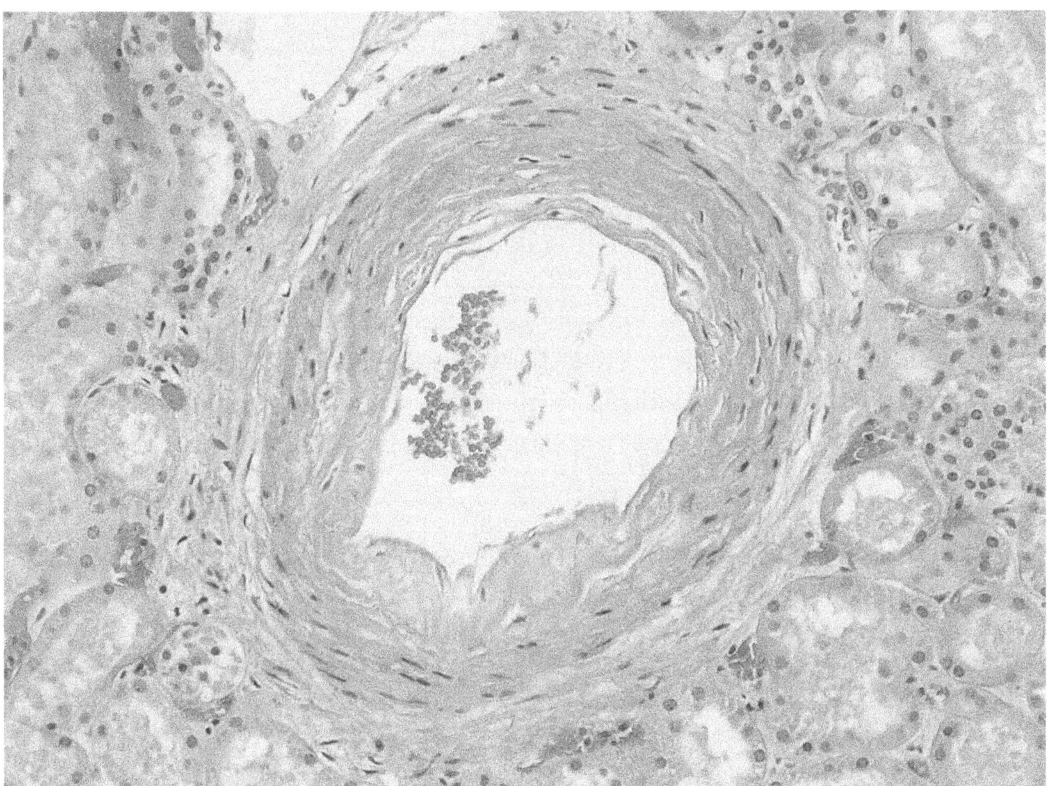

Figure 23.5: Hypertensive nephrosclerosis — arcuate artery. Marked medial hypertrophy and fibrous intimal thickening of an arcuate artery with concentric laminar narrowing of the lumen (onion-skin change in severe/malignant hypertension). The adjacent parenchyma shows tubular atrophy and interstitial fibrosis. H&E, ×200. (Source: Mikael Häggström, Wikimedia Commons, CC0.)

Thrombotic Microangiopathies

The thrombotic microangiopathies (TMAs) are a group of disorders characterised by endothelial injury leading to thrombosis of arterioles and capillaries, microangiopathic haemolytic anaemia, thrombocytopenia, and organ damage. The kidney is a principal target organ. The two classic TMAs are haemolytic uraemic syndrome (HUS) and thrombotic thrombocytopenic purpura (TTP), though the clinical and pathological features overlap.

Definition: Most common TMA in children. D+HUS: Shiga toxin-producing E. coli O157:H7.

Pathogenesis: E. coli O157:H7 → Shiga toxin → Endothelial injury → Platelet activation + Fibrin deposition → Microthrombi → MAHA + Thrombocytopenia + AKI

Key finding: Fibrin thrombi in glomerular capillaries/arterioles + schistocytes on smear. Supportive care; avoid antibiotics.

Exam yield: ★★★ HIGH

Atypical HUS: Complement mutations (Factor H/I, MCP, C3, Factor B) → Uncontrolled alternative complement activation → Endothelial TMA.

Treatment/DDx: Eculizumab (anti-C5 mAb). TTP: ADAMTS13 deficiency → ultra-large vWF multimers → platelet thrombi (neurological).

Exam yield: ★★★ HIGH — HUS vs TTP vs atypical HUS comparison.

Integration: *TMAs connect to haemostatic disorders and DIC (see Chapter 4), complement biology (see Chapter 5), and vascular endothelial pathology (see Chapter 13). For platelet biology and coagulation cascade details, see Volume 1.*

Quick Recall: Renal Vascular Diseases

Benign nephrosclerosis: Hyaline arteriolosclerosis; finely granular kidney; HTN and DM.

Malignant HTN: Onion-skin hyperplastic arteriolosclerosis; fibrinoid necrosis; flea-bitten kidney.

Typical HUS: E. coli O157:H7; Shiga toxin; children; fibrin thrombi; triad of MAHA + thrombocytopenia + AKI.

Atypical HUS: Complement mutations; eculizumab.

TTP: ADAMTS13 deficiency; platelet thrombi; pentad; plasma exchange.

Renal Neoplasms

Renal neoplasms encompass a diverse group of benign and malignant tumours arising from the renal parenchyma, collecting system, and mesenchymal elements. Renal cell carcinoma (RCC) accounts for approximately 85% of primary malignant renal neoplasms in adults, while Wilms tumour (nephroblastoma) is the most common renal malignancy of childhood. The WHO 5th Edition Classification of Urinary and Male Genital Tumours (2022) has significantly expanded the classification of renal tumours, incorporating molecularly defined entities.

WHO 5th Edition Classification (2022): Renal Tumours (Selected)

Renal cell tumours:

Clear cell renal cell carcinoma
Multilocular cystic renal cell neoplasm of low malignant potential
Papillary renal cell carcinoma
Chromophobe renal cell carcinoma
Collecting duct carcinoma
Renal medullary carcinoma
MiT family translocation renal cell carcinomas (TFE3-rearranged; TFEB-altered)
Fumarate hydratase-deficient renal cell carcinoma
Succinate dehydrogenase-deficient renal cell carcinoma
Clear cell papillary renal cell tumour
ELOC-mutated renal cell carcinoma
Acquired cystic disease-associated renal cell carcinoma
Eosinophilic solid and cystic (ESC) renal cell carcinoma

Metanephric tumours: Metanephric adenoma

Oncocytic and chromophobe tumours: Oncocytoma; Chromophobe RCC

Mesenchymal tumours: Angiomyolipoma (classic, epithelioid)

Embryonal tumours: Nephroblastoma (Wilms tumour)

Clear Cell Renal Cell Carcinoma

Definition: Most common RCC (70–80%). Proximal tubular origin. VHL loss (chr 3p25) in >90%.

Pathogenesis: VHL loss → HIF-α stabilisation → ↑VEGF, ↑PDGF, ↑TGF-α, ↑EPO → Angiogenesis + Proliferation + Erythrocytosis

Gross: Golden-yellow, well-circumscribed cortical mass (lipid + glycogen). Haemorrhage, necrosis, cystic change.

Microscopy: Clear cells (lipid/glycogen dissolved in processing), distinct membranes, solid nests/acini/tubules.

Key finding: Clear cells + arborising sinusoidal vascular network. Higher grade = eosinophilic. Sarcomatoid/rhabdoid = Grade 4.

IHC: CK7−, CD10+, CA-IX+ (diffuse membranous box-like), PAX8+, vimentin+.

Grading: WHO/ISUP: G1 (no nucleoli ×400), G2 (visible ×400), G3 (visible ×100), G4 (extreme/sarcomatoid/rhabdoid).

Metastasis: Renal vein → IVC → right atrium. Late metastases: bone, brain, thyroid, skin.

Exam yield: ★★★ HIGH

The WHO/ISUP grading system (replacing the older Fuhrman system) grades RCC based on nucleolar prominence: Grade 1 (absent/inconspicuous nucleoli at ×400), Grade 2 (conspicuous nucleoli at ×400 but not at ×100), Grade 3 (conspicuous nucleoli at ×100), and Grade 4 (extreme nuclear pleomorphism, giant cells, or any sarcomatoid/rhabdoid differentiation). This grading system applies to clear cell and papillary RCC; chromophobe RCC uses a separate system.

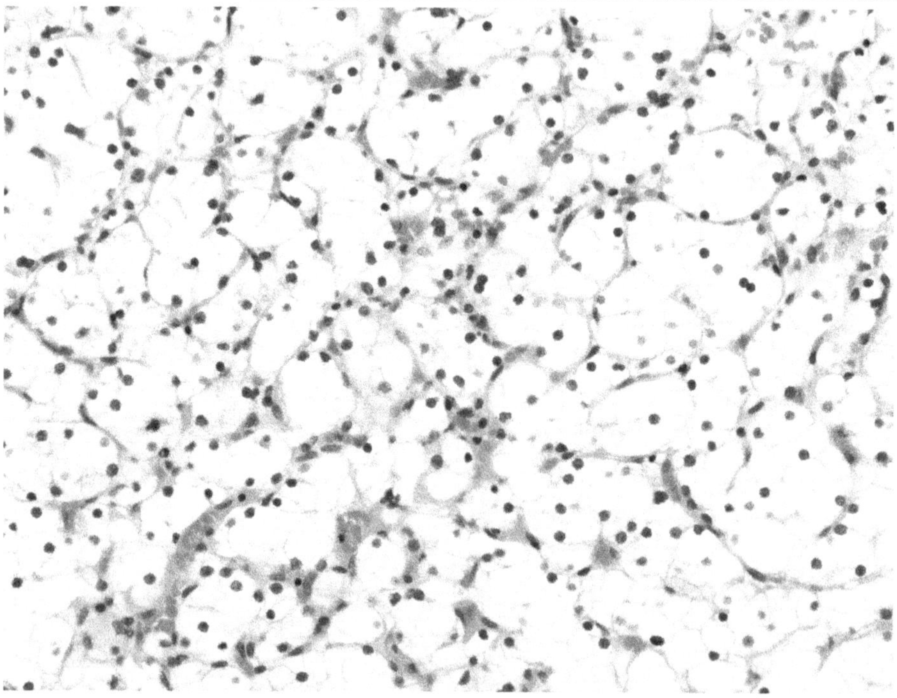

Figure 23.6: Clear cell renal cell carcinoma. Nests of cells with abundant clear cytoplasm (glycogen/lipid dissolved), round central nuclei, and prominent sinusoidal thin-walled vasculature (H&E, high power). (Source: Nephron, Wikimedia Commons, CC BY-SA 3.0.)

Papillary Renal Cell Carcinoma

Definition: Second most common RCC (10–15%). Proximal tubule origin.

Microscopy: Papillary/tubular architecture. Cuboidal to columnar, basophilic cytoplasm. Trisomy 7, 17; loss of Y.

Key finding: Foamy macrophages in papillary cores + psammoma bodies. CK7+, AMACR+. WHO 5th Ed: no Type 1/2 separation required.

Key DDx: Papillary adenoma (<1.5 cm, grade 1–2, no capsule) = benign.

Exam yield: ★★★ *HIGH*

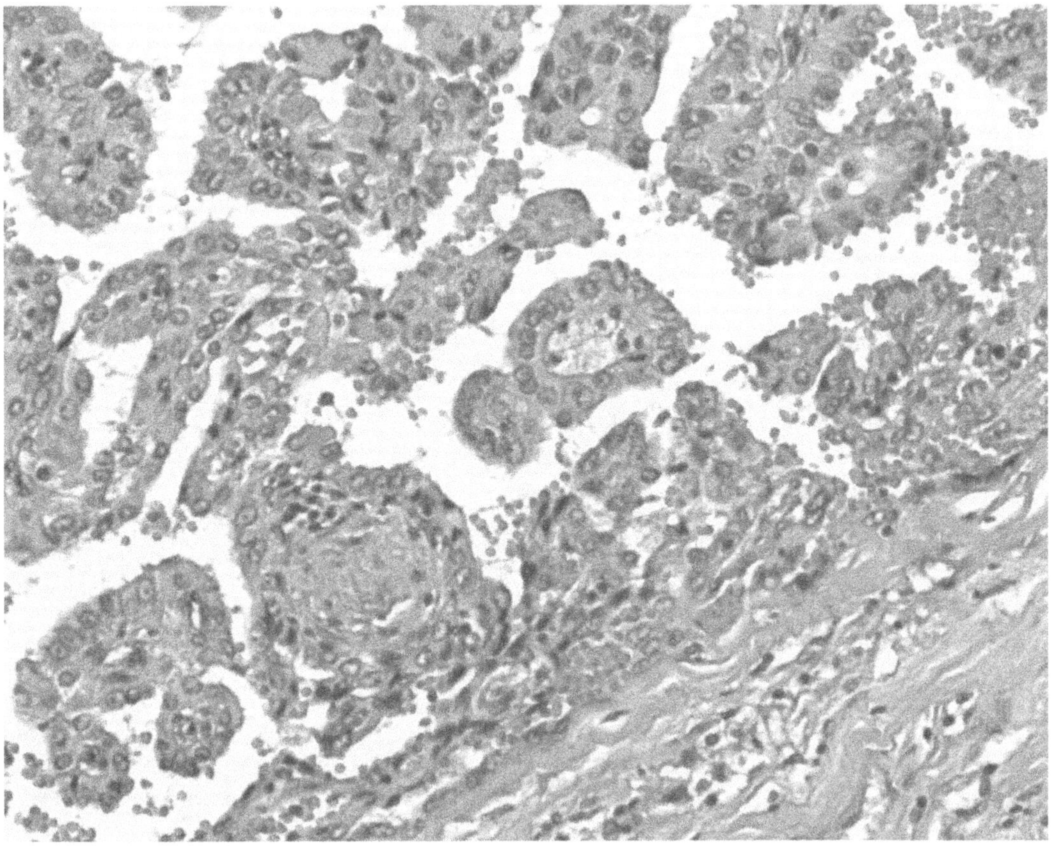

Figure 23.7: Papillary renal cell carcinoma. Papillary architecture with fibrovascular cores lined by cuboidal to columnar epithelial cells showing moderate nuclear atypia. H&E. (Source: Nephron, Wikimedia Commons, CC BY-SA 3.0.)

Definition: ~5% of RCCs. Intercalated cell origin. Multiple whole-chromosome losses.

Microscopy: Pale fluffy cytoplasm, prominent membranes ("plant cell"), perinuclear haloes ("fried-egg"), raisinoid nuclei.

Key finding: Plant-cell appearance + Hale colloidal iron diffuse cytoplasmic positivity. CK7+, CD117+, CA-IX−.

Exam yield: ★★★ *HIGH*

Oncocytoma

Definition: Benign (3–7% of renal tumours). Intercalated cell origin.

Gross: Mahogany-brown cut surface, central stellate scar.

Microscopy: Uniform round oncocytes (granular eosinophilic cytoplasm, mitochondria-packed), nests/tubules/sheets. No papillary, no necrosis, no vascular invasion.

Key finding: CK7− (vs chromophobe CK7+) — the single most useful discriminating marker. CD117+, vimentin−.

Exam yield: ★★★ HIGH

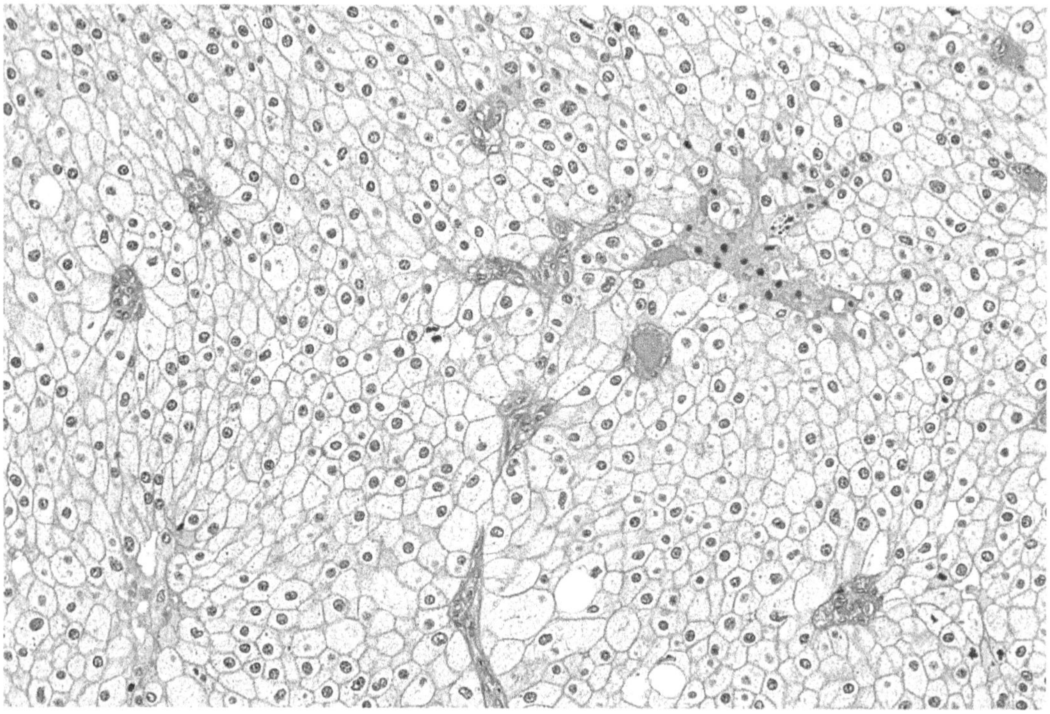

Figure 23.8: Chromophobe renal cell carcinoma. Sheets of large polygonal cells with pale flocculent cytoplasm and prominent cell membranes (plant-cell appearance), perinuclear haloes, and wrinkled (raisinoid) nuclei. H&E, intermediate magnification. (Source: Nephron, Wikimedia Commons, CC BY-SA 3.0.)

The Pathologist's Eye: Oncocytoma vs Chromophobe RCC

At the microscope, both tumours show eosinophilic cells. Chromophobe RCC typically has more prominent cell membranes (plant-cell appearance), perinuclear haloes, irregular nuclear contours with raisinoid wrinkling, and binucleation. Oncocytoma has round, regular nuclei with smooth contours, uniform cytoplasmic granularity, and no perinuclear halo. On needle biopsy, if the differential remains unresolved, the term "oncocytic renal neoplasm" may be used with a recommendation for excision. Birt-Hogg-Dubé syndrome should be considered when hybrid oncocytic/chromophobe tumours are encountered.

Marker	Clear Cell RCC	Papillary RCC	Chromophobe RCC	Oncocytoma
CK7	Negative	Positive/focal	Positive (diffuse)	Negative (or focal)
CD10	Positive	Positive (luminal)	Negative	Negative
CA-IX	Positive (membranous)	Negative/focal	Negative	Negative
CD117	Negative	Negative	Positive	Positive

Vimentin	Positive	Positive	Negative	Negative
AMACR	Negative	Positive	Negative	Negative
PAX8	Positive	Positive	Positive	Positive
CK20	Negative	Negative	Negative	Negative

MiT Family Translocation Renal Cell Carcinomas

Definition: TFE3/TFEB fusions (MiTF family). Young patients. Papillary/variable architecture.

Key finding: CK/EMA weak/negative but PAX8+, HMB45+, Melan-A+, cathepsin K+. Nuclear TFE3/TFEB IHC; FISH gold standard.

Exam yield: ★★ MODERATE

Fumarate Hydratase-Deficient and SDH-Deficient RCC

FH-Deficient RCC: WHO 5th Ed molecularly defined entity. HLRCC syndrome. Aggressive; requires early IHC detection.

Pathogenesis: FH loss → Fumarate accumulation → Prolyl hydroxylase inhibition → HIF stabilisation (pseudohypoxia)

Key finding: Eosinophilic inclusion-like nucleoli with perinucleolar halo. IHC: FH loss + 2SC gain.

SDH-Deficient RCC: SDH subunit loss (SDHB most common). Paraganglioma-pheo syndromes. Flocculent pale inclusions. SDHB IHC loss.

Exam yield: ★★★ HIGH

Collecting Duct Carcinoma and Renal Medullary Carcinoma

Collecting Duct Ca: Rare, aggressive. Irregular angulated tubules in desmoplastic stroma, high grade, medullary.

Renal Medullary Ca: Highly aggressive; young patients with sickle cell trait.

Key finding: INI1/SMARCB1 loss on IHC in sickle cell trait patient. Median survival <12 months.

Exam yield: ★★★ HIGH — Sickle trait + INI1 loss = renal medullary Ca.

Wilms Tumour (Nephroblastoma)

Definition: Most common childhood renal malignancy (peak 2–5y). Embryonal tumour from nephrogenic blastema.

Syndromes: WAGR (WT1 del 11p13), Denys-Drash (WT1 point mutation, DMS), Beckwith-Wiedemann (11p15.5, organomegaly).

Pathogenesis: WT1/WT2 alteration → Failed blastema differentiation → Nephrogenic rests (precursor) → Triphasic tumour

Key finding: Triphasic — blastemal (small round blue cells) + epithelial (abortive tubules/glomeruloid) + stromal (fibrous/myxoid/heterologous).

IHC/Prognosis: WT1+ (epithelial/blastemal), CK+ (epithelial), desmin+ (blastema). Favourable (>85% cure) vs unfavourable (diffuse anaplasia).

Exam yield: ★★★ HIGH

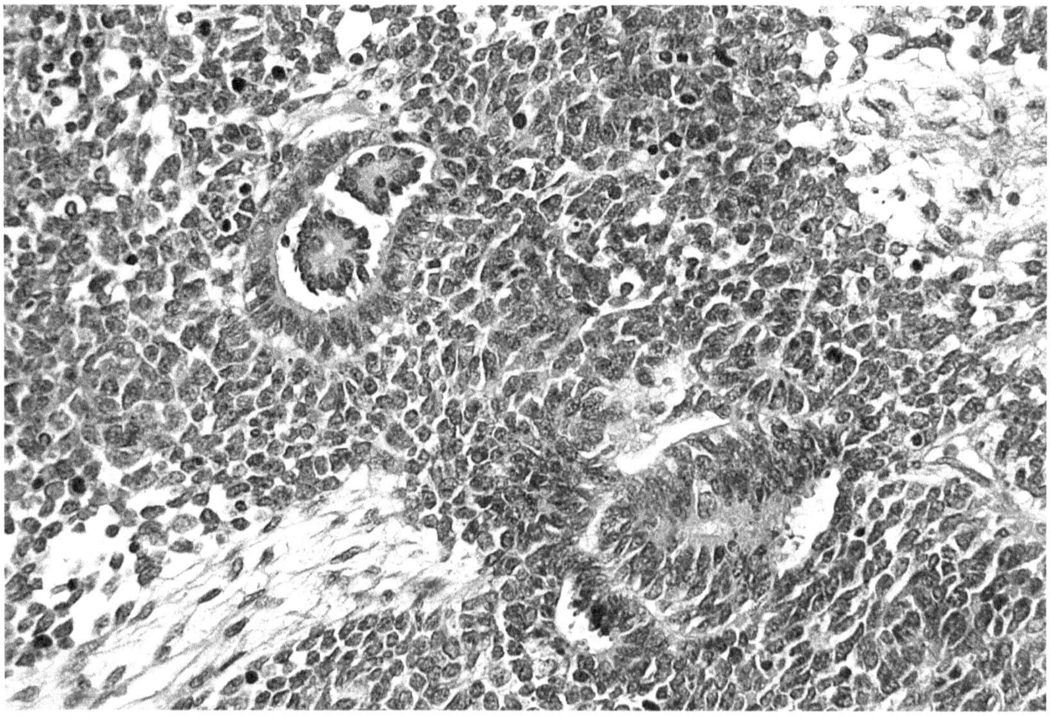

Figure 23.9: Wilms tumour (nephroblastoma). High-magnification view showing the classical triphasic pattern: undifferentiated blastemal cells (small round blue cells), abortive epithelial tubules, and primitive mesenchymal stroma. H&E. (Source: Nephron, Wikimedia Commons, CC BY-SA 3.0.)

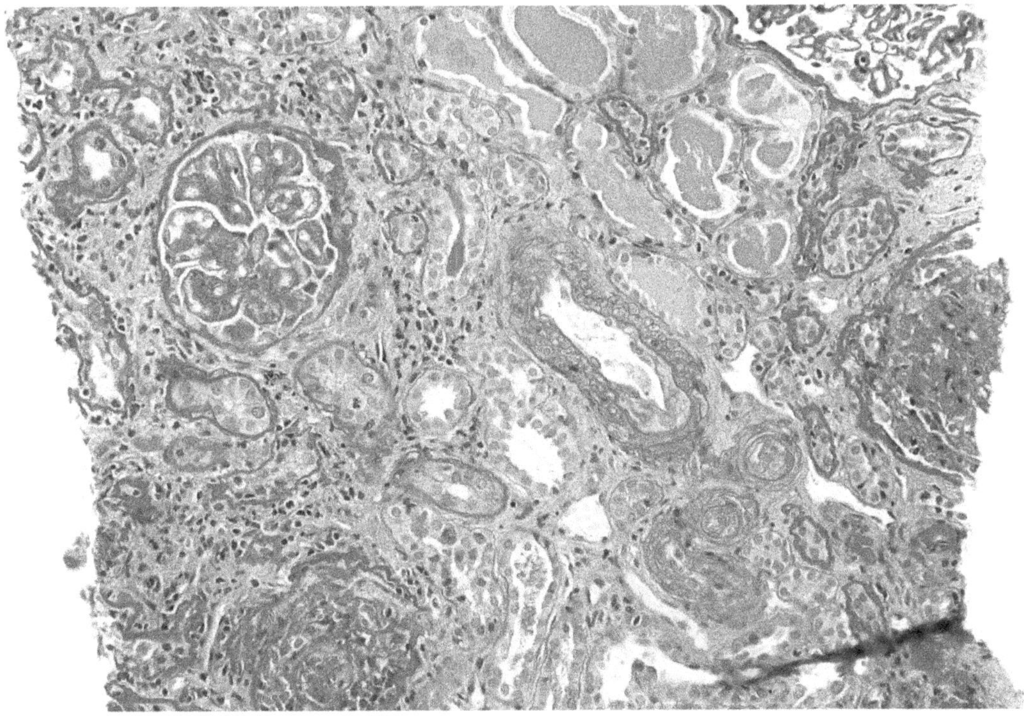

Figure 23.10: Thrombotic microangiopathy. Renal cortex (PAS) showing the spectrum of TMA changes: an ischaemic wrinkled glomerulus (upper left) with retracted capillary tuft; arterioles with luminal occlusion by fibrinoid material and fragmented red cells; and ischaemic tubular injury. These features correspond to HUS/TTP/atypical HUS, where endothelial injury produces microthrombi in arterioles and glomerular capillaries. (Source: Nephron, Wikimedia Commons, CC BY-SA 3.0.)

Angiomyolipoma

Definition: Benign PEComa: thick-walled vessels + smooth muscle + fat. 80% sporadic; 20% TSC (bilateral).

Key finding: HMB45+, Melan-A+, SMA+. Epithelioid variant = only subtype with malignant potential.

Exam yield: ★★ MODERATE

Quick Recall: Renal Neoplasms

Clear cell RCC: Most common RCC; VHL loss; yellow mass; clear cells + arborising vasculature; CA-IX+; grade by WHO/ISUP.

Papillary RCC: Second most common; papillary/tubular; AMACR+; foamy macrophages; trisomy 7, 17.

Chromophobe RCC: Plant-cell appearance; CK7+, CD117+; Hale colloidal iron diffusely positive; good prognosis.

Oncocytoma: Benign; mahogany brown + central scar; CK7 negative; CD117+.

MiT translocation RCC: Young patients; TFE3/TFEB; melanocytic markers positive; epithelial markers weak/negative.

Wilms tumour: 2-5 years; triphasic (blastema + epithelial + stroma); WT1+; WAGR, DDS, BWS syndromes.

Renal medullary carcinoma: Sickle cell trait; INI1/SMARCB1 loss; aggressive.

Staging of Renal Cell Carcinoma

TNM Stage	Description	Approximate 5-Year Survival
pT1a	Tumour ≤4 cm, limited to kidney	95%
pT1b	Tumour >4 cm but ≤7 cm, limited to kidney	90%
pT2a	Tumour >7 cm but ≤10 cm, limited to kidney	80%
pT2b	Tumour >10 cm, limited to kidney	70%
pT3a	Invades perirenal fat, renal sinus fat, or renal vein	60%
pT3b	Extends into IVC below diaphragm	40-50%
pT3c	Extends into IVC above diaphragm or invades IVC wall	30-40%
pT4	Invades beyond Gerota fascia or adrenal gland (contiguous)	10-20%

Renal Transplant Pathology

Definition: Gold standard for diagnosing rejection, drug toxicity, recurrent disease, BK nephropathy.

AMR: AMR: DSA + C4d in peritubular capillaries (IF/IHC) + microvascular inflammation (PTC/glomerulitis).

TCMR: TCMR: Tubulitis (t-score) + interstitial inflammation (i-score). Vascular: intimal arteritis (v-score).

Key finding: C4d in peritubular capillaries (AMR); tubulitis (TCMR). Chronic AMR → transplant glomerulopathy (GBM duplication).

Other: CNI toxicity (arteriolar hyalinosis, isometric vacuolisation, striped fibrosis). BK nephropathy (ground-glass nuclei, SV40+).

Exam yield: ★★★ HIGH

Quick Recall: Renal Transplant Pathology

AMR: DSA + C4d in peritubular capillaries + microvascular inflammation (peritubular capillaritis/glomerulitis).

TCMR: Tubulitis + interstitial inflammation; vascular rejection = intimal arteritis.

CNI toxicity: Arteriolar hyalinosis (nodular, unlike HTN hyaline), isometric vacuolisation, striped fibrosis.

BK nephropathy: Ground-glass nuclei; SV40 IHC positive; mimics rejection on biopsy.

Exam Pitfall: BK Nephropathy vs Acute Rejection

BK polyomavirus nephropathy and acute T-cell mediated rejection share interstitial inflammation and tubulitis, and distinguishing them is clinically critical because their treatments are opposite: rejection requires increased immunosuppression, while BK nephropathy requires reduced immunosuppression. SV40 immunohistochemistry must be performed on every transplant biopsy showing tubulitis to exclude BK nephropathy before diagnosing rejection.

Recent Advances

Banff 2019 Kidney Meeting Report — refined T-cell-mediated and antibody-mediated rejection criteria. The Banff 2019 Kidney Meeting Report consolidated more than two decades of Banff classification updates and clarified criteria for chronic active T-cell-mediated rejection, borderline rejection, and antibody-mediated rejection in renal allografts (Loupy et al. American Journal of Transplantation 2020; 20: 2318–2331; PMID 32463180). Chronic active T-cell-mediated rejection is now defined by interstitial fibrosis with tubulitis (IFTA + i-IFTA + t-IFTA) and is distinguished from acute T-cell-mediated rejection by the chronic background. Borderline lesions are addressed by re-examining the threshold for interstitial inflammation (i0 versus i1) in light of evidence that even low-grade infiltrates can progress to overt rejection. Antibody-mediated rejection criteria were extended to incorporate biopsies showing microvascular inflammation (peritubular capillaritis plus glomerulitis) in the absence of C4d staining or detectable donor-specific antibodies, with a supportive role for molecular diagnostics (Banff Human Organ Transplant gene panel and Molecular Microscope). Reporting implication: native and allograft renal biopsies are reported with full Banff lesion scores (i, t, v, g, ptc, c4d, ah, ci, ct, cv, cg, mm) and an integrated diagnostic statement that specifies category (1 normal, 2 antibody-mediated, 3 borderline, 4 T-cell-mediated, 5 IFTA, 6 other), permitting standardised international comparison.

The WHO 5th Edition (2022) classification of renal tumours has introduced several molecularly defined entities that reshape diagnostic practice. FH-deficient RCC, SDH-deficient RCC, ELOC-mutated RCC, eosinophilic solid and cystic (ESC) RCC, and ALK-rearranged RCC are now recognised as distinct categories. These additions emphasise the importance of IHC screening (FH, SDHB, ALK) in eosinophilic renal tumours that do not fit classic categories. The concept of "oncocytic renal neoplasm of low malignant potential, NOS" provides a diagnostic safety net for tumours with borderline oncocytoma/chromophobe features.

Targeted therapies for RCC have expanded considerably. Combination immunotherapy (nivolumab plus ipilimumab) and tyrosine kinase inhibitor-immunotherapy combinations (cabozantinib-nivolumab, lenvatinib-pembrolizumab) are now first-line for advanced clear cell RCC. Belzutifan, a HIF-2α inhibitor, has been approved for VHL-associated RCC, representing a direct translation of the VHL-HIF molecular pathway into therapy. Adjuvant pembrolizumab after nephrectomy for high-risk RCC has shown disease-free survival benefit (KEYNOTE-564 trial).

In tubulointerstitial disease, the recognition of IgG4-related kidney disease as a distinct clinicopathological entity has improved diagnostic accuracy and therapeutic responses to corticosteroids and rituximab. Biomarkers such as KIM-1 (kidney injury molecule-1) and NGAL (neutrophil gelatinase-associated lipocalin) are being validated for early detection of ATI, potentially replacing serum creatinine as more sensitive and specific indicators of tubular injury. Liquid biopsy approaches using circulating tumour DNA (ctDNA) and cell-free DNA methylation patterns are emerging for non-invasive monitoring of RCC recurrence and minimal residual disease (see Chapter 37, Chapter 41).

Approach to the Histopathology Slide

Renal mass/nephrectomy specimen: Systematic approach: (1) Identify the architecture: solid nests, papillary, tubular, cystic, or mixed. (2) Assess the cytoplasm: clear, eosinophilic/granular, or basophilic. (3) Evaluate the vasculature: arborising sinusoidal network (clear cell RCC) or inconspicuous. (4) Look for specific features: psammoma bodies (papillary RCC), perinuclear haloes (chromophobe), central scar (oncocytoma), triphasic pattern (Wilms). (5) Check the grade: nucleolar prominence (WHO/ISUP). (6) Assess for sarcomatoid or rhabdoid features (grade 4).

Renal biopsy (non-tumour): Evaluate tubules for simplification, brush border loss, and casts (ATI). Look for interstitial inflammation with eosinophils (drug-induced TIN) versus neutrophils in tubular lumina (pyelonephritis). Check arterioles for hyaline deposits (nephrosclerosis) or onion-skinning (malignant HTN). Look for fibrin/platelet thrombi in glomerular capillaries (TMA). In transplant biopsies, quantify tubulitis (t-score), interstitial inflammation (i-score), and peritubular capillaritis (ptc-score) per Banff criteria.

The Pathologist's Eye: Fat-Containing Renal Mass

When a renal mass contains fat on imaging, the differential diagnosis includes angiomyolipoma (most common), clear cell RCC with osseous metaplasia containing fatty marrow, liposarcoma (extremely rare in kidney), and Wilms tumour with lipomatous stroma. On biopsy, HMB45 positivity in the smooth muscle component confirms AML. Do not mistake an AML for a sarcoma based on the smooth muscle component alone; the key is to identify all three components (vessels, smooth muscle, fat) and confirm with HMB45/Melan-A.

Ultra High-Yield Chapter Summary

Topic	Must Remember
ATI (ATN)	Most common cause of AKI; ischaemia or nephrotoxins; tubular simplification, muddy brown casts; reversible if BM intact
Drug-induced TIN	Antibiotics, NSAIDs, PPIs; immune-mediated; interstitial eosinophils + tubulitis; withdraw offending drug
Analgesic nephropathy	Chronic NSAID combinations; papillary necrosis + chronic TIN; risk of TCC of pelvis
Acute pyelonephritis	E. coli ascending infection; neutrophilic tubulitis and microabscesses; predisposed by reflux, obstruction, DM
Chronic pyelonephritis	Irregular cortical scars + blunted calyces; thyroidisation; reflux or obstruction
ADPKD	PKD1/PKD2; polycystin/cilium; bilateral massive cysts; liver cysts + berry aneurysms; tolvaptan
ARPKD	PKHD1; collecting duct cysts; congenital hepatic fibrosis; neonatal/infantile
Nephronophthisis	Ciliopathy; most common genetic cause of childhood ESRD; corticomedullary cysts
Benign nephrosclerosis	HTN; hyaline arteriolosclerosis; finely granular kidney
Malignant HTN	Onion-skin hyperplastic arteriolosclerosis; fibrinoid necrosis; flea-bitten kidney
TMA (HUS/TTP)	HUS: E. coli O157:H7, fibrin thrombi, children; TTP: ADAMTS13, platelet thrombi; atypical HUS: complement, eculizumab
Clear cell RCC	Most common RCC; VHL loss; HIF-VEGF; yellow mass; arborising vasculature; CA-IX+, CK7-; WHO/ISUP grading
Papillary RCC	Second most common; papillary/tubular; AMACR+, CK7+; foamy macrophages; trisomy 7, 17

Chromophobe RCC	Intercalated cells; plant-cell appearance; CK7+, CD117+; Hale colloidal iron+; good prognosis
Oncocytoma	Benign; mahogany brown + central scar; CK7-; CD117+; HMB45-
MiT translocation RCC	TFE3/TFEB fusions; young patients; melanocytic markers+; CK/EMA weak/negative
FH-deficient RCC	HLRCC; pseudohypoxia; eosinophilic inclusion-like nucleoli; FH loss + 2SC gain on IHC
Renal medullary carcinoma	Sickle cell trait; INI1/SMARCB1 loss; highly aggressive
Wilms tumour	2-5 years; triphasic (blastema + epithelial + stroma); WT1+; WAGR, DDS, BWS; nephrogenic rests
AML	PEComa family; vessels + smooth muscle + fat; HMB45+; TSC association; epithelioid variant is malignant
AMR (transplant)	DSA + C4d + microvascular inflammation (PTC/glomerulitis)
TCMR (transplant)	Tubulitis + interstitial inflammation; intimal arteritis = vascular rejection
BK nephropathy	Ground-glass nuclei; SV40+; mimics rejection; reduce immunosuppression
WHO 5th Ed new entities	FH-deficient, SDH-deficient, ELOC-mutated, ESC, ALK-rearranged RCC; belzutifan for VHL-RCC

Table 23.1: Differential Diagnosis of Cystic Renal Diseases

Disease	Inheritance	Pathology	Clinical	Gene
ADPKD	AD	Bilateral large kidneys; cortical + medullary cysts	Adult onset; HTN, haematuria, renal failure by 60s; liver cysts, berry aneurysms	PKD1 (85%), PKD2
ARPKD	AR	Bilateral enlarged; fusiform collecting duct dilatation	Neonatal/infantile; congenital hepatic fibrosis; Potter sequence if severe	PKHD1
Acquired cystic	None	Multiple cortical cysts in	Dialysis patients (>3 yrs); risk of	N/A

		atrophic kidneys	RCC (papillary type)	
Medullary sponge	Sporadic	Dilated medullary collecting ducts (Swiss cheese)	Recurrent UTIs, nephrolithiasis; benign course	Unknown
Simple cyst	None	Thin-walled, clear fluid, cortical	Incidental; no malignant potential; Bosniak I	N/A

Table 23.2: WHO 5th Edition (2022) Renal Tumour Classification -- Key Changes

Change	Old (WHO 4th)	New (WHO 5th)	Exam Significance
Grading	Fuhrman (4-tier)	ISUP nucleolar (1-4)	Grade 4 = rhabdoid/sarcomatoid; ISUP now universal
New entity: Eosinophilic solid and cystic (ESC) RCC	Not recognised	TSC1/TSC2-mutated; women; indolent	Must distinguish from chromophobe/oncocytoma
TFE3/TFEB-rearranged	Xp11 translocation RCC	MiT family translocation RCC (expanded)	TFE3 IHC; young patients; may mimic clear cell
FH-deficient RCC	Hereditary leiomyomatosis-associated	FH-deficient RCC (stand-alone entity)	FH loss + 2SC positivity; aggressive; young patients
Papillary RCC	Type 1 and Type 2	Papillary RCC (unified); type no longer required	IHC: AMACR+, CK7+; grading predicts behaviour
Clear cell papillary RCT	Tumour, not carcinoma	Clear cell papillary renal cell tumour	Indolent; CK7+, CA-IX (cup-shaped); no 3p loss

In tubulointerstitial nephritis, the key diagnostic thinking is that the interstitium tells the story that the glomerulus misses. Drug-induced AIN shows eosinophils + granulomas in the interstitium with relatively normal glomeruli -- the LM pattern is interstitial, not glomerular.

For renal tumour classification, the diagnostic thinking shift in WHO 5th Edition is: morphology alone is insufficient. Molecular/IHC subtyping (FH, TFE3, SDH) now defines entities that were previously lumped under unclassified RCC.

[CLASSIFICATION ALGORITHM: Fig 23.X -- Tubulointerstitial Nephritis Approach. Flowchart: Acute vs Chronic -> Acute: drug-induced (eosinophils, granulomas) vs infection-related vs autoimmune. Chronic: reflux, analgesic, metabolic (urate, oxalate), heavy metals. Source: Author's original.]

Chapter 24: Male Genital Tract and Lower Urinary Tract Pathology

THE BIG PICTURE

This chapter covers the pathology of the prostate, testis, penis, and scrotal contents. Benign prostatic hyperplasia and prostatic adenocarcinoma are among the most common conditions in surgical pathology, while testicular germ cell tumours represent one of the most curable malignancies in medicine. The Gleason grading system (now ISUP Grade Groups) for prostatic carcinoma, the interpretation of prostatic needle biopsies with IHC, and the WHO 5th Edition classification of testicular tumours are fundamental to postgraduate examinations. Urothelial carcinoma of the urinary bladder — the dominant malignancy of the lower urinary tract — is addressed in this chapter together with urothelial CIS, the WHO 5th Edition classification, AJCC 8th TNM staging, and variant histologies with treatment implications.

High-yield topics in this chapter: Benign prostatic hyperplasia; Prostatic intraepithelial neoplasia (PIN) and intraductal carcinoma; Interpretation of prostatic needle biopsies (benign mimics, ASAP, minimal carcinoma); Prostatic adenocarcinoma (Gleason grading, Grade Groups, IHC, staging); Testicular germ cell tumours (classification, seminoma, non-seminomatous GCTs, serum markers); GCNIS; Testicular biopsy in male infertility; Penile carcinoma and HPV.

The prostate gland generates more surgical pathology specimens than almost any other organ, and the distinction between benign mimics and carcinoma on needle biopsy remains one of the most challenging and consequential calls in diagnostic practice. Testicular tumours, though relatively uncommon, provide a masterclass in embryological differentiation, with each histological subtype recapitulating a specific stage of germ cell development. This chapter covers the spectrum from hyperplasia through intraepithelial neoplasia to high-grade malignancy across the male genital tract.

24.1 Benign Prostatic Hyperplasia

Definition: Nodular hyperplasia of stroma + glands in periurethral (transition) zone. ~50% by age 60, ~90% by 85.

Pathogenesis: Testosterone → 5α-reductase 2 → DHT → AR activation → Paracrine growth factors → Stromal + epithelial proliferation

Gross: Enlarged prostate, well-defined nodules in transition zone compressing urethra.

Microscopy: Glandular: dilated glands with double layer (columnar secretory + basal). Stromal: fibromuscular. Corpora amylacea.

Key finding: Basal cell layer PRESENT (vs carcinoma: ABSENT). p63/HMWCK confirm.

Clinical: LUTS. Treatment: finasteride, tamsulosin, TURP.

Exam yield: ★★★ HIGH

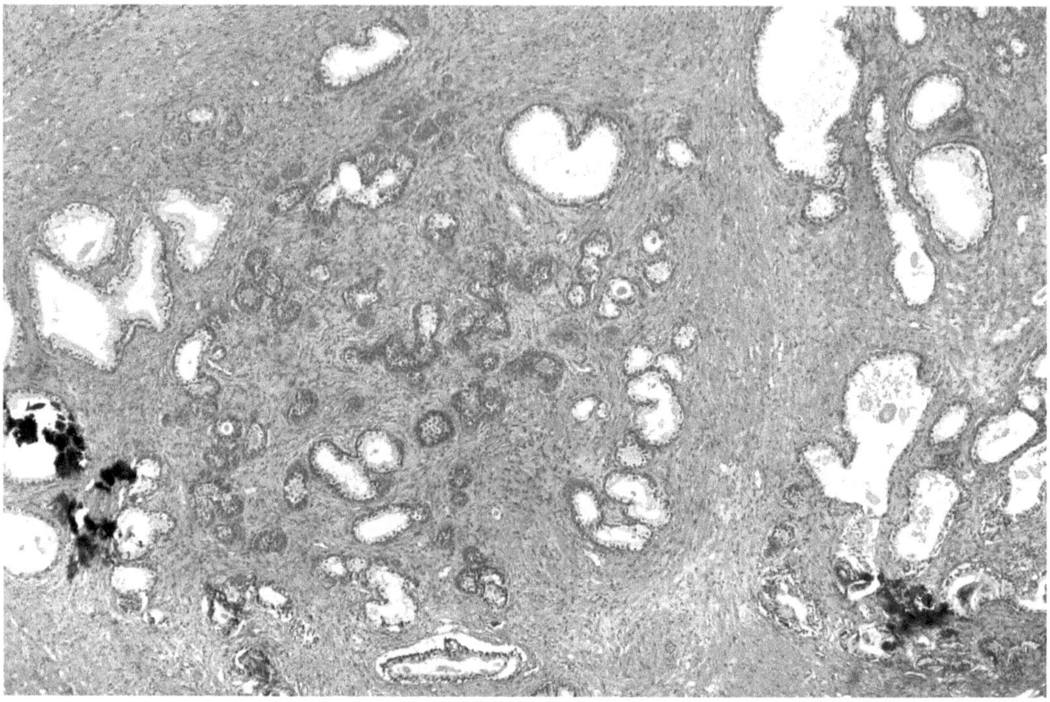

Figure 24.1: Benign prostatic hyperplasia. Nodular proliferation of prostatic glands and stroma with preserved double-layered epithelium (columnar secretory cells overlying a continuous basal cell layer) and corpora amylacea within gland lumina. H&E. (Source: Nephron, Wikimedia Commons, CC BY-SA 3.0.)

24.2 Prostatic Intraepithelial Neoplasia

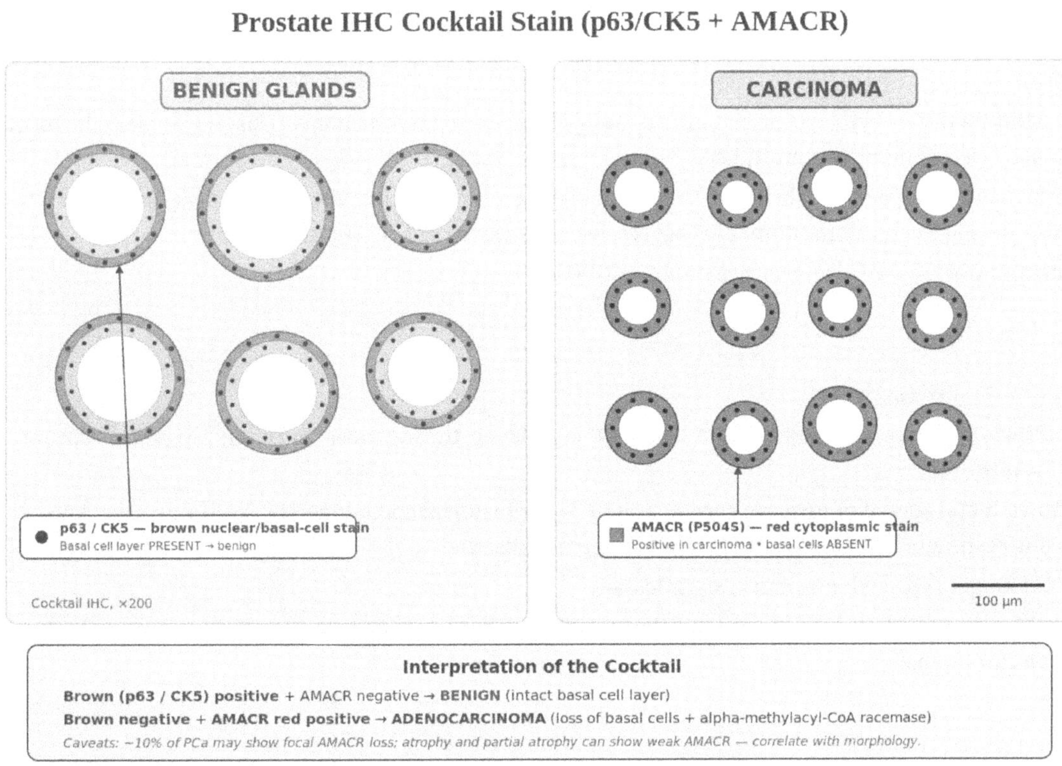

Figure 24.2: Prostate IHC cocktail stain — schematic diagram. Basal cell markers (p63, HMWCK) mark benign glands (brown); AMACR (P504S, red) marks carcinoma; absence of both basal-cell stain and presence of AMACR defines the IHC signature of prostatic adenocarcinoma. (Source: Author's original.)

Definition: Accepted precursor of prostatic adenocarcinoma. Cytologically atypical cells lining pre-existing glands.

Microscopy: Nuclear enlargement, prominent nucleoli, hyperchromasia. Four patterns: tufting (~70%), micropapillary, cribriform, flat.

Key finding: Patchy but present basal cell layer — cardinal feature distinguishing HGPIN from invasive Ca. AMACR often positive.

Management: ~25–30% Ca on repeat biopsy. Re-biopsy 6–12 months if multifocal (>2 cores). LGPIN no longer reported.

Exam yield: ★★★ HIGH

Definition: Intraductal spread of high-grade Ca into pre-existing ducts. Distinct from HGPIN.

Microscopy: Dense cribriform/solid, fills entire lumen, comedonecrosis, marked atypia. Basal layer retained.

Key finding: Dense cribriform filling entire lumen + comedonecrosis + retained basal layer. Almost always with adjacent invasive Ca (Gleason 4/5).

Exam yield: ★★★ HIGH

Exam Pitfall: HGPIN vs Intraductal Carcinoma of Prostate (IDC-P)

Both retain a basal cell layer. Confusing them is a critical error because their clinical implications differ dramatically.

HGPIN: Mild-moderate cytologic atypia; tufting/micropapillary; no comedonecrosis; no dense cribriform; repeat biopsy in 6-12 months if multifocal.

IDC-P: Marked atypia; dense cribriform/solid; comedonecrosis common; virtually always associated with high-grade invasive carcinoma; mandates aggressive rebiopsy or radical treatment.

Key discriminator: IDC-P fills the entire lumen, HGPIN does not.

Quick Recall: PIN and IDC-P

HGPIN: Precursor lesion; cytologic atypia + patchy basal layer; tufting most common; AMACR+; repeat biopsy if multifocal.

IDC-P: Intraductal spread of invasive carcinoma; dense cribriform/comedonecrosis; retains basal layer but fills entire lumen; near-certain marker of high-grade disease.

LGPIN: No longer reported; no clinical significance.

Basal cell layer rule: Present in both HGPIN and IDC-P (differentiating from invasive carcinoma); absent in invasive carcinoma.

24.3 Prostatic Adenocarcinoma

Definition: Most common male malignancy. Peripheral zone (70%). TMPRSS2-ERG fusions (~50%), PTEN loss, TP53 (late).

Pathogenesis: AR activation → Proliferation → TMPRSS2-ERG fusion → PTEN loss → PI3K/AKT → High-grade → TP53/RB1 loss → Castration resistance

Microscopy: Small infiltrative glands, angulated lumina, amphophilic cytoplasm, prominent nucleoli.

Key finding: Loss of basal cells (p63−/HMWCK−) + AMACR+. Perineural invasion = pathognomonic of malignancy.

Ancillary: Intraluminal blue mucin, crystalloids, collagenous micronodules, glomeruloid projections.

Grading: GG1 (3+3): discrete glands. GG2 (3+4): minor fused. GG3 (4+3): predominant fused. GG4 (8): pattern 4 dominant. GG5 (9–10): pattern 5.

Exam yield: ★★★ HIGH

24.3.1 Histomorphology and Diagnostic Features

Microscopically, acinar adenocarcinoma consists of small, infiltrative glands with a **single cell layer** (loss of the basal cell layer is the histological hallmark). Glands are angulated, have sharp luminal contours, and are lined by cells with enlarged nuclei containing prominent nucleoli and amphophilic cytoplasm. Diagnostic clues on biopsy include intraluminal blue-tinged mucin (mucinous secretions), pink amorphous crystalloids, collagenous micronodules (mucinous fibroplasia), glomeruloid intraluminal projections, and perineural invasion. Perineural invasion is pathognomonic of malignancy in prostate biopsies (benign glands do not invade nerves) and predicts extraprostatic extension.

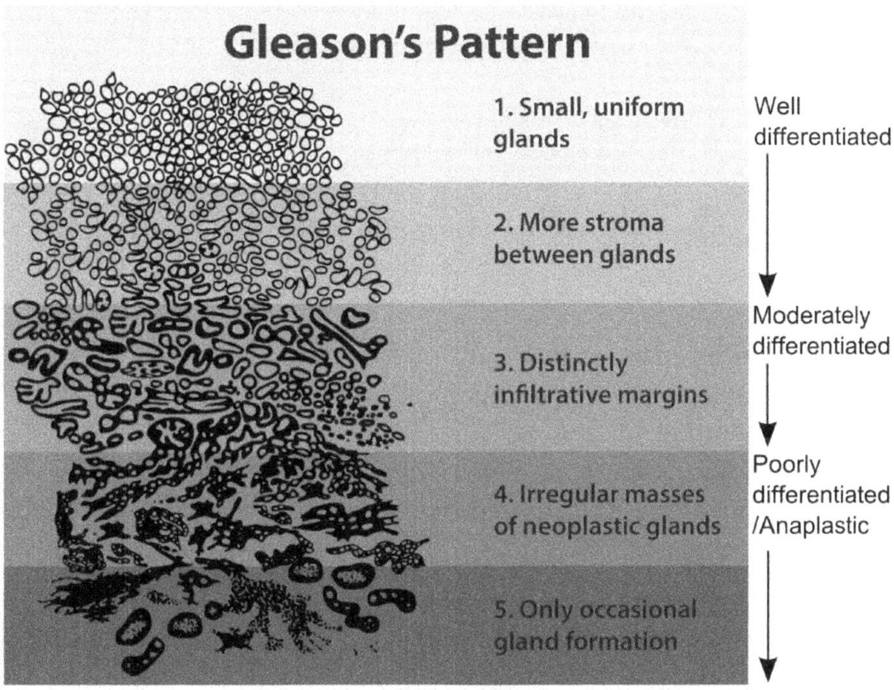

Figure 24.3: Gleason's five architectural patterns of prostatic adenocarcinoma (schematic). Pattern 1: small uniform glands, well differentiated. Pattern 2: more stroma between glands. Pattern 3: distinctly infiltrative margins, moderately differentiated. Pattern 4: irregular masses of neoplastic glands, poorly differentiated. Pattern 5: only occasional gland formation, anaplastic. After Donald Gleason (1966). (Source: Gleasonscore.jpg, Wikimedia Commons, Public Domain — NIH/SEER.)

24.3.2 Gleason Grading and ISUP Grade Groups

Table 24.1: WHO 5th Edition (2022): Key Updates in Prostate Tumour Classification

Entity/Update	WHO 5th Edition Recommendation
ISUP Grade Groups	GG1 (Gleason 3+3=6), GG2 (3+4=7), GG3 (4+3=7), GG4 (4+4/3+5/5+3=8), GG5 (4+5/5+4/5+5=9-10). ISUP GG is standard; Gleason score reported alongside.
Intraductal carcinoma (IDC-P)	Distinct entity; NOT graded as Gleason pattern. Report separately. Often

	associated with BRCA2, high-grade/volume disease.
Cribriform pattern	Cribriform architecture = Gleason pattern 4 (minimum ISUP GG2). No longer acceptable as pattern 3.
Acinar adenocarcinoma variants	Atrophic, pseudohyperplastic, microcystic, foamy gland patterns retained; all grade as pattern 3 if architecture qualifies.
Neuroendocrine tumours	Treatment-emergent neuroendocrine carcinoma (t-NEPC) recognised; distinct from de novo small cell carcinoma.
Grading after therapy	Post-treatment specimens: treatment effect grading system replaces Gleason.

The Gleason grading system, modified at the 2014 and 2019 ISUP consensus conferences, grades prostatic carcinoma based on architectural pattern at low magnification. Pattern 3 consists of well-formed, separate, non-fused glands infiltrating the stroma. Pattern 4 encompasses poorly formed glands, fused glands, cribriform glands, and glomeruloid structures. Pattern 5 represents loss of glandular differentiation: single cells, cords, solid sheets, and comedonecrosis. Patterns 1 and 2 are rarely diagnosed and should not be assigned on needle biopsy.

The Gleason score is the sum of the primary (most prevalent) and secondary (second most prevalent) patterns. When three patterns are present on biopsy, the primary pattern plus the highest-grade pattern are reported (e.g., 3+5=8, not 3+4=7). The ISUP Grade Group system translates Gleason scores into a more intuitive 1-to-5 framework.

ISUP Grade Group	Gleason Score	Pattern Description	Clinical Significance
1	3+3 = 6	Only well-formed discrete glands	Indolent; active surveillance candidate
2	3+4 = 7	Predominantly well-formed + minor poorly formed/fused/cribriform	Intermediate favourable
3	4+3 = 7	Predominantly poorly formed/fused/cribriform + minor well-formed	Intermediate unfavourable
4	4+4=8; 3+5=8; 5+3=8	Predominantly pattern 4 or mixture with pattern 5	High risk
5	4+5=9; 5+4=9;	Pattern 5 predominant or high-grade	Very high risk; poor

	5+5=10	combinations	prognosis

Viva hook: "Why was the Grade Group system introduced alongside the Gleason score?" The traditional Gleason score of 6 was misleading to patients, as it implied a mid-range cancer on a 2-to-10 scale. Grade Group 1 (Gleason 6) correctly conveys this is the lowest grade of clinically detected cancer. Grade Groups 2 (3+4) and 3 (4+3) have significantly different prognoses despite both summing to Gleason 7, justifying their separation.

24.3.3 Immunohistochemistry in Prostatic Biopsy

The diagnostic IHC panel for problematic prostate biopsies uses basal cell markers (p63, CK903) and AMACR (P504S); in carcinoma, basal markers are absent and AMACR is positive (see Quick Recall box and Figure 24.3).

For metastatic settings, NKX3.1 (nuclear, highly sensitive and specific for prostatic origin), PSA, and PSAP confirm prostatic origin. NKX3.1 retains expression even in poorly differentiated and treatment-resistant tumours where PSA may be lost.

24.3.4 Staging of Prostatic Carcinoma

TNM Stage	Description	Approximate 10-Year Survival
pT2	Organ-confined (no extraprostatic extension)	95%
pT3a	Extraprostatic extension (EPE)	75-80%
pT3b	Seminal vesicle invasion	50-60%
pT4	Invasion of bladder neck, external sphincter, rectum, levator, or pelvic wall	30-40%
N1	Regional lymph node metastasis	Variable; systemic therapy
M1a	Non-regional lymph nodes	M1 overall: 30% 5-year
M1b	Bone metastases (most common distant site)	Predominantly osteoblastic
M1c	Other distant sites	

Key prognostic parameters in the pathology report include: Gleason score/Grade Group, tumour volume and percentage of cores involved, extraprostatic extension (EPE), seminal vesicle invasion (SVI), surgical margin status (positive margins predict biochemical recurrence), lymphovascular invasion, and perineural invasion. The distinction from Ch 7 is that Gleason grading is architecture-based and specifically relevant to prostate; no other organ system uses this grading paradigm.

24.4 Interpretation of Prostatic Needle Biopsies

The interpretation of prostatic needle biopsies is a cornerstone of surgical pathology practice and a frequently examined topic (W-2025 SAQ). The diagnostic challenge centres on distinguishing small foci of adenocarcinoma from benign mimics, recognising precursor lesions (HGPIN, IDC-P), and appropriately reporting equivocal findings.

24.4.1 Benign Mimics of Prostatic Carcinoma

Several benign conditions produce small glandular proliferations on needle biopsy that can be mistaken for adenocarcinoma. Recognising these mimics is essential to avoid overdiagnosis.

Benign Mimic	Key Distinguishing Features	Basal Layer	AMACR
Atrophy (simple and proliferative)	Small crowded glands with scant cytoplasm; lobular arrangement preserved; no nuclear atypia or prominent nucleoli	Present (may be attenuated)	Negative (rarely weak focal)
Adenosis (atypical adenomatous hyperplasia)	Small crowded glands in a lobular configuration; merges with surrounding benign glands; minimal atypia	Patchy (may require IHC)	May be weakly positive
Basal cell hyperplasia	Nests of small basaloid cells; may have nucleoli; solid or cribriform	Prominent (p63/CK903 strongly positive)	Usually negative
Seminal vesicle/ejaculatory duct epithelium	Bizarre degenerative nuclear atypia; golden-brown lipofuscin pigment; no mitoses	Present	Negative
Post-atrophic hyperplasia	Small glands with scant cytoplasm in a lobular pattern; adjacent to atrophic glands	Present	Negative
Radiation atypia	Cytoplasmic vacuolisation; nuclear enlargement without nucleolar	Present	Variable (not reliable post-

	prominence; stromal fibrosis		treatment)
Nephrogenic adenoma (urethra/bladder neck)	Small tubules lined by hobnail cells; can occur in prostatic urethra	PAX8 positive; p63 negative	Often positive (misleading)

The distinction between adenosis (AAH) and well-differentiated carcinoma rests on three features: adenosis maintains a lobular architecture with glands merging imperceptibly into surrounding benign glands, retains at least a patchy basal cell layer on IHC, and lacks significant cytological atypia. Carcinoma infiltrates as isolated glands between benign glands, completely lacks the basal layer, and shows nuclear enlargement with prominent nucleoli.

24.4.2 Atypical Small Acinar Proliferation (ASAP)

Definition: Small atypical focus insufficient for Ca diagnosis (too few glands, equivocal IHC, borderline).

Key finding: ~40% Ca on repeat biopsy (stronger indication than HGPIN). Re-biopsy 3–6 months, MRI-guided.

Exam yield: ★★★ HIGH

24.4.3 Minimal Adenocarcinoma on Biopsy

For minimal adenocarcinoma (single/few glands), diagnosis requires integration of architecture, cytology, ancillary features (intraluminal mucin, crystalloids, perineural invasion), and confirmatory IHC (absent basal cells, positive AMACR). Report: cores involved, percentage, Gleason/Grade Group, and ancillary findings.

24.4.4 Reporting Requirements for Prostatic Needle Biopsy

A complete prostatic biopsy report should include: number of cores submitted and number positive for carcinoma; maximum percentage and linear extent (mm) of carcinoma in each positive core; Gleason score and ISUP Grade Group; presence of perineural invasion; presence of extraprostatic tissue involvement; presence of HGPIN, IDC-P, or ASAP; and any benign findings (BPH, inflammation, atrophy). The percentage of pattern 4 should be recorded for Grade Group 2 tumours, as this informs active surveillance eligibility.

The Pathologist's Eye: Three Traps in Prostate Biopsy Reporting

1. Atrophy masquerading as carcinoma: Proliferative atrophy with small crowded glands can alarm the unwary. Look for the lobular pattern, scant cytoplasm (not amphophilic), and absence of nucleolar prominence. If uncertain, p63 and AMACR resolve most cases.

2. Seminal vesicle epithelium mistaken for high-grade carcinoma: The bizarre nuclear atypia of seminal vesicle epithelium is degenerative (lipofuscin-laden), not neoplastic. It lacks mitotic activity and has golden-brown pigment. PAX8 positivity and PSA negativity confirm seminal vesicle origin.

3. Overcalling AMACR in benign glands: AMACR can be weakly positive in adenosis, partial atrophy, and nephrogenic adenoma. Never diagnose carcinoma on AMACR positivity alone; always require concordant absence of basal markers and supporting morphological features.

Quick Recall: Prostatic Biopsy Interpretation

Basal cell markers (p63, HMWCK): Present in benign glands, HGPIN, IDC-P, BPH; absent in invasive carcinoma.

AMACR: Positive in ~80% of carcinomas; also positive in HGPIN, some adenosis, nephrogenic adenoma. Never diagnostic alone.

ASAP: Suspicious but not diagnostic; ~40% carcinoma on repeat biopsy; re-biopsy in 3-6 months.

Minimal carcinoma: Even one gland sufficient for diagnosis if morphological + IHC criteria met.

Benign mimics checklist: Atrophy, adenosis, basal cell hyperplasia, seminal vesicle, radiation effect.

Report must include: Cores +ve/total, %, Gleason/Grade Group, perineural invasion, EPE, HGPIN/IDC-P/ASAP.

Fig 24.2 — Approach to Prostate Needle Biopsy

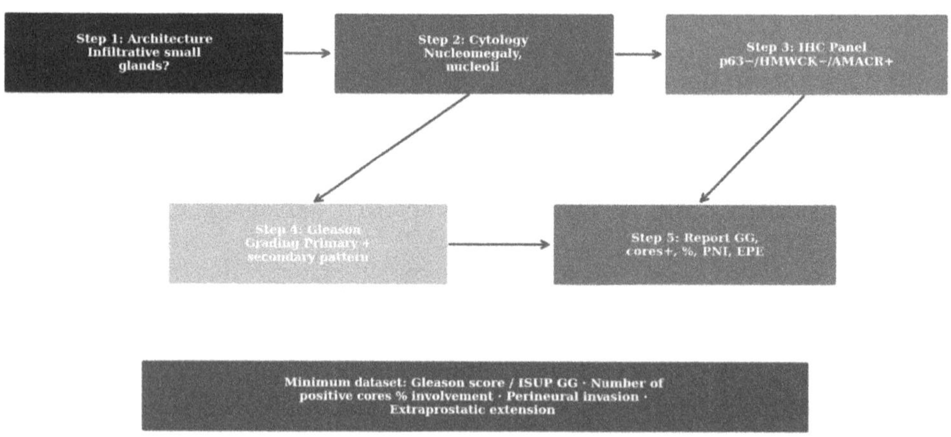

Figure 24.4: Approach to prostate needle biopsy. Five-step diagnostic workflow: architecture, cytology, IHC panel (p63-/HMWCK-/AMACR+), Gleason grading, reporting minimum dataset. (Source: Author's original.)

Integration: Prostatic biopsy interpretation connects to IHC principles (see Chapter 36), molecular pathology (TMPRSS2-ERG fusion detection, see Chapter 37), and neoplasia grading systems (see Chapter

7). The concept of loss of the basal cell layer as evidence of invasion parallels breast pathology (myoepithelial cell loss in invasive vs in-situ carcinoma, see Chapter 26).*

24.5 Diseases of the Testis

24.5.1 Cryptorchidism

Definition: Undescended testis; ~3% full-term neonates. Most descend by 3 months.

Pathogenesis: Elevated temperature → Germ cell loss + tubular atrophy → 4–8× GCT risk (even post-orchiopexy). GCNIS in 2–5%.

Exam yield: ★★ MODERATE

24.5.2 Testicular Germ Cell Tumours

Testicular germ cell tumours (GCTs) account for approximately 95% of all testicular neoplasms. They occur predominantly in young men (15 to 40 years) and are among the most curable solid malignancies, with overall cure rates exceeding 95% due to their exceptional sensitivity to cisplatin-based chemotherapy. Risk factors include cryptorchidism, prior GCT, family history, and disorders of sex development (particularly those with Y-chromosome material).

WHO 5th Edition Classification (2022): Testicular Germ Cell Tumours

GCNIS-derived (postpubertal) tumours: Seminoma; Embryonal carcinoma; Yolk sac tumour (postpubertal type); Choriocarcinoma; Teratoma (postpubertal type); Mixed germ cell tumour.

Non-GCNIS-derived tumours: Spermatocytic tumour (older men); Prepubertal-type teratoma; Prepubertal-type yolk sac tumour.

Definition: Precursor of all postpubertal GCTs. Atypical germ cells replacing spermatogonia along BM.

Microscopy/IHC: Clear cytoplasm, enlarged nuclei, prominent nucleoli. OCT3/4+, PLAP+, D2-40+, CD117+. Isochromosome 12p.

Significance: In ~90% adjacent to tumour; ~5% contralateral testis.

Exam yield: ★★★ HIGH

Primordial germ cell → GCNIS (gain of 12p, isochromosome 12p) → Seminoma or Non-seminomatous GCT

Definition: Most common GCT (~50%). Peak 4th decade.

Gross: Homogeneous, lobulated, cream-white to tan mass.

Microscopy: Large uniform polygonal cells, clear cytoplasm (glycogen), distinct membranes, central round nuclei.

Key finding: Clear cells + fibrous stroma with lymphocytes (± granulomas). OCT3/4+, CD117+, SALL4+; CD30−, AFP−.

Markers: AFP always normal (elevated = not pure seminoma). hCG mildly ↑ in 10–15%. LDH ↑.

Exam yield: ★★★ HIGH

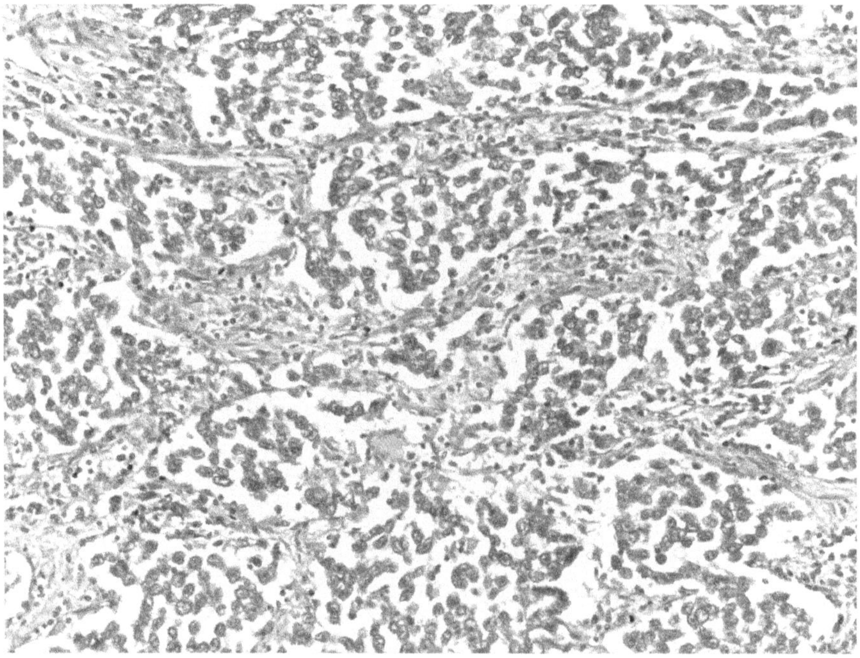

Figure 24.5: Seminoma. Sheets of large, uniform, polygonal cells with abundant clear cytoplasm (glycogen-rich), distinct cell membranes, central round nuclei with prominent nucleoli, and characteristic fibrous septa infiltrated by lymphocytes. H&E, 20×. (Source: Calicut Medical College, Wikimedia Commons, CC BY-SA 4.0.)

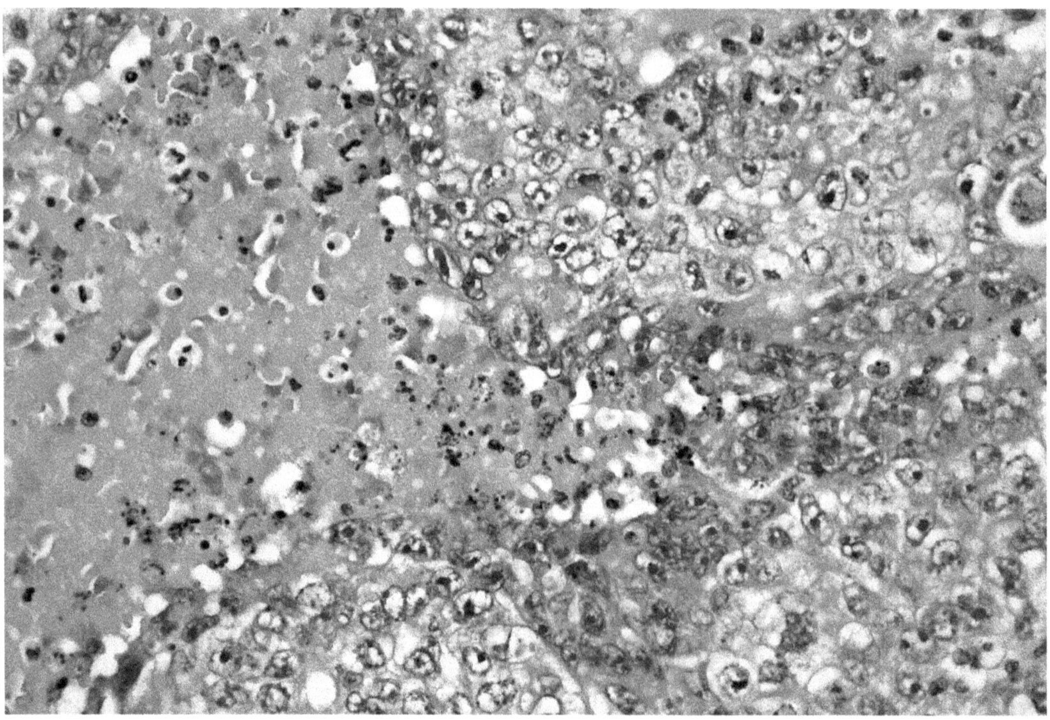

Figure 24.6: Embryonal carcinoma (non-seminomatous germ cell tumour). Pleomorphic cells with indistinct cell borders, large nuclei with prominent nucleoli, and areas of necrosis (left). CD30 and OCT3/4 positive; cytokeratin positive. (Source: Nephron, Wikimedia Commons, CC BY-SA 3.0.)

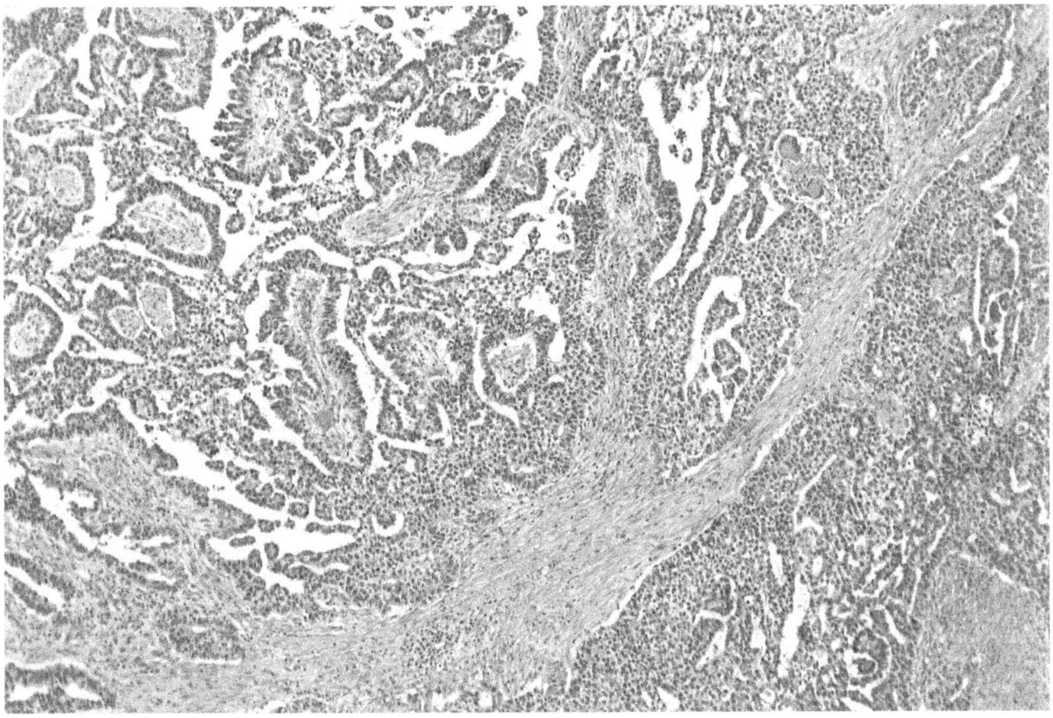

Figure 24.6B: Yolk sac tumour (testis, H&E, low-to-intermediate magnification). Reticular and microcystic architecture composed of loose, anastomosing chords and cords of primitive epithelial tumour cells with vacuolated cytoplasm forming a labyrinthine pattern. Slender fibrovascular septa traverse the tumour. The pattern is characteristic of postpubertal yolk sac tumour; Schiller-Duval bodies (when present, not seen in this field) consist of a central capillary surrounded by a glomeruloid mantle of tumour cells projecting into a cystic space. AFP is markedly elevated in serum and tumour cytoplasm and hyaline globules; Glypican-3 and SALL4 are positive; OCT3/4 is negative. (Source: Nephron, Wikimedia Commons, CC BY-SA 3.0.)

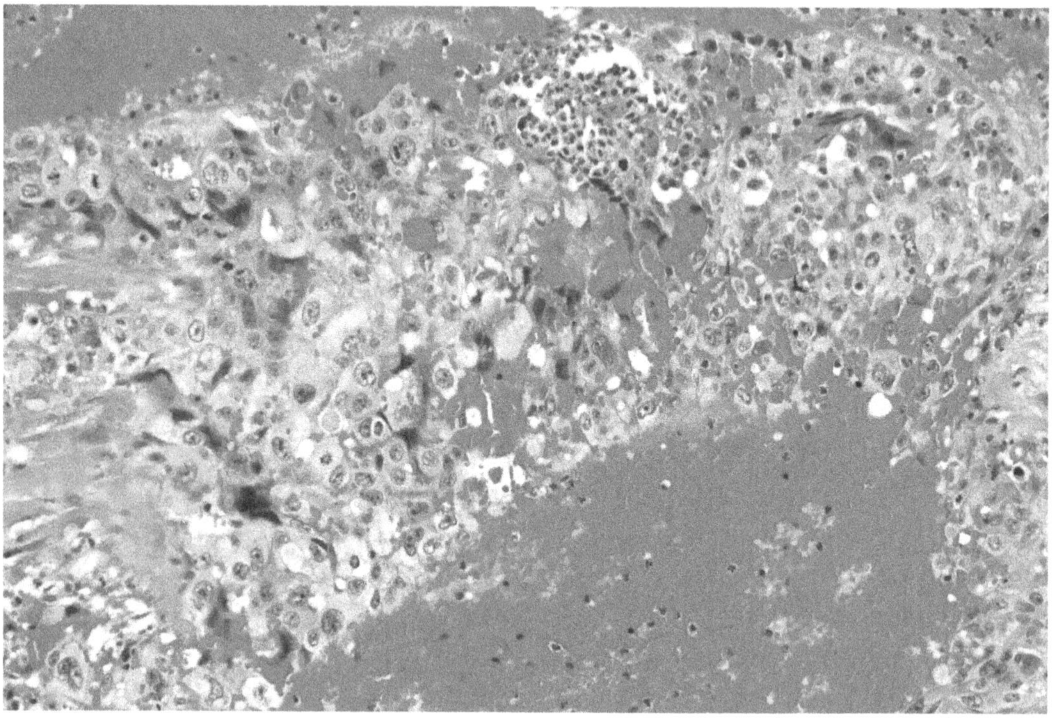

Figure 24.6C: Choriocarcinoma (testis, H&E, high magnification). Biphasic neoplasm composed of two trophoblastic populations against a background of extensive haemorrhage: mononucleated cytotrophoblasts (smaller cells with clear cytoplasm and distinct cell borders, centre-left) admixed with larger, multinucleated syncytiotrophoblasts (eosinophilic, irregular nuclei). Vascular invasion and early haematogenous spread are characteristic. Serum β-hCG is markedly elevated; β-hCG IHC is positive in syncytiotrophoblasts; SALL4 is positive; OCT3/4 and AFP are negative. (Source: Nephron, Wikimedia Commons, CC BY-SA 3.0.)

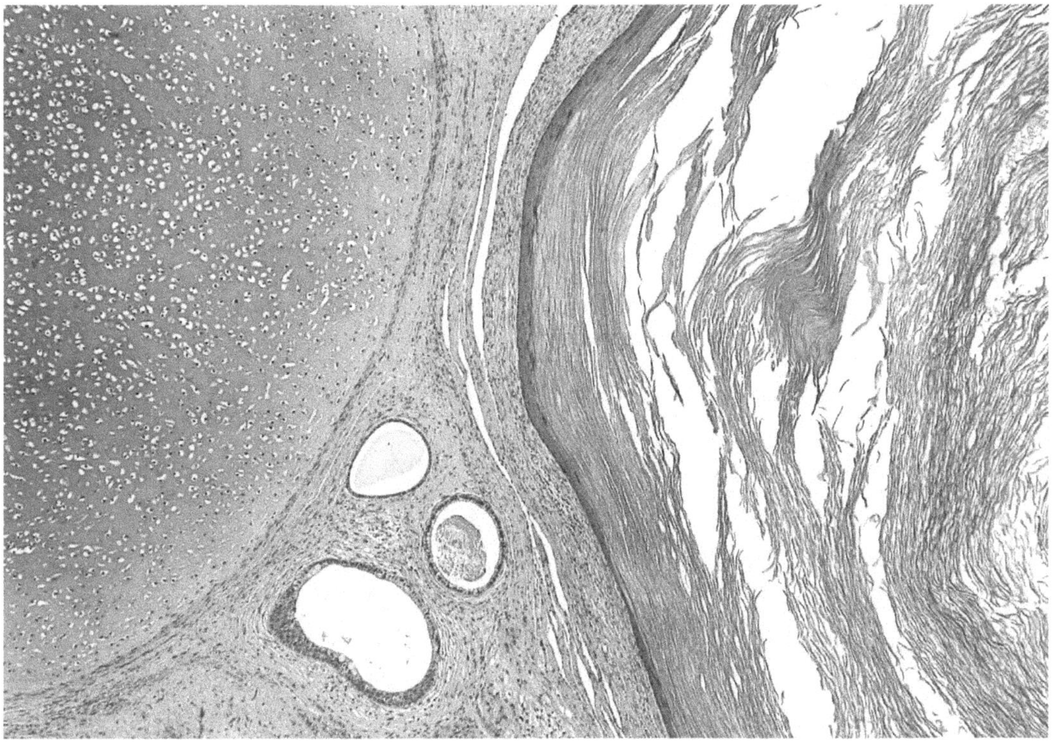

Figure 24.6D: Teratoma (testis, H&E, low magnification). Mature teratoma showing multiple somatic tissue elements derived from more than one germ-cell layer: hyaline cartilage (left, basophilic matrix with chondrocytes in lacunae) representing mesodermal differentiation, mature glandular structures (lower centre) representing endodermal differentiation, and keratinising squamous epithelium with anucleate keratin lamellae (right) representing ectodermal differentiation. In postpubertal patients, all teratomas (whether mature or immature) are GCNIS-derived and treated as malignant; in prepubertal children, mature teratoma is benign. (Source: Nephron, Wikimedia Commons, CC BY-SA 3.0.)

Definition: Most aggressive pure GCT. Primitive pleomorphic cells, solid/glandular/papillary.

Key finding: OCT3/4+, CD30+ (membranous), SALL4+; CD117−. CD30 = key discriminator from seminoma.

Exam yield: ★★★ HIGH

Microscopy: Diverse patterns: reticular/microcystic, solid, papillary, hepatoid.

Key finding: Schiller-Duval body (papilla with central vessel). Hyaline globules (PAS+). Glypican-3+, AFP markedly ↑, SALL4+; OCT3/4−.

Exam yield: ★★★ HIGH

Key finding: Biphasic cytotrophoblasts + syncytiotrophoblasts, extensive haemorrhage/necrosis. hCG markedly ↑. Early haematogenous spread.

Exam yield: ★★★ HIGH

Table 24.2: Immunohistochemistry and Serum Marker Panel for Testicular Germ Cell Tumours

Marker	Seminoma	Embryonal Ca	Yolk Sac Tumour	Choriocarcinoma	Teratoma
SALL4	Positive	Positive	Positive	Positive	– / focal
OCT3/4	Positive	Positive	Negative	Negative	Negative
CD117 (c-KIT)	Positive	Negative	Negative	Negative	Negative
CD30	Negative	Positive (membrane)	Negative / focal	Negative	Negative
Glypican-3	Negative	Negative	Positive	Focal (syncytio)	Negative
D2-40 (podoplanin)	Positive	Variable	Negative	Negative	Negative
AFP (IHC)	Negative	– / focal	Positive (cytoplasm, hyaline globules)	Negative	– (+ if YS elements)
β-hCG (IHC)	Rare (syncytio)	Rare	Negative	Positive (syncytio)	Negative
AFP (serum)	Normal (always)	Normal / mildly ↑	Markedly ↑	Normal	Normal
β-hCG (serum)	Normal / mildly ↑ (~15%)	Normal / mildly ↑	Normal	Markedly ↑	Normal
LDH (serum)	Often ↑	↑	↑	↑	Normal

Exam Pitfall: Elevated AFP in a 'Seminoma'

If serum AFP is elevated in a patient with a testicular tumour that appears morphologically to be pure seminoma, **treat and manage as a non-seminomatous GCT**.

Possible explanations: occult yolk sac tumour component not sampled by the sections examined, or a mixed GCT.

Never ignore elevated AFP in this setting. Conversely, mild hCG elevation (due to syncytiotrophoblast giant cells) is acceptable in pure seminoma.

Quick Recall: Testicular GCTs

GCNIS: Precursor of postpubertal GCTs; OCT3/4+, D2-40+, CD117+; isochromosome 12p.

Seminoma: Most common; clear cells + lymphocytic stroma; AFP always normal; OCT3/4+, CD117+.

Embryonal Ca: Most aggressive pure GCT; CD30+; OCT3/4+.

Yolk sac tumour: Schiller-Duval bodies; AFP markedly elevated; Glypican-3+.

Choriocarcinoma: Biphasic trophoblasts; haemorrhagic; hCG markedly elevated.

Mixed GCT: ~40% of testicular GCTs; specify all components and percentages.

24.5.3 Sex Cord-Stromal Tumours

Definition: Most common sex cord-stromal tumour (~5%). Endocrine effects: gynaecomastia (adults), precocious puberty (children).

Microscopy: Large polygonal eosinophilic cells.

Key finding: Reinke crystalloids — eosinophilic rod-shaped inclusions (pathognomonic, 25-40%). Inhibin+, calretinin+, Melan-A+.

Prognosis: Most benign. Large cell calcifying Sertoli cell tumour: Carney complex, Peutz-Jeghers.

Exam yield: ★★ MODERATE

Testicular biopsy for infertility is indicated to evaluate azoospermia (distinguishing obstructive from non-obstructive causes) and assess spermatogenesis. The biopsy requires **Bouin fixation** (not formalin, which causes tubular shrinkage artefact). Histological patterns include: normal spermatogenesis (confirms obstructive azoospermia), hypospermatogenesis (reduced but present spermatogenesis), maturation arrest (spermatogenesis halts at a specific stage, commonly spermatocyte level), Sertoli cell-only syndrome (complete absence of germ cells; Klinefelter syndrome, chemotherapy, cryptorchidism), and tubular sclerosis/atrophy. Johnsen scoring (1 to 10 scale based on the most advanced germ cell type present) provides semiquantitative assessment.

The Pathologist's Eye: Testicular Biopsy Pitfalls

Fixation artefact: Formalin causes tubular shrinkage, artificial basement membrane thickening, and nuclear pyknosis that may be misinterpreted as tubular atrophy. Always insist on Bouin fixation for infertility biopsies.

GCNIS screening: In cryptorchid patients, routinely stain for OCT3/4 or PLAP to detect GCNIS. Cryptorchid testes harbour GCNIS in 2-5% of cases.

Report must include: Mean tubular diameter, basement membrane thickness, interstitial Leydig cell status, presence/absence of GCNIS, and Johnsen score.

24.6 Diseases of the Penis

24.6.1 Inflammatory and Non-Neoplastic Conditions

Phimosis (inability to retract the foreskin) and balanitis (inflammation of the glans) are common non-neoplastic conditions. Balanitis xerotica obliterans (genital lichen sclerosus) produces a white, sclerotic, scarring process on the glans and prepuce that may cause phimosis. It is characterised histologically by epidermal atrophy, hyalinisation of the upper dermis, and a band-like lymphocytic infiltrate. Lichen sclerosus is a recognised risk factor for differentiated PeIN and SCC (HPV-independent pathway).

Peyronie disease is fibromatosis of the tunica albuginea of the penis, producing fibrous plaques that cause penile curvature. It is analogous to superficial fibromatoses elsewhere (palmar/Dupuytren, plantar/Ledderhose). The plaques show dense collagenous tissue with variable cellularity and occasional chronic inflammation. It is not premalignant.

24.6.2 Penile Squamous Cell Carcinoma

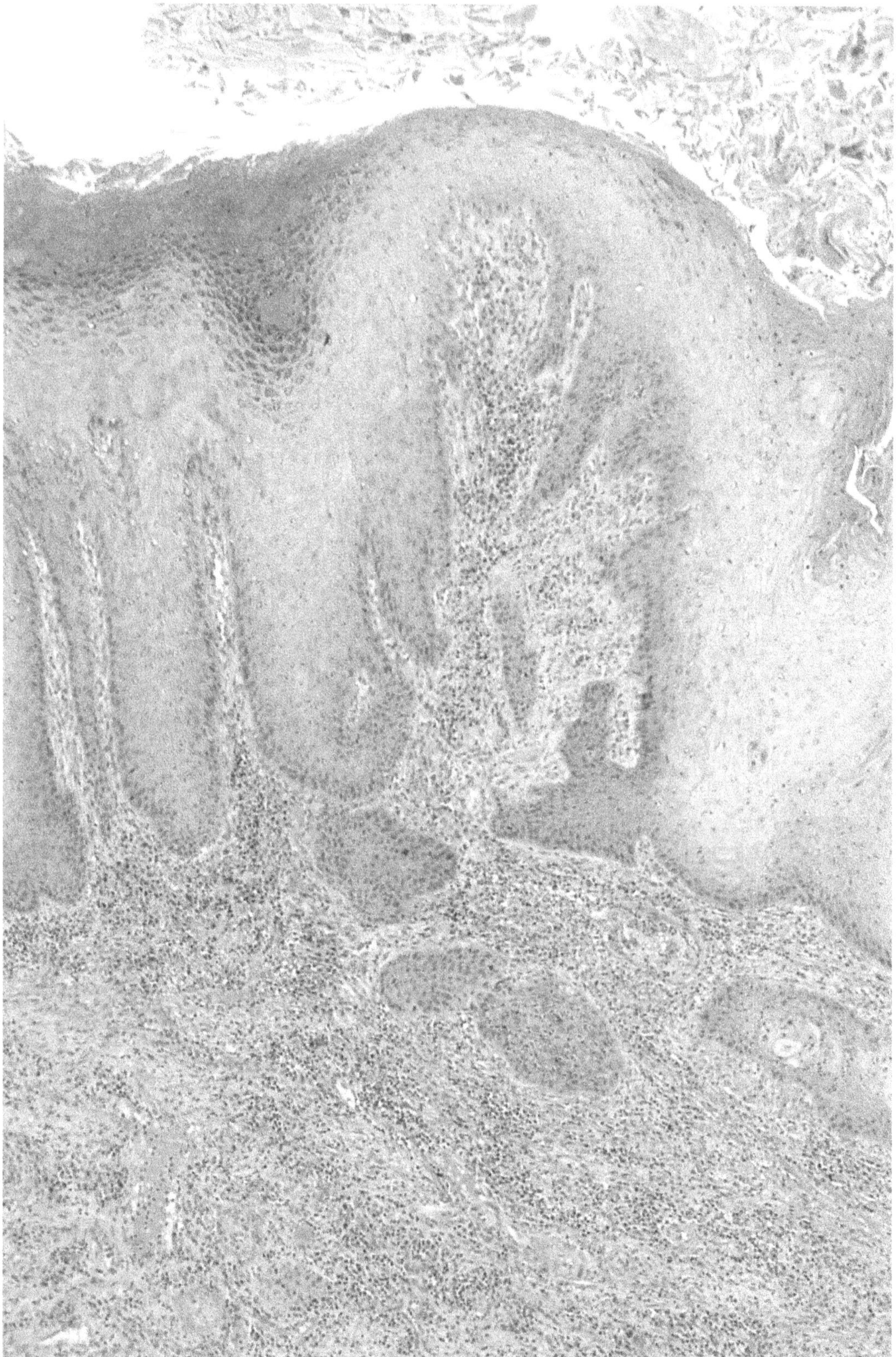

Figure 24.7: Squamous cell carcinoma of the penis. Low-magnification view showing keratinising invasive squamous cell carcinoma arising from the epidermis with irregular nests infiltrating the underlying dermis and a brisk chronic inflammatory infiltrate at the invasive front. H&E. (Source: Nephron, Wikimedia Commons, CC BY-SA 3.0.)

Definition: Most common penile malignancy. Risks: no circumcision, phimosis, lichen sclerosus, HPV 16/18 (30–50%).

Pathogenesis: HPV-dependent (undifferentiated PeIN, p16+, basaloid/warty) vs HPV-independent (differentiated PeIN, lichen sclerosus, p16−, usual/verrucous).

Subtypes: Usual type (most common), basaloid, warty, verrucous (Buschke-Lowenstein: exophytic, HPV−, rarely metastatic), sarcomatoid.

Key finding: p16+ (HPV-driven, better prognosis) vs p16−. Verrucous Ca: broad pushing margin, bulbous rete (vs condyloma: koilocytic, no deep invasion).

Prognosis: Inguinal LN metastasis = most important prognostic factor.

Exam yield: ★★★ HIGH

Viva hook: "A 2-year-old boy presents with a painless, solid testicular mass. Serum AFP is markedly elevated. What is the most likely diagnosis, and how does management differ from an adult with the same findings?" Answer: Prepubertal-type yolk sac tumour. In children, this is a non-GCNIS-derived tumour with an excellent prognosis after orchidectomy alone (no adjuvant chemotherapy required for Stage I). In an adult, yolk sac tumour is GCNIS-derived, almost always a component of a mixed GCT, and requires cisplatin-based chemotherapy for stages beyond Stage I.

Integration: HPV biology and E6/E7 oncoproteins connect to cervical pathology (Chapter 25), oropharyngeal carcinoma (Chapter 17), and neoplasia biology (Chapter 6). p16 IHC as a surrogate for HPV is discussed in Chapter 36. The dual HPV-dependent and HPV-independent pathways in penile carcinoma parallel the two pathways of vulvar SCC (Chapter 25).*

24.7 Lower Urinary Tract Pathology

The lower urinary tract — renal pelvis, ureter, urinary bladder, and urethra — is lined almost entirely by urothelium (transitional epithelium), a single epithelial surface over a field that extends from the calyces to the proximal urethra. Its unifying histological identity explains the "field-defect" biology of urothelial carcinoma: multifocal, synchronous and metachronous tumours at any point along the urinary tract in a single patient. Urothelial carcinoma is the dominant malignancy of this system and the focus of most exam questions; squamous and glandular carcinomas, and rare mesenchymal lesions, are far less common but must be recognised for morphological and aetiological reasons.

Normal Urothelium

Histology. The normal urothelium is a specialised stratified epithelium three to seven cells thick, depending on bladder distension. Three compartments are recognised: a single layer of basal cells resting on the basement membrane, several layers of intermediate (pear-shaped) cells, and a superficial layer of umbrella cells — large, often binucleate cells with a luminal glycosaminoglycan-rich apical membrane (the asymmetric unit membrane containing uroplakins). The umbrella cell layer is the functional barrier to urine permeability, and its loss or attenuation is an early and diagnostically useful sign of neoplastic transformation.

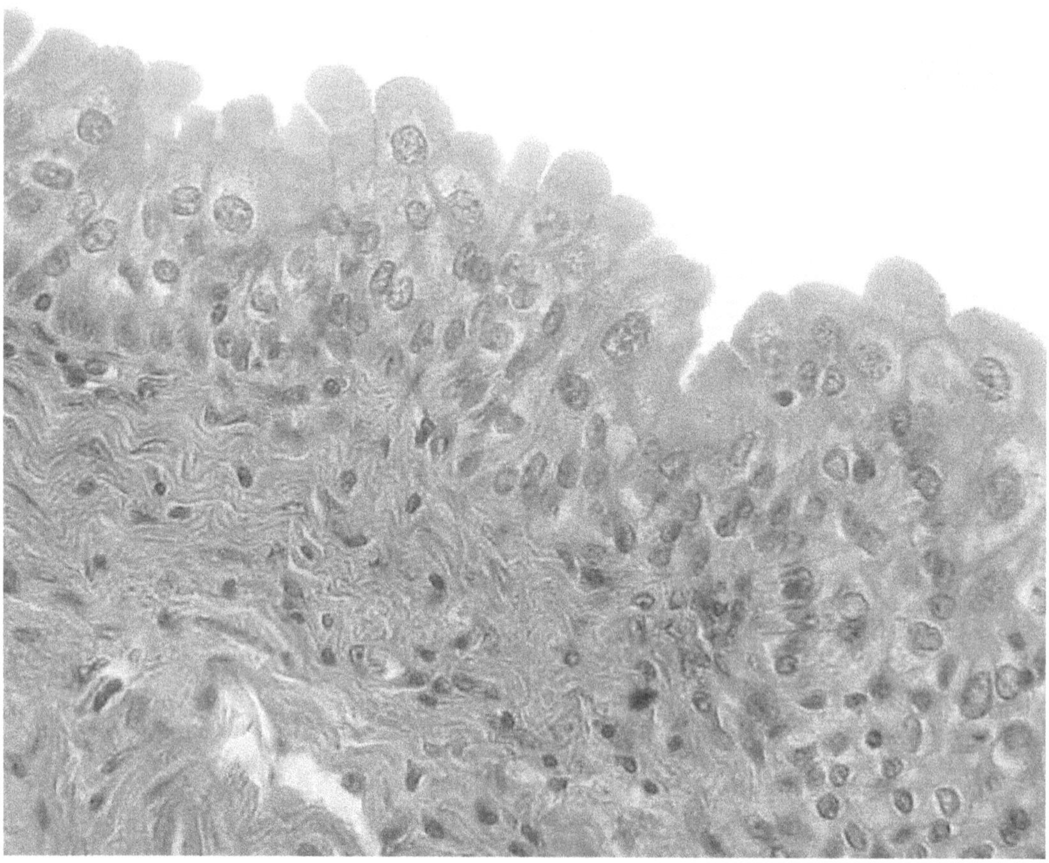

Figure 24.8: Normal urothelium. Three to seven cell layers with flattened umbrella cells at the luminal surface, pear-shaped intermediate cells, and a single basal layer resting on an intact basement membrane. The asymmetric unit membrane rich in uroplakins forms the impermeable luminal barrier. (H&E, intermediate magnification.) Compare with the atypia and architectural loss in Figures 24.10 and 24.11. (Source: Polarlys, Wikimedia Commons, CC BY-SA 3.0.)

Urothelial Neoplastic Spectrum and WHO 5th Edition (2022) Classification

Urothelial neoplasia follows two biologically and molecularly distinct pathways. Approximately 70-80 percent of bladder tumours present as papillary, non-muscle-invasive lesions carrying FGFR3 or HRAS activating mutations; they have a high local recurrence rate but low progression to muscle invasion. The remaining 20-30 percent arise from flat urothelial carcinoma in situ (CIS) through a TP53 and RB1 pathway and carry a much higher risk of muscle invasion and metastasis. The WHO 5th Edition (2022) preserves the 2016/2004 four-tier architecture — papilloma, PUNLMP, low-grade papillary urothelial carcinoma, and high-grade papillary urothelial carcinoma — while folding in molecular subtyping (luminal, basal, neuroendocrine-like) that is now informing treatment selection.

Table 24.3: WHO 5th Edition (2022) Classification of Non-Invasive Urothelial Neoplasms

Entity	Architecture / cytology	Recurrence / progression
Urothelial papilloma	Delicate papillae lined by urothelium of normal thickness, normal polarity; umbrella cells preserved; no cytological atypia.	Recurrence less than 10 percent; progression negligible. True benign neoplasm.
Papillary urothelial neoplasm of low malignant potential (PUNLMP)	Papillae with thickened urothelium, preserved polarity, minimal cytological atypia; normal or slightly increased mitoses limited to basal layers.	Recurrence 25-35 percent; progression to higher-grade disease 4-5 percent.
Low-grade papillary urothelial carcinoma (LG-PUC)	Clear architectural and cytological atypia — variation in polarity, nuclear enlargement, occasional pleomorphism; mitoses in any layer but sparse.	Recurrence 50-60 percent; progression to high-grade or invasion 10-15 percent.
High-grade papillary urothelial carcinoma (HG-PUC)	Marked architectural disorder — loss of polarity, cellular discohesion; severe cytological atypia, frequent mitoses at all levels, often atypical; umbrella cells lost.	Recurrence 60-80 percent; progression to muscle invasion 15-40 percent within 5 years.
Urothelial carcinoma in situ (CIS) — flat lesion	Full-thickness severe cytological atypia in a flat (non-papillary) urothelium; large pleomorphic nuclei, prominent nucleoli, discohesion; may be inconspicuous on cystoscopy (erythematous mucosa or normal-looking).	High risk of progression to muscle-invasive disease (50-80 percent over 5 years if untreated); intravesical BCG is standard of care.

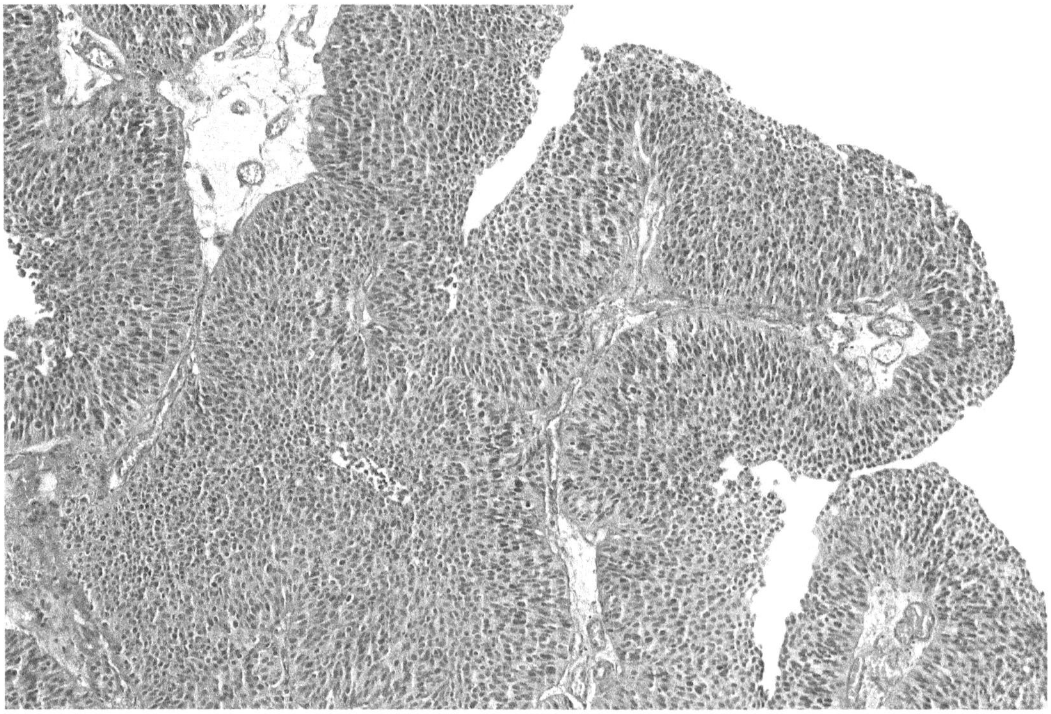

Figure 24.9: Low-grade papillary urothelial carcinoma (H&E, intermediate magnification). Slender branching fibrovascular cores are covered by thickened but orderly urothelium with mild nuclear enlargement and hyperchromasia, preserved polarity, and rare basal mitoses. Umbrella cells may still be identifiable at the surface. (Source: CoRus13, Wikimedia Commons, CC0.)

Diagnostic pearl: The single most reliable low-power feature separating LG-PUC from PUNLMP is loss of polarity — nuclei orient randomly rather than perpendicular to the basement membrane. On a biopsy that is ambiguous, a diagnosis of LG-PUC is preferred over PUNLMP for a tumour that recurs repeatedly, because the clinical behaviour guides management more than the borderline morphology.

High-Grade Papillary Urothelial Carcinoma

High-grade papillary urothelial carcinoma shows fused, irregular papillae with loss of the umbrella cell layer, marked nuclear pleomorphism, coarse chromatin, prominent nucleoli, and frequent atypical mitoses extending through the full thickness of the urothelium. Discohesion is a hallmark. The biopsy must be examined for muscularis propria (detrusor) invasion — the single most important staging criterion — and for lymphovascular invasion.

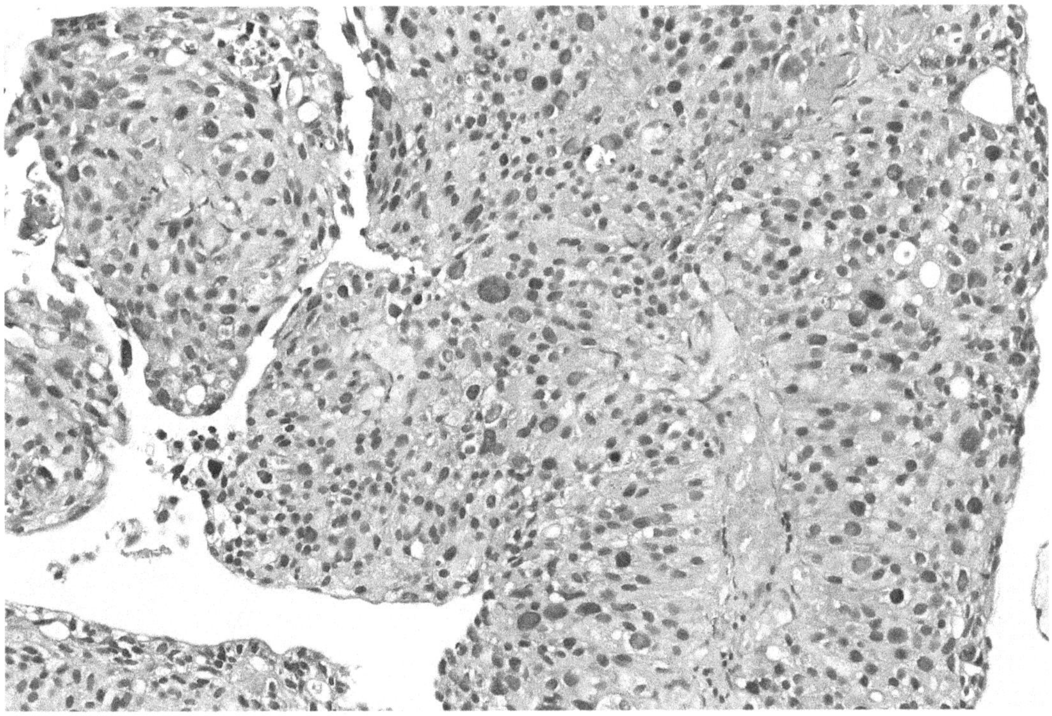

Figure 24.10: High-grade papillary urothelial carcinoma (H&E, high magnification). Disorganised papillae with fusion, loss of polarity, severe nuclear pleomorphism, prominent nucleoli, and scattered mitotic figures including atypical forms. The umbrella cell layer is absent. Compare with Figure 24.9. (Source: CoRus13, Wikimedia Commons, CC0.)

Urothelial Carcinoma In Situ — the Flat Lesion

Definition and biology. Urothelial CIS is a flat, non-papillary full-thickness high-grade dysplasia of the urothelium. Cystoscopically it may appear as velvety erythematous patches or as apparently normal mucosa — hence the role of random bladder biopsies and narrow-band imaging. Histologically the urothelium shows severe cytological atypia from base to surface: enlarged nuclei (four to five times lymphocyte size), coarse chromatin, prominent nucleoli, and frequent mitoses. Cellular discohesion is characteristic and results in positive urine cytology. CIS is biologically distinct from papillary carcinoma — it arises through the TP53 and RB1 pathway, has a much higher risk of muscle-invasive progression (50-80 percent over 5 years), and is managed with intravesical BCG immunotherapy, often combined with repeat biopsy-based surveillance.

Primary vs secondary CIS. Primary CIS occurs without a concurrent papillary tumour; secondary CIS is found adjacent to or within a papillary tumour and upstages the prognosis. Concomitant CIS with a papillary urothelial carcinoma is an indication for more intensive therapy and closer surveillance. IHC: strong and diffuse CK20 positivity (not confined to umbrella cells as in normal urothelium), p53 overexpression or null pattern, loss of CD44 (which is retained in reactive urothelium).

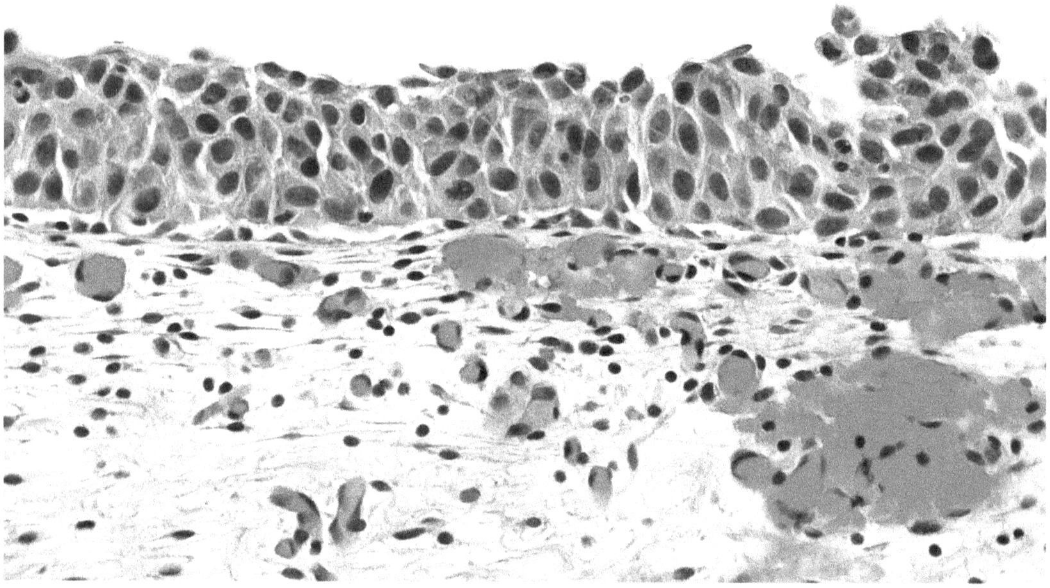

Figure 24.11: Urothelial carcinoma in situ (H&E, high magnification). Flat urothelium with full-thickness severe cytological atypia — enlarged hyperchromatic nuclei, prominent nucleoli, discohesion — but without papillary architecture. Adjacent normal-appearing mucosa in a biopsy specimen is the common gross appearance; CIS is often clinically occult until urine cytology flags it. (Source: Nephron, Wikimedia Commons, CC BY-SA 3.0.)

Invasive Urothelial Carcinoma and AJCC 8th Edition TNM Staging

Invasion through the basement membrane defines urothelial carcinoma. Depth of invasion drives therapy: non-muscle-invasive (Ta, T1, CIS) disease is managed by transurethral resection plus intravesical therapy (BCG for high-risk; mitomycin C for intermediate); muscle-invasive disease (T2 and above) requires radical cystectomy with pelvic lymphadenectomy, frequently preceded by neoadjuvant cisplatin-based chemotherapy. Distinguishing pT1 (lamina propria invasion) from pT2 (detrusor muscle invasion) is the single most consequential call on a TURBT specimen; adequate muscularis propria in the specimen is essential, and if absent a repeat resection is indicated. Do not confuse the thin smooth muscle fascicles of the muscularis mucosae (within the lamina propria) with the thick bundles of muscularis propria (the detrusor).

Table 24.4: AJCC 8th Edition (2017) T Categories for Urinary Bladder Carcinoma

T category	Depth of invasion	Clinical implication
Ta	Non-invasive papillary carcinoma.	Intravesical BCG for high-grade; surveillance cystoscopy.
Tis	Carcinoma in situ, flat high-grade dysplasia.	Intravesical BCG; if refractory, radical cystectomy.

T1	Tumour invades lamina propria (subepithelial connective tissue).	High-risk non-muscle-invasive; consider BCG plus early cystectomy for T1 high-grade. Substaging (T1a/b/c by muscularis mucosae) is prognostically useful but not part of AJCC.
T2a / T2b	Invades superficial (T2a inner half) or deep (T2b outer half) muscularis propria.	Muscle-invasive disease. Neoadjuvant cisplatin-based chemotherapy then radical cystectomy; or chemoradiation in selected bladder-preservation candidates.
T3a / T3b	Extends into perivesical soft tissue microscopically (3a) or macroscopically (3b).	Radical cystectomy; adjuvant therapy based on nodal status and margins.
T4a / T4b	Invades prostate stroma, seminal vesicles, uterus, or vagina (4a); or pelvic or abdominal wall (4b).	Locally advanced; multimodal therapy; T4b generally unresectable.

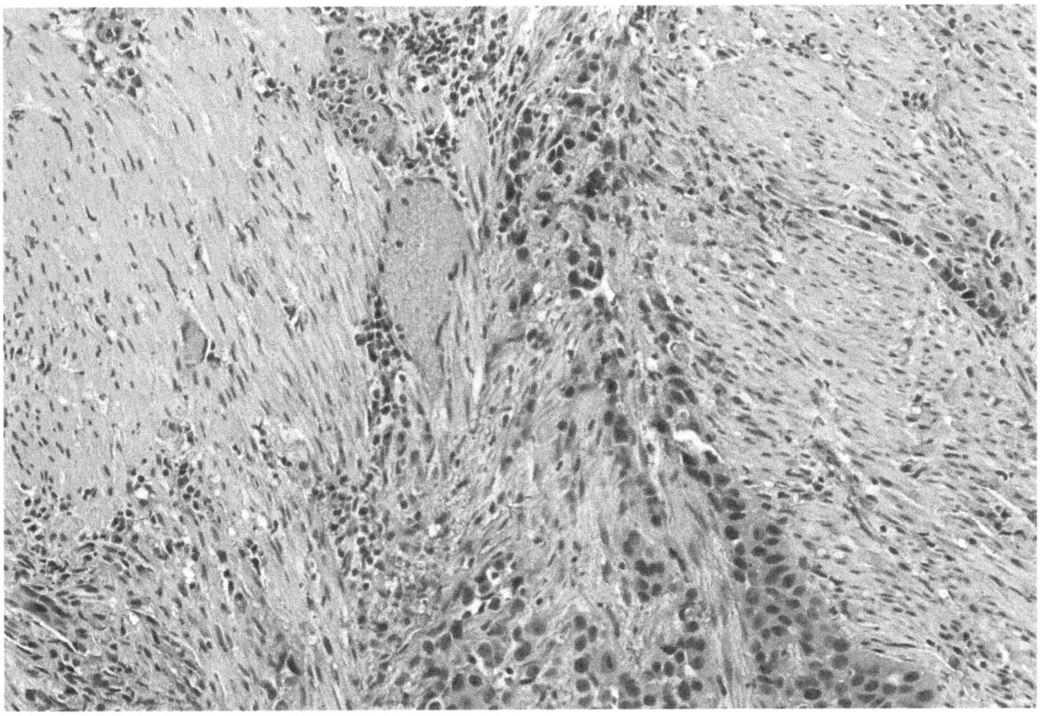

Figure 24.12: Invasive urothelial carcinoma, muscle-invasive (H&E, intermediate magnification). Irregular nests of urothelial tumour cells dissect between thick smooth muscle bundles of the muscularis propria (detrusor). Distinguishing detrusor from the thin muscularis mucosae of the lamina propria is the critical assessment and determines pT2 vs pT1 staging. Lymphovascular invasion, when present, should be documented separately. (Source: Nephron, Wikimedia Commons, CC BY-SA 3.0.)

Variant Histologies of Urothelial Carcinoma

The WHO 5th Edition recognises numerous morphological variants of urothelial carcinoma, several of which alter treatment or trigger molecular testing. Recognition on biopsy is essential — the variant component may be focal and clinically under-appreciated. Any variant component requires explicit reporting with an approximate percentage, because pure or predominant variants may prompt neoadjuvant chemotherapy even in the absence of muscle invasion.

Table 24.5: Clinically Significant Variants of Urothelial Carcinoma (WHO 5th Edition 2022)

Variant	Morphology / immunoprofile	Clinical consequence
Micropapillary	Small avascular tufts of tumour cells within lacunar spaces; reverse polarity; MUC1 apical staining reversed.	Aggressive; high rate of upstaging; early cystectomy preferred even for T1 disease.
Plasmacytoid	Discohesive single cells resembling plasma cells; eccentric nuclei, eosinophilic cytoplasm; loss of E-cadherin (CDH1); cytokeratin-positive.	Extremely aggressive, diffuse peritoneal spread; often misdiagnosed as lymphoma or metastatic carcinoma.
Sarcomatoid	Biphasic with epithelial component plus malignant spindle cell / sarcomatoid component; cytokeratin focally positive in spindle component; GATA3 helpful.	Poor prognosis; managed as high-grade UC with aggressive local and systemic therapy.
Nested	Bland small tubules and nests infiltrating the lamina propria and muscularis propria; deceptively banal on superficial biopsy.	Misdiagnosed as benign (von Brunn nests, nephrogenic adenoma); aggressive behaviour at presentation.
Lymphoepithelioma-like	Syncytial sheets of large undifferentiated cells in dense lymphoplasmacytic stroma; EBV generally negative (unlike nasopharyngeal LELC).	Paradoxically chemo-responsive; good prognosis when pure.
Small cell / neuroendocrine	Sheets of small round blue cells with moulded nuclei, scant cytoplasm, and neuroendocrine markers (synaptophysin, chromogranin, INSM1) positivity.	Aggressive; treated like small cell lung carcinoma (platinum-etoposide chemotherapy).

Non-Urothelial Carcinomas of the Bladder

Squamous cell carcinoma. Approximately 5 percent of bladder carcinomas are pure squamous cell carcinoma. In regions endemic for Schistosoma haematobium (Egypt, parts of sub-Saharan Africa), chronic schistosomal cystitis drives the majority of bladder cancers and squamous histology predominates. Outside Schistosoma-endemic regions, squamous cell carcinoma of the bladder is infrequent and usually arises on a background of chronic inflammation (long-term indwelling catheters in spinal-cord-injured patients, bladder stones, recurrent infections). Pure squamous histology requires keratinisation or intercellular bridges and absence of urothelial component; a tumour with any urothelial differentiation is classified as urothelial carcinoma with squamous differentiation (more common, different prognosis).

Adenocarcinoma. Primary adenocarcinoma of the bladder accounts for less than 2 percent of cases and is classified by origin as urachal (midline dome, often producing mucin and signet-ring cells, requires partial cystectomy with umbilectomy) or non-urachal (trigone, may arise from metaplasia in chronic irritation or bladder exstrophy). Histological patterns include intestinal, mucinous (colloid), signet-ring, and clear cell (mesonephric-like) types. Differential with metastatic colorectal adenocarcinoma is critical — CK7 positivity and CK20 plus CDX2 patterns, together with imaging and clinical correlation, are the typical discriminators.

Molecular Pathways and Therapeutic Implications

The two biological pathways of bladder neoplasia have distinct molecular signatures. The papillary, non-muscle-invasive pathway is driven predominantly by activating mutations in FGFR3 (approximately 60-80 percent of low-grade papillary tumours) and HRAS, with retention of p53 and Rb. FGFR3 inhibitors such as erdafitinib are now approved for advanced urothelial carcinoma with susceptible FGFR2 or FGFR3 alterations. The flat CIS / muscle-invasive pathway is characterised by TP53 mutations (approximately 50 percent), RB1 loss, and genomic instability with frequent chromosomal aneuploidy. Molecular subtyping (luminal, basal, neuroendocrine-like) is emerging as a therapy-selection framework: basal-squamous tumours respond best to neoadjuvant chemotherapy while luminal tumours may be candidates for checkpoint inhibition (pembrolizumab, atezolizumab, nivolumab) or antibody-drug conjugates such as enfortumab vedotin (Nectin-4) and sacituzumab govitecan (Trop-2).

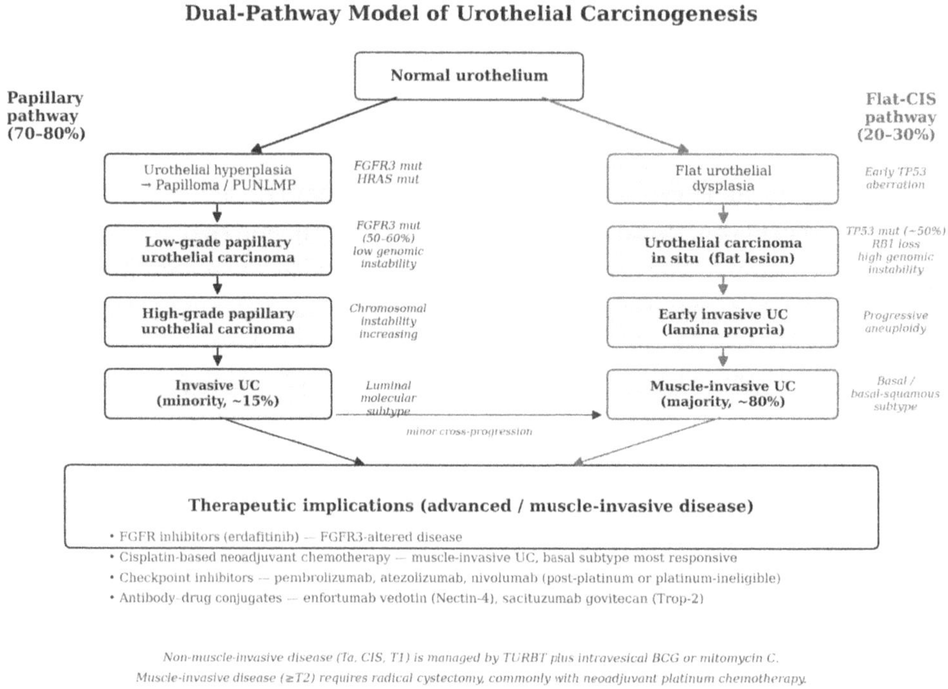

Figure 24.13: The dual-pathway model of urothelial carcinogenesis. FGFR3 and HRAS mutations drive the indolent papillary pathway (PUNLMP → LG-PUC → HG-PUC), which frequently recurs but infrequently progresses to muscle invasion. TP53 and RB1 inactivation drive the flat CIS pathway, which progresses rapidly to muscle-invasive and metastatic disease. Selected actionable alterations are shown for each branch. (Source: Author’s original.)

Ureteral and Urethral Pathology

Urothelial carcinoma of the upper tract (renal pelvis and ureter) shares biology with bladder urothelial carcinoma but has two distinctive associations worth remembering. First, Balkan endemic nephropathy and aristolochic acid exposure (historically from traditional herbal preparations; ongoing in parts of Asia) drive high-incidence upper-tract urothelial carcinoma with distinctive TP53 mutational signatures. Second, Lynch syndrome (especially MSH2 mutation) carries an elevated risk of upper-tract urothelial carcinoma, and mismatch-repair IHC (MLH1, PMS2, MSH2, MSH6) should be considered in young patients or those with a suggestive family history. Urethral carcinoma is uncommon; in men it is typically squamous (often HPV-associated, distal) or urothelial (proximal), whereas in women it is more often adenocarcinoma (clear cell subtype arising in urethral diverticulum) or squamous.

Exam point: A young patient with painless haematuria and an upper-tract urothelial carcinoma should raise two specific considerations — aristolochic acid exposure through traditional herbal remedies, and Lynch syndrome (MSH2 mutation especially). Reflex mismatch-repair IHC is justified in this demographic. For bladder urothelial carcinoma, the single most testable point is the pT1 versus pT2 distinction on TURBT: know the histological landmarks of muscularis mucosae (thin, fragmented, within lamina propria) versus muscularis propria (thick, organised detrusor bundles), and know that if muscularis propria is absent from the TURBT specimen, a re-resection is mandated before staging can be finalised.

24.8 Recent Advances

WHO 5th edition classification of tumours of the urinary system and male genital organs — Part A. The 2022 fifth-edition WHO classification of urogenital tumours introduced site-specific revisions across renal, penile, and testicular pathology, with direct implications for the surgical-pathology report (Moch et al. European Urology 2022; 82: 458–468; PMID 35853783). For renal tumours, a molecularly driven classification was added alongside the morphological scheme, introducing SMARCB1-deficient medullary renal cell carcinoma, TFEB-altered renal cell carcinoma, ALK-rearranged renal cell carcinoma, ELOC-mutated renal cell carcinoma, and the morphologically defined eosinophilic solid and cystic renal cell carcinoma as discrete entities. Penile squamous cell carcinomas are now grouped as either human-papillomavirus-associated or human-papillomavirus-independent, simplifying the prior multiplicity of morphological subtypes and emphasising the prognostic significance of HPV status. Testicular tumour nomenclature is largely retained, with continued use of germ cell neoplasia in situ as the precursor of most germ cell tumours; the term primitive neuroectodermal tumour has been replaced by embryonic neuroectodermal tumour to separate these tumours unambiguously from Ewing sarcoma, and carcinoid has been redesignated neuroendocrine tumour, with most testicular examples reclassified as prepubertal-type testicular neuroendocrine tumour. A new chapter on tumours of the scrotum has been introduced. Reporting implication: contemporary urological surgical specimens should map findings to the WHO 5 entity and incorporate molecular diagnostics where the entity is molecularly defined.

Molecular subtypes and targeted therapy in prostate cancer. Genomic analyses have identified ETS fusion-positive (TMPRSS2-ERG), SPOP-mutant, FOXA1-mutant, and IDH1-mutant molecular subtypes. BRCA2 germline mutations confer significantly increased prostate cancer risk and predict sensitivity to PARP inhibitors (olaparib, rucaparib), now approved for metastatic castration-resistant prostate cancer with homologous recombination repair (HRR) deficiency. PSMA PET-CT has transformed staging, and lutetium-177 PSMA radioligand therapy (VISION trial) offers a new treatment paradigm for PSMA-expressing metastatic disease.

Artificial intelligence in Gleason grading. AI-assisted Gleason grading of prostate biopsies has shown pathologist-level accuracy in multicentre studies, with systems (Paige Prostate, PathAI) approved or in regulatory pathways. AI reliably detects Gleason pattern 4 and quantifies percentage of pattern 4, which is critical for active surveillance decisions. Integration into clinical workflows is accelerating globally (see Chapter 38).

MicroRNA liquid biopsy for GCTs. Serum miR-371a-3p has emerged as a highly sensitive (>90%) and specific biomarker for active testicular GCT, outperforming AFP and hCG for detection and monitoring of both seminomatous and non-seminomatous tumours. The WHO 5th Edition classification has refined the separation of GCNIS-derived (postpubertal) from non-GCNIS-derived (prepubertal) tumours, which has direct implications for staging and follow-up intensity.

24.9 Approach to the Histopathology Slide

Prostate needle biopsy: (1) Scan at low power for small, crowded glands with infiltrative pattern. (2) Assess for loss of basal cell layer (single cell lining). (3) Look for amphophilic cytoplasm, prominent nucleoli, intraluminal blue mucin, crystalloids, perineural invasion. (4) Assign Gleason pattern and Grade Group. (5) If equivocal, order p63/HMWCK + AMACR. (6) Check for HGPIN, IDC-P, or ASAP in adjacent tissue.

Orchidectomy for GCT: (1) Identify tumour type(s) by architecture and cytology. (2) Look for clear cells + lymphocytic stroma (seminoma), primitive pleomorphic cells + CD30 pattern (embryonal), Schiller-Duval bodies (yolk sac), biphasic trophoblasts (choriocarcinoma), or differentiated tissues (teratoma). (3) Check for GCNIS in adjacent tubules. (4) Assess for lymphovascular invasion, rete testis invasion, and tunica involvement for staging. (5) If mixed, estimate percentage of each component.

International Frameworks

ISUP/WHO Prostate Cancer Grade Group system (2014/2016). Validated in a multi-institutional cohort of 20,845 radical prostatectomy and 5,501 radiotherapy patients across seven academic centres, the Grade Group system collapses Gleason scores into five prognostic tiers with stepwise hazard ratios for biochemical recurrence relative to Grade Group 1: 1.9 (Group 2, Gleason 3+4=7), 5.1 (Group 3, Gleason 4+3=7), 8.0 (Group 4, Gleason 8), and 11.7 (Group 5, Gleason 9–10). Two design benefits address long-standing clinical confusion: the lowest grade is renumbered as 1 rather than 6 (mitigating overtreatment of low-risk disease), and the prognostic distinction between Gleason 3+4 and 4+3 is made explicit. Reporting requirement: contemporary prostate biopsy and prostatectomy reports should record both the Gleason score and the corresponding Grade Group, and for biopsies with multiple cores both the highest individual core grade and an overall grade should be reported, with percentage of pattern 4 quantified in 5–10% increments to inform active-surveillance decisions. Citation: Epstein JI, et al. Eur Urol 2016;69(3):428–435. PMID 26166626.

Ultra High-Yield Chapter Summary

<table>
<tr><th>Topic</th><th>Must Remember</th></tr>
<tr><td>BPH</td><td>Transition zone; DHT/5-alpha reductase; nodular glandular + stromal hyperplasia; basal layer intact</td></tr>
<tr><td>HGPIN</td><td>Precursor to carcinoma; cytologic atypia + patchy basal layer; tufting most common; ~25-30% subsequent Ca risk</td></tr>
<tr><td>IDC-P</td><td>Intraductal spread of high-grade Ca; dense cribriform/comedonecrosis; basal layer retained; near-certain high-grade invasive disease</td></tr>
<tr><td>Prostatic adenocarcinoma</td><td>Peripheral zone; small infiltrative glands; absent basal layer; TMPRSS2-ERG; perineural invasion</td></tr>
<tr><td>Gleason/Grade Groups</td><td>GG1 (3+3) to GG5 (5+5); architecture-based; never assign pattern 1-2 on biopsy; % pattern 4 for GG2</td></tr>
<tr><td>Prostate IHC panel

IHC Panel: Prostate Needle Biopsy
<table><tr><th>Marker</th><th>Basal Cells</th><th>Carcinoma</th></tr></table></td><td>p63/HMWCK absent + AMACR positive = carcinoma; ERG for fusion; NKX3.1 for metastatic origin</td></tr>
</table>

p63	Positive (nuclear)	Negative
HMWCK (34betaE12)	Positive (cytoplasmic)	Negative
AMACR (P504S)	Negative/weak	Positive (granular cytoplasmic)
ERG	Negative	Positive in ~50% (TMPRSS2-ERG fusion)
NKX3.1	Positive	Positive (retained)
PIN4 cocktail	p63+/HMWCK+ (brown) + AMACR- (red)	p63-/HMWCK- + AMACR+ (red)

Essential/Desirable: Prostatic Adenocarcinoma (Needle Biopsy)

Essential: Absent basal cells (p63 negative, HMWCK negative); AMACR positive; Gleason pattern assignment; ISUP Grade Group.

Desirable: Perineural invasion; percentage pattern 4; cribriform morphology; ERG positivity; extraprostatic extension; lymphovascular invasion.

Prostate staging	pT2 organ-confined; pT3a EPE; pT3b SVI; M1b bone (osteoblastic) most common distant site
ASAP	Atypical small acinar proliferation; ~40% Ca on repeat biopsy; re-biopsy in 3-6 months
Benign mimics	Atrophy, adenosis, basal cell hyperplasia, seminal vesicle, post-atrophic hyperplasia, radiation
Cryptorchidism	4-8x increased GCT risk; screen for GCNIS with OCT3/4
GCNIS	Precursor of postpubertal GCTs; OCT3/4+, D2-

	40+, CD117+; isochromosome 12p
Seminoma	Most common GCT; clear cells + lymphocytic stroma; AFP always normal; OCT3/4+, CD117+
Embryonal carcinoma	Most aggressive pure GCT; primitive cells; CD30+; OCT3/4+
Yolk sac tumour	Schiller-Duval bodies; AFP elevated; Glypican-3+
Choriocarcinoma	Biphasic trophoblasts; haemorrhage; hCG markedly elevated
Mixed GCT	~40% of testicular GCTs; specify all components and percentages
Leydig cell tumour	Reinke crystalloids; gynaecomastia; usually benign; inhibin+
Testicular biopsy	Bouin fixation; Sertoli cell-only, maturation arrest, hypospermatogenesis; Johnsen score
Penile SCC	HPV 16/18; PeIN; verrucous carcinoma
PARP inhibitors	Olaparib/rucaparib for BRCA2-mutant mCRPC; HRR deficiency testing
miR-371a-3p	Serum microRNA for active GCT; superior to AFP/hCG
AI Gleason grading	Pathologist-level accuracy; quantifies % pattern 4; regulatory approval progressing

Table 24.6: WHO 5th Edition (2022) Prostate -- ISUP Grade Groups

ISUP GG	Gleason Score	Pattern	Prognosis
GG1	3+3=6	Individual discrete glands	Indolent; active surveillance candidate
GG2	3+4=7	Predominantly discrete glands + minor fused	Favourable intermediate risk

GG3	4+3=7	Predominantly fused/cribriform + minor discrete	Unfavourable intermediate; cribriform = poor outcome
GG4	4+4=8, 3+5=8, 5+3=8	Fused/cribriform/glomeruloid or very poorly formed	High risk
GG5	4+5=9, 5+4=9, 5+5=10	Solid sheets/cords/single cells/necrosis	Very high risk; consider neoadjuvant therapy

Key WHO 5th Edition changes: IDC-P (intraductal carcinoma of prostate) now formally recognised as high-grade pattern associated with BRCA2 mutations and adverse outcome. Cribriform pattern is assigned to Gleason pattern 4 regardless of size. Cribriform-only Gleason 3+4 behaves like 4+3, mandating clinical vigilance.

Table 24.7: IHC Panel for Prostate Biopsy

Marker	Basal cells	Carcinoma	Role
p63	+ (nuclear)	- (lost)	Basal cell marker; loss supports carcinoma
HMWCK (34betaE12)	+ (cytoplasmic)	- (lost)	Basal cell marker; patchy in atrophy/HGPIN
AMACR (P504S)	-/focal	+++ (granular cytoplasmic)	Positive in carcinoma, HGPIN, nephrogenic adenoma
ERG	-	+ in ~50% (TMPRSS2-ERG fusion)	Highly specific for carcinoma when positive
NKX3.1	+	+	Prostate lineage marker; useful for metastatic CUP
PIN-4 cocktail	p63+/HMWCK+/AMACR-	p63-/HMWCK-/AMACR+	Triple stain; single slide for small foci

Essential and Desirable Diagnostic Criteria: Prostatic Adenocarcinoma

ESSENTIAL: Infiltrating small glands/acini lacking basal cells (p63-/HMWCK-); nuclear atypia (prominent nucleoli); AMACR+; ISUP Grade Group assignment

DESIRABLE: ERG positivity (supports TMPRSS2-ERG fusion); percentage of core involved; perineural invasion; extraprostatic extension; IDC-P presence

PITFALL: Atrophy, adenosis (atypical adenomatous hyperplasia), and partial atrophy can mimic low-grade carcinoma. Patchy basal cell staining does not exclude benign -- use cocktail staining and correlation with H&E.

The cardinal diagnostic thinking in prostate pathology: a focus of small glands suspicious for carcinoma must be evaluated with a triple approach: (1) loss of basal cells (p63/HMWCK), (2) positive AMACR, and (3) architectural infiltration. No single marker is sufficient; the diagnosis is always a synthesis.

Cribriform architecture in prostate is always significant. In the post-WHO 5th Edition era, any cribriform pattern is Gleason 4, and cribriform-only GG2 behaves like GG3. This single architectural pattern drives both grading and clinical management.

[MORPHOLOGY: Fig 24.X -- Gleason/ISUP Patterns Illustrated. Layout: 5-panel. Pattern 3 (discrete glands), Pattern 4 (fused/cribriform/glomeruloid), Pattern 5 (sheets/cords/comedonecrosis). Annotated with Grade Group assignments. Source: Author's original.]

Index

Page references point to the primary discussion of each topic. Where an entity is treated across multiple chapters, the most substantive locations are cited. Cross-references direct the reader to the preferred index term, or to the companion volume (Volume 2B) where coverage lies outside the scope of this volume.

A

B

C

D

E

F

G

H

I

J

K

L

M

N

O

P

I

J

K

L

M

N

O

P

R

S

T

U

V

W

X

Y

Z

Also from Vayden

A focused list of postgraduate and examination titles published by Vayden Academic Press, Mumbai.

USMLE Step 1 Pathology

Pathway to USMLE: Pathology — three-volume comprehensive textbook (Volume 1: General Pathology • Volume 2: Systemic Pathology I • Volume 3: Systemic Pathology II)

Pathology in Patterns — rapid-revision companion to the Pathway series

USMLE Vignettes in Pathology — two-volume vignette workbook with stepwise reasoning (Volume 1 • Volume 2)

FRCPath Part 1

FRCPath First Paper: Haematology — two-volume preparation set (Volume 1 • Volume 2)

FRCPath First Paper: Histopathology — two-volume preparation set (Volume 1 • Volume 2)

Integrated Pathology — Postgraduate Reference

Volume 1: Haematopathology and Transfusion Medicine

Volume 2B: Specialised Systems, Cytopathology, and Applied Laboratory Pathology — *companion to the present volume*

All titles available from Amazon worldwide and direct from www.vaydenpress.com.

Errata and Corrections

Pathology evolves; printed text does not. WHO classifications are revised, AJCC editions supersede one another, immunohistochemistry panels are refined, and molecular criteria shift. A textbook of this scope, written by a single author, will inevitably contain errors of fact, classification, image attribution, or interpretation. Those errors matter, and the publisher is committed to correcting them.

If you identify an error in this volume — a diagnostic threshold, an IHC marker, a WHO subtype, an AJCC stage, a figure attribution, or a typographical slip — please write to the publisher with the page number, the location on the page, and a brief description of the correction. Where possible, cite the source supporting the proposed change.

SUBMIT CORRECTIONS

publishing@vaydenpress.com

Subject: Errata — Integrated Pathology, Volume 2A

Verified corrections will be incorporated into subsequent printings of this volume and posted, with acknowledgement to the reader who reported them, on the public errata page at **www.vaydenpress.com/errata**. Readers who hold an earlier printing are encouraged to consult the errata page periodically.

The author thanks every reader who takes the time to report an error. A textbook is improved by its readers as much as by its writer.

Vayden Academic Press • Mumbai • 2026

www.ingramcontent.com/pod-product-compliance
Lightning Source LLC
Chambersburg PA
CBHW082233240926
51846CB00014B/1370
9788168673007